MEDICAL RADIOLOGY
Diagnostic Imaging

Editors:
A. L. Baert, Leuven
K. Sartor, Heidelberg

Ali Guermazi (Ed.)

Imaging of Kidney Cancer

With Contributions by

R. Abo-Kamil · D. W. Barker · E. D. Billingsley · J. A. S. Brookes · R. F. J. Browne · J. Y. Byun
J. A. Choi · J.-M. Correas · N. S. Curry · R. El-Galley · I. El-Hariry · E. K. Fishman · T. Fujimori
D. A. Gervais · A. Guermazi · P. F. Hahn · O. Hélénon · G. M. Israel · H. Ito · H. S. Kang
K. A. Kim · L. H. Lowe · Y. Miaux · T. Miyazaki · P. R. Mueller · C. G. C. Ooi · C. M. Park
U. Patel · J.-P. Pelage · E. S. Pretorius · S. D. Qanadli · S. Restrepo · S. H. Rha · S. E. Rha
C. Schiepers · S. Sheth · A. K. Singh · E. M. Taboada · M. Takahashi · S. Tomita
W. C. Torreggiani · T. Ueda · Y. Ueda · S. K. Yoon · R. J. Zagoria

Series Editor's Foreword by
A. L. Baert

Foreword by
M. A. Bosniak

With 487 Figures in 1033 Separate Illustrations, 195 in Color and 30 Tables

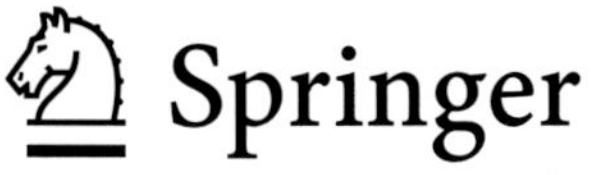 Springer

ALI GUERMAZI, MD
Senior Radiologist
Scientific Director, Oncology Services
Department of Radiology Services
Synarc Inc.
575 Market Street, 17th Floor
San Francisco, CA 94105
USA

MEDICAL RADIOLOGY · Diagnostic Imaging and Radiation Oncology
Series Editors: A. L. Baert · L. W. Brady · H.-P. Heilmann · M. Molls · K. Sartor

Continuation of Handbuch der medizinischen Radiologie
Encyclopedia of Medical Radiology

Library of Congress Control Number: 2005923492

ISBN 3-540-21129-2 Springer Berlin Heidelberg New York
ISBN 978-3-540-21129-7 Springer Berlin Heidelberg New York

Springer is part of Springer Science+Business Media

http//www.springeronline.com
© Springer-Verlag Berlin Heidelberg 2006
Printed in Germany

Medical Editor: Dr. Ute Heilmann, Heidelberg
Desk Editor: Ursula N. Davis, Heidelberg
Production Editor: Kurt Teichmann, Mauer
Cover-Design and Typesetting: Verlagsservice Teichmann, Mauer

Printed on acid-free paper – 21/3151xq – 5 4 3 2 1 0

Series Editor's Foreword

Radiological imaging studies are playing an increasingly important role in the modern management of malignant neoplasms of the kidney with respect to both diagnosis and therapy.

This book offers its readers a complete and comprehensive overview of kidney cancer in all its various manifestations, from the common renal cell carcinoma to much rarer malignant neoplasms of the kidney, and describes in minute detail the impact of modern radiological imaging on the diagnosis and therapy of these lesions. Several chapters are dedicated to the emerging field of minimally invasive percutaneous treatment of some forms of kidney cancer.

The collaboration of many internationally renowned experts has resulted in top-quality, up-to-date, well-written and exhaustive chapters on all main topics.

I would like to congratulate Dr. Ali Guermazi, a prominent oncological radiologist, for his judicious choice of contributing authors and for producing another standard reference work on oncologic imaging in our series "Medical Radiology: Diagnostic Imaging". This outstanding book will certainly meet with great interest not only from general and sub-specialized radiologists but also from medical oncologists, urologists and pediatricians. They will all greatly benefit from its contents for a better management of their patients. I am confident that it will meet the same success with the readers as the previous volumes published in this series.

Leuven
ALBERT L. BAERT

Foreword

"Imaging of Kidney Cancer", edited by Dr. Ali Guermazi, summarizes the present status of detecting, diagnosing, treating, and helping plan the treatment of renal cancer. It reviews the current histologic classification of renal neoplasms and updates the present use of the many modalities used in diagnosis and staging of these tumors. The text presents the imaging findings in the various types of renal neoplasms and pseudoneoplasms, including renal cell carcinoma, sarcoma, lymphoma, and neoplasms of the collecting system, as well as pediatric renal cancer and unusual and less common neoplasms. This is truly a global effort, with contributors from around the world. The authors demonstrate extensive experience in their fields and the reader is treated to a number of differing approaches and a diversity of opinions.

For radiologists in training as well as for the practicing radiologist and urologist, this book defines the present state of the art, updates what is currently known in the field and will become a valuable reference source. For older radiologists (such as myself) it can also serve to make one marvel at the advances that have taken place in this field over the past 50 years, and to reminisce about the changes in imaging and treatment of kidney cancer that have occurred in one's lifetime in radiology. For those not familiar with the progression of imaging events and the changes in treatment that have occurred in the diagnosis and treatment of renal cancer over this time, I would like to describe my own personal experience and memories on this journey as a radiologist with particular interest in the imaging of renal masses[1]. Sometimes to appreciate the present and to contemplate the future, one must look to the past.

In 1956, when I started my residency in radiology, the most effective way of diagnosing a renal mass was by nephrotomography, a technique that had just been described 2 years earlier (EVANS et al. 1954). Prior to nephrotomography, intravenous urography (often called intravenous pyelography or just IVP) was the least invasive way to evaluate the urinary tract and detect renal masses. Because urograms did not visualize the kidneys adequately in many cases, urologists frequently resorted to retrograde pyelography to diagnose a renal mass since the technique provided superior demonstration of the collecting system structures. Urography and retrograde pyelography could detect a mass if it displaced the collecting system structures or was large enough to create a density associated with the contour of the kidney, but it could not separate a cyst from a tumor unless the lesion contained calcification or it invaded the collecting system structures.

Renal mass puncture at that time was occasionally helpful but it was invasive and successful only on very large lesions. Also there was a high percentage of failed attempts because of difficulties in localization, and false-positive and -negative results were common. Often the decision to operate on a patient was based on the "clinical triad" of a palpable mass, hematuria, and flank pain. "Exploratory surgery" was frequently performed for diagnosis and treatment. Benign cysts were often discovered and unroofed or the kidney had to be removed if the diagnosis of cyst could not be established for certain at surgery. Nephroto-

---

[1] For information about uroradiology in the first half of the twentieth century, the articles by ELKIN (1990) and POLLACK (1996) are of interest.

mography therefore was a significant advance in the diagnosis of a renal mass. Nephroto-mography was essentially intravenous urography but with a much higher dose of intrave-nous contrast medium delivered rapidly through a large-bore needle (12 gauge) and with tomograms taken during the nephrogram phase. This allowed a high level of contrast agent in the bloodstream, giving a dense nephrogram and therefore superior visualization of the parenchyma of the kidney. Masses could then be seen as dense (tumor) or lucent (cyst, if it had sharp margination and a thin wall). The technique was made possible by the introduction of contrast material that was significantly less toxic than previously available materials[2]. Nephrotomography was actually a major advance over what had been available for renal mass diagnosis and it made differentiation of cyst and solid tumor possible, particularly in larger lesions. Although the technique was quite successful in a number of medical centers, it suffered from false negatives (in hypovascular lesions), making clinicians wary of the results. Also, the examination often was not well performed by radiologists. They were not used to inserting large-bore needles into veins, or did not want to do a cut-down on an antecubital vein so that a large amount of contrast could be delivered rapidly to achieve the necessary density for a successful nephrogram. Because of this, some studies were poorly performed and the technique never achieved full acceptance by urologists. "Exploratory surgery" was still common, although somewhat less so than before the introduction of nephrotomography.

The next major step in the diagnosis of a renal mass came with the introduction of renal angiography, which could be performed safely by radiologists in the radiology department. Abdominal aortography had previously been performed by surgeons as it required an arterial cutdown on the femoral artery and insertion of a catheter into the aorta. Because the procedure was significantly invasive, it was rarely used in renal mass diagnosis. Visualization of the aorta and renal arteries was performed by some urologists with translumbar aortography, another significantly invasive procedure which also suffered from considerable morbidity and low diagnostic accuracy, except in hypervascular neoplasms. However, in 1953, SELDINGER devised a method of putting a catheter into the aorta percutaneously. Eventually the renal arteries and all the branches of the aorta were selectively catheterized. This procedure was greatly aided by the introduction of image intensification for fluoroscopy. (It should be remembered that prior to this development, red goggles were needed for fluoroscopy, which was performed in a darkened room). Arteriography was also enhanced by the introduction of rapid film changes and power injectors. The initial work using the Seldinger technique was performed by Swedish radiologists (O. Olssen and E. Boijsen) in the 1950s. (Many of us traveled to Sweden to learn their techniques). Arteriography was quickly adopted and practiced around the world. By the 1960s the technique was well established and added stature to the specialty of radiology because with it, diagnoses that could not be made preoperatively became possible in the kidneys, of course, and the rest of the body as well. Radiologists gained the appreciation of their clinical colleagues and were considered more than just "film readers"[3]. The diagnostic accuracy of differentiating renal cyst from tumor with selective arteriography was high (in the range of 95%). But since angiography could not be performed on everyone with a renal mass, nephrotomography (although modified by introducing contrast by bolus and drip infusion, or just

---

[2] Introduced in 1955, the diatriozate compounds, led by diatriozate sodium (Hypaque) were much better tolerated by patients than the previously used acetriozate sodium (Urokon). In fact, nephrotomography was originally performed with 90% Hypaque which had to be warmed to lessen its viscosity so that it could be injected rapidly.

[3] The ability to perform selective arteriography in the radiology department transformed the specialty of radiology, in my opinion. It was a great advance for the specialty because radiologists gained added respect from their clinical colleagues, who became more dependent on them. It also stimulated top-class medical students to enter the specialty and led to the field of cardiovascular radiology and subsequently to interventional radiology as we know it today.

drip infusion through a smaller-bore needle) was still needed to triage renal masses so that angiography could be reserved for questionable cases or cases more likely to be tumor. Arteriography was readily embraced by urologists as it enabled preoperative visualization of the vascular anatomy of the kidney, which greatly aided the surgical approach, as well as providing improved preoperative staging of malignancy.

Another technique, ultrasound, was developed in the late 1960s and early 1970s and proved to be an important modality in the triage of renal masses. Imaging with ultrasound started with A mode, advanced to B mode, and progressed to "real time" and gray scale with continuous improvement in accuracy as instrumentation advanced. The technique, like all others, had limitations, and its accuracy was highly dependent on the experience, persistence, and ability of the individual performing the study, but ultrasound was able to separate simple benign cysts from other masses that required more study. As ultrasound developed, its ability to clearly and accurately diagnose a simple cyst (by far the most common renal mass) without contrast injections or radiation exposure was in itself a great contribution to renal mass evaluation[4].

In the 1970s, with the invention of computed tomography (CT) by Sir Godfrey Hounsfield (HOUNSFIELD 1980; ISHERWOOD 2005), we witnessed the greatest advance in imaging of the body since the discovery of X-rays by Wilhelm Roentgen in 1895. CT was initially applied to the brain and shortly thereafter to the body as well. Some machines were available in the middle and late 1970s, but by the 1980s the technology was available in most sizable hospitals around the world. In the years since its introduction, CT has been continuously updated and improved. CT scans of the body on the early units (e.g., second-generation body scanner; EMI 5005) obtained single axial slices of 13 mm thickness in 27 seconds per slice. An examination took up to an hour to perform because of the constraints of tube cooling, reconstruction time, and disc storage space. Now, of course, with multidetector-row CT (MDCT) an axial slice of less than 1 mm can be obtained in less than 1 second and an entire scan of the abdomen can be obtained in much less time than it took to get a single slice on the early scanners. (The introduction of non-ionic contrast agents further expanded the value and use of CT.) With the discovery of CT, the computer age and radiography were joined and modern radiology was born[5].

The introduction of magnetic resonance (MR) imaging was a further great advance in imaging of the body[6]. Its rapid development and use were, to a great extent, helped by the "concepts of digital data acquisition, sophisticated interactive display systems and powerful image processing" that were used in the development of CT (ISHERWOOD 2005). MR imaging has continued to improve since its introduction with the use of higher field magnets, surface coils, and advances in pulse sequences. The technique has already proven to be even more important than CT for imaging many areas of the body. The future of MR imaging seems almost limitless, with the introduction of more powerful magnets, the development of functional imaging, including perfusion- and diffusion-weighted MR imaging techniques, and spectroscopy. At this time, CT remains the most important technique in imaging of the kidney for renal cancer, although MR imaging has a significant role since it eliminates the use of ionizing radiation and iodinated contrast medium. MR imaging is valuable in staging renal cancer and, because of its direct multiplanar imaging

---

[4] Ultrasound with cyst puncture was frequently used by some radiologists to diagnose renal cysts, but cyst puncture as well as nephrotomography quickly became obsolete as CT equipment became available. However, tomography remained an essential part of the urogram (GOLDMAN and SANDLER 2000).

[5] With the introduction of CT and its continued development, the roles of intravenous urography and retrograde pyelography have continuously lessened. Conventional intravenous urography is now only occasionally used as an independent examination but is being incorporated into CT urography, which has become even more feasible with the introduction of MDCT (MR urography can also be performed).

[6] The Nobel Prize in Medicine in 2003 was presented to Paul C. Lauterbur and Peter Mansfield for their part in the development of MR imaging (PARTAIN 2004).

ability, provides an excellent roadmap for surgical removal or ablation of renal lesions (MDCT scanners can provide excellent resolution in interpolated planes as well). Because of its superior contrast resolution, MR imaging can also be helpful in evaluating some renal mass cases which are inconclusive on CT.

These great advances in imaging have resulted in advances in the detection, diagnosis, and treatment of diseases throughout the body and certainly in renal cancer as well. We now detect many more cancers of the kidney before they have metastasized, which increases the cure rate. These advances in imaging have been vital in the progress of the treatment of renal cancer from "exploratory surgery" to radical nephrectomy and then to nephron-sparing partial nephrectomy. Laparoscopic nephrectomy and laparoscopic partial nephrectomy have developed into increasingly useful procedures, and tumor ablation techniques (including percutaneous image-guided tumor ablation) are available in appropriate cases.

The rest of the story of the imaging of kidney cancer is modern radiology and is covered fully and illustrated beautifully in the pages of this book.

This review of the history of imaging in the diagnosis of renal cancer over the past 50 years is my own personal perspective. Others might view some aspects somewhat differently (GOLDMAN and SANDLER 2000). I have been fortunate to have practiced radiology during the introduction and development of all of these techniques from nephrotomography (BOSNIAK and FAEGENBURG 1965) through renal arteriography (BOSNIAK et al 1968; EVANS and BOSNIAK 1971) and computed tomography (BOSNIAK 1986; BOSNIAK 1991) to MR imaging (ISRAEL and BOSNIAK 2004). It is important for us to remember that while the technology available to us is continuously improving, we must be careful not to rely solely on the technology to do the job for us but to take the time and make the effort to perform the highest-quality examinations possible with the equipment available. We owe this to those who developed these modalities, to the specialty of radiology, to our clinical colleagues, and, most of all, to our patients.

New York

MORTON A. BOSNIAK
Professor Emeritus of Radiology
New York University Medical Center

References

Bosniak MA (1986) The current radiological approach to renal cysts. Radiology 158:1–10

Bosniak MA (1991) The small (<3.0 cm) renal parenchymal tumor: detection, diagnosis and controversies. Radiology 179:307–317

Bosniak MA (1968) Renal arteriography in patients with metastatic renal cell carcinoma. Its use as a substitute for histopathologic biopsy. JAMA 203:249–254

Bosniak MA, Faegenburg D (1965) The thick-wall sign: an important finding in nephrotomography. Radiology 84:692–697

Elkin M (1990) Stages in the growth of uroradiology. Radiology 175:297–306

Evans JA, Bosniak MA (1971) Atlas of tumor radiology: the kidney. Yearbook, Chicago

Evans JA, Dubilier W, Montrith JC (1954) Nephrotomography: a preliminary report. AJR Am J Roentgenol 71:213–223

Goldman SM, Sandler CM (2000) Genitourinary imaging: the past 40 years. Radiology 215:313–324

Hounsfield GN (1980) Computed medical imaging. Nobel Lecture, December 8, 1979. J Comput Assist Tomogr 4:665–674

Isherwood I (2005) Sir Godfrey Hounsfield. In memoriam. Radiology 234:975–976

Israel GM, Bosniak MA (2004) MR imaging of cystic renal masses. Magn Reson Imaging Clin N Am 12:403–412

Partain CL (2004) The 2003 Nobel prize for MRI; significance and impact. J Magn Reson Imaging 20:173–174

Pollack HM (1996) Uroradiology. In: McClennan BL (ed) Radiology centennial. Radiology Centennial, Reston, VA, pp195–253

Seldinger SI (1953) Catheter replacement of the needle in percutaneous arteriography. A new technique. Acta Radiol 39:368–376

Preface

Until recently, surgical resection was considered the only option for treatment of kidney cancer, especially renal cell carcinoma. The disease is relatively resistant to both radiotherapy and chemotherapy, and although alternative systemic therapies such as interleukin-2 immunotherapy and interferon have shown promise, objective response rates are still quite low. Minimally invasive therapies have piqued the interest of researchers by showing significant improvements in treatment and management of kidney cancer. These techniques currently are seen as the most promising new approaches for treating renal cell carcinoma and its complications. Although progress has been frustratingly slow at times, the combination of new treatments and imaging techniques is improving the prognosis.

Regardless of type or treatment, management of kidney cancer depends substantially on the effective use of imaging. This is true at all stages, from initial diagnosis to follow up. During the course of the disease, any or all of the available imaging modalities may play a role. These include the older methods of plain film and angiography, the more recent such as ultrasound, CT and MR imaging, as well as the newest, particularly PET and PET/CT. Each has its advantages – and disadvantages – all of which are discussed in detail.

Much discussion is also given to kidney cancer subtypes, with complete histological descriptions, numerous illustrations of surgical specimens and microscopic views, and thorough descriptions of the radiological and pathological correlations. Techniques of minimally invasive surgery, including laparoscopic nephron-sparing surgery, transarterial embolization and radiofrequency ablation, are covered in depth.

Each of these issues is discussed by authors selected for their prominence in their specialty, and the list of authors represents a deep and broad combination of experience and learning. This is the most complete and most current volume available on the subject.

Many people have helped me to bring this project to fruition; without their assistance, which I gratefully acknowledge, this book would have never been published. I want especially to thank Professor Albert Baert, who supported my idea and made its realization possible. This volume is the second I have edited in the series he supervises, and when I first approached him about the appropriateness of such a book on kidney cancer, he said yes without hesitation. I am most grateful to Professor Baert for his support and encouragement.

I am also grateful to the authors, many of whom I now count among my friends, who have made working on this volume really enjoyable. I should not forget my two guardian angels, David Breazeale for his unconditional editorial assistance, and Ursula Davis for always being there to answer my questions, and for her endless patience.

Finally, I would like to thank my wife Noura who no longer believes me when I tell her "this is the last book I am going to edit". I would like to dedicate this volume to my daughter Dorra, my son Elias, and my parents for their love during the time I spent working on the book. I also would like to thank my friends for their unconditional support.

San Francisco   Ali Guermazi

"Geometry is useful because it enlightens the intelligence of the man who cultivates it and gives him the habit of thinking exactly"

Abu Abdullah Muhammad Ibn Musa Al-Khawarizmi (Algorizm) 770-840

"Knowledge is the conformity of the object and the intellect"

Abul Waleed Muhammad Ibn Ahmed Ibn Rushd (Averroes) 1126-1198

"Human subtlety will never devise an invention more beautiful, more simple or more direct than does Nature, because in her inventions, nothing is lacking and nothing is superfluous"

Leonardo da Vinci 1452-1519

Contents

List of Abbreviations

AML	Angiomyolipoma
CNR	Contrast-to-noise ratio
efgre	enhanced fast gradient recalled echo
FDA	Food and Drug Administration
FDG	Fluorine 18 fluorodeoxyglucose
FLASH	Fast low-angle shot
FSE	Fast spin echo
FSPGR	Fast spoiled gradient-recalled
GRE	Gradient recalled echo
HASTE	Half-Fourier acquisition single-shot turbo spin echo
HU	Hounsfield Units
IVC	Inferior vena cava
MIP	Maximum intensity projection
MR	Magnetic resonance
MRA	Magnetic resonance angiography
MRU	Magnetic resonance urography
MRV	Magnetic resonance venography
PET	Positron emission tomography
RCC	Renal cell carcinoma
RF	Radiofrequency
ROI	Region of interest
SE	Spin echo
SNR	Signal-to-noise ratio
SSFSE	Single-shot fast spin echo
TCC	Transitional cell carcinoma
TSA	Turbo spin echo
VIBE	Volumetric interpolated breath-hold examination

1 Histopathological Classification

Shigeki Tomita, Yoshihiko Ueda and Takahiro Fujimori

CONTENTS

1.1
Introduction

Among all benign and malignant tumors, few are the result of kidney cancer. Cancer of the kidney accounts for only about 3% of all cancers in adults, with about 36,000 cases expected in the United States in 2004 (Jemal et al. 2004).

S. Tomita, MD, PhD
Assistant Professor of Pathology, Department of Surgical and Molecular Pathology, Dokkyo University School of Medicine; Department of Surgical Pathology, Dokkyo University Hospital, 880 Kitakobayashi, Mibu, Shimo-tsuga, Tochigi 321-0293, Japan
Y. Ueda, MD, PhD
Professor and Chairman, Department of Pathology, Koshigaya Hospital, Dokkyo University School of Medicine, 2-1-50 Minami-Koshigaya, Koshigaya, Saitama 343-8555, Japan
T. Fujimori, MD, PhD
Professor and Chairman, Department of Surgical and Molecular Pathology, Dokkyo University School of Medicine; Director, Department of Surgical Pathology, Dokkyo University Hospital, 880 Kitakobayashi, Mibu, Shimo-tsuga, Tochigi 321-0293, Japan

The first description of a renal cell carcinoma, in 1883, appears to have been hypernephroma (Grawitz 1883). More recently, investigators have developed a classification system for renal tumors based on cytological appearance, architectural features and presumed cellular origin in the renal tubular system (Colvin 2003; Delahunt and Eble 2002; Kovacs et al. 1997). Recently, a revised pathological classification of kidney tumors has been proposed (Takahashi et al. 2003; Zambrano et al. 1999). Hereditary kidney tumors are associated with genetic disorders, and the same genetic abnormalities are thought to be involved in sporadic kidney cancers (Nagashima et al. 2004).

Herein we describe the World Health Organization (WHO) classification of renal tumors based on pathology (Eble et al. 2004), and discuss relevant issues in arriving at the correct differential diagnosis based on morphological findings.

1.2
Histopathological Classification

Kidney tumors are classified as benign or malignant depending on their histopathological features. Papillary/tubulopapillary adenoma, oncocytic adenoma, and metanephric adenoma are classified as benign. Conventional (clear cell) renal cell carcinoma, papillary renal cell carcinoma, chromophobe renal cell carcinoma, collecting duct carcinoma, cyst-associated renal cell carcinoma, sarcomatoid renal cell carcinoma, and renal medullary carcinoma are classified as malignant (Table 1.1).

Early attempts to develop a classification system of kidney cancers met with limited success (Delahunt and Eble 1998). The first worldwide classification of kidney cancer, the Mainz classification, was based solely on morphological criteria (Thoenes et al. 1986). The WHO has developed a new classification system for kidney cancer based on morphology and molecular findings (Eble et al. 2004).

Table 1.1. Histological classification of kidney tumors. *RCC* renal cell carcinoma

Malignant tumors
Conventional (clear cell) RCC
Papillary renal cell carcinoma
Chromophobe RCC
Collecting duct RCC
Renal cell carcinoma, unclassified
Others: Cyst-associated carcinoma RCC
Sarcomatoid RCC (Spindle RCC)
Granular cell carcinoma
Renal medullary carcinoma
Benign tumors
Papillary/tubulopapillary adenoma
Renal oncocytoma
Metanephric adenoma

1.2.1
Conventional Clear Cell Carcinoma

Renal cell carcinoma (RCC) accounts for 2% of all cancers. Clear cell carcinoma accounts for about 80–90% of all RCC. Generally, patients with RCC are men (by a ratio of 4:1) diagnosed in their sixth decade. Renal cell carcinoma usually presents with micro/macro-hematuria, costal vertebral pain, and abdominal mass (MOTZER et al. 1996); however, patients rarely present with this classical triad. Weight loss, anemia, thrombocytosis (INOUE et al. 2004), and abnormal hormone production (ALTAFFER and CHENAULT 1979) are common. Renal cell carcinoma may present with hypertension caused by rennin secretion (HOLLIFIELD et al. 1975), and polycythemia as the result of erythropoietin secretion (OKABE et al. 1985).

Macroscopic findings of typical clear cell RCC show a rounded, whitish-yellow, sometimes tanbrown or gray, solid, well-circumscribed tumor with focal hemorrhage and necrosis (Fig. 1.1a). A pseudocapsule is often formed by compressed normal parenchyma. Multiple nodules may be present. Cystic change can be marked, and occasionally tumors are seen as small yellow nodules on the inner surface of benign cyst. The size may range from less than 1 cm to more than 25 cm.

Microscopic findings show the usual pattern is predominantly clear cells in an alveolar architecture (Fig. 1.1b). The tumor cells are generally homogenous and characteristically possess clear cytoplasm due to abundant lipid and glycogen (Fig. 1.2). Some of the tumor cells may be eosinophilic or contain granular cytoplasm. Focal dysplastic areas can be seen in adjacent normal tubules. The tumor frequently causes hyalinization and hemorrhage. Immunohistochemically, RCC shows reactivity to keratin (CK8, 18, and 19; BANNER et al. 1990; LANGNER et al. 2004), epithelial membrane antigen (EMA), and vimentin (WALDHERR and SCHWECHHEIMER 1985). The tumor cells are negative for col-

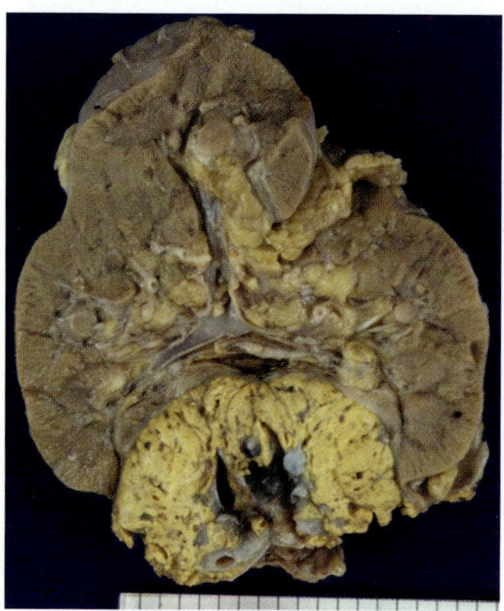
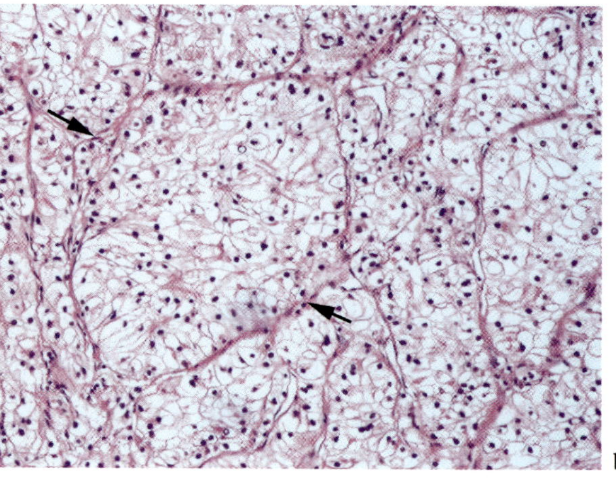

Fig. 1.1a,b. Conventional clear cell carcinoma in a 55-year-old man. **a** Macroscopic view shows a rounded, whitish-yellow, solid, well-circumscribed tumor with focal hemorrhage and necrosis. **b** Microscopic examination shows typical pattern is predominantly proliferation of clear cells, due to abundant lipid and glycogen in an alveolar architecture (*arrows*) (Hematoxylin and eosin stain; original magnification, ×100).

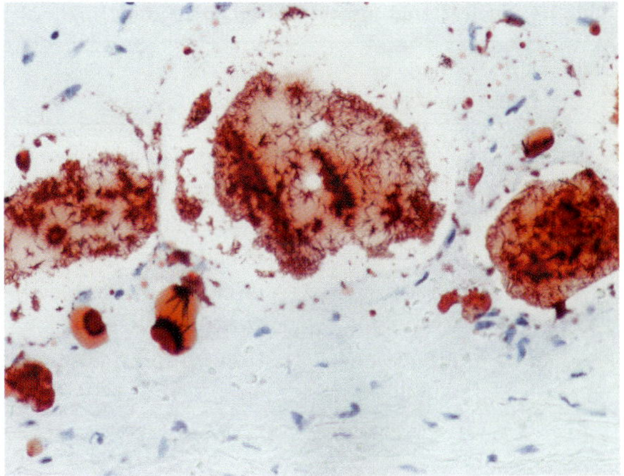

Fig. 1.2. Small conventional clear cell carcinoma in a 42-year-old woman. Microscopic examination shows positive stain for neutral lipid in frozen section (oil red O stain; original magnification, ×200).

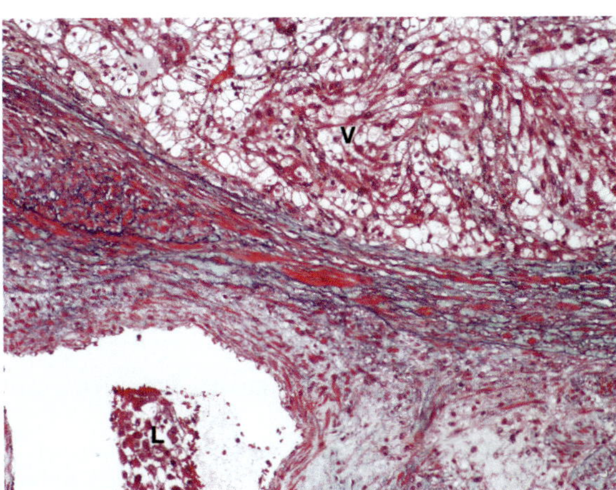

Fig. 1.3. Renal cell carcinoma in a 63-year-old man. Microscopic examination shows that the tumor involves the lymphatic (*L*) and venous (*V*) channels (Elastica Masson stain; original magnification, ×100).

loidal iron, HMB45, and lectin. The tumor tends to invade the renal vein and the inferior vena cava with metastases especially to the lung, bone, liver, and brain (Fig. 1.3; Bukowski et al. 2004).

It is usually not difficult to diagnose clear cell carcinoma, but the possibility of an adrenal rest should be excluded. Distinguishing clear cell carcinoma from adrenal cortical tumor may be difficult; immunohistochemical investigation with CD10 or RCC antigen expression can help. It is important to distinguish between primary and secondary clear cell tumor with vimentin, CD10, and RCC antigen (McGregor et al. 2001).

Prognoses vary depending on tumor size, tumor stage, nuclear grade, DNA content, and proliferation markers. The size of the primary tumor correlates with the likelihood of distant metastases. One rare case of a very small (<3 cm) tumor that had metastasized, as confirmed at autopsy, has been reported (Hellsten et al. 1981). Recently, an increasing number of small renal tumors have been revealed by CT, ultrasound, and MR imag-

ing. Patients diagnosed with renal tumor are classified by tumor stage, with the stage based on surgical material. We use two staging systems: the Robson system is simple and has four stages (Table 1.2; Robson et al. 1967). It is used mainly by urologists. The TNM staging system is more complex but provides more information (Fig. 1.4; Table 1.3; Ficarra et al. 2004; Guinan et al. 1997). It is used by both urologists and pathologists. Tumors can also be graded according to nuclear size, shape, and nucleoli, all of which are considered prognostic factors. The most widely used nuclear grading system is that of Fuhrman et al. (1982; Fig. 1.5; Table 1.4). In the Fuhrman system, there is a distinct prognostic difference between grade-I/II and grade-III/IV tumors. A correlation has been reported between DNA content (ploidy) and nuclear grading. Proliferation markers [Ki-67, nucleolar organizer regions (AgNORs), S-phase fraction, and proliferating cell nuclear antigen (PCNA)] have all been reported to correlate with the prognosis (Srigley et al. 1997).

Table 1.2. Tumor staging system of RCC (Robson criteria)

Stage I	Stage II	Stage III	Stage IV
Tumor confined to the kidney	Perirenal fat involvement but confined to Gerota's fascia	A: Gross renal vein or inferior vena cava involvement	A: Involvement of adjacent organs other than adrenal gland
		B: Lymphatic involvement C: Vascular and lymphatic involvement and metastasis to regional lymph nodes	B: Distant metastases

Table 1.3. The TNM tumor staging system of RCC. (From Guinan et al. 1997)

TNM clinical classification

T: primary tumor
- TX: primary tumor cannot be assessed
- T0: no evidence of primary tumor
- T1: tumor 7.0 cm or less in greatest dimension, limited to the kidney
- T2: tumor more than 7.0 cm in greatest dimension, limited to the kidney
- T3: tumor extends into major veins or invades adrenal gland or perinephric tissues but not beyond Gerota's fascia
    - T3a: tumor invades adrenal gland or perinephric tissues but not beyond Gerota's fascia
    - T3b: tumor grossly extends into renal vein(s) or vena cava below diaphragm
    - T3c: tumor grossly extends into vena cava above diaphragm
- T4: tumor invades beyond Gerota's fascia

N: regional lymph nodes
- NX: regional lymph nodes cannot be assessed
- N0: no regional lymph node metastasis
- N1: metastasis in a single regional lymph node
- N2: metastasis in more than one regional lymph node

M: distant metastasis
- MX: distant metastasis cannot be assessed
- M0: no distant metastasis
- M1: distant metastasis

Other classifications

pTNM pathological classification:
pT, pN, and pM categories correspond to the T, N, and M categories

Histopathological grading:
- GX: grade of differentiation cannot be assessed
- G1: well differentiated
- G2: moderately differentiated
- G3–G4: poorly differentiated/undifferentiated

Stage grouping:
- Stage I: T1, N0, M0
- Stage II: T2, N0, M0
- Stage III: T1, N1, M0
             T2, N1, M0
             T3, N0 or N1, M0
- Stage IV: T3, N0 or N1, M0
             Any T, N2, M0
             Any T, any N, M1

Table 1.4. Nuclear grading system (Fuhrman grade)

Grade	Size (cm)	Shape of nuclei	Nucleoli
1	10	Round, uniform	Inconspicuous or absent nucleoli
2	15	Slightly irregular	Evident at high power (×400)
3	20	Obviously irregular	Prominent, large at low power (×100)
4	> 20	Bizarre, often multilobed	Heavy chromatin clump

1.2.2
Special Types of Renal Cell Carcinoma

1.2.2.1
Papillary Renal Cell Carcinoma

Papillary RCC is the second most common type of renal tubular tumor in the elderly, accounting for about 10% of all RCC. Papillary RCC is also known as "chromophil RCC" or "tubulopapillary carcinoma." Thoenes et al. (1986) first and Amin et al. (1997) more recently have developed a set of histological criteria for papillary RCC. The male-to-female ratio is 8:1. The prognosis is better than for conventional RCC.

Macroscopic findings of papillary RCC show a rounded, heterogeneous, gray-tan, solid, well-circumscribed tumor with hemorrhage and fibrous capsule (Fig. 1.6a). The tumor size can be less than 20 cm. It is often multiple and bilateral.

Microscopic findings show that papillary RCC is characterized by papillary, tubular, and tubulopapillary growth with several cell patterns over at least 50% of its area (Fig. 1.6b). Thoenes et al. (1986) further divided papillary RCC into eosinophilic, basophilic, and duophilic. Recently, Delahunt and Eble (1997) classified papillary RCC as type 1 or type 2. Type 1 has a papillary pattern of small cells with scant basophilic cytoplasm and low-grade nuclear atypia (grades 1–2). Type 2 is composed of large cells with abundant eosinophilic cytoplasm with large nuclei (grades 3–4). Foamy macrophages and neutrophils are common in the stroma adjacent the tumor. Hemosiderin, glomeruloid papillae, psammoma bodies, edema, and foamy macrophages are common in type 1, but not in type 2. Immunohistochemically, type 1 (80%) and type 2 (20%) tumors show reactivity for Kerain (CK7). Assessment of tumor growth kinet-

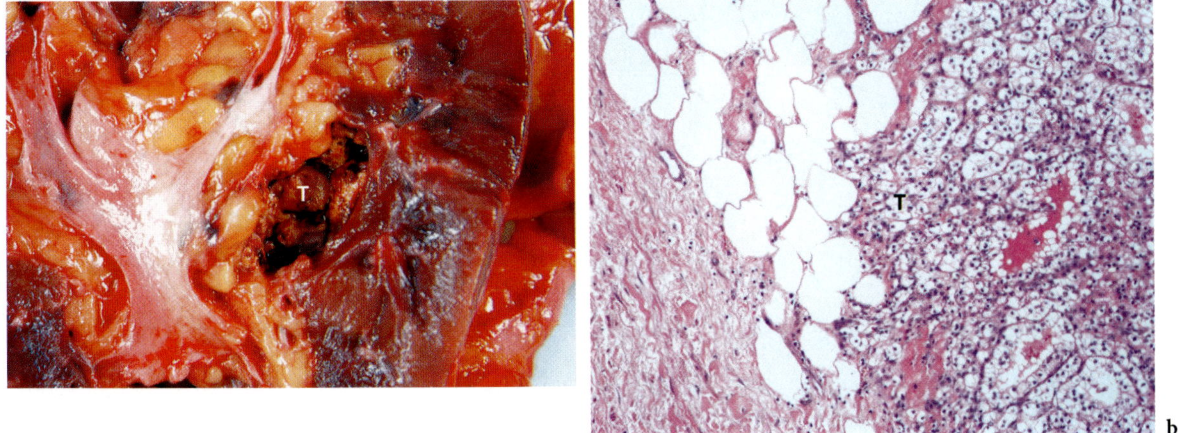

Fig. 1.4a,b. Renal cell carcinoma in a 60-year-old man. **a** Macroscopic view shows the tumor extending into the perinephric tissue (*T*; pT3 tumor). **b** Microscopic examination shows the tumor (*T*) involving the fatty tissue in sinus renalis (hematoxylin and eosin stain; original magnification, ×80).

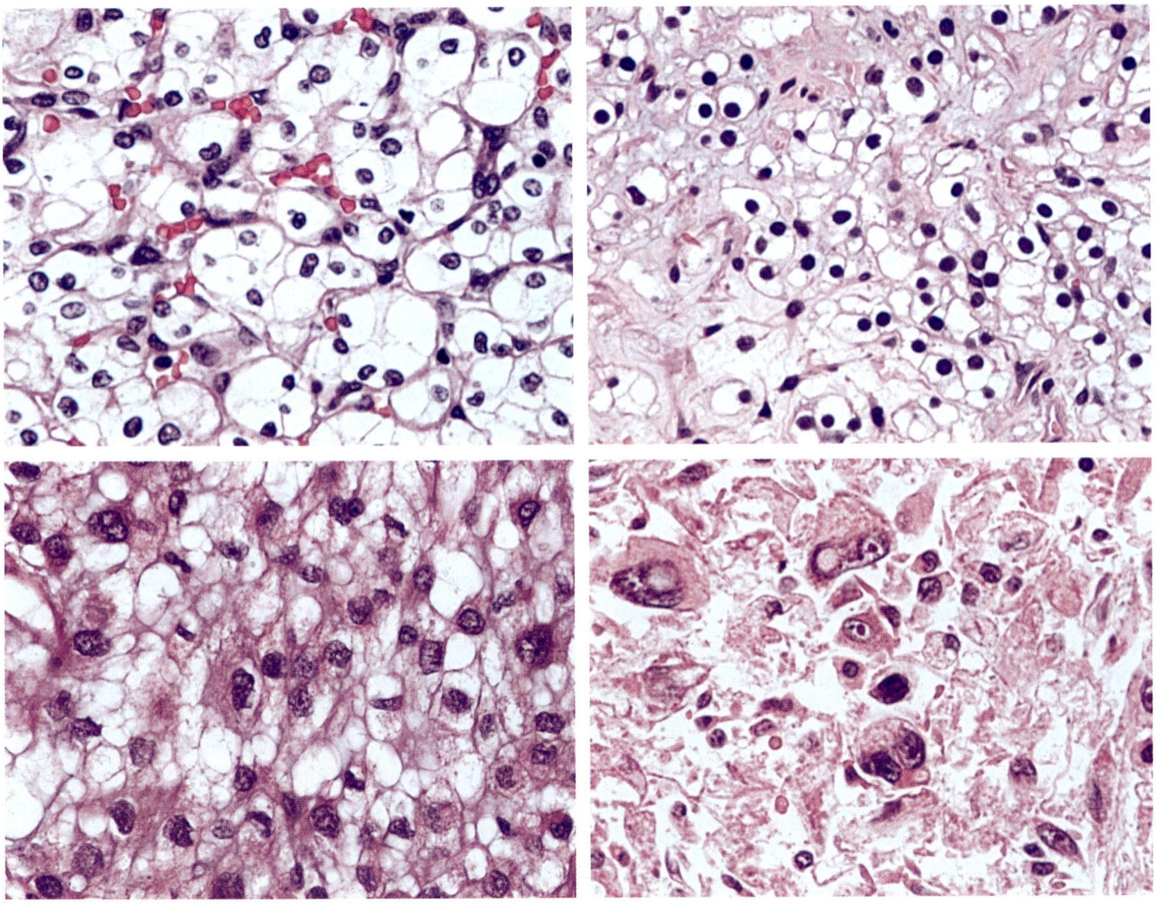

Fig. 1.5a-d. Different grades for renal cell carcinoma by Fuhrman nuclear grading system. **a** Microscopic examination of grade 1 shows the regular, uniform nuclei comparable in size to the red blood cells (hematoxylin and eosin stain; original magnification, ×400). **b** Microscopic examination of grade 2 shows the nuclei varying in size, generally larger than in the grade-1 tumor cells. The chromatins are hyperconcentrated and the nucleoli are frequently visible (hematoxylin and eosin stain; original magnification, ×400). **c** Microscopic examination of grade 3 shows the large nuclei with hyperchromatin along with marked variability in size and shape. The nucleoli are large and conspicuous (hematoxylin and eosin stain; original magnification, ×400). **d** Microscopic examination of grade 4 shows tumor cells exhibiting large pleomorphic nuclei with chromatin clumping and conspicuous nucleoli (hematoxylin and eosin stain; original magnification, ×400).

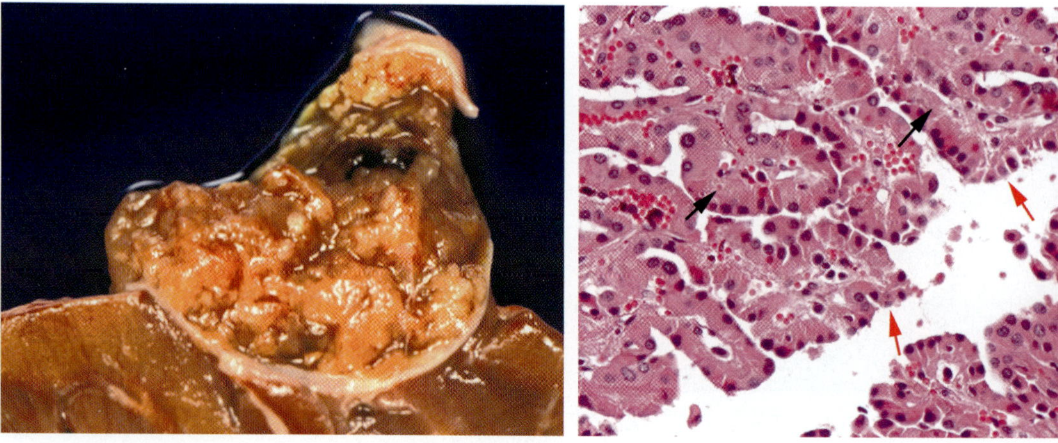

Fig. 1.6a,b. Papillary renal cell carcinoma in a 67-year-old man. **a** Macroscopic view shows a rounded, heterogeneous, gray-tan, solid, well-circumscribed tumor with hemorrhage and fibrous capsule. **b** Microscopic examination shows papillary, tubular, tubulo-papillary growth (*red arrows*) with eosinophilic cells (*black arrows*) (Hematoxylin and eosin stain; original magnification, ×200).

ics showed significant mean AgNOR scores and Ki-67 indices between the two histological types (DELAHUNT et al. 2001).

It is important to distinguish between benign and malignant renal tumors with papillary projection. Surgical pathologists use a standard protocol to make the distinction: (a) papillary, tubular, or tubulopapillary projection; (b) less than 5 mm in diameter; (c) does not histologically resemble clear cell, chromophobe, or collecting duct RCC (DELAHUNT and EBLE 1997). Collecting duct RCC is stained with lectin-binding protein [*Ulex europaeus* agglutinin-I (UEA-I), anti-keratin MA903] and expresses high molecular weight keratins, but papillary RCC is negative for these markers.

1.2.2.2
Chromophobe Renal Cell Carcinoma

THOENES et al. first described chromophobe RCC in 12 patients in 1985. It was first recognized in a non-human experimental tumor in 1974 (BANNASCH et al. 1974), but it was not established as a variant of human RCC until 2004 (PEYROMAURE et al. 2004). Chromophobe RCC accounts for less than 6% of renal carcinomas and has a favorable prognosis (CHEVILLE et al. 2003). It affects men and women equally. Chromophobe RCC usually presents symptoms (e.g., abdominal mass) similar to conventional RCC. Immunohistochemical, enzyme histochemical, and ultrastructural findings suggest that the intercalating cells of the collecting duct are the counterpart cells of chromophobe RCC.

Macroscopic findings of chromophobe RCC show a rounded, homogenous, gray-beige, solid, well-circumscribed tumor without hemorrhage or necrosis (Fig. 1.7a). Single nodules may be present. Cystic and hyalinization changes are uncommon. Tumor size may vary. Radiologically, chromophobe RCC tumors are hypovascular, with less prominent vascularity than conventional RCC.

Microscopic findings of chromophobe RCC consist of a solid or glandular growth pattern of large cells with pale/clear cytoplasm called "pale cells" and small cells with eosinophilic cytoplasm called "eosinophilic cells" (Fig. 1.7b). Mixtures of these patterns also occur. The cell membranes are prominent in the solid or glandular pattern (COCHAND-PRIOLLET et al. 1997). These cells have little lipid or glycogen compared with conventional RCC. The nuclei are irregular and small, and appear hyperchromatic with a perinuclear halo. Chromophobe RCC usually is lower nuclear grade (grades 1–2). Ultrastructurally, chromophobe RCC commonly reveals numerous micro-cystic vesicles and mitochondria (THOENES et al. 1985). Immunohistochemically and enzyme histochemically, pale cells and eosinophilic cells stain with colloidal iron (Fig. 1.7c; THOENES et al. 1985) and show reactivity to keratin (CK18 and CK9; THOENES et al. 1988), EMA, and paxillin (KURODA et al. 2001). The tumor cells are negative for vimentin, CD10, and RCC antigen (AVERY et al. 2000).

The main differential diagnosis is between oncocytoma and conventional RCC. Colloidal iron stain can distinguish chromophobe RCC from oncocytoma and conventional RCC. CD10, RCC antibody,

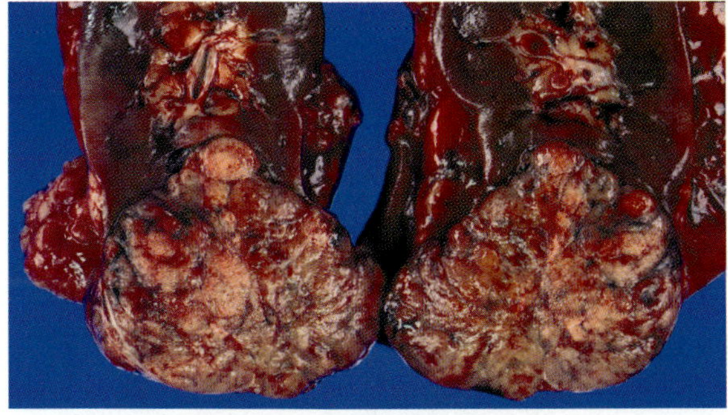

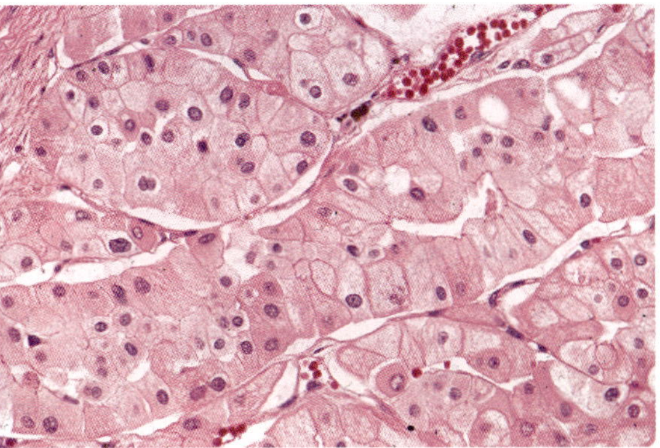

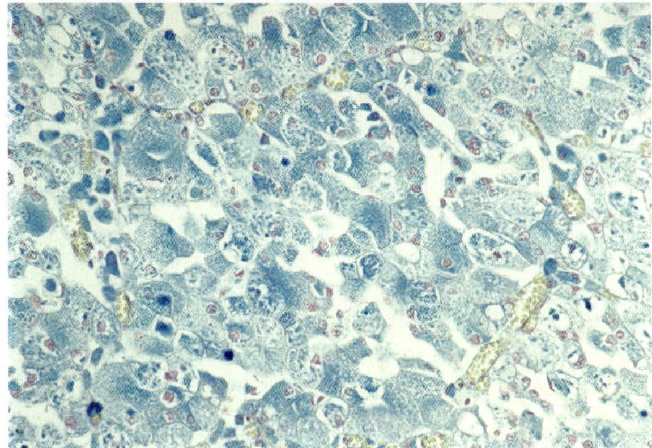

Fig. 1.7a-c. Chromophobe renal cell carcinoma in a 65-year-old man. **a** Macroscopic view shows a rounded, homogenous, gray-beige, solid, well-circumscribed tumor without hemorrhage or necrosis. **b** Microscopic examination shows the solid and glandular growth pattern with "pale cell" and "eosinophilic cell" with perinuclear halo (hematoxylin and eosin stain; original magnification, ×200). **c** Microscopic examination shows positive stain for colloidal iron in cytoplasm (colloidal iron stain; original magnification, ×200).

and vimentin are usually negative, and cytokeratin 18 is expressed in chromophobe RCC. On the other hand, CD10 is positive for conventional RCC, RCC antibody, and negative for vimentin.

1.2.2.3
Collecting Duct Carcinoma

Collecting duct carcinoma, also known as Bellini duct carcinoma, is a rare variant of RCC, representing less than 3% of all malignant renal tumors. The tumor arises from or differentiates from the epithelium of the collecting duct, which is also known as Bellini's duct. In 1976 MANCILLA-JIMENEZ et al. first reported that collecting duct carcinoma is a form of RCC that arises from the collecting ducts. Some pathologists have suggested that collecting duct carcinoma is distinct from other types of RCC.

Collecting duct carcinoma occurs twice as often in men as in women. Initial presentation consists of hematuria and pain. An abdominal mass indicates an advanced metastatic stage (SRIGLEY and EBLE 1998). Advanced collecting duct carcinoma may be manifested by fever and leukocytosis caused by tumor-derived inflammatory cytokines (NAGASHIMA et al. 2004). Approximately half of all patients die within 2 years. There is no effective therapy.

Macroscopic findings of collecting duct carcinoma show a solid, white-gray tumor with invasive growth to the renal capsule, spreading to the perirenal fat (Fig. 1.8a). The tumor is usually located in the medulla or central portion of the kidney, and ranges in size from 2.5 to 12 cm. It is often necrotic and shows micro-cystic changes.

Microscopic findings show that collecting duct carcinoma is characterized by papillary, tubulopapillary, cystic, glandular, and solid patterns of tubules with desmoplastic reaction (Fig. 1.8b). Sarcomatoid/spindle cell changes may be present (KENNEDY et al. 1990). The tumor cells have a marked nuclear atypia with eosinophilic cytoplasm and a hobnail appearance. Tumor-producing mucin may be identified. A dysplastic epithelium adjacent to the tumor also secretes mucin. These tumor cells are surrounded by desmoplastic and inflammatory stroma with many neutrophils. Immunohistochemically, collecting duct carcinoma shows reactivity to EMA and high molecular weight keratins (CK19, 34betaE12) and stains with lectin [Arachis hypogaea (PNA) and soybean agglutinin (SBA)], UEA-I (DIMOPOULOS et al. 1993).

Differential diagnosis is sometimes difficult, as macroscopically collecting duct carcinoma resembles papillary RCC. Papillary RCC is positive for lectin-binding proteins from the proximal or distal

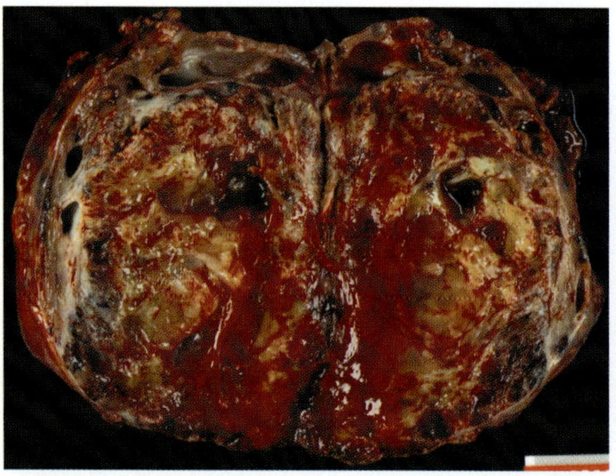
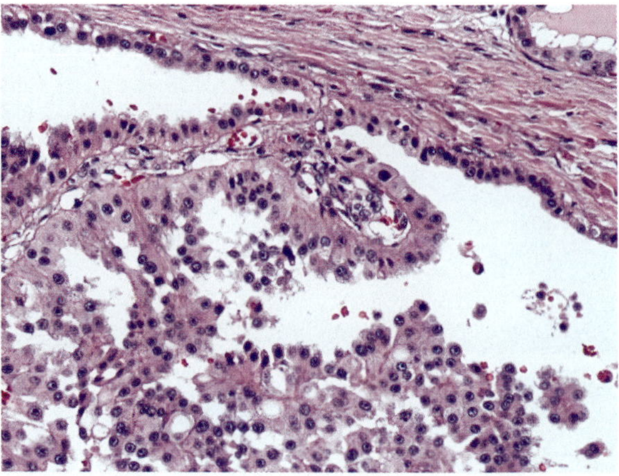

a

b

Fig. 1.8a,b. Collecting duct renal cell carcinoma in a 33-year-old woman. **a** Macroscopic view shows a solid tumor with invasive growth to the renal capsule and spread to perirenal tissue. **b** Microscopic examination shows papillary, tubulopapillary, cystic patterns of tubules (hematoxylin and eosin stain; original magnification, ×200).

nephron, but collecting duct carcinoma is positive only for proteins from the distal nephron.

1.2.3
Other Renal Cancers

1.2.3.1
Cyst-Associated Renal Cell Carcinoma

Cyst-associated renal cell carcinoma (also known as multilocular cystic RCC) is an uncommon neoplasm, accounting for only a few rare cases out of all renal tumors (Fig. 1.9a). PERLMANN et al. (1928) first described cyst-associated RCC with a lymphangioma containing a small population of clear cells. The tumor appeared to be a distinct subtype of RCC with characteristic gross and microscopic features. Since then, HARTMAN et al. (1986) have suggested mechanisms by which renal cells may present carcinoma as a cystic lesion. The classification of RCC in Japan lists cyst-associated RCC rather than multilocular cystic RCC. Its etiology and behavior is uncertain, and it may be difficult to distinguish from predominantly cystic neoplasms of the kidney. Histologically, cyst-associated RCC are well-demarcated multicystic lesions containing variably sized aggregates of neoplastic clear cells with low-grade atypia (grade 1). The cyst walls are densely fibrotic and the lining is often devoid of epithelium (Fig. 1.9b). Recently, using immunohistochemistry and lectin histochemistry, it has been demonstrated that cyst-associated RCC originates from the epithelium between the distal convoluted

tubule and the collecting duct (IMURA et al. 2004). With surgery the prognosis is excellent.

However, there are many patients with long-term hemodialysis in Japan. Long-term hemodialysis frequently causes the renal tubules to dilate, and leads to malignant tumors including RCC associated with acquired cystic kidney disease (ISHIKAWA 1991). It is also known that RCC occurs as atypical cysts in patients with autosomal-dominant polycystic kidney disease (ADPKD; Fig. 1.10; KEITH et al. 1994). It is difficult to distinguish between ADPKD-related RCC and non-related RCC, and diagnosis of ADPKD may require investigation of the patient's family medical history. It has been suggested that an RCC in ADPKD is sarcomatoid change more often than not (ISHIKAWA and KOVACS 1993).

1.2.3.2
Sarcomatoid Renal Cell Carcinoma

Sarcomatoid RCC was first described by FARROW et al. in 1968 (Fig. 1.11a). These tumors make up less than 5% of all RCC. They have also been known as spindle cell carcinoma, anaplastic carcinoma, or carcinosarcoma. Sarcomatoid RCC is characterized by marked cytological atypia (nuclear grade 4; Fig. 1.11b) and contains enlarged pleomorphic or malignant spindle cells resembling those in sarcoma (Fig. 1.11c–e; CHEVILLE et al. 2004; PERALTA-VENTURINA et al. 2001). The aggressive behavior of sarcomatoid RCC generally leads to a poor prognosis; however, sarcomatoid RCC was not included in a recent classification scheme, because a sarcomatoid component can

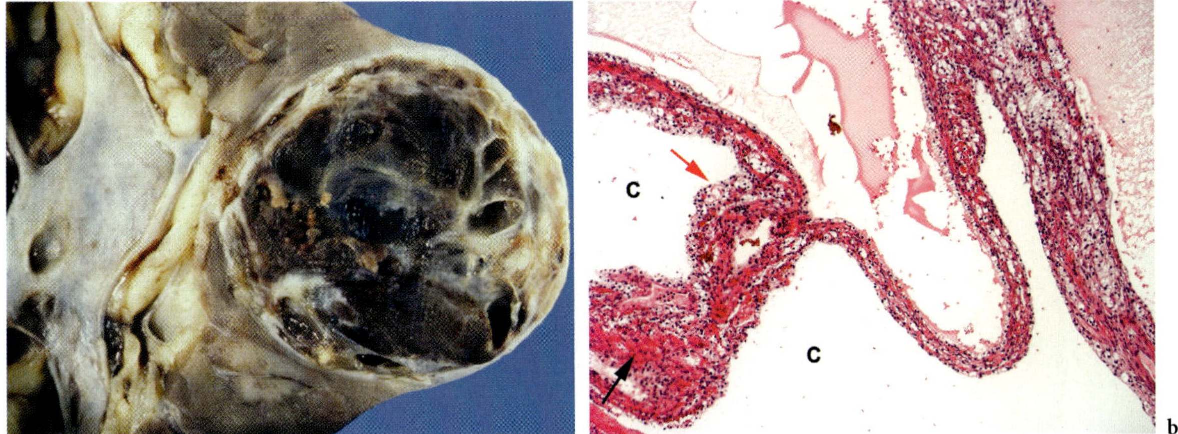

Fig. 1.9a,b. Cyst-associated renal cell carcinoma in a 65-year-old man. **a** Macroscopic view shows a multiloculated tumor with subdividing thin septa into various-sized loculi. **b** Microscopic examination shows multicystic lesions (*C*) containing variably sized aggregates of neoplastic clear cells (*red arrow*) with fibrotic stroma (*black arrow*) (Hematoxylin and eosin stain; original magnification, ×80).

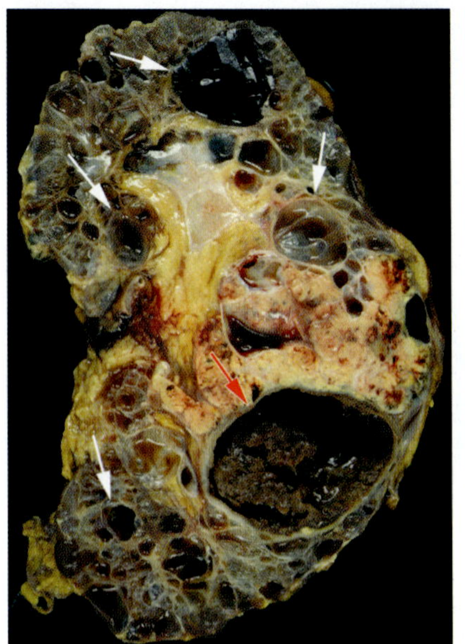

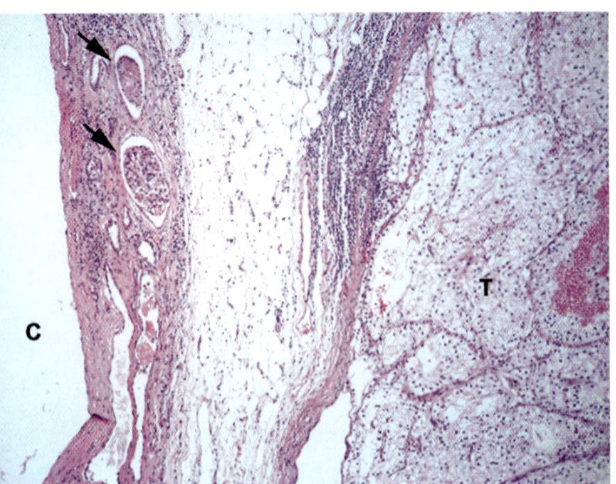

Fig. 1.10a,b. Autosomal-dominant polycystic kidney disease in a 54-year-old man with hematoma. **a** Macroscopic view shows multicystic lesions (*white arrows*) with a rounded hematoma (*red arrow*). **b** Microscopic examination shows the tumor cells of renal cell carcinoma (*T*) are adjacent to cystic lesion (*C*) with intact glomeruli (*arrows*) (Hematoxylin and eosin stain; original magnification, ×80).

occur in all histological subtypes of RCC, especially chromophobe RCC (AKHTAR et al. 1997).

RCC was eliminated from a recently proposed classification (REUTER and PRESTI 2000), and the term is no longer used in pathological diagnosis.

1.2.3.3
Granular Renal Cell Carcinoma

Histologically, granular RCC appears granular because of the abundant eosinophilic cytoplasm and mitochondria in its cells. The only point of distinction between granular RCC and conventional RCC is the granular appearance, and distinguishing between granular RCC with low-grade nuclear atypia and benign oncocytoma is difficult. Granular

1.2.3.4
Renal Medullary Carcinoma

In 1995 DAVIS et al. first described renal medullary carcinoma in conjunction with the sickle cell trait and sickle cell hemoglobin disease. Grossly, tumors range from 4 to 12 cm in diameter and are located in the medulla. Histologically, the tumor resembles a reticular, yolk-sac tumor or an adenoid cystic carcinoma.

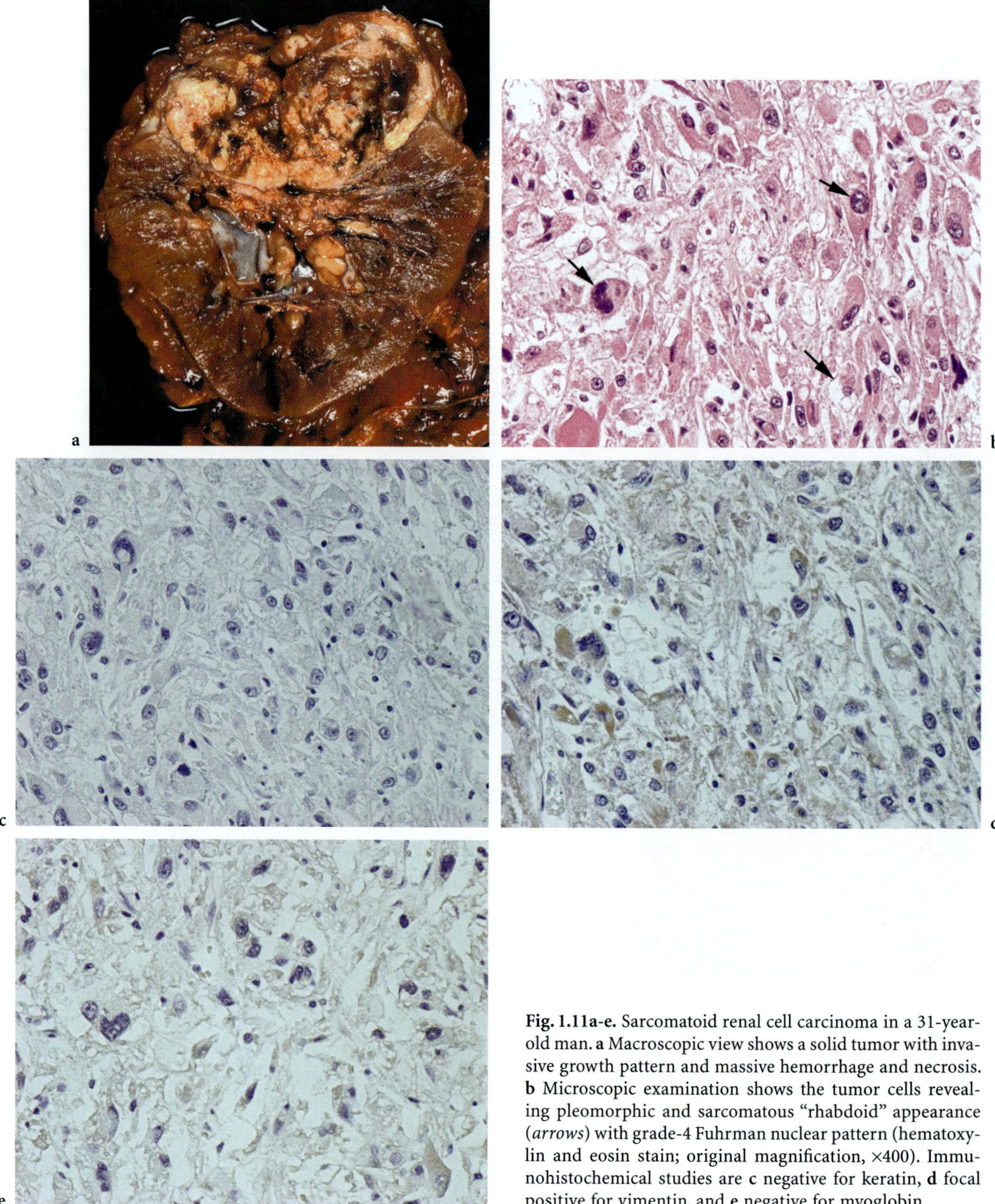

Fig. 1.11a-e. Sarcomatoid renal cell carcinoma in a 31-year-old man. **a** Macroscopic view shows a solid tumor with invasive growth pattern and massive hemorrhage and necrosis. **b** Microscopic examination shows the tumor cells revealing pleomorphic and sarcomatous "rhabdoid" appearance (*arrows*) with grade-4 Fuhrman nuclear pattern (hematoxylin and eosin stain; original magnification, ×400). Immunohistochemical studies are **c** negative for keratin, **d** focal positive for vimentin, and **e** negative for myoglobin.

Peripheral satellites in the cortex and perirenal tissue with venous and lymphatic invasion are common. The tumor has a desmoplastic stroma with inflammatory cells and lymphoid follicles. Its cells react to the same stains as collecting duct carcinoma. The tumor is aggressive (SWARTZ et al. 2002).

1.3
Cytology

Renal cell carcinoma can be diagnosed with urine cytology. The RCC tumor cells may contain neutral lipids that stain with oil red O or Sudan IV (Fig. 1.12a). The specimen should consist of fresh, unfixed material since lipids dissolve in alcohol. Cytological examination of urine is simple and safe. Urine cytology is primarily for the diagnosis of symptomatic patients. The most common symptom of RCC is gross or micro-hematuria, but voided urine rarely yields adequate material for cytological examination, as tumor cells are not present until an advanced stage (Fig. 1.12b–d). Several investigators have suggested that retrograde catheterization with brush/lavage and fine-needle aspiration biopsy gives better results (Bibbo et al. 1974; Truong et al. 1999).

1.4
Genetic and Molecular Events in Renal Cell Carcinoma

Recent advances in genetic and molecular research have associated some types of RCC with distinct genetic and molecular abnormalities.

The von Hippel-Lindau (VHL) disease is an autosomal-dominant hereditary syndrome. Patients with VHL disease frequently develop conventional RCC (Gnarra et al. 1996). Conventional RCC has a loss of chromosome 3 and loss of function of *VHL* gene mutation (Gnarra et al. 1994). Hypermethylation of the *VHL* gene has been found in conventional RCC (Herman et al. 1994). Abnormalities of the *VHL* gene lead to dysfunction of the hypoxia-inducible factors–VHL protein-elongin B-C (HIF–VBC) complex pathway (Morris et al. 2004). Duplication and trisomy of chromosome 5q (Kovacs 1993) and

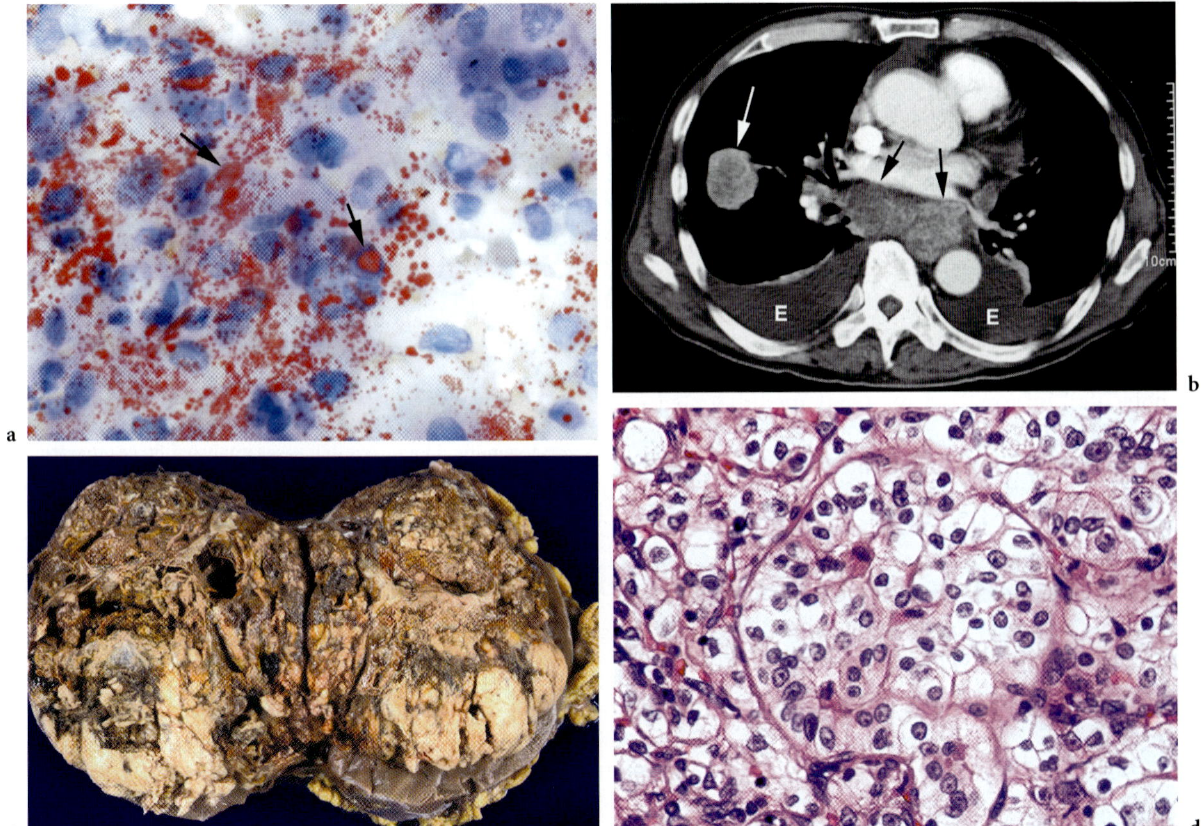

Fig. 1.12a-d. Metastatic renal cell carcinoma in a 63-year-old man. **a** Cytological study shows positive stain (*arrows*) for neutral lipid obtained from pleural effusion (Oil red O stain; original magnification, ×400). **b** Axial contrast-enhanced CT scan shows a large metastasis (*white arrow*) in the right lung associated with a large subcarinal lymph node (*black arrows*) and bilateral pleural effusion (*E*). **c** Macroscopic view of the resected renal neoplasm shows a large, solid tumor with invasive growth to the renal capsule. **d** Microscopic examination shows typical features of renal cell carcinoma consistent with conventional clear cell carcinoma (hematoxylin and eosin stain; original magnification, ×400).

allelic loss of chromosomes 8p, 9p, 11p, 13q, 14q, and 17p (ANGLARD et al. 1991) have been described in conventional RCC.

On the other hand, papillary RCC has trisomy and tetrasomy of chromosomes 7 and 17 (BENTZ et al. 1996). There are gains on chromosome 20 and losses of chromosome 17p and Y chromosome (DIJKHUIZEN et al. 1996). Translocations between chromosome X and 1 or 17 have been observed in 60–70% of papillary RCC (HEIMANN et al. 2001; TONK et al. 1995). Loss of heterozygosity on chromosomes 6p, 9p, 11q, 14q, and 21q (THRASH-BINGHAM et al. 1995), and the *MET* gene mutations (SCHMIDT et al. 1997), have been identified in papillary RCC.

Chromophobe RCC carcinoma has a loss of multiple chromosomes and monosomes of chromosomes 1, 2, 6, 10, 13, 17, and 20 (NAGY et al. 2004). Birt-Hogg-Dubé (BHD) syndrome has been characterized by skin tumor, pneumothorax, and renal tumor (NICKERSON et al. 2002). This renal tumor was recognized as chromophobe RCC. The *BHD* gene, located in chromosome 1p42, is reported to be a tumor suppressor gene for chromophobe RCC (OKIMOTO et al. 2004).

Cytogenetically, collecting duct RCC shows a homogeneous chromosome alteration pattern with multiple numerical and structural aberrations (mean 11.1, range 7–15) and continuous involvement of chromosomes 1 and X or Y, both as translocations and deletion/monosomy (ANTONELLI et al. 2003). Loss of heterozygosity of 1q, 2q, 6p, 8p, 13q, and 21q has been described in this RCC (FOGT et al. 1998).

To our knowledge, there is little genetic and molecular information on renal medullary carcinoma. Recently, YANG et al. (2004) reported the gene expression profiles of two renal medullary carcinomas using micro-arrays containing a 21,632 cyclic DNA clone.

A good genetic and molecular marker of RCC is needed, and several investigators are working to identify markers that can differentiate the subtypes (BOER et al. 2001; BRUDER et al. 2004; LAM et al. 2004).

1.5
Conclusion

Management strategies for patients with kidney cancer are progressing significantly, based on advances in basic research and the growing number of clinical trials. Numerous classifications have been proposed, with varying degrees of acceptance, based on morphological and molecular futures; therefore, to arrive at the correct differential diagnosis, it is essential for the pathologist and radiologist to provide effective histological and imaging information to the urologist.

References

Akhtar M, Tulbah A, Kardar AH, Ali MA (1997) Sarcomatoid renal cell carcinoma: the chromophobe connection. Am J Surg Pathol 21:1188–1195

Altaffer LF 3rd, Chenault OW Jr (1979) Paraneoplastic endocrinopathies associated with renal tumors. J Urol 122:573–577

Amin MB, Corless CL, Renshaw AA, Tickoo SK, Kubus J, Schultz DS (1997) Papillary (chromophil) renal cell carcinoma: histomorphologic characteristics and evaluation of conventional pathologic prognostic parameters in 62 cases. Am J Surg Pathol 21:621–635

Anglard P, Tory K, Brauch H et al. (1991) Molecular analysis of genetic changes in the origin and development of renal cell carcinoma. Cancer Res 51:1071–1077

Antonelli A, Portesi E, Cozzoli A et al. (2003) The collecting duct carcinoma of the kidney: a cytogenetical study. Eur Urol 43:680–685

Avery AK, Beckstead J, Renshaw AA et al. (2000) Use of antibodies to RCC and CD10 in the differential diagnosis of renal neoplasms. Am J Surg Pathol 24:203–210

Bannasch P, Schacht U, Storch E (1974) Morphogenesis and micromorphology of epithelial tumors of the kidney of nitrosomorpholine intoxicated rats. I. Induction and histology. Z Krebsforsch Klin Onkol Cancer Res Clin Oncol 81:311–331

Banner BF, Burnham JA, Bahnson RR et al. (1990) Immunophenotypic markers in renal cell carcinoma. Mod Pathol 3:129–134

Bentz M, Bergerheim US, Li C et al. (1996) Chromosome imbalances in papillary renal cell carcinoma and first cytogenetic data of familial cases analyzed by comparative genomic hybridization. Cytogenet Cell Genet 75:17–21

Bibbo M, Gill WB, Harris MJ et al. (1974) Retrograde brushing as a diagnostic procedure of ureteral, renal pelvic and renal calyceal lesions. A preliminary report. Acta Cytol 18:137–141

Boer JM, Huber WK, Sultmann H et al. (2001) Identification and classification of differentially expressed genes in renal cell carcinoma by expression profiling on a global human 31,500-element cDNA array. Genome Res 11:1861–1870

Bruder E, Passera O, Harms D et al. (2004) Morphologic and molecular characterization of renal cell carcinoma in children and young adults. Am J Surg Pathol 28:1117–1132

Bukowski RM, Negrier S, Elson P (2004) Prognostic factors in patients with advanced renal cell carcinoma: development of an international kidney cancer working group. Clin Cancer Res 10:6310S–6314S

Cheville JC, Lohse CM, Zincke H et al. (2003) Comparisons of outcome and prognostic features among histologic subtypes of renal cell carcinoma. Am J Surg Pathol 27:612–624

Cheville JC, Lohse CM, Zincke H et al. (2004) Sarcomatoid

renal cell carcinoma: an examination of underlying histologic subtype and an analysis of associations with patient outcome. Am J Surg Pathol 28:435-441

Cochand-Priollet B, Molinie V, Bougaran J et al. (1997) Renal chromophobe cell carcinoma and oncocytoma. A comparative morphologic, histochemical, and immunohistochemical study of 124 cases. Arch Pathol Lab Med 121:1081–1086

Colvin RB (2003) Renal parenchymal tumors: classification and new entities. Mark EJ, Young RH, Harris NL (eds) Current concepts in surgical pathology. Harvard Medical School, Boston, pp 59–80

Davis CJ Jr, Mostofi FK, Sesterhenn IA (1995) Renal medullary carcinoma. The seventh sickle cell nephropathy. Am J Surg Pathol 19:1–11

Delahunt B, Eble JN (1997) Papillary renal cell carcinoma: a clinicopathologic and immunohistochemical study of 105 tumors. Mod Pathol 10:537–544

Delahunt B, Eble JN (1998) Renal tumours: the new order. N Z Med J 111:307-309

Delahunt B, Eble JN (2002) Renal cell neoplasia. Pathology 34:13–20

Delahunt B, Eble JN, McCredie MR et al. (2001) Morphologic typing of papillary renal cell carcinoma: comparison of growth kinetics and patient survival in 66 cases. Hum Pathol 32:590–595

Dijkhuizen T, Van den Berg E, Van den Berg A et al. (1996) Chromosomal findings and p53-mutation analysis in chromophilic renal-cell carcinomas. Int J Cancer 68:47–50

Dimopoulos MA, Logothetis CJ, Markowitz A et al. (1993) Collecting duct carcinoma of the kidney. Br J Urol 71:388–391

Eble JN, Sauter G, Epstein JI et al. (2004) WHO classification of tumours. In: Eble JN, Sauter G, Epstein JI (eds) Tumours of the urinary system and male genital organs. IARC Press, Lyon, France

Farrow GM, Harrison EG Jr, Utz DC (1968) Sarcomas and sarcomatoid and mixed malignant tumors of the kidney in adults. Cancer 22:556–563

Ficarra V, Novara G, Galfano A et al. (2004) Neoplasm staging and organ-confined renal cell carcinoma: a systematic review. Eur Urol 46:559–564

Fogt F, Zhuang Z, Linehan WM et al. (1998) Collecting duct carcinomas of the kidney: a comparative loss of heterozygosity study with clear cell renal cell carcinoma. Oncol Rep 5:923–926

Fuhrman SA, Lasky LC, Limas C (1982) Prognostic significance of morphologic parameters in renal cell carcinoma. Am J Surg Pathol 6:655–663

Gnarra JR, Tory K, Weng Y et al. (1994) Mutations of the VHL tumour suppressor gene in renal carcinoma. Nat Genet 7:85–90

Gnarra JR, Duan DR, Weng Y et al. (1996) Molecular cloning of the von Hippel-Lindau tumor suppressor gene and its role in renal carcinoma. Biochim Biophys Acta 1242:201–210

Grawitz PA (1883) Die Enstehung von Nierentumoren aus Nebennierengewebe. Arch Klin Chir 30:824–830

Guinan P, Sobin LH, Algaba F et al. (1997) TNM staging of renal cell carcinoma: Workgroup No. 3. Union International Contre le Cancer (UICC) and the American Joint Committee on Cancer (AJCC). Cancer 80:992–993

Hartman DS, Davis CJ Jr, Johns T et al. (1986) Cystic renal cell carcinoma. Urology 28:145–153

Heimann P, El Housni H, Ogur G et al. (2001) Fusion of a novel gene, RCC17, to the TFE3 gene in t(X;17)(p11.2;q25.3)-bearing papillary renal cell carcinomas. Cancer Res 61:4130-4135

Hellsten S, Berge T, Wehlin L (1981) Unrecognized renal cell carcinoma. Clinical and pathological aspects. Scand J Urol Nephrol 15:273–278

Herman JG, Latif F, Weng Y et al. (1994) Silencing of the VHL tumor-suppressor gene by DNA methylation in renal carcinoma. Proc Natl Acad Sci USA 91:9700–9704

Hollifield JW, Page DL, Smith C et al. (1975) Renin-secreting clear cell carcinoma of the kidney. Arch Intern Med 135:859–864

Imura J, Ichikawa K, Takeda J et al. (2004) Multilocular cystic renal cell carcinoma: a clinicopathological, immuno- and lectin histochemical study of nine cases. APMIS 112:183–191

Inoue K, Kohashikawa K, Suzuki S et al. (2004) Prognostic significance of thrombocytosis in renal cell carcinoma patients. Int J Urol 11:364–367

Ishikawa I (1991) Uremic acquired renal cystic disease. Natural history and complications. Nephron 58:257–267

Ishikawa I, Kovacs G (1993) High incidence of papillary renal cell tumours in patients on chronic haemodialysis. Histopathology 22:135–139

Jemal A, Tiwari RC, Murray T et al. (2004) Cancer statistics, 2004. CA Cancer J Clin 54:8–29

Keith DS, Torres VE, King BF et al. (1994) Renal cell carcinoma in autosomal dominant polycystic kidney disease. J Am Soc Nephrol 4:1661–1669

Kennedy SM, Merino MJ, Linehan WM et al. (1990) Collecting duct carcinoma of the kidney. Hum Pathol 21:449–456

Kovacs G (1993) Molecular cytogenetics of renal cell tumors. Adv Cancer Res 62:89–124

Kovacs G, Akhtar M, Beckwith BJ et al. (1997) The Heidelberg classification of renal cell tumours. J Pathol 183:131–133

Kuroda N, Guo L, Toi M et al. (2001) Paxillin: application of immunohistochemistry to the diagnosis of chromophobe renal cell carcinoma and oncocytoma. Appl Immunohistochem Mol Morphol 9:315–318

Lam JS, Belldegrun AS, Figlin RA (2004) Tissue array-based predictions of pathobiology, prognosis, and response to treatment for renal cell carcinoma therapy. Clin Cancer Res 10:6304S–6309S

Langner C, Wegscheider BJ, Ratschek M et al. (2004) Keratin immunohistochemistry in renal cell carcinoma subtypes and renal oncocytomas: a systematic analysis of 233 tumors. Virchows Arch 444:127–134

Mancilla-Jimenez R, Stanley RJ, Blath RA et al. (1976) Papillary renal cell carcinoma: a clinical, radiologic, and pathologic study of 34 cases. Cancer 38:2469–2480

McGregor DK, Khurana KK, Cao C et al. (2001) Diagnosing primary and metastatic renal cell carcinoma: the use of the monoclonal antibody "renal cell carcinoma marker". Am J Surg Pathol 25:1485–1492

Morris MR, Maina E, Morgan NV et al. (2004) Molecular genetic analysis of FIH-1, FH, and SDHB candidate tumour suppressor genes in renal cell carcinoma. J Clin Pathol 57:706–711

Motzer RJ, Bander NH, Nanus DM (1996) Renal-cell carcinoma. N Engl J Med 335:865–875

Nagashima Y, Inayama Y, Kato Y et al. (2004) Pathological and molecular biological aspects of the renal epithelial neoplasms, up-to-date. Pathol Int 54:377–386

Nagy A, Buzogany I, Kovacs G (2004) Microsatellite allelotyping differentiates chromophobe renal cell carcinomas from renal oncocytomas and identifies new genetic changes. Histopathology 44:542–546

Nickerson ML, Warren MB, Toro JR et al. (2002) Mutations in a novel gene lead to kidney tumors, lung wall defects, and benign tumors of the hair follicle in patients with the Birt-Hogg-Dube syndrome. Cancer Cell 2:157–164

Okabe T, Urabe A, Kato T et al. (1985) Production of erythropoietin-like activity by human renal and hepatic carcinomas in cell culture. Cancer 55:1918–1923

Okimoto K, Sakurai J, Kobayashi T et al. (2004) A germ-line insertion in the Birt-Hogg-Dube (BHD) gene gives rise to the Nihon rat model of inherited renal cancer. Proc Natl Acad Sci USA 101:2023–2027

Peralta-Venturina M de, Moch H et al. (2001) Sarcomatoid differentiation in renal cell carcinoma: a study of 101 cases. Am J Surg Pathol 25:275–284

Perlmann S (1928) Ubereinen Fall von Lymphangioma cysticum der Niere. Virchows Arch Pathol Anat Physiol Klin Med 268:524–535

Peyromaure M, Misrai V, Thiounn N et al. (2004) Chromophobe renal cell carcinoma: analysis of 61 cases. Cancer 100:1406–1410

Reuter VE, Presti JC Jr (2000) Contemporary approach to the classification of renal epithelial tumors. Semin Oncol 27:124–137

Robson CJ, Churchill BM, Anderson W (1967) The results of radical nephrectomy for renal cell carcinoma. J Urol 101:297–301

Schmidt L, Duh FM, Chen F et al. (1997) Germline and somatic mutations in the tyrosine kinase domain of the MET proto-oncogene in papillary renal carcinomas. Nat Genet 16:68–73

Srigley JR, Eble JN (1998) Collecting duct carcinoma of kidney. Semin Diagn Pathol 15:54–67

Srigley JR, Hutter RV, Gelb AB et al. (1997) Current prognostic factors–renal cell carcinoma: Workgroup No. 4. Union Internationale Contre le Cancer (UICC) and the American Joint Committee on Cancer (AJCC). Cancer 80:994–996

Swartz MA, Karth J, Schneider DT et al. (2002) Renal medullary carcinoma: clinical, pathologic, immunohistochemical, and genetic analysis with pathogenetic implications. Urology 60:1083–1089

Takahashi M, Yang XJ, Sugimura J et al. (2003) Molecular subclassification of kidney tumors and the discovery of new diagnostic markers. Oncogene 22:6810–6818

Thoenes W, Storkel S, Rumpelt HJ (1985) Human chromophobe cell renal carcinoma. Virchows Arch B Cell Pathol Incl Mol Pathol 48:207–217

Thoenes W, Storkel S, Rumpelt HJ (1986) Histopathology and classification of renal cell tumors (adenomas, oncocytomas and carcinomas). The basic cytological and histopathological elements and their use for diagnostics. Pathol Res Pract 181:125–143

Thoenes W, Storkel S, Rumpelt HJ et al. (1988) Chromophobe cell renal carcinoma and its variants: a report on 32 cases. J Pathol 155:277–287

Thrash-Bingham CA, Salazar H, Freed JJ et al. (1995) Genomic alterations and instabilities in renal cell carcinomas and their relationship to tumor pathology. Cancer Res 55:6189–6195

Tonk V, Wilson KS, Timmons CF et al. (1995) Renal cell carcinoma with translocation (X;1). Further evidence for a cytogenetically defined subtype. Cancer Genet Cytogenet 81:72–75

Truong LD, Todd TD, Dhurandhar B et al. (1999) Fine-needle aspiration of renal masses in adults: analysis of results and diagnostic problems in 108 cases. Diagn Cytopathol 20:339–349

Waldherr R, Schwechheimer K (1985) Co-expression of cytokeratin and vimentin intermediate-sized filaments in renal cell carcinomas. Comparative study of the intermediate-sized filament distribution in renal cell carcinomas and normal human kidney. Virchows Arch A Pathol Anat Histopathol 408:15–27

Yang XJ, Sugimura J, Tretiakova MS et al. (2004) Gene expression profiling of renal medullary carcinoma: potential clinical relevance. Cancer 100:976–985

Zambrano NR, Lubensky IA, Merino MJ et al. (1999) Histopathology and molecular genetics of renal tumors toward unification of a classification system. J Urol 162:1246–1258

2 Ultrasound and Doppler in Kidney Cancer

OLIVIER HÉLÉNON and JEAN-MICHEL CORREAS

CONTENTS

2.1
Introduction

Imaging of kidney cancer relies mainly on computed tomography (CT) which is the gold standard for detecting and characterizing renal neoplasms and staging renal cell carcinoma (RCC). Although ultrasound (US) has a poor sensitivity in detecting small renal lesions, it plays a key role in the early diagnosis of kidney cancer because of its widespread use in the evaluation of the abdomen. Moreover,

O. HÉLÉNON, MD
Professor and Chairman, Department of Radiology, Necker University Hospital, 149 rue de Sèvres, 75743 Paris Cedex 15, France
J.-M. CORREAS, MD, PhD
Associate Professor and Vice-Chairman, Department of Radiology, Necker University Hospital, 149 rue de Sèvres, 75743 Paris Cedex 15, France

despite its limitations in providing a complete evaluation of renal cancer before planning treatment, US can provide additional diagnostic information in some selected renal masses that remain equivocal after CT. Recent technical improvements of gray-scale imaging have increased US performance, especially in the detection of small renal tumors. The diagnostic accuracy of US also benefits from recent advances in the use of US contrast agents (USCA). Besides some diagnostic and therapeutic procedures that can benefit from US guidance, intraoperative US remains the only available method that allows renal-parenchymal-sparing surgery. The use of US and Doppler in the diagnosis of kidney cancer and its current role in the differential diagnosis and preoperative assessment of RCC are discussed.

2.2
Ultrasound Detection of Kidney Cancer

2.2.1
Increased Incidental Detection of RCC

One of the most useful clinical benefits of US is increased early detection of RCC. Because US is routinely used for examination of the abdomen, which includes evaluation of the kidneys, the detection rate of RCC in asymptomatic patients has increased dramatically. Renal cell carcinoma is found incidentally in 0.18–0.80% of asymptomatic patients undergoing abdominal US (LEVINE and KING 2000). Up to 83% of asymptomatic renal tumors are detected this way (SIEMER et al. 2000).

Tumors detected at initial screening are significantly smaller (mean 5.5 cm) and at a lower local tumor stage than those found in symptomatic patients (mean 7.8 cm; SIEMER et al. 2000). Approximately 30% of all RCC tumors detected on US are 3 cm or less in diameter. Early detection has led to an improved prognosis and overall survival rate in patients with RCC.

2.2.2
Detection of Small RCC

Accurate detection of small renal neoplasms (3 cm or less) relies on the high sensitivity of contrast-enhanced CT. Comparison of CT and US shows that CT depicts more and smaller masses than US. Computed tomography detects 75% of masses 10–15 mm in size, whereas US finds only 28%; with larger masses, 15–20 mm, CT detects 100% and US 58%. One hundred percent of larger masses, 25–30 mm, are found equally well with both techniques (Jamis-Dow et al. 1996).

Thus, US is inadequate for screening for renal tumors, especially in patients with hereditary renal kidney cancer (in von Hippel-Lindau disease or hereditary papillary RCC). Contrast-enhanced CT is usually required in such cases; however, in such a young patient population, the lack of ionizing radiation that US offers is a significant consideration, and the cost-to-benefit ratio can be optimized by using a follow-up strategy based on both US and CT. On the other hand, in the general population, incidental finding of a small solid renal mass on US is common and usually requires a CT examination to characterize the tumor tissue.

In addition to technical and anatomical factors, and to operator skill, which can affect US performance, the ability of US to detect renal carcinomas depends mainly on the size, location, and echogenicity of the tumor. Ultrasound is least effective at detecting two types of renal tumors: small isoechoic intraparenchymal tumors (those that are non-contour-deforming) and tumors of polar origin with extrarenal growth that may be obscured by bowel gas. Among small RCC, 23–46% of solid tumors are iso- or hypoechoic compared with normal renal cortex (Fig. 2.1; Forman et al. 1993; Jinzaki et al. 1998; Yamashita et al. 1992). A hyperechoic pattern (relative to renal cortex echogenicity) is more common, occurring in up to 48% of all RCC. On the other hand, the majority of small benign tumors are hyperechoic (94% of small angiomyolipomas) and easily depicted on US; therefore, despite the increased detection of small hyperechoic renal carcinomas, most renal tumors overlooked on US are small RCC.

Recent technical improvements in gray-scale imaging have increased US detection of small renal tumors. Harmonic B-mode tissue imaging is now widely used, as it offers better contrast resolution and fewer artifacts on gray-scale images. In addition to superior characterization of cystic renal masses, this modality may help depict small slightly hypo- or hyperechoic solid masses (Schmidt et al. 2003; Hélénon et al. 2001). It also provides better delineation of kidney margins, allowing a more confident diagnosis of small subcapsular isoechoic tumors responsible for a capsular bulging.

Color Doppler, with either conventional velocity or power mode, seems not to increase significantly the detection rate of small renal tumors. The presence of a color-coded rim, due to renal blood vessels that arise outside the lesion and surround it (Fig. 2.2), points strongly to a diagnosis of small isoechoic intraparenchymal tumors. Such a finding is better seen on power Doppler US images.

Ultrasound contrast agents (USCA) have improved the ability of US to assess intrarenal vascularity. They provide significant cortical signal enhancement after intravenous administration on both color Doppler and gray-scale images obtained

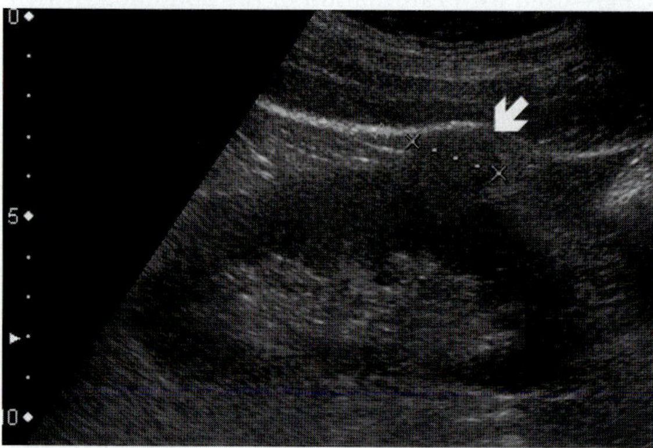
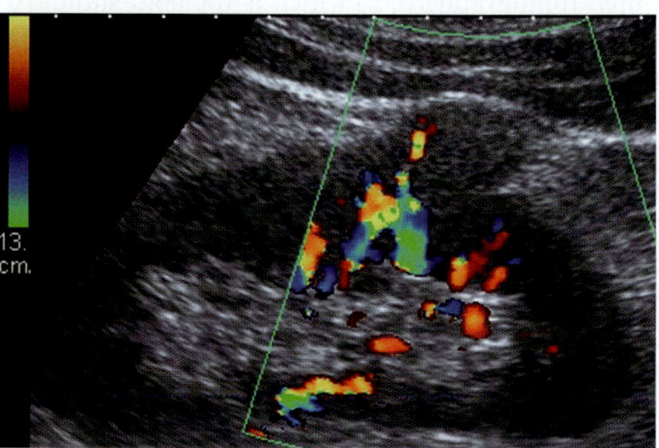

Fig. 2.1a,b. Small asymptomatic renal cell carcinoma in a 56-year-old man. **a** Longitudinal US image shows isoechoic, homogeneous, solid renal mass responsible for capsular bulging (*arrow*). **b** Tumor vascularity on color Doppler exhibits a penetrating vascular distribution.

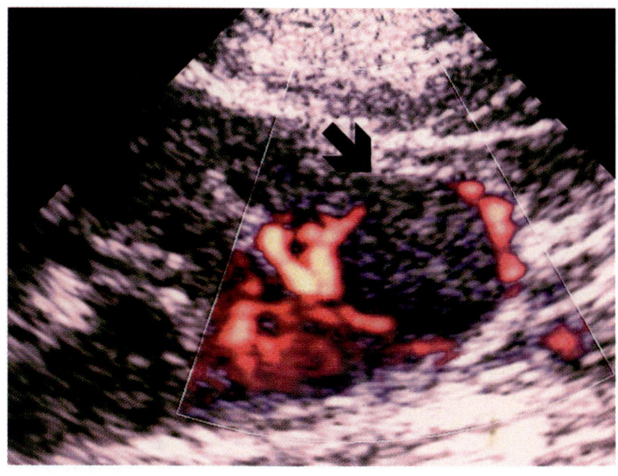

Fig. 2.2. Small isoechoic intraparenchymal renal neoplasm in a 68-year-old woman. Transverse power Doppler US image shows hypovascular, round lesion (*arrow*) surrounded by normal renal vessels.

with dedicated imaging sequences. The detection of small renal masses, especially those that exhibit an isoechoic pattern, can be improved with USCA, since the normal renal vascular architecture is altered. At peak enhancement, small masses may appear as round cortical defects underlined by the massive blood flow enhancement seen in the normal surrounding vessels on postcontrast color Doppler images (Correas et al. 1999). The same effect can be achieved with B-mode non-linear imaging. Despite the significant increase in the detection rate of small renal tumors, contrast-enhanced US is still less sensitive than CT or MR imaging.

2.3
US Diagnosis of Solid RCC

The goals of imaging in characterizing solid renal tumors are: (a) to differentiate renal tumors from normal variants or pseudotumors which may mimic a neoplasm; and (b) to differentiate benign and malignant renal tumors, especially angiomyolipoma, from non-fatty renal tumors which should be removed. Although several features of gray-scale US can help differentiate benign from malignant renal neoplasms, CT is always mandatory to best characterize the tumor.

Gray-scale US features exhibited by solid renal tumors do not provide definitive tissue characterization since there is a considerable overlap in echogenicity among renal tumors (Forman et al. 1993; Jinzaki et al. 1997; Jinzaki et al. 1998; Siegel

et al. 1996; Yamashita et al. 1992; Yamashita et al. 1993); however, several features are advocated as significant for the differential diagnosis of solid tumors. Although not pathognomonic, some findings that correlate with the gross appearance of the tumor on histopathological examination can help differentiate malignant from benign tumors.

Although demonstration of vascularity within a renal mass using color Doppler may ensure the diagnosis of a renal neoplasm (provided that a pseudotumor has been ruled out), a lack of demonstrable blood flow within the lesion does not exclude a renal tumor, especially a carcinoma. Color Doppler and contrast-enhanced US can add some information to that obtained by gray-scale US, which can be useful for the differential diagnosis of solid tumors. A power-Doppler-based classification of tumor vascular architecture before and after USCA administration has been reported by Jinzaki et al. (1998).

2.3.1
Large RCC

Large RCC typically show a heterogeneous pattern on US, caused by intratumoral hypoechoic necrotic areas, which is sometimes associated with scattered calcifications (Fig. 2.3). Large RCC also often exhibit lobulated contours with poorly visualized irregular interfaces and adjacent normal renal parenchyma. A large solid heterogeneous tumor that displays such features and that disrupts normal kidney anatomy is highly suggestive of RCC. On Doppler US, the

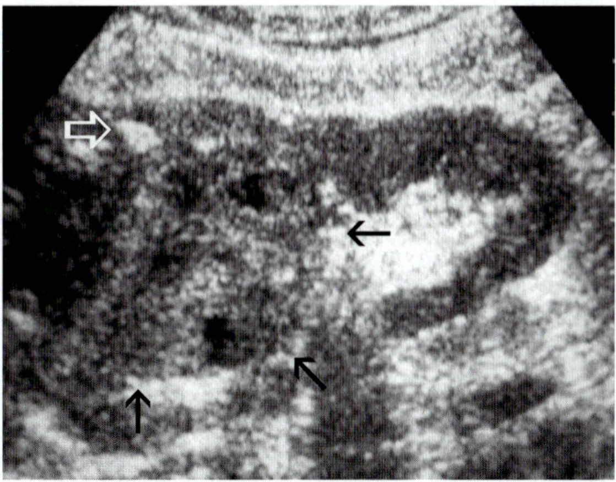

Fig. 2.3. Large renal cell carcinoma in a 72-year-old man. Longitudinal gray-scale US image shows a large heterogeneous solid renal mass (*black arrows*) that disrupts the normal kidney anatomy. Note the presence of intratumoral calcifications (*white arrow*).

presence of intratumoral arteriovenous shunting also indicates RCC. Such a finding is best characterized by spectral analysis of vessels exhibiting a high-velocity signal on color Doppler image (Fig. 2.4); however, even this finding is not a defini-

tive diagnostic criterion for RCC, since angiomyolipoma (AML) can exhibit the same pattern. The use of microbubbles may help to reveal necrotic areas within a large RCC on postcontrast US. Typically, the solid tumor tissue surrounding non-enhanced hypoechoic areas with irregular margins exhibits early contrast enhancement (Fig. 2.5).

On the other hand, the association of a large renal tumor and venous tumor invasion strongly suggests malignancy and RCC regardless of the gray-scale appearance of the lesion.

2.3.2
Small RCC

About 30% of small RCC appear as markedly hyperechoic masses (i.e., equal to or greater than the echogenicity of the renal sinus) and may mimic AML (FORMAN et al. 1993). The presence of an anechoic rim or small intratumoral cysts can suggest RCC on gray-scale US (Fig. 2.6; YAMASHITA et al. 1993); however, the usefulness of these findings for differ-

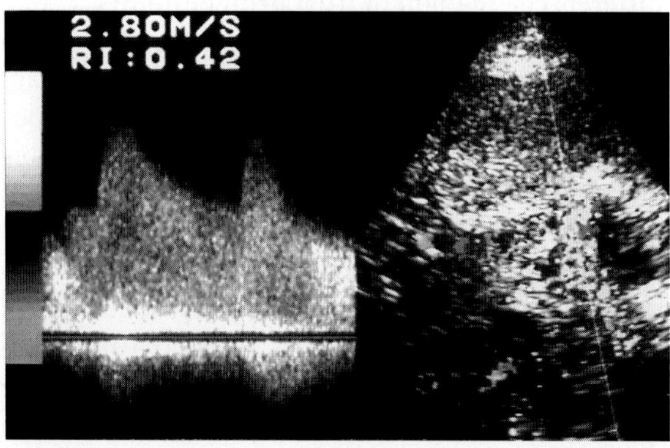

Fig. 2.4. Large renal cell carcinoma in a 76-year-old woman. Spectral analysis of duplex Doppler obtained from intratumoral vessels shows high systolic–diastolic velocities with low resistive index (RI=0.42) indicating the presence of an intratumoral arteriovenous shunt.

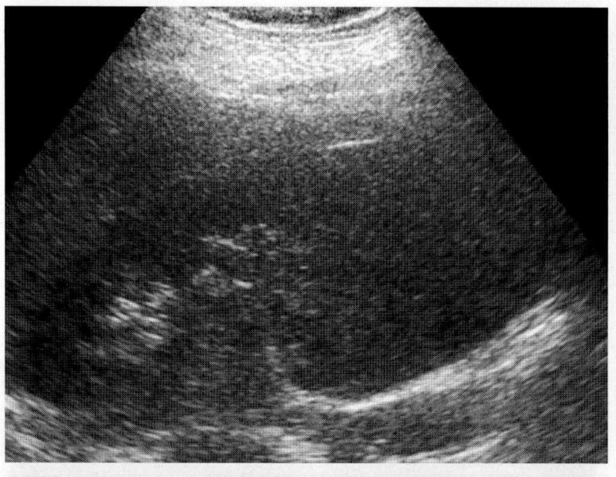

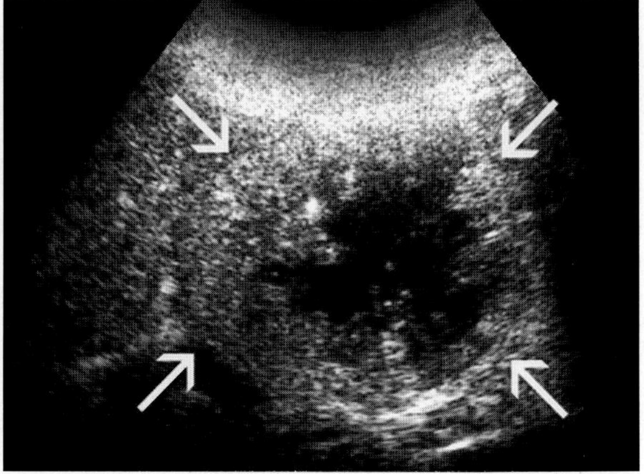

a

b

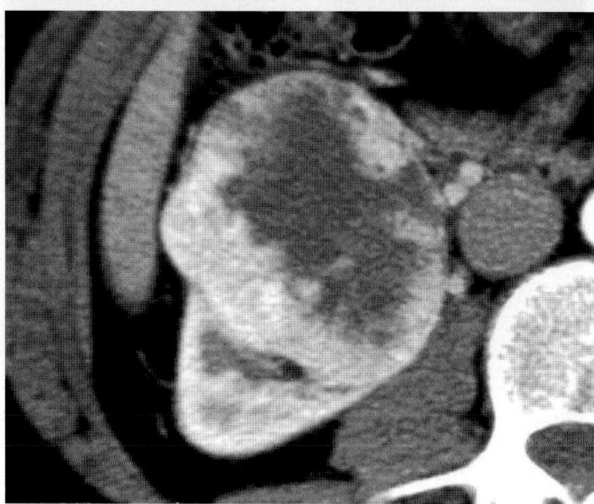

c

Fig. 2.5a-c. Typical large renal cell carcinoma in a 77-year-old man. a Pre- and b postcontrast gray scale US images show heterogeneous contrast enhancement (*arrows*) with central non-enhancing necrotic areas. c Axial contrast-enhanced CT scan shows the typical appearance of a large necrotic renal cell carcinoma of the right kidney.

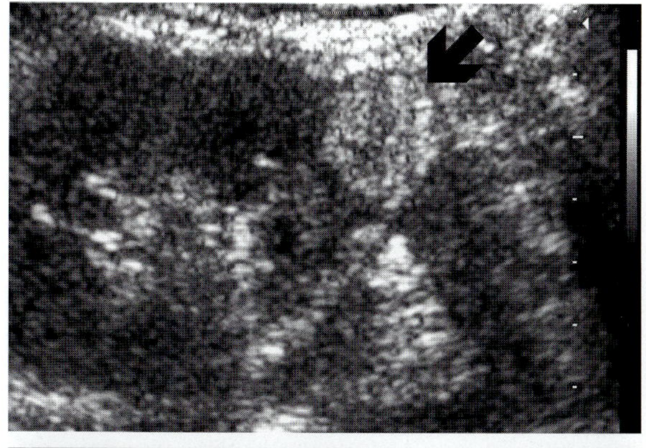

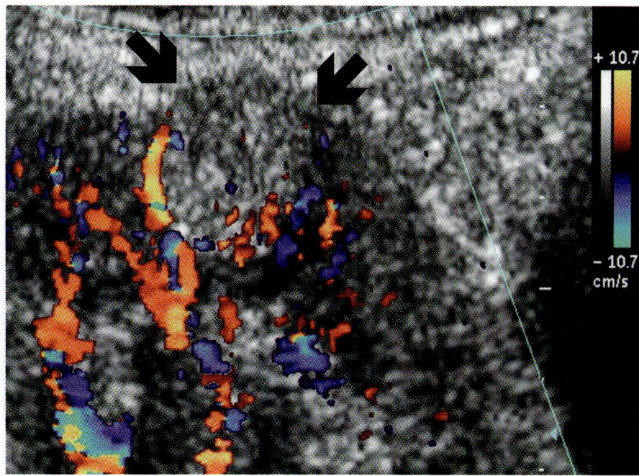

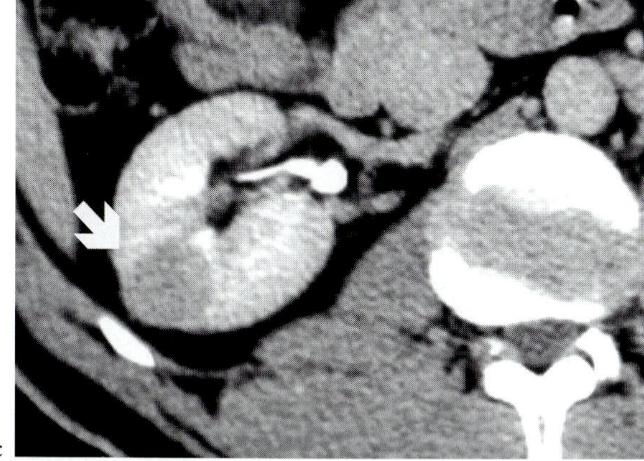

Fig. 2.6a-c. Small renal cell carcinoma in a 56-year-old man. **a** Transverse US image shows hyperechoic tumor with hypoechoic rim (*arrow*) which suggests malignancy. **b** Transverse color Doppler US image shows a mixed, penetrating, and peripheral vascular distribution (*arrows*). **c** Axial contrast-enhanced CT scan shows a small histologically proved renal cell carcinoma of the right kidney (*arrow*).

ential diagnosis has not been established since their detection rate varies considerably among investigators, from 8 to 84% for RCC and 12 to 31% for AML (JINZAKI et al. 1998; SIEGEL et al. 1996; YAMASHITA et al. 1993; YAMASHITA et al. 1992).

The vascular distribution seen on power Doppler US can provide useful information in addition to that of gray-scale US for the diagnosis of RCC. The classification reported in the work of JINZAKI et al. (1998) categorizes tumor vascular architecture into five patterns based on the appearance of the vascular distribution on power Doppler US: pattern 0, no signal; pattern 1, intratumoral and focal signals; pattern 2, penetrating vessels; pattern 3, peripheral vascular distribution; and pattern 4, mixed, penetrating and peripheral (Fig. 2.6b). Among the 64 small renal neoplasms in the study, no RCC exhibited patterns 0, 1, or 2, whereas all the 26 RCC but only 20% of AML were associated with patterns 3 or 4. Although not specific enough for a definitive diagnosis, such power Doppler patterns may suggest malignancy, particularly when they are combined with gray-scale data. Although a small, homogeneous, markedly hyperechoic and well-delineated tumor with vascularity patterns 0–2 strongly indi-

cates a small AML, CT or MR imaging are still necessary to confirm the presence of intratumoral fat typical of AML.

2.4
US Diagnosis of Cystic RCC

The diagnosis of cystic RCC relies on the demonstration of vascularity within the solid components (thick, irregular walls or septations and mural nodules) of a cystic renal mass. Typically, based on CT findings, such a lesion falls into category IV of the Bosniak classification which is 100% specific for malignancy (CURRY et al. 2000). Ultrasound appears to be very sensitive to intracystic septations and mural nodules (Fig. 2.7). In cases of RCC with cystic degeneration due to massive necrosis, US usually shows inhomogeneous fluid content with internal echoes suggestive of malignancy (Fig. 2.8). The US depiction of vascularity within the solid tumor components using color Doppler with appropriate low-flow settings also strongly suggests the neoplastic nature of the lesion. The use of USCA may improve the US depiction of

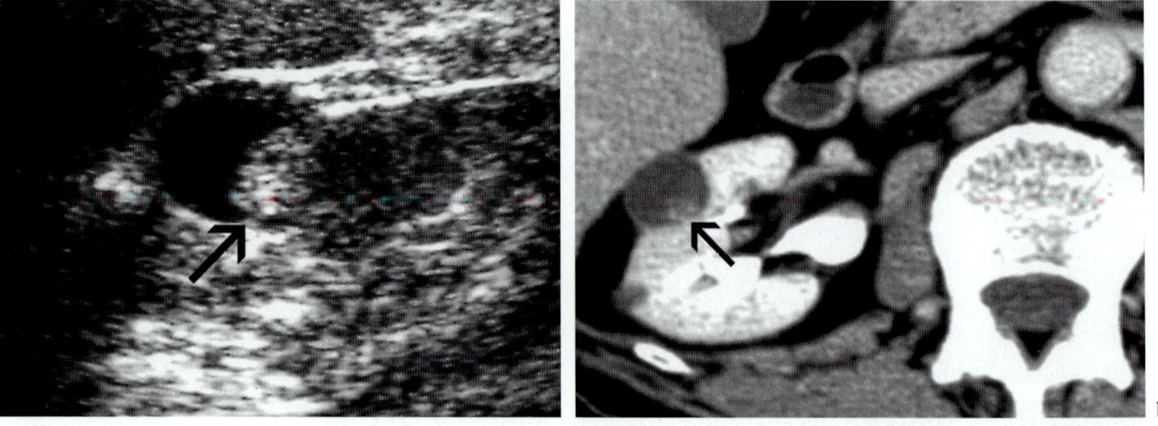

Fig. 2.7a,b. Cystic renal cell carcinoma in a 73-year-old man. **a** Longitudinal US image shows a cystic renal mass of the right kidney with solid mural nodule (*arrow*). **b** Axial contrast-enhanced CT scan confirms the typical cystic renal cell carcinoma (category IV) appearance with contrast-enhanced tumor tissue component (*arrow*).

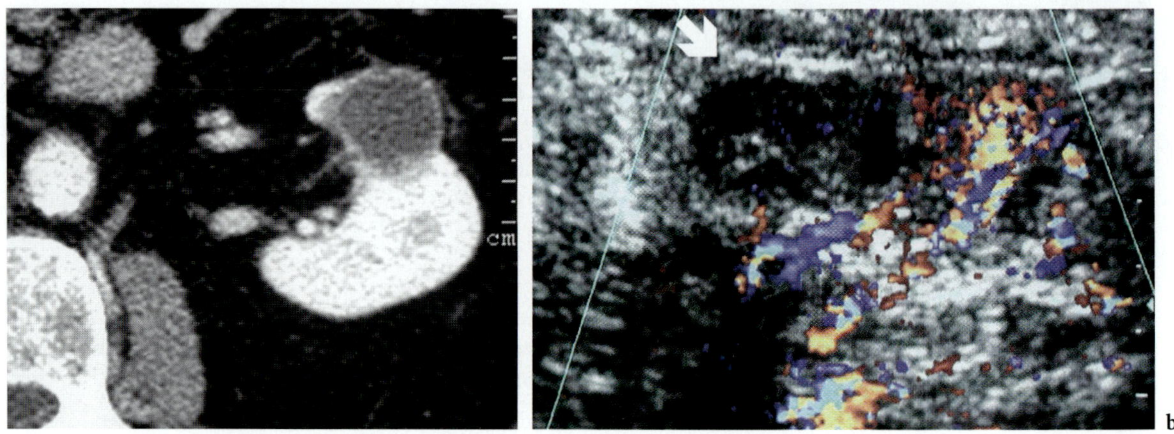

Fig. 2.8a,b. Atypical pseudocystic renal cell carcinoma in a 65-year-old man. **a** Axial contrast-enhanced CT scan shows indeterminate Bosniak type-III left renal mass with thick regular wall. **b** Transverse color Doppler US image shows cystic mass with echoic heterogeneous content and thick irregular peripheral wall which suggests necrotic renal tumor (*arrow*).

vascularity on contrast-enhanced power Doppler US (Kim et al. 1999) or on gray-scale contrast imaging which provides better spatial resolution (Fig. 2.9; Robbin et al. 2003). As a result, most typical cystic RCC (i.e., category IV of the Bosniak classification) shown with CT also exhibit an appearance on US that is strongly indicative of malignancy.

Small RCC with intrinsic cystic growth that are Bosniak category III, and multiloculated cystic neoplasms with thin septations or thicker but uniform septations, are categorized as indeterminate cystic renal masses on CT or US. Contrast enhancement of the wall and/or the septations, usually assessed with CT or MR imaging, is the key criterion in determining whether the lesion should be excised surgically or merely followed. When US is used for follow-up,

USCA may help to better characterize the lesion by demonstrating significant enhancement with microbubbles (Robbin 2001).

2.5
Differential Diagnosis

2.5.1
Solid Pseudotumors

Several normal variants can appear as a focal renal mass on US and may be mistaken for a renal neoplasm, especially by inexperienced operators. Although some inflammatory renal masses can

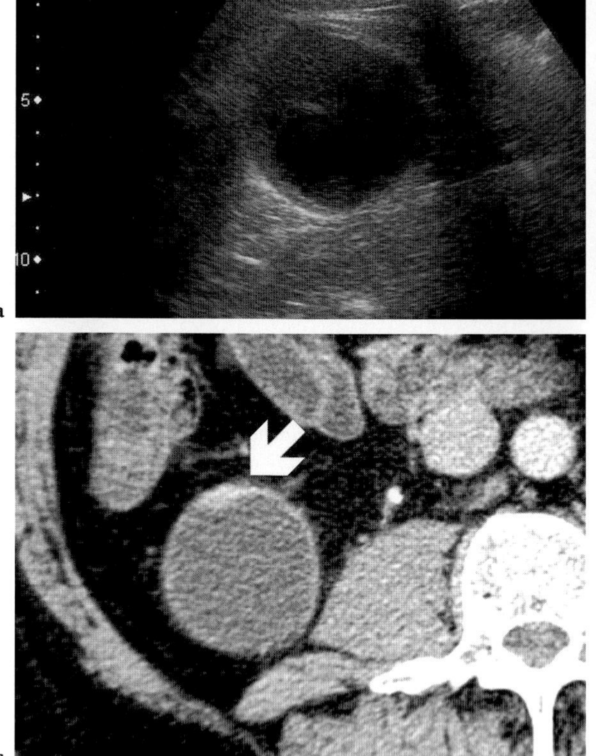

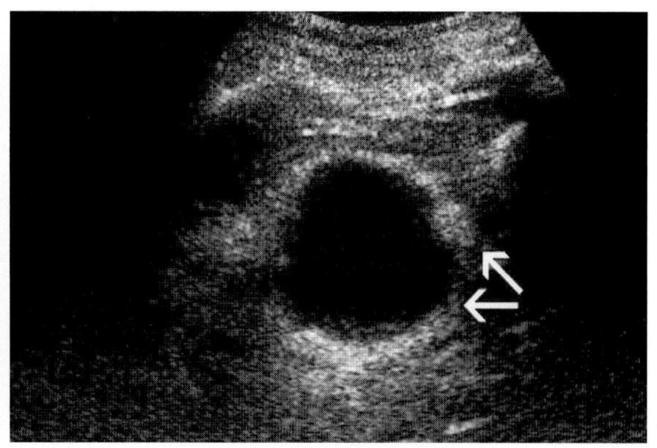

Fig. 2.9a-c. Cystic renal cell carcinoma in a 52-year-old man. a Transverse US image shows a cystic right renal mass with uniform thick wall (Bosniak category III). b Transverse contrast-enhanced B-mode non-linear US image shows obvious contrast enhancement of the wall (*arrows*). c Axial contrast-enhanced CT scan demonstrates a complex cystic mass with a small mural nodule (*arrow*) which strongly suggests malignancy.

mimic renal neoplasms, such masses are usually associated with a clinical history that suggests their infectious origin and prompts follow-up imaging during treatment.

2.5.1.1
False Hyperechoic Tumors

Some cortical defects containing fat can mimic a small subcapsular hyperechoic tumor on US. Such a finding may be related to a normal variant known as the junctional parenchymal defect (YEH et al. 1992), or to a postoperative defect packed with retroperitoneal fat (PAPANICOLAOU et al. 1988). Criteria that may help in avoiding unnecessary workups are the presence of a junctional parenchymal hyperechoic line associated with the parenchymal notch in the first case (Fig. 2.10), and a history of partial renal resection in the latter case.

On the other hand, renal sinus fat can make diagnosing a hyperechoic parenchymal tumor difficult. Some fatty tissue arising from the renal sinus may be located at the corticomedullary junction and can

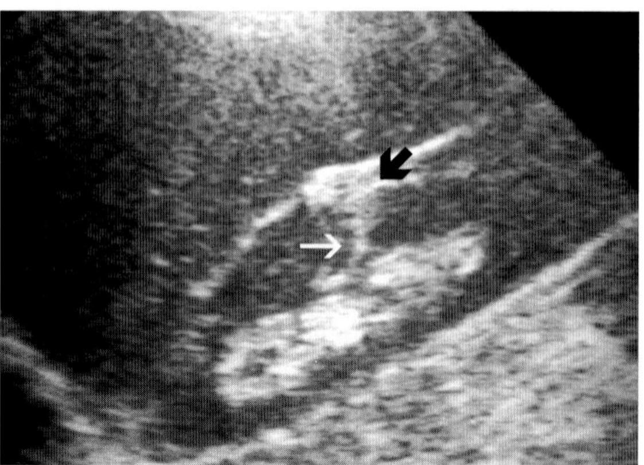

Fig. 2.10. Junctional parenchymal defect in a 52-year-old woman. Longitudinal US image of the right kidney shows that the parenchymal defect is mimicking a small hyperechoic subcapsular renal neoplasm (*black arrow*). Typically, a hyperechoic intraparenchymal line (*white arrow*) connects the parenchymal notch to renal sinus.

mimic a round hyperechoic mass within the deep cortex. Conversely, the intrasinusal growth of a hyperechoic neoplasm may prevent tumor identification while mimicking sinus lipomatosis.

2.5.1.2
Lobar Dysmorphism and Fetal Lobations

Lobar dysmorphisms are well-known variants that can mimic a renal tumor with sinus growth. Typical gray-scale US features include a well-defined mass arising from the deep renal parenchyma, which is isoechoic compared with the renal cortex; a homogeneous pattern; and the presence of a hypoechoic Malpighi's pyramid in the case of junctional lobar dysmorphism (Fig. 2.11; YEH et al. 1992). Color Doppler US may increase confidence in diagnosing such variants by demonstrating a normal vasculature which consists of normal segmental and interlobar blood vessels that arise outside the lesion and surround it before reaching the neighboring corticomedullary junction. Arcuate branches can also be seen within the mass, especially in cases of junctional dysmorphism.

Diagnosis of pseudotumoral fetal lobation also can benefit from color Doppler US demonstration of a normal cortical vascular distribution compared with the surrounding renal parenchyma (JINZAKI et al. 1998).

2.5.2
Solid Benign Neoplasms

2.5.2.1
Angiomyolipoma

As noted above, on US some hyperechoic RCC can be confused with benign AML. In addition to the US criteria that indicate a small hyperechoic RCC, findings that suggest a small AML may help to differentiate the tumors (Fig. 2.12): a markedly hyperechoic lesion (iso- or hyperechoic compared with renal sinus); a homogeneous pattern with sharp margins; shadowing, seen in 21–33% of AML; on power Doppler an intratumoral focal vascular flow corresponding to Jinzaki's pattern 1; or penetrating vascular flow corresponding to pattern 2 (HÉLÉNON et al. 1997; JINZAKI et al. 1998; SIEGEL et al. 1996). Contrary to previous reports, the echogenicity of AML seems not to correlate with the amount of intratumoral fat (HÉLÉNON et al. 1997); however, in a series of six AML with minimal fat, JINZAKI et al. (1998) found homogeneous isoechogenicity on US in all six cases. Although a markedly hyperechoic homogeneous lesion is highly suggestive of AML, it is not pathognomonic and requires CT confirmation. A renal tumor with such a suggestive US pattern should prompt careful CT examination or

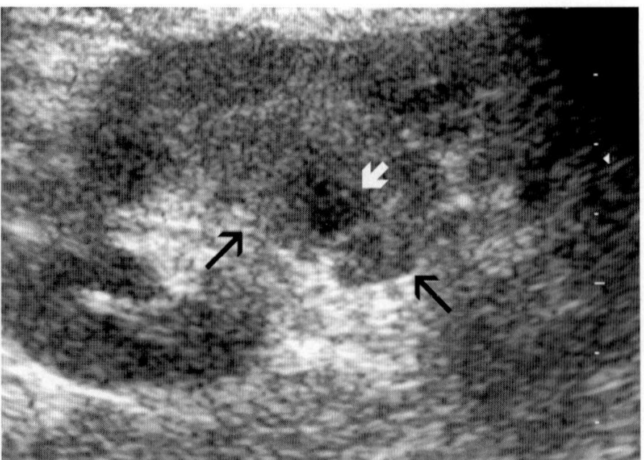

Fig. 2.11. Junctional lobar dysmorphism in a 46-year-old man. Longitudinal US image shows lobar portion of renal parenchyma with renal sinus development consisting of renal cortex (*black arrows*) and medulla (*white arrow*).

repeat examination, using a dedicated CT scanning protocol including precontrast thin (3 mm or less) sections (Fig. 2.12c). On the other hand, small AML with atypical US appearance include slightly hyperechoic lesions (not as echogenic as renal sinus fat) which account for 29% of AML, and lesions that are iso- or hypoechoic compared with renal parenchyma, which account for 6% of AML (JINZAKI et al. 1997).

Although large AML often have a hyperechoic appearance that may suggest the diagnosis on US, a heterogeneous pattern is also seen, which is indicative of hemorrhagic changes within the tumor.

Two variations of US tissue characterization, ultrasonic frequency dependent attenuation (TANIGUCHI et al. 1997), and relative gray-scale value measurements (compared with renal cortex; SIM et al. 1999) have been evaluated for their efficacy in the diagnosis of solid renal tumors. Both techniques show some promise in differentiating hyperechoic RCC from AML.

2.5.2.2
Oncocytoma

There are no reports of a US pattern that can reliably differentiate oncocytomas from RCC. Although tumor homogeneity may suggest a small oncocytoma, it is of no help in making the differential diagnosis because of the considerable overlap in degrees of homogeneity among small renal tumors, including RCC.

On the other hand, some patterns found on CT in the diagnosis of large oncocytomas are also seen

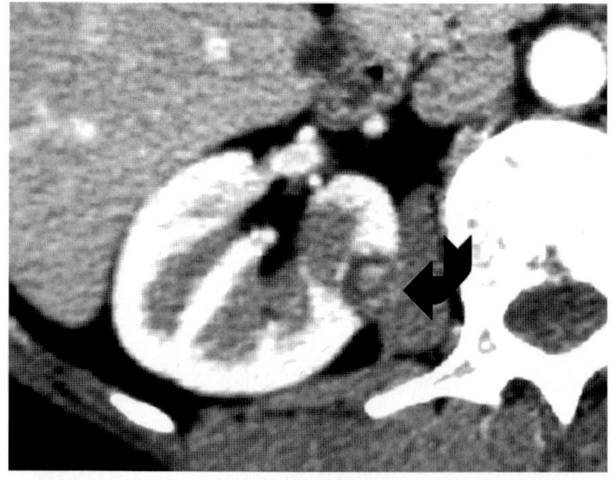

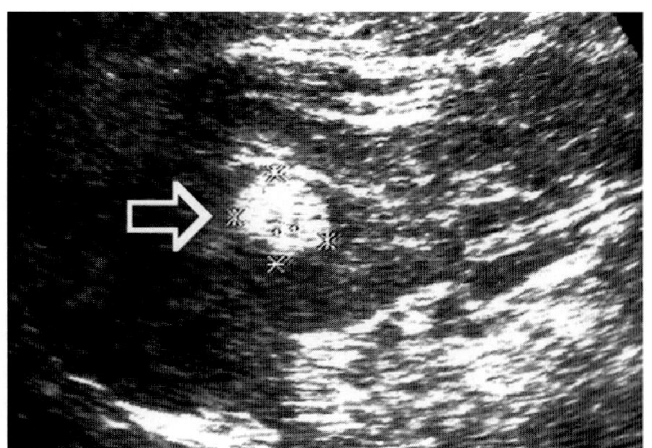

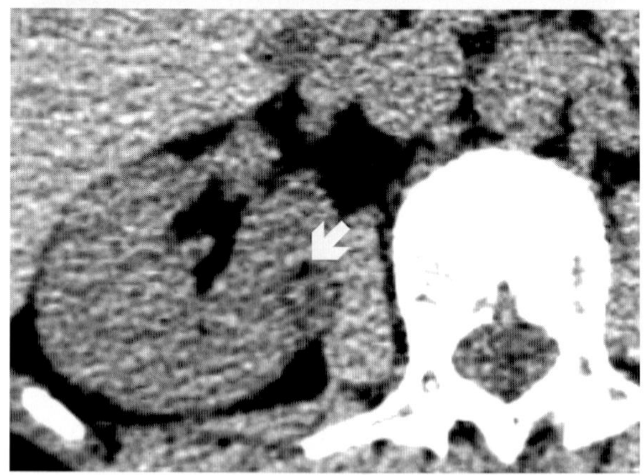

Fig. 2.12a-c. Small atypical angiomyolipoma with minimal fat component in a 49-year-old man. **a** Axial contrast-enhanced CT scan using a standard protocol of 5-mm slice thickness shows a small neoplasm of the right kidney (*arrow*) without obvious intratumoral fat. **b** Transverse US image shows suggestive hyperechoic pattern (*arrow*) that prompted a repeat CT examination using thinner collimation. **c** Axial unenhanced CT scan using 3-mm slice thickness clearly demonstrates a tiny intratumoral island of fat tissue (*arrow*) which prevented surgery.

on US but with a lower detection rate and with lower confidence. The central scar seen in large oncocytomas produces a stellate hypoechoic area on US (Goiney et al. 1984). A spoked-wheel distribution of tumor vessels also can be demonstrated on color Doppler with or without the association of a central hypoechoic scar. Both US criteria are seen in only a small percentage of large oncocytomas and cannot help differentiate RCC from benign oncocytoma because of poor specificity.

2.5.3
Bleeding Renal Tumors

Renal neoplasms can be responsible for spontaneous bleeding, including subcapsular hematoma or more extensive retroperitoneal bleeding, which may prevent tumor identification and characterization. Such circumstances should prompt screening for renal tumors, especially RCC (Fig. 2.13). The differential diagnosis between RCC and AML in patients with a hemorrhagic renal tumor relies on CT dem-

onstration of recognizable intratumoral fat. Associated intratumoral false aneurysm is an unusual complication that may occur within a hemorrhagic AML (Lapeyre et al. 2002). Such a finding on color Doppler US or CT favors a diagnosis of AML rather than RCC, since it has only been reported in hemorrhagic AML (Lapeyre et al. 2002).

2.5.4
Secondary Renal Neoplasms

Other renal neoplasms that can mimic the appearance of RCC on US include transitional cell carcinomas with renal parenchymal invasion, renal metastases, and lymphoma. Percutaneous needle biopsy may be indicated, depending on CT findings (Fig. 2.14) and a suggestive clinical history. Percutaneous needle biopsy provides proper histological diagnosis that is critical for appropriate treatment planning (nephroureterectomy in case of transitional cell carcinoma or chemotherapy in case of metastases or lymphoma) which differs from

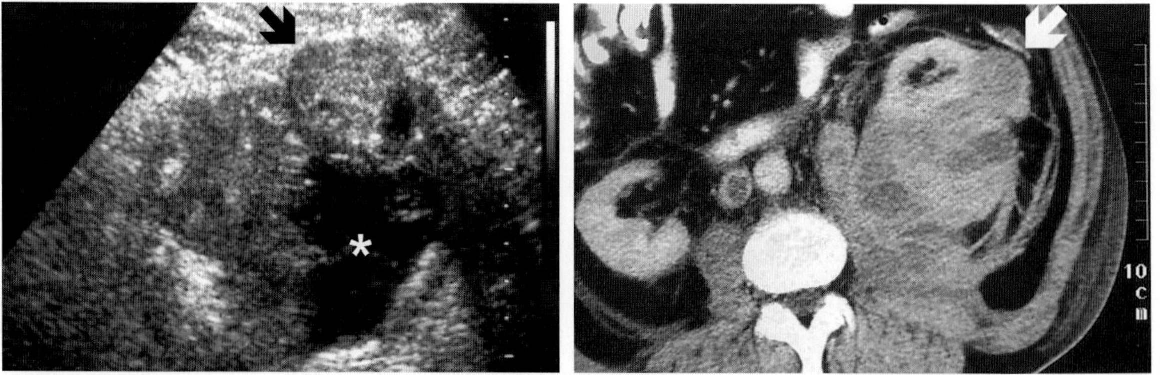

Fig. 2.13a,b. Small, bleeding renal cell carcinoma in a 64-year-old man. **a** Transverse US image of the left kidney shows a small solid mass (*arrow*) associated with perirenal blood collection (*asterisk*). **b** Axial contrast-enhanced CT scan confirms the small renal neoplasm (*arrow*) with perirenal hemorrhage.

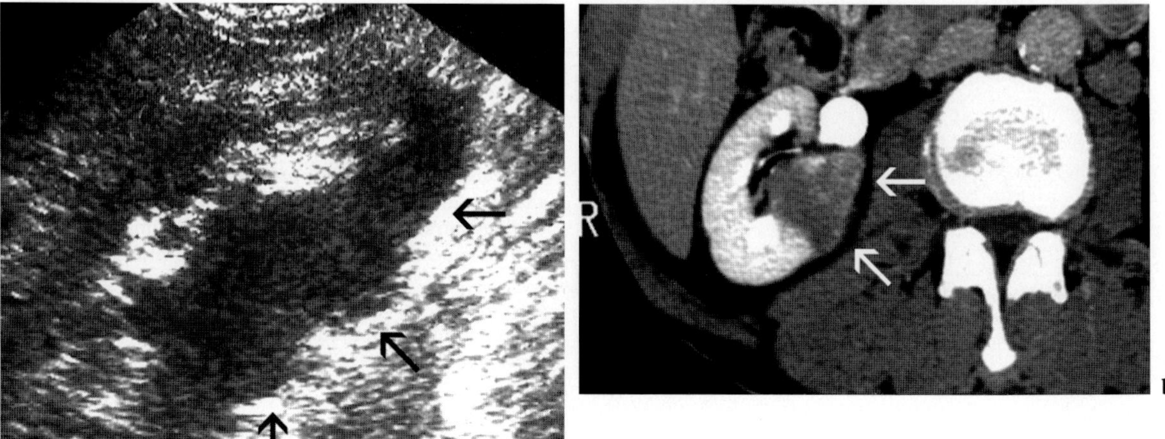

Fig. 2.14a,b. Renal lymphoma in a 59-year-old woman. **a** Longitudinal US image of the right kidney shows focal hypoechoic infiltration of the renal parenchyma (*arrows*). **b** Axial contrast-enhanced CT scan confirms the presence of an infiltrative lesion (*arrows*) which prompted percutaneous biopsy.

standard surgery for RCC. Ultrasound guidance has several advantages over CT in renal tumor percutaneous biopsy: it provides real time follow-up of the procedure, kidney and renal lesions can be targeted while moving with respiration; it can be performed using a dedicated US mobile unit; and it can be used intraoperatively or combined with another imaging technique such as CT.

2.5.5
Complex Cysts

The Bosniak classification of cystic renal masses is based on CT findings and requires careful use of CT with contrast administration (BOSNIAK 1986). The Bosniak criteria, however, can be applied to certain cystic masses seen on gray-scale US, especially to rule out a cystic tumor that meets the criteria of a type-2 lesion (minimally complicated cyst). All other complex cystic masses should be considered suspicious and require CT or MR imaging with contrast administration. Nonlinear US modalities, such as harmonic and pulse-inversion imaging, have recently improved the ability of gray-scale US to characterize complex cystic lesions. Ultrasound criteria that strongly suggest a cystic or pseudocystic renal neoplasm include a thick irregular peripheral wall; the presence of echoic mural nodule(s) (Figs. 2.7-2.9); the presence of multiple thick septa; heterogeneous and thick content; and demonstration of vascular flow signal within the solid component of the lesion on color Doppler US or postcontrast cyst wall enhancement after USCA administration.

On CT, category III (indeterminate cystic masses) often poses difficult diagnostic problems with cystic neoplasms. Conversely, categories II and IV are without doubt benign minimally complicated cysts and cystic/necrotic RCC. Gray-scale US can provide useful additional information that may help differentiate benign complex cysts from some atypical renal tumors that belong to category III.

Category-III complex cysts, resulting mostly from intracystic hemorrhage or infection, include those with regular thick walls and/or septations, with or without postcontrast enhancement of the walls. High density values within a cyst suggest benign hemorrhage when the mass is of small size, with CT numbers typically higher than 50 HU. Cysts also appear homogeneous and sharply marginated on pre- and postcontrast scans with no change after contrast administration (lack of enhancement). Hyperdense RCC are rare tumors that can mimic hyperdense complex cysts, but tumor vascularity usually is obvious on postcontrast CT images. Small hypovascularized tumors (mostly tubulopapillary RCC) also can mimic a spontaneously hyperdense cyst, as postcontrast enhancement can remain undetectable or only minimally visible (Fig. 2.15). In addition, the artifactual increase in density values of renal cysts on contrast-enhanced CT images may contribute to equivocal CT findings (Bae et al. 2000; Coulam et al. 2000; Heneghan et al. 2002); therefore, an isodense (>20, <50 HU) renal mass that does not exhibit substantial postcontrast enhancement should be viewed as a possible hypovascularized tumor (especially when the CT technique is inadequate, i.e., without delayed cuts). This finding should prompt US examination since hyperdense cysts are anechoic in about 30–50% of cases. Atypical isodense complex cysts on CT with such a US appearance require no further workup.

The RCC with massive necrosis also can exhibit a category-III pattern with thick, regular-enhancing walls. Such pseudocystic RCC often exhibit a homogeneous, isodense, non-enhancing content quite similar to the fluid content of a complex cyst on CT. Ultrasound is often helpful in characterizing tumor content that presents a heterogeneous echoic appearance, which is consistent with necrosis often associated with a thicker and more irregular wall compared with its appearance on CT (Fig. 2.8).

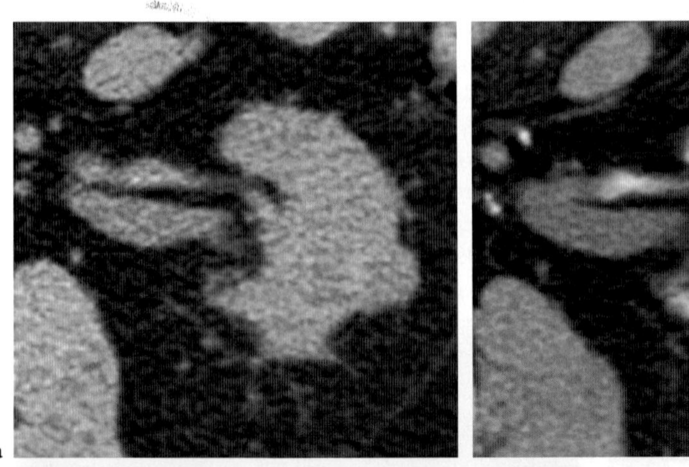
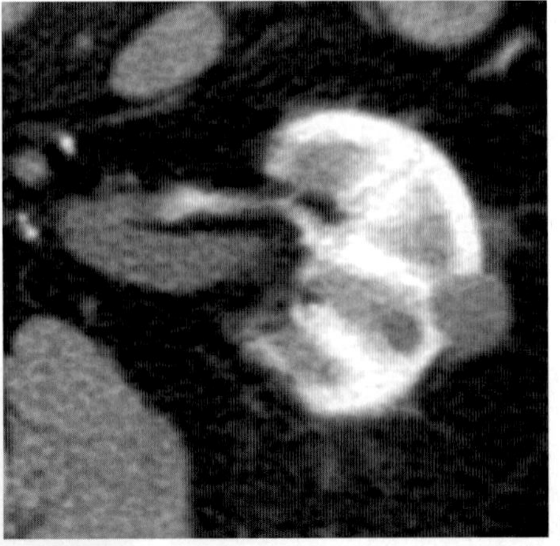
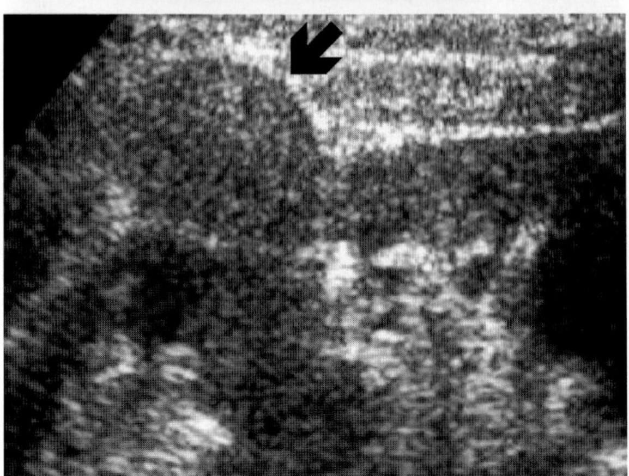

Fig. 2.15a–c. Small hypovascular renal neoplasm in a 52-year-old man. a Axial unenhanced and b contrast-enhanced CT scans of the left kidney show an equivocal postcontrast variation of the renal tumor density (+12 HU). c Transverse US image demonstrates a solid renal tumor (*arrow*) with homogeneous pattern. This tumor yielded papillary renal cell carcinoma at histology.

2.6
US Preoperative Tumor Staging

Ultrasound can provide useful information in addition to CT when staging RCC, especially in the assessment of venous invasion. Accurate preoperative evaluation of a T3b renal cancer is crucial for patient management. The cranial extent of a tumor thrombus from the involved renal vein is often poorly evaluated on CT because of the inhomogeneous contrast filling of the inferior vena cava (IVC) on early and intermediate (30–120 s) postcontrast scans. Although delayed cuts show homogeneous enhancement of the IVC lumen, in most cases the contrast level is insufficient to identify accurately the enhanced tumor thrombus. An additional step is often required. Although MR imaging has become the gold standard for this purpose, US can be performed first since it is highly accurate in assessing IVC involvement, provided that the examination is technically adequate (Bos and MENSIK 1998; HÉLÉNON et al. 1998). The tumor thrombus is seen as a solid echoic mass lying within the venous lumen, often responsible for a venous enlargement and more or less surrounded by color flow (Fig. 2.16). The upper limit of the tumor thrombus within the intrahepatic IVC should be accurately localized with respect to the hepatic veins and right atrium.

The presence of neovascularity indicates tumor thrombus; however, an associated bland thrombus, often located cranially and/or below the level of the renal veins, is difficult to differentiate from tumor tissue. The patient should also be screened, with cau-

tion, for an invaded retro-aortic left renal vein especially when the RCC is on the left side and the infrarenal IVC has thrombosed, or when the main hilar pre-aortic renal vein is not seen. Such a variation in the renal vein in conjunction with venous tumor invasion may be responsible for a false-negative result on CT, because of the lack of normal infrarenal venous system enhancement on early postcontrast images.

The use of USCA may improve tumor thrombus assessment in difficult cases by demonstrating flow contrast enhancement within the patent IVC distal to the thrombus. In addition, contrast agents have the potential to better characterize the tumor vascularity which may help differentiate tumor from bland thrombus.

2.7
US Intraoperative Tumor Evaluation

From a therapeutic point of view, renal-parenchymal-sparing surgery and nonsurgical modalities can benefit from US guidance. Intraoperative US remains the only available modality that may help remove a small renal tumor deeply located within the renal cortex or sinus (Fig. 2.17). It may identify additional tumors, after visible lesions have been removed, in up to 25% of patients suffering from hereditary renal cancer such as von Hippel-Lindau disease and hereditary papillary renal carcinomas (CHOYKE et al. 2001).

The development of percutaneous treatment using radio-frequency interstitial tissue ablation

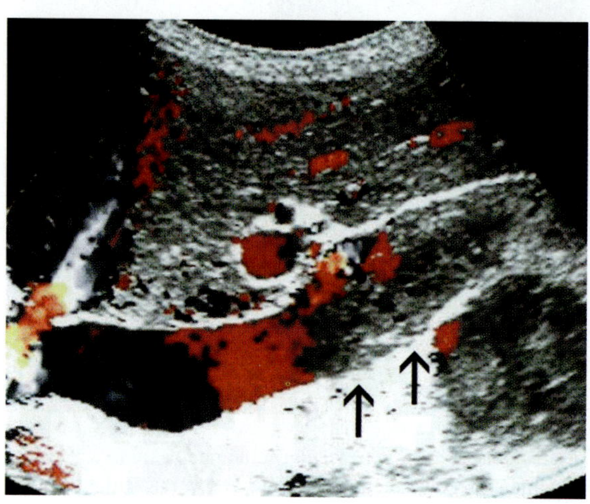

Fig. 2.16. Renal cell carcinoma in an 83-year-old woman with inferior vena cava invasion. Longitudinal color Doppler US image of the inferior vena cava shows tumor thrombus (*arrows*) with accurate delineation of the cranial extent.

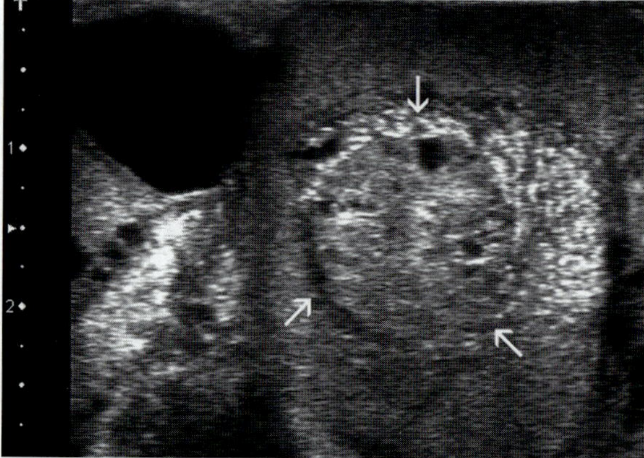

Fig. 2.17. Intraoperative ultrasound of renal cell carcinoma in a 42-year-old woman with von Hippel-Lindau disease. Longitudinal intraoperative US image performed with 12-MHz probe shows the delineation of the small solid renal tumor (*arrows*) located deeply within the renal parenchyma (medulla). Note the presence of a simple cyst originating from the subcapsular cortex.

likely will benefit from US guidance and contrast-enhanced US intraoperative evaluation of tumor vascularity (Fig. 2.18; ROBBIN et al. 2003). Advantages of US over CT include real-time needle placement, multiple scanning planes, and the ability to perform multiple contrast-enhanced evaluations of residual tumor tissue using a small bolus of contrast agent without nephrotoxicity.

2.8
Conclusion

Ultrasound plays a key role in screening renal cancer in asymptomatic patients. With the exception of large solid RCC with venous invasion, most renal tumors remain indeterminate on US and require CT for accurate characterization; however, US may help charac-

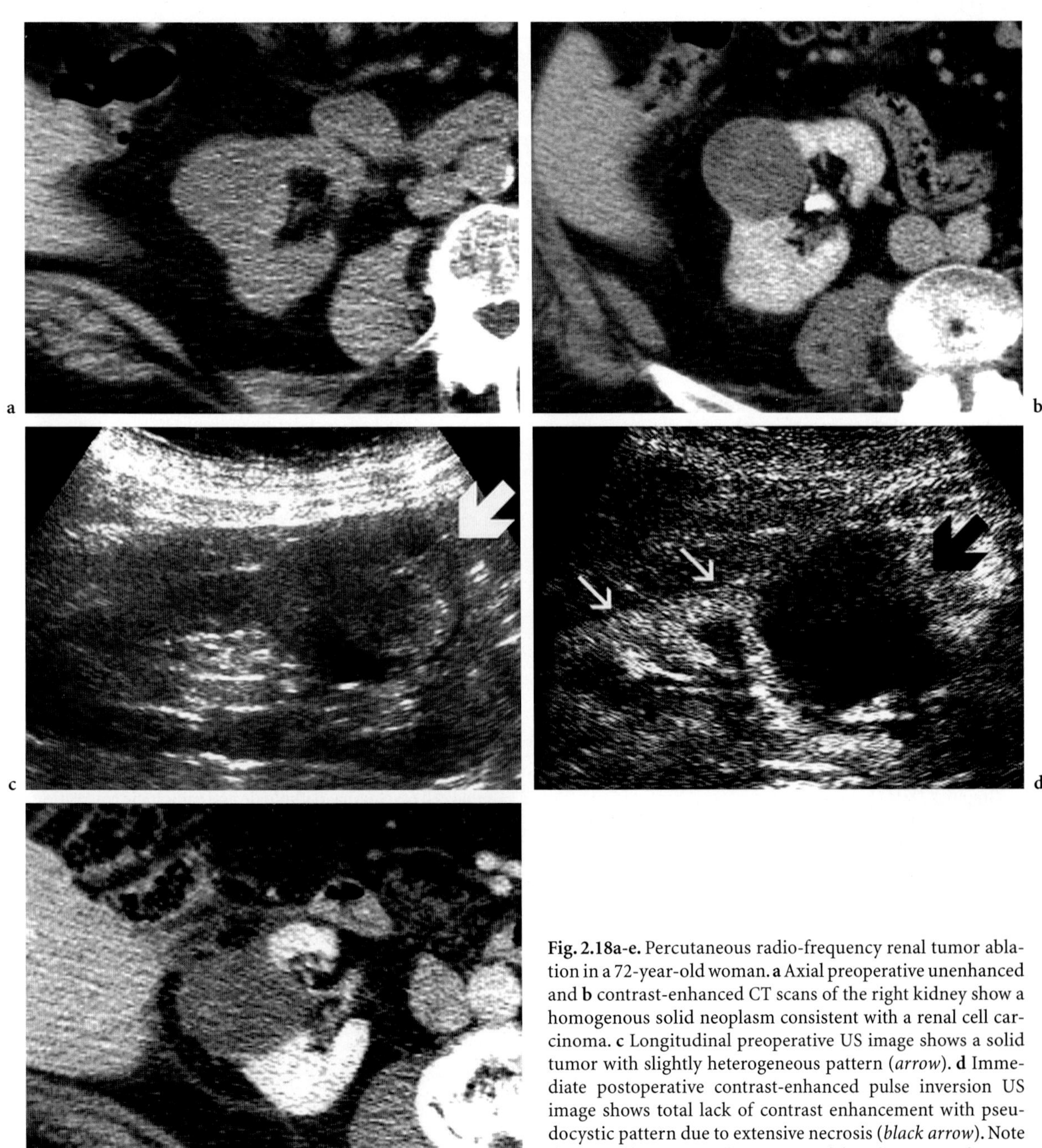

Fig. 2.18a-e. Percutaneous radio-frequency renal tumor ablation in a 72-year-old woman. **a** Axial preoperative unenhanced and **b** contrast-enhanced CT scans of the right kidney show a homogenous solid neoplasm consistent with a renal cell carcinoma. **c** Longitudinal preoperative US image shows a solid tumor with slightly heterogeneous pattern (*arrow*). **d** Immediate postoperative contrast-enhanced pulse inversion US image shows total lack of contrast enhancement with pseudocystic pattern due to extensive necrosis (*black arrow*). Note the normal contrast enhancement of the adjacent renal cortex (*white arrows*). **e** Axial contrast-enhanced CT scan confirms the lack of enhanced residual tumor tissue.

terize cystic RCC that remain equivocal on CT. Recent technical improvements in gray-scale imaging have increased the accuracy of US in the diagnosis and staging of kidney cancer. Intraoperative evaluation of radio-frequency tumor ablation also can benefit from recent advances in the use of US contrast agents.

References

Bae KT, Heiken JP, Siegel CL, Bennett HF (2000) Renal cysts: Is attenuation artifactually increased on contrast-enhanced CT images? Radiology 216:792–796

Bos SD, Mensik HJ (1998) Can duplex Doppler ultrasound replace computerized tomography in staging patients with renal cell carcinoma? Scand J Urol Nephrol 32:87–91

Bosniak MA (1986) The current radiological approach to renal cyst. Radiology 158:1–10

Choyke PL, Pavlovich CP, Daryanani KD, Hewitt SM, Lineham WM, Walther MM (2001) Intraoperative ultrasound during renal parenchymal sparing surgery for hereditary renal cancers: a 10-year experience. J Urol 165:397–400

Correas JM, Hélénon O, Moreau JF (1999) Contrast-enhanced ultrasonography of native and transplanted kidney diseases. Eur Radiol 9 (Suppl 3):394–400

Coulam CH, Sheafor DH, Leder RA et al. (2000) Evaluation of pseudoenhancement of renal cysts during contrast-enhanced CT. Am J Roentgenol 174:493–498

Curry NS, Cochran ST, Bissada NK (2000) Cystic renal masses: accurate Bosniak classification requires adequate renal CT. Am J Roentgenol 175:339–342

Forman HP, Middleton WD, Melson GL, McLennan BL (1993) Hyperechoic renal cell carcinomas: increase in detection at US. Radiology 188:431–434

Goiney RC, Goldenberg L, Cooperberg PL (1984) Renal oncocytoma: sonographic analysis of 14 cases. Am J Roetgenol 143:1001–1004

Hélénon O, Merran S, Paraf F et al. (1997) Unusual fat-containing tumors of the kidney: a diagnostic dilemma. RadioGraphics 17:129–144

Hélénon O, Correas JM, Chabriais J et al. (1998) Renal vascular Doppler imaging: clinical benefits of power mode. RadioGraphics 18:1441–1454

Hélénon O, Correas JM, Ballayeguier C et al. (2001) Ultrasound of renal tumors. Eur Radiol 11:1890–1901

Heneghan JP, Spielmann AL, Sheafor DH et al. (2002) Pseudoenhancement of simple renal cysts: a comparison of single and multidetector helical CT. J Comput Assist Tomogr 26:90–94

Jamis-Dow CA, Choyke PL, Jennings SB, Linehan WM, Thakore KN, Walther MM (1996) Small (≤ 3 cm) renal masses: detection with CT versus US and pathologic correlation. Radiology 198:785–788

Jinzaki M, Tanimoto A, Narimatsu Y et al. (1997) Angiomyolipoma: imaging findings in lesions with minimal fat. Radiology 205:497–502

Jinzaki M, Okhuma K, Tanimoto A et al. (1998) Small solid renal lesions: usefulness of power Doppler US. Radiology 209:549–550

Kim AY, Kim SH, Kim YJ, Lee IH (1999) Contrast-enhanced power Doppler sonography for differentiation of cystic renal lesions: preliminary study. J Ultrasound Med 18:581–588

Lapeyre F, Correas JM, Ortonne N, Balleyguier C, Hélénon O (2002) Color Doppler imaging of pseudoaneurysm in bleeding angiomyolipomas. Am J Roentgenol 179:145–147

Levine E, King BF (2000) Adult malignant renal parenchymal neoplasms. In: Pollack HM, McClennan BL (eds) Clinical urography. Saunders, Philadelphia, pp 1440–1559

Papanicolaou N, Harbury OL, Pfister RC (1988) Fat-filled postoperative renal cortical defects: sonographic and CT appearance. Am J Roentgenol 151:503–505

Robbin ML (2001) Ultrasound contrast agents: a promising future. Radiol Clin North Am 39:399–414

Robbin ML, Lockhart ME, Barr RG (2003) Renal imaging with ultrasound contrast: current status. Radiol Clin North Am 41:963–978

Schmidt T, Hohl C, Haage P et al. (2003) Diagnosis accuracy of phase-inversion tissue harmonic imaging versus fundamental B-mode sonography in the evaluation of focal lesions of the kidney. Am J Roengenol 180:1639–1647

Siegel CL, Middleton WD, Teefey SA, McClennan BL (1996) Angiomyolipoma and renal cell carcinoma: US differentiation. Radiology 198:789–793

Siemer S, Uder M, Humke U et al. (2000) Value of ultrasound in early diagnosis of renal cell carcinomas. Urologe 39:149–153

Sim JS, Seo CS, Kim SH et al. (1999) Differentiation of small hyperechoic renal cell carcinoma from angiomyolipoma: computer-aided tissue echo quantification. J Ultrasound Med 18:261–264

Taniguchi N, Itoh K, Nakamura S, Obayashi T, Kawai F, Nakamura M (1997) Differentiation of renal cell carinomas from angiomyolipomas by ultrasonic frequency dependent attenuation. J Urol 157:1242–1245

Yamashita Y, Takahashi M, Watanabe O et al. (1992) Small renal cell carcinoma: pathologic and radiologic correlation. Radiology 184:493–498

Yamashita Y, Ueno S, Makita O et al. (1993) Hyperechoic renal tumors: anechoic rim and intratumoral cysts in US differentiation of renal cell carcinoma from angiomyolipoma. Radiology 188:179–182

Yeh HS, Halton KP, Shapiro RS, Rabinowitz JG, Mitty HA (1992) Junctional parenchyma: revised definition of hypertrophic column of Bertin. Radiology 185:725–732

3 CT in Kidney Cancer

SHEILA SHETH and ELLIOT K. FISHMAN

CONTENTS

S. SHETH, MD
Associate Professor of Radiology and Pathology, Johns Hopkins University School of Medicine, Director, Biopsy Service, Department of Radiology, Johns Hopkins Hospital, 600 North Wolfe Street, HAL B176D, Baltimore, MD 21287, USA
E. K. FISHMAN, MD, FACR
Professor of Radiology and Oncology, Johns Hopkins University School of Medicine, Director, Diagnostic Radiology and Body CT, Department of Radiology, Johns Hopkins Outpatient Center, 601 North Caroline Street, Room 3254, Baltimore, MD 21287, USA

3.1 Introduction

The past two decades have witnessed significant changes in the presentation, diagnosis, and management of renal tumors. With the widespread use of cross-sectional imaging, over one-third of renal cell carcinomas (RCC) are discovered serendipitously, and the majority of these incidental tumors are stage T1 lesions (LESLIE et al. 2003). Paralleling this clinical-stage migration, there is a growing trend for more limited surgical resection, such as adrenal-sparing radical nephrectomy, laparoscopic nephrectomy, or partial, nephron-sparing, nephrectomy (RUSSO 2000). Computed tomography (CT) plays a central role in the evaluation of a patient with a suspected renal mass, not only in the detection but also in the characterization of the mass. Renal lesions are among the most common incidental findings on ultrasound or abdominal CT (CARRIM and MURCHISON 2003). The vast majority are cysts that do not require any further management. If, however, the mass is not obviously a simple cyst, it becomes critical to differentiate between minimally complicated cysts, which can be observed. and potentially malignant lesions which require surgical removal. In patients with solid renal masses, CT is an essential tool for staging and surgical planning.

In this chapter we review state-of-the art CT techniques for evaluation of the kidneys. We discuss CT protocols best suited for detection of small renal tumors, emphasize important findings pertinent to characterization of renal masses, and briefly outline CT strategies for staging malignant renal tumors.

3.2 CT Techniques

3.2.1 Phases of Renal Enhancement

Single and multidetector CT (MDCT) have dramatically refined the diagnostic evaluation of renal pathology by allowing rapid image acquisition through the entire kidney during various phases of contrast enhancement and excretion following the administration of a single bolus of intravenous iodinated contrast medium.

Four distinct phases of renal enhancement can be imaged depending on acquisition time (Fig. 3.1). The timing of these phases varies with the speed of intravenous contrast injection. We routinely inject 100–120 ml of non-ionic contrast in a large antecubital vein at a rate of 3 ml/s:

1. The arterial phase. During this short phase, which occurs at about 15–25 s after the initiation of intravenous contrast injection, there is maximum opacification of the renal arteries. The renal veins also usually opacify in the late arterial phase. This phase is important for imaging potential renal donors or patients with suspected renal arterial pathology.
2. The corticomedullary phase (also called angionephrographic or late arterial phase; CMP/AP). This phase starts at about 25–70 s after the initiation of intravenous contrast injection. There is intense enhancement of the renal cortex due to preferential arterial flow to the cortex and glomerular filtration of the contrast material, while the medulla remains relatively less enhanced. This phase provides information about the vascularity of solid renal masses and is also the best phase for maximum opacification of the renal veins.
3. The nephrographic phase (also called the parenchymal venous phase; NP/VP) begins at 80–120 s. In this phase the contrast filters through the glomeruli into the collecting ducts and provides

homogeneous enhancement of the normal renal parenchyma. This is the best phase for the detection of subtle parenchymal lesions.
4. The excretory phase (EP) starts at 180 s. Excretion of the contrast material allows opacification of the calyces, renal pelves, and ureters, while the intensity of the nephrogram progressively declines. We routinely acquire excretory phase images at 240 s to ensure opacification of the ureter (Fig. 3.1).

For evaluation of renal masses, a minimum of three acquisition sequences are required for detection as well as characterization of renal lesions. An initial series of unenhanced scans through the kidneys should be part of every protocol for evaluation of a suspected renal mass: it provides a baseline to measure the enhancement within the lesion after the administration of intravenous contrast. This enhancement characteristic is very important in distinguishing hyperdense cysts from solid tumors.

Our protocol for imaging a patient with a suspected renal mass follows.

Studies are performed using a 16-row-detector CT scanner (Siemens Sensation 16 scanner, Siemens Medical Solutions, Malvern, Pa.):

1. Precontrast image acquisition through the kidneys with 16×0.75-mm detector collimation, 0.75-mm slice thickness, 12 mm per rotation table speed, 5-mm reconstruction increment.
2. Late arterial phase (AP) acquisition through the kidney obtained 25 s after the start of injection of 120 ml iohexol at an injection rate of 3 ml/s with 16×0.75-mm detector collimation, 0.75-mm slice

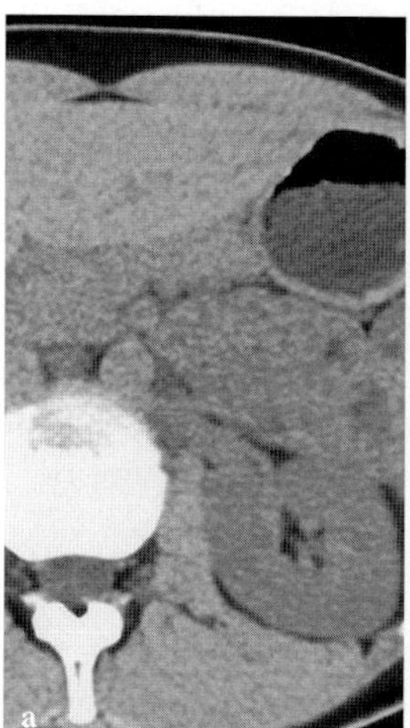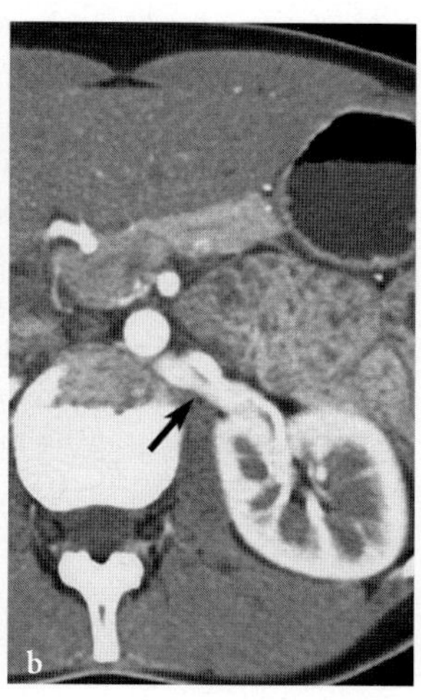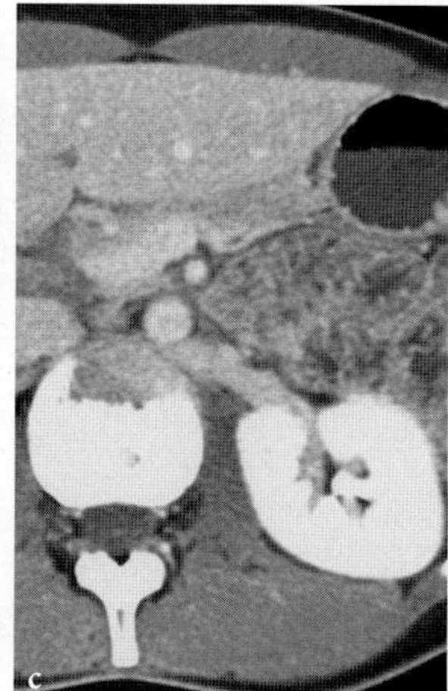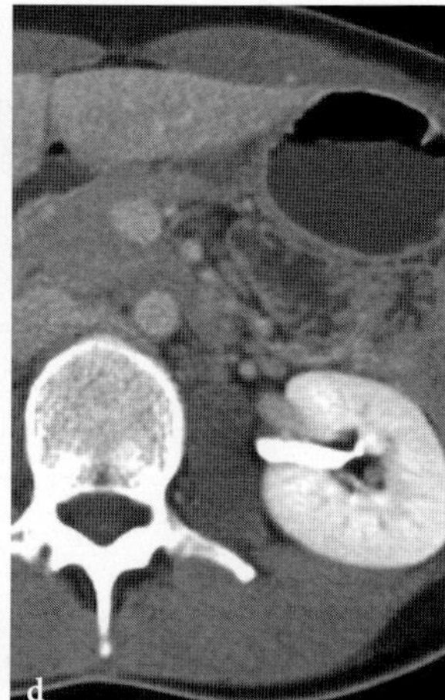

Fig. 3.1a-d. Phases of renal enhancement at CT in a 42-year-old woman with history of hematuria. **a** Axial precontrast CT scan. **b** Axial contrast-enhanced corticomedullary (late arterial phase [AP]) CT scan. Note excellent opacification of the retro-aortic left renal vein (*arrow*). **c** Axial contrast-enhanced nephrographic (parenchymal venous phase [VP]) CT scan. **d** Axial contrast-enhanced excretory phase (EP) CT scan.

thickness, 12-mm per rotation table speed, and 0.5-mm reconstruction increment. This phase depicts the renal arterial anatomy as well as the status of the renal vein, critical information for tumor staging as well as planning for surgery.

3. Delayed (excretory) phase (EP) acquisition through the abdomen and pelvis obtained after 180 to 240 s with 16×0.75-mm detector collimation, 0.75-mm slice thickness, 12 mm per rotation table speed, and 0.5-mm reconstruction increment.

We usually limit image acquisition to three sequences to minimize radiation to the patients. An additional venous phase (VP) acquisition (obtained at 55 s, with same scanning parameters as the arterial phase) can be added in select circumstances.

3.2.2
Advantages of Multidetector CT

Several advantages of multidetector CT over older-generation single-detector CT are well documented in the literature. It allows faster data acquisition times (average 2.6 times for a four-detector-row CT) when compared with single-detector CT, with no loss in image quality. Very rapid data acquisition times are possible because of short gantry rotation times (0.5 s) combined with multiple detectors providing increased coverage along the z axis (Hu et al. 2000; Foley 2003). Timing of the contrast bolus can thus be optimized to evaluate the arterial and venous supply of the kidney as well as the renal parenchyma and collecting system, and images of the entire kidneys and collecting systems can be generated during multiple phases of parenchymal enhancement and contrast excretion. Another advantage of MDCT is improved z-axis spatial resolution. The 16-detector-row scanners combine rapid data acquisition with narrow collimation. Thinner collimation greatly improves the quality of three-dimensional (3D) data sets and allows generation of excellent 3D images of the renal arteries and veins and the collecting system, comparable to those of conventional angiography and urography.

3.2.3
Post-Processing Techniques

Efficient interactive workstations are essential to handle the high number of images generated with MDCT and to generate reconstructed images sim-

ulating conventional angiographic or urographic images. Maximum intensity projection (MIP), multiplanar reconstruction, and volume-rendering (VR) techniques have been shown to be very effective. Volume rendering uses attenuation information from the entire data set by assigning shades of gray to varying attenuation values. It allows the viewer to interact with the data sets in real time, obviating the need for complex editing (Rubin 2001). It is invaluable in planning surgical management. Urologists find the interactive display of a 3D model of the affected kidney and its vascular supply particularly helpful before considering partial (nephron-sparing) nephrectomy, undertaking venous thrombectomy, and for planning extensive resection to remove a locally invasive renal cell or transitional cell cancer.

3.3
Detection and Characterization of Renal Masses

3.3.1
Detection of Renal Masses

Unlike the renal parenchyma, renal masses do not contain functioning renal nephrons. After the patient receives intravenous iodinated contrast, renal lesions exhibit varying degree of enhancement depending on their vascularity. Vascular tumors display maximum enhancement in the AP; however, in the delayed phases (VP and EP), almost all renal masses have lower attenuation than the homogeneously enhancing surrounding normal renal tissue. Many studies have demonstrated that the VP is more sensitive than the AP for the detection of small (<3 cm) renal lesions (Fig. 3.2; Cohan et al. 1995; Kopka et al. 1997; Szolar et al. 1997; Yuh and Cohan 1999). In one study that examined 295 lesions smaller than 3 cm, 84 more renal masses were seen in the VP than in the AP. This increased conspicuity was due to a statistically significant higher difference in attenuation values between the small lesions and the renal parenchyma in the VP, compared with the AP (Szolar et al. 1997). The difference was most striking for the smallest lesions (<1.1 cm) and those located in the medullary portion of the kidney (Cohan et al. 1995; Szolar et al. 1997). The AP was associated with a higher number of false-negative results as well as false-positive results. A small hypervascular solid tumor

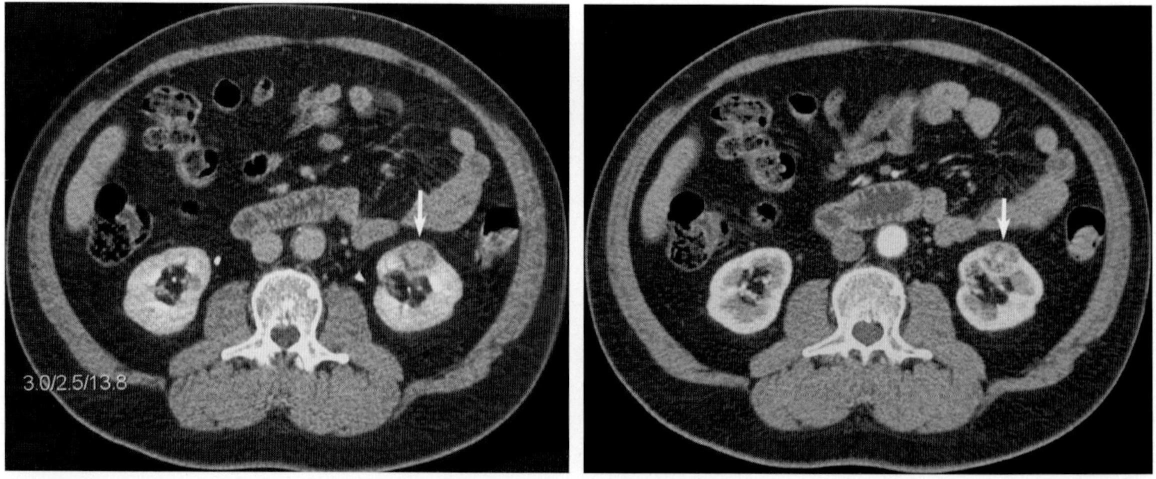

Fig. 3.2a,b. Incidental renal mass in a 58-year-old man. **a** Axial contrast-enhanced CT scan in the EP shows a 2.5-cm mass in the left kidney (*arrow*). **b** Axial contrast-enhanced CT scan in the AP shows the mass is subtle and could be mistaken for an unenhanced medulla (*arrow*). The patient underwent nephron-sparing surgery for a conventional renal cell carcinoma.

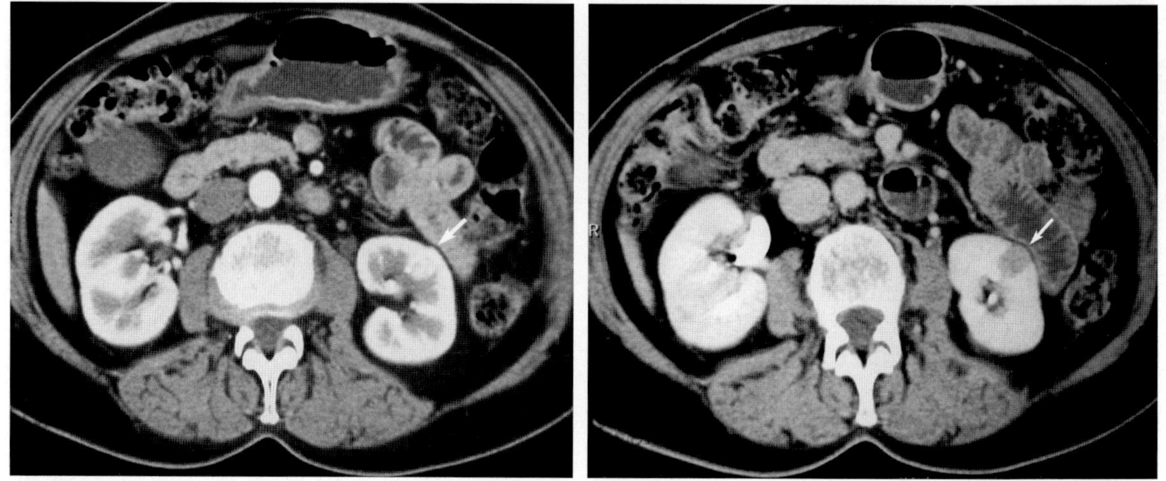

Fig. 3.3a,b. Incidental renal mass in a 64-year-old woman. **a** Axial contrast-enhanced CT scan in the AP shows a small hypervascular mass (*arrow*) in the mid portion of the left kidney which is barely visible. **b** Axial contrast-enhanced CT scan in the EP clearly shows a 2-cm mass (*arrow*) which is hypodense to the renal parenchyma in this phase. Partial left nephrectomy was performed and pathology revealed a small angiomyolipoma.

may enhance to the same degree as the renal cortex and may be mistaken for normal parenchyma on the AP (Fig. 3.3). A more common source of error (false negative) occurs when a centrally located mass is mistaken for the normal hypoenhancing medulla. On the other hand, mistaking a heterogeneously enhancing medulla for a solid tumor is a potential cause of a false-positive diagnosis.

Many of the additional small lesions detected on the VP have been shown to be clinically insignificant renal cysts (Fig. 3.4) or are too small to characterize (COHAN et al. 1995), although it appears that a significant number of small solid renal tumors are only detected on this phase. While many original reports have compared the AP with the VP, which delayed imaging sequence is most useful is still an unanswered question. One major advantage of image acquisition in the early EP is visualization of the collecting system and its relationship with central tumors, critical information if nephron-sparing surgery is to be considered. A recent study comparing VP and EP concluded that although VP images were more esthetically pleasing, both phases were equally effective in detecting and characterizing renal lesions (YUH et al. 2000).

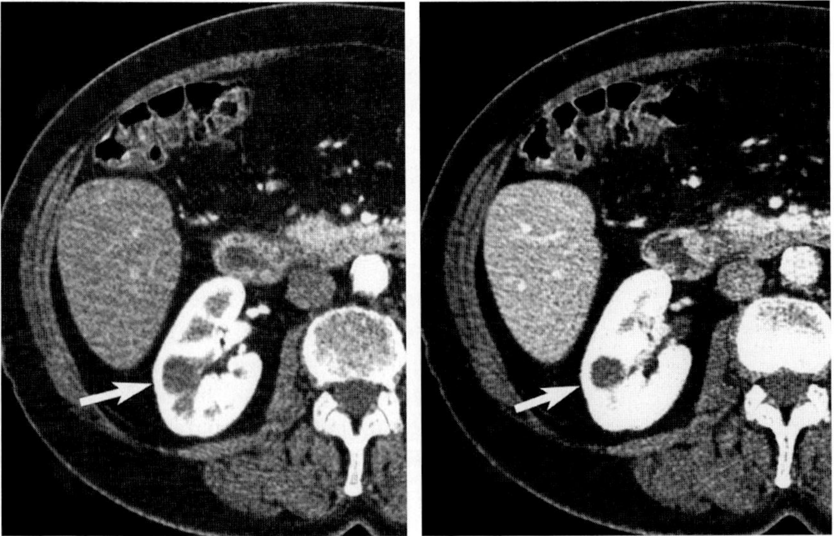

Fig. 3.4a,b. Small cyst in a 58-year-old man. **a** Axial contrast-enhanced CT scan in the VP clearly shows a small cyst (*arrow*) in the right kidney. **b** Axial contrast-enhanced CT scan in the AP shows that the cyst is much more subtle (*arrow*) and could be mistaken for the normal medulla.

3.3.2
Characterization of Renal Masses

Once a renal mass is detected, it is critical to accurately characterize it and to differentiate clinically insignificant renal cysts from solid and potentially malignant renal tumors. Renal cysts are fluid filled, and because they are avascular lesions, they demonstrate no enhancement after intravenous contrast administration. In contrast, RCC have a rich vascular supply and enhance significantly after contrast; thus, accurate measurement of the degree of enhancement in renal masses is critical to distinguish complex cysts from solid and potentially malignant lesions.

3.3.3
Concept of Significant Enhancement

Objective determination of lesion enhancement involves measurement of attenuation values within the mass before and after intravenous contrast. These quantitative data are obtained from operator-defined regions of interest (ROI) in various acquisitions sequences. Enhancement values of more than 10–12 Hounsfield units (HU) above pre-contrast measurements are considered significant. For these data to be reliable, it is important to pay careful attention to technical details, particularly when dealing with small lesions. The ROI should

be placed in similar portions of the lesion, while all imaging parameters remain unchanged between the pre-contrast and post-contrast scans. If nodularity or wall thickening is present, their enhancement should be assessed. In small lesions, retrospective reconstruction over thinner intervals is helpful to avoid partial-volume averaging. Small cysts may demonstrate post-contrast "pseudo-enhancement" caused by beam-hardening artifacts, although this rarely exceeds the 10-HU threshold (COULAM et al. 2000).

In addition to these technical considerations, it is crucial to choose the optimal imaging sequence to measure the degree of enhancement. Most published studies agree that the VP or EP are more accurate than the AP in assessing the degree of enhancement of renal masses (BIRNBAUM et al. 1996; KOPKA et al. 1997; SZOLAR et al. 1997; YUH and COHAN 1999). Enhancement of solid renal tumors is time dependent and is greater in the VP compared with the AP. Some RCC enhance slowly over time and would be wrongly classified as non-enhancing if the AP were used.

Delayed scans can also be used in lieu of pre-contrast scans to characterize an incidental renal lesion detected on a routine contrast-enhanced CT. MACARI and BOSNIAK (1999) have suggested that measurement of the washout of contrast in a lesion at 15 min allows differentiation between hyperdense cysts and renal neoplasms. In their study, there was no change in the attenuation of high-density cysts between the initial contrast CT and the 15-min delayed images. In comparison, all lesions that proved to be neoplasms at surgery or on follow-up studies demonstrated decreased attenuation or "de-enhancement" of at least 15 HU on delayed CT, attributed to the washout of contrast from the vascular bed of the tumor (MACARI and BOSNIAK 1999).

3.4
Renal Cystic Lesions

Renal cysts are among the most common renal lesions detected on cross-sectional imaging; the majority are isodense to water (attenuation values of <20 HU) and easily diagnosed, although some renal cysts do not fulfill the established diagnostic criteria and can prove difficult to define. Since its publication in 1986, the Bosniak classification of renal cysts has been widely used to classify these lesions and to separate cystic lesions that can be safely followed from those requiring surgical resection (BOSNIAK 1986; CURRY et al. 2000):

1. Simple renal cysts. These cysts are classified as Bosniak category I, are homogeneous and isodense to water on pre-contrast images (<20 HU), do not enhance post-contrast, and display an imperceptible wall, a sharp interface with the adjacent renal parenchyma, and no septations or calcifications (Fig. 3.5). No further work-up or follow-up is necessary.

2. Minimally complicated cysts. These cysts belong to Bosniak category II, and contain one or two thin septa or thin wall calcifications, or may be hyperdense on pre-contrast images (homogeneously high attenuation; Figs. 3.6, 3.7). The wall is thin and they do not show enhancement post-contrast. These lesions are clearly benign and most are presumed to represent hemorrhagic cysts (SUSSMAN et al. 1984). A separate category IIF includes lesions that are slightly more complex and require careful follow-up.

3. Indeterminate cystic lesions. These cysts comprise Bosniak category III and, although some prove benign at pathology, surgery is usually indicated because some RCC may be classified in this category. The cystic mass may be multilocular or may have thick septations or a uniformly thick wall or calcifications (Fig. 3.8).

4. Potentially malignant cystic masses. Lesions in Bosniak category IV are potentially malignant. The wall may be focally thick and enhancing, and enhancing nodules may be present within the mass or near the wall (Fig. 3.9).

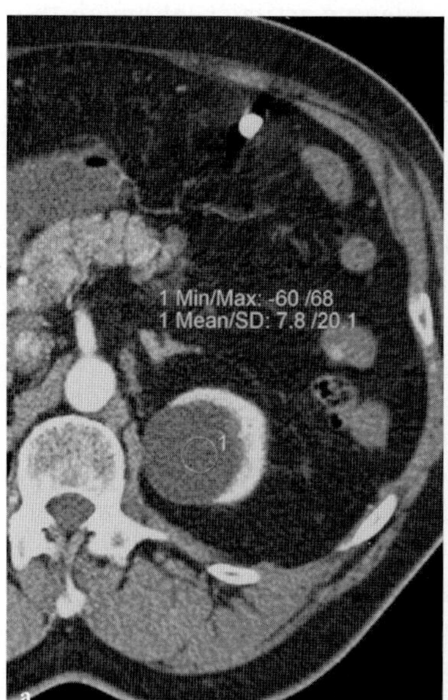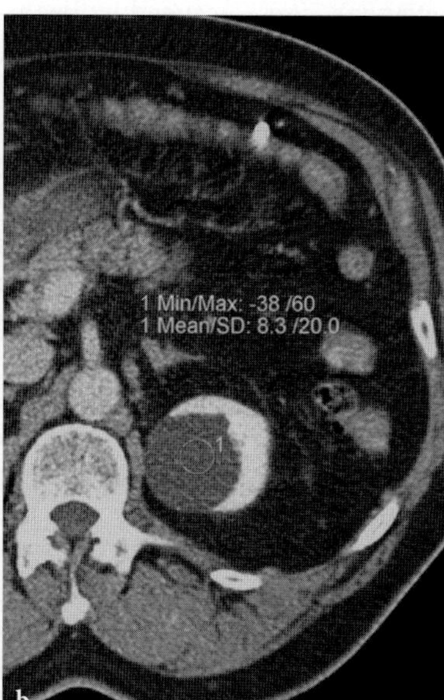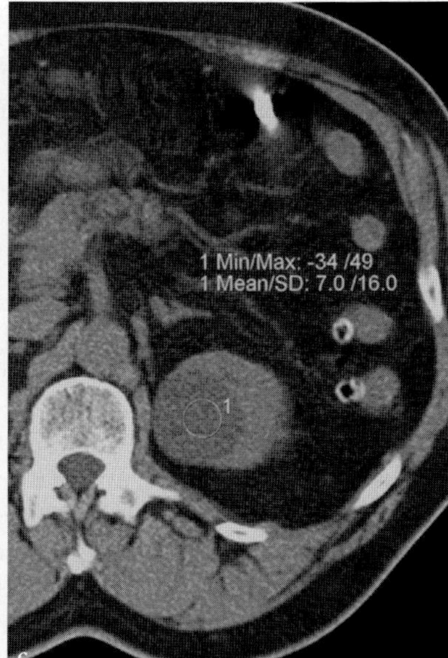

Fig. 3.5a-c. Simple renal cyst in a 65-year-old woman with an indeterminate left renal mass on ultrasound. **a** Axial precontrast CT scan shows a lesion in the left kidney. The lesion has water attenuation. **b** Axial contrast-enhanced CT scan in the AP shows no significant enhancement in the lesion. Note that the cyst has thin walls and no septation. **c** Axial contrast-enhanced CT scan in the EP confirms the absence of enhancement. This is a typical Bosniak I renal cyst.

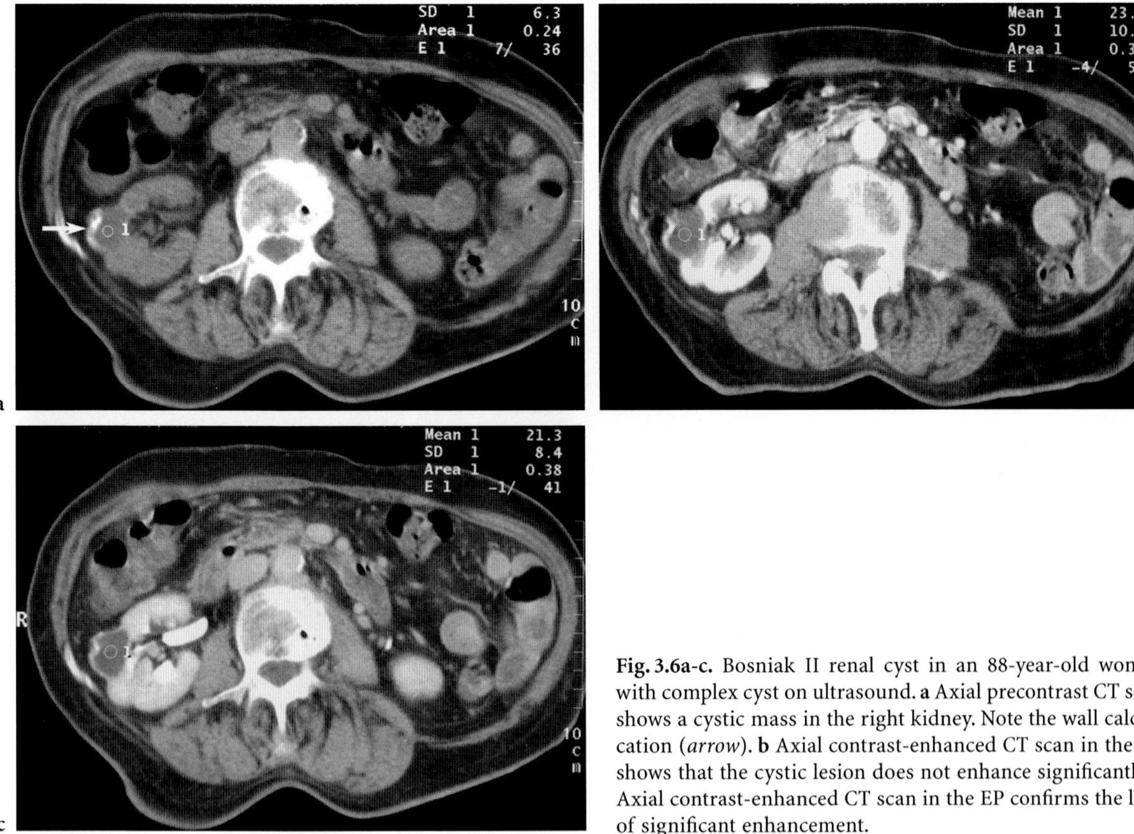

Fig. 3.6a-c. Bosniak II renal cyst in an 88-year-old woman with complex cyst on ultrasound. **a** Axial precontrast CT scan shows a cystic mass in the right kidney. Note the wall calcification (*arrow*). **b** Axial contrast-enhanced CT scan in the AP shows that the cystic lesion does not enhance significantly. **c** Axial contrast-enhanced CT scan in the EP confirms the lack of significant enhancement.

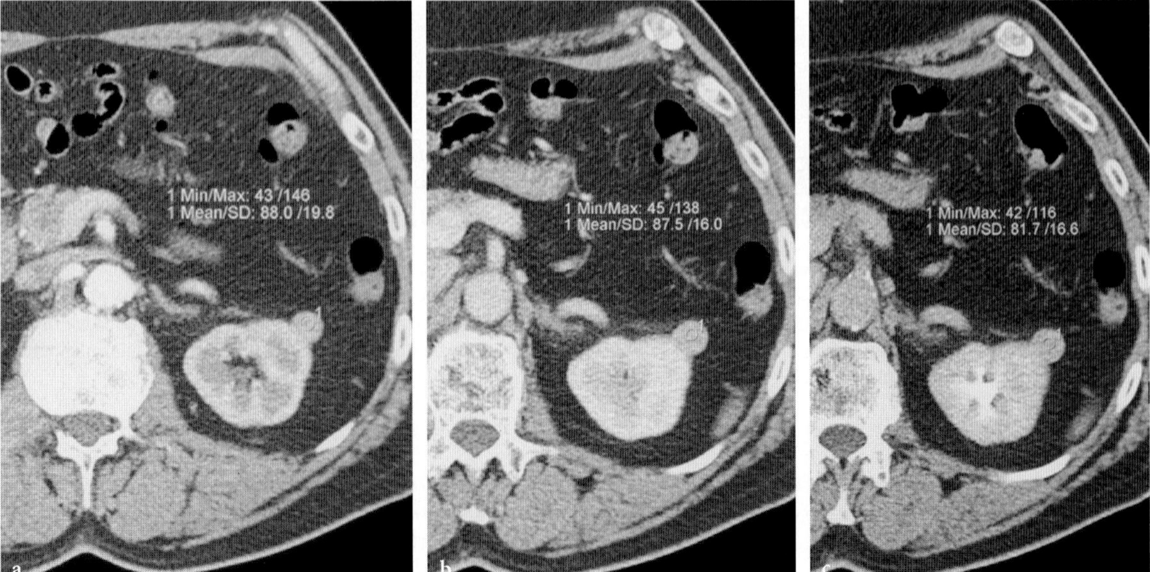

Fig. 3.7a-c. Incidental hyperdense cyst in a 60-year-old man. **a** Axial contrast-enhanced CT scan in the AP shows a hyperdense (88 HU) 1.5-cm exophytic lesion in the left kidney. **b** Axial contrast-enhanced CT scan in the VP shows no change in attenuation of the lesion. **c** Axial contrast-enhanced CT scan in the delayed phase shows no significant de-enhancement in the lesion (82 HU), confirming that this is a hyperdense cyst.

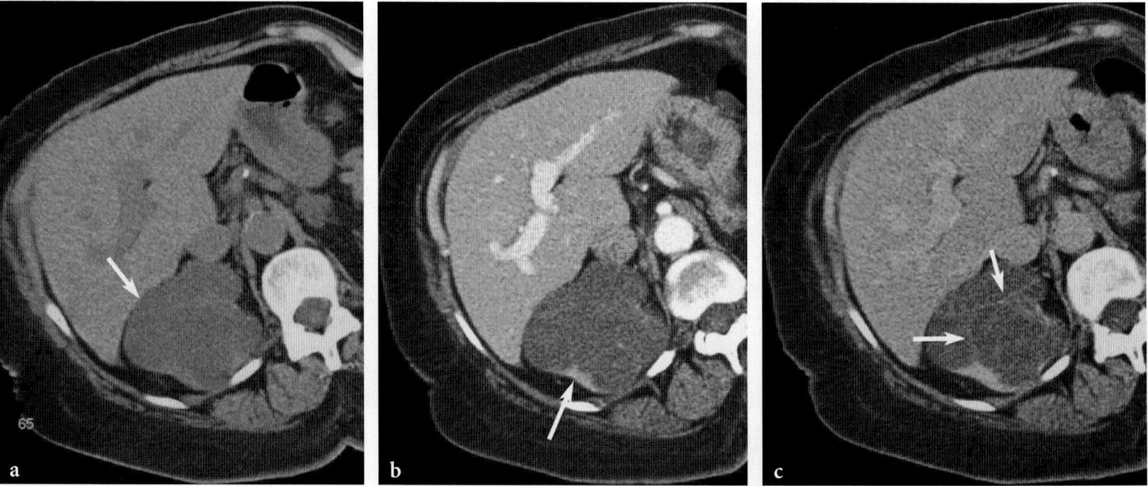

Fig. 3.8a-c. Bosniak III renal cyst in a 78-year-old woman. **a** Axial precontrast CT scan shows a cystic mass in the right kidney (*arrow*). **b** Axial contrast-enhanced CT scan in the AP shows enhancement in the wall (*arrow*). **c** Axial contrast-enhanced CT scan in the EP shows enhancement in the wall as well as thin, enhancing septations (*arrows*). The patient elected to "watch and wait" because of comorbid conditions. The lesion has been stable in size for 18 months.

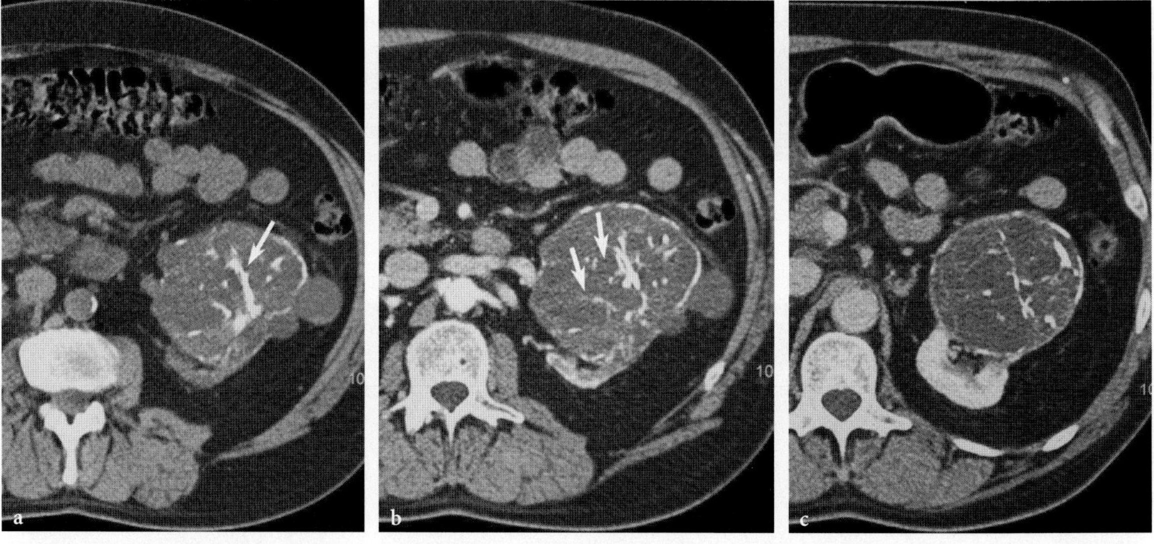

Fig. 3.9a-c. Incidental renal mass discovered on chest CT in a 68-year-old man. **a** Axial precontrast CT scan shows a 10-cm cystic mass with chunky calcifications in the left kidney (*arrow*). **b** Axial contrast-enhanced CT scan in the AP shows subtle areas of septal enhancement (*arrows*). Note that the left renal vein is normal. **c** Axial contrast-enhanced CT scan in the nephrographic phase (VP) shows similar findings. The patient underwent a radical left nephrectomy. Pathology revealed a cystic multilocular renal cell carcinoma, Fuhrman grade 2.

3.5
Renal Cell Carcinoma

3.5.1
Conventional Renal Cell Carcinoma

Conventional RCC arise from the convoluted tubules of the renal cortex and present as a solid expansile mass bulging and distorting the renal contour. They appear as a soft tissue mass, often of slightly higher attenuation than the normal renal parenchyma, with attenuation values of 20 HU or greater on precontrast CT. While the majority of RCC are solitary, approximately 5% are multifocal (RICHSTONE et al. 2004). Small-to-moderate size RCC usually have well-defined margins due to the presence of a pseudo-capsule formed by compressed surrounding renal tissue and fibrotic reaction. Calcifications are detected in up to 30% of tumors. After intravenous contrast, RCC exhibit significant enhancement above pre-contrast measurements, typically over 100 HU in the AP and 60 HU in the delayed phase (Figs. 3.10, 3.11). Small (3 cm or less) tumors usually have a homogenous appearance (Fig. 3.12) and show enhancement, whereas larger lesions tend to be more heterogeneous, due to intra-tumoral hemorrhage or necrosis. Another important finding recently described is that abnormal tumor vessels cause a relatively rapid washout of contrast from the tumor resulting in rapid de-enhancement (MACARI and BOSNIAK 1999). This pattern is characteristic of the most common type of RCC, the conventional (or clear cell) tumor which accounts for approximately 70% of renal malignancies.

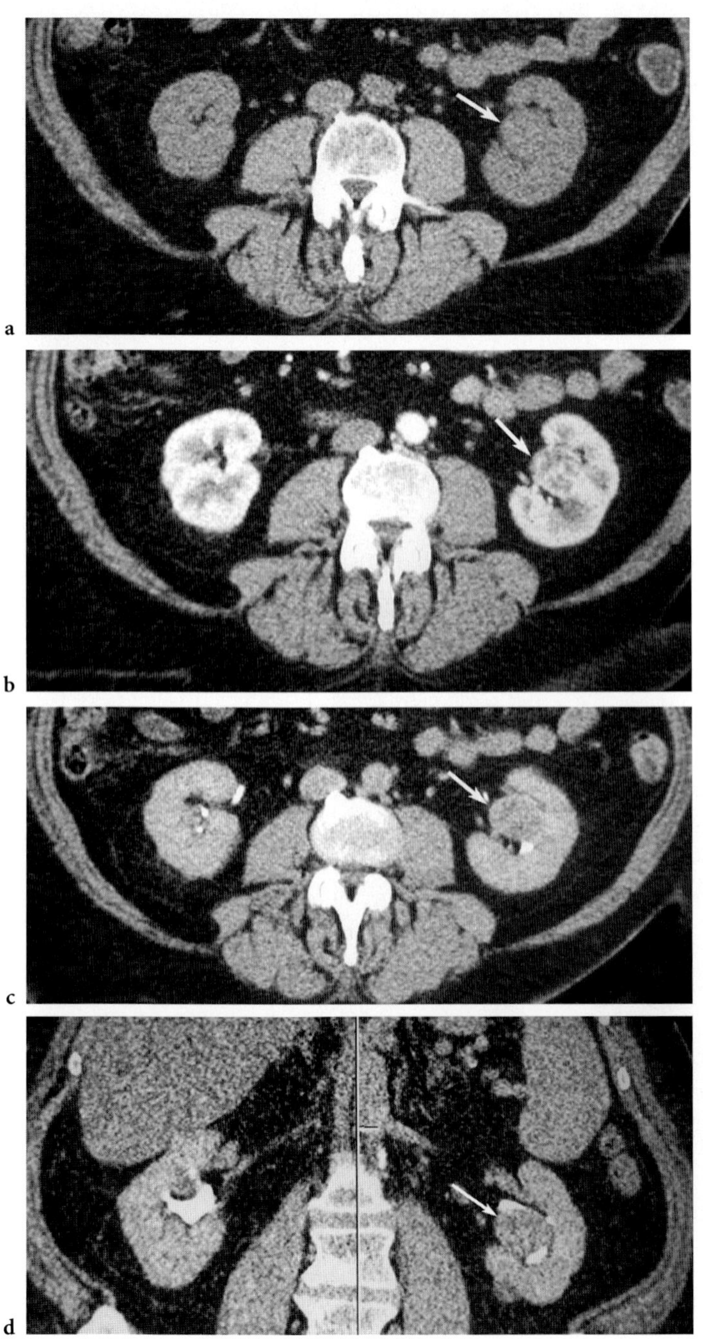

Fig. 3.10a-d. Small left renal cell carcinoma in a 61-year-old woman with history of partial right nephrectomy for renal cell carcinoma. a Axial unenhanced CT scan shows a 3-cm centrally located soft tissue mass (56 HU) in the left kidney (*arrow*). b Axial contrast-enhanced CT scan in the AP shows significant enhancement within the mass (98 HU; *arrow*). c Axial contrast-enhanced CT scan shows that the mass (63 HU; *arrow*) is distorting the collecting system. d Coronal-reconstruction CT image in the EP confirms the distortion of the collecting system by the mass (*arrow*). Although the location of the mass would favor a transitional cell carcinoma, its vascularity is suggestive of a renal cell carcinoma. A conventional renal cell carcinoma (Fuhrman grade 2) was found at nephrectomy.

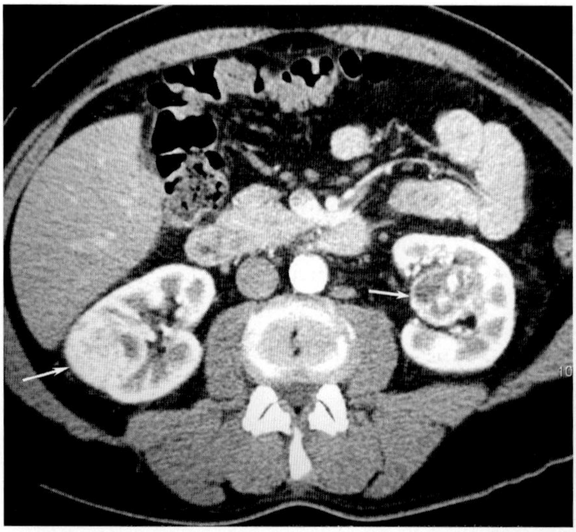

Fig. 3.11a-c. Bilateral renal cell carcinomas in a 70-year-old man presenting with right upper quadrant pain. **a** Axial contrast-enhanced CT scan in the AP shows hypervascular masses in both kidneys (*arrows*). The mass in the left kidney extends into the renal hilum. **b** Axial contrast-enhanced CT scan in the VP shows the same findings (*arrows*). **c** Axial contrast-enhanced CT scan in the EP shows that the masses (*arrows*) are abutting the collecting system. Partial right and radical left nephrectomy revealed bilateral conventional renal cell carcinoma. (With permission from SHETH et al. 2001)

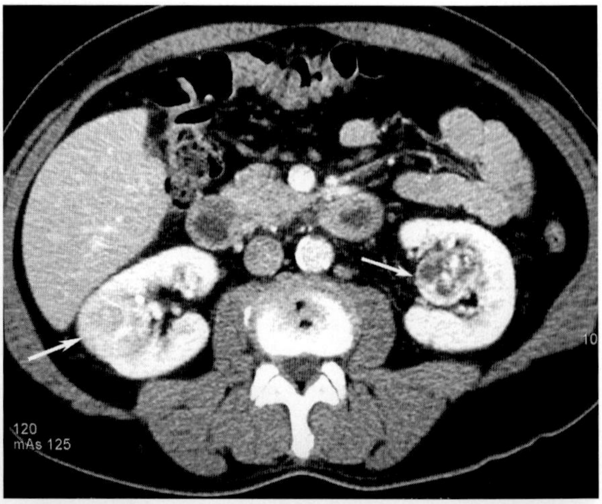

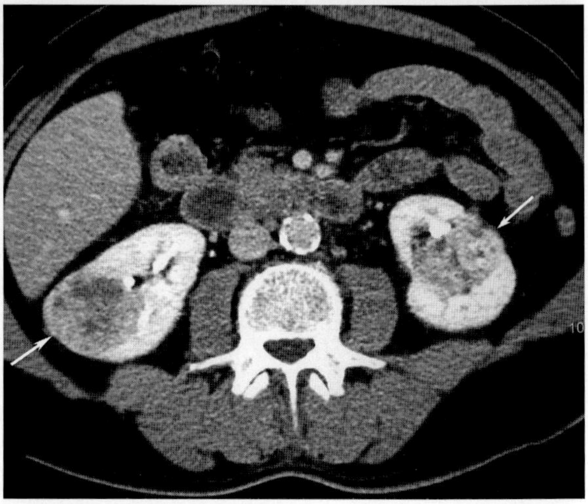

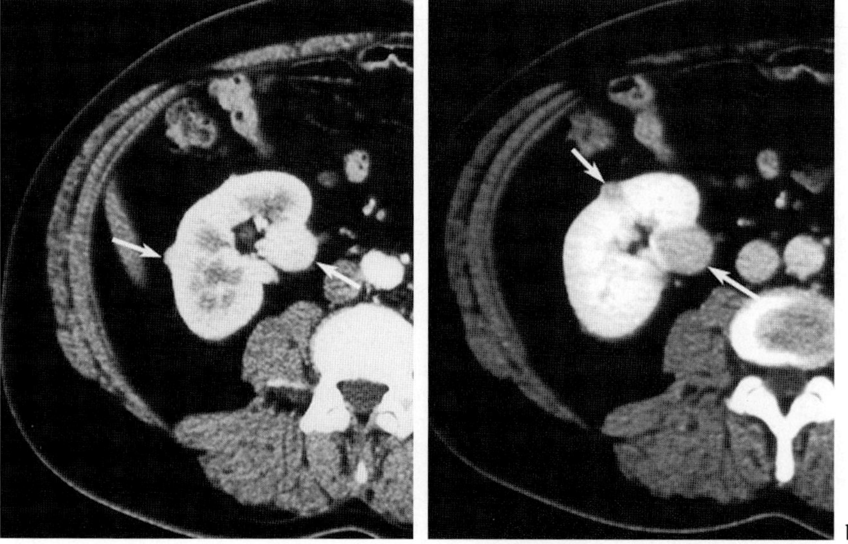

Fig. 3.12a,b. Multiple small renal cell carcinomas in a 52-year-old man. **a** Axial contrast-enhanced CT scan in the AP shows multiple small homogeneously enhancing masses in the right kidney (*arrows*). **b** Axial contrast-enhanced CT scan in the VP shows that the masses (*arrows*) are hypodense to the normal renal parenchyma. Note that the smaller lesions are more clearly seen.

3.5.2
Papillary and Chromophobe Renal Cell Carcinoma

Papillary RCC are associated with a better prognosis, reaching 80–90% 5-year survival. They comprise about 20% of RCC. Chromophobe cancers have the most favorable outcome with over 90% 5-year survival. By contrast, the rare (<1% of renal cell cancers) collecting duct carcinoma is associated with the worst prognosis with 5-year mortality reaching 95%. In a recently published retrospective review, KIM et al. (2002) attempted to determine whether CT appearance and enhancement patterns correlated with the histological type of tumor. In their study, degree of enhancement was the most useful parameter. Most conventional carcinomas enhanced strongly in the AP and delayed phases and large masses were heterogeneous. By contrast, chromophobe tumors showed weak and homogeneous enhancement. Papillary cancers tend to exhibit a more gradual enhancement (Figs. 3.13, 3.14; JINZAKI et al. 2000).

3.5.3
Collecting Duct Cancer

Collecting duct carcinomas are rare, aggressive cancers presumably arising from the collecting ducts of Bellini in the renal medulla. Tumor growth follows an infiltrative pattern, with the underlying normal renal tissues used as scaffolding for the invasive growth. This diagnosis can be suggested on CT, if the tumor is centered in the medullary portion of the kidney and infiltrates the renal parenchyma, with poorly defined transition and preservation of the reniform shape of the kidney (PICKHARDT et al. 2001). The prognosis is poor.

3.6
Differential Diagnosis of Solid Renal Masses

Careful analysis of CT appearance and attenuation values is often useful in differentiating RCC from other benign or malignant renal tumors; however, if imaging findings are equivocal, image-guided percutaneous biopsy is invaluable in achieving the correct diagnosis (NEUZILLET et al. 2004).

3.6.1
Benign Renal Tumors

3.6.1.1
Renal Oncocytoma

Renal oncocytomas are histologically benign solid vascular neoplasms of the kidney. They vary in size

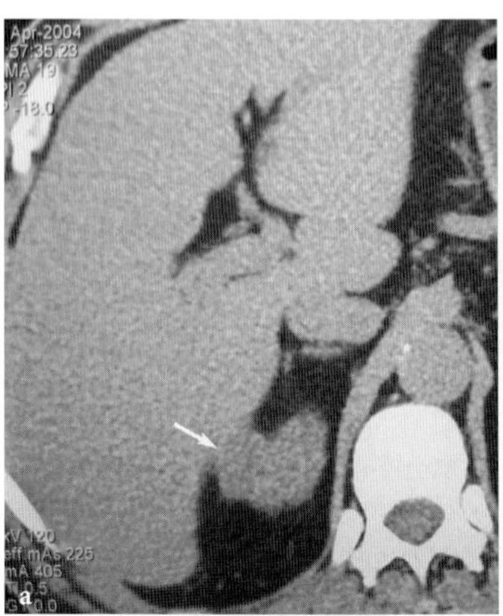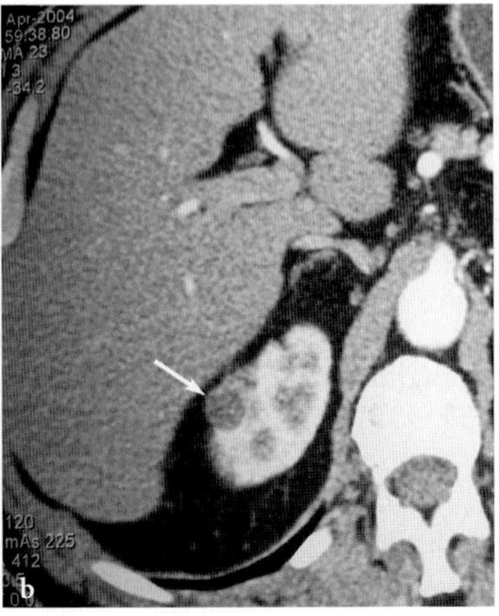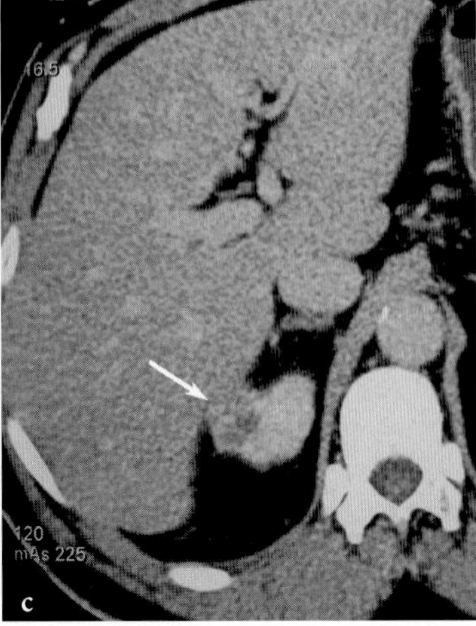

Fig. 3.13a-c. Incidental renal cell carcinoma in a 62-year-old man with history of staghorn calculus. **a** Axial precontrast CT scan shows a 2.5-cm exophytic soft tissue mass (*arrow*) in the upper pole of the right kidney. Region of interest (ROI) reading was 33.3 HU. **b** Axial contrast-enhanced CT scan in the AP shows the mass (*arrow*). The ROI reading was 33.6 HU. **c** Axial contrast-enhanced CT scan in the early EP shows enhancement within the mass (*arrow*). The ROI reading was 73.2 HU. Partial right nephrectomy revealed a papillary renal cell carcinoma.

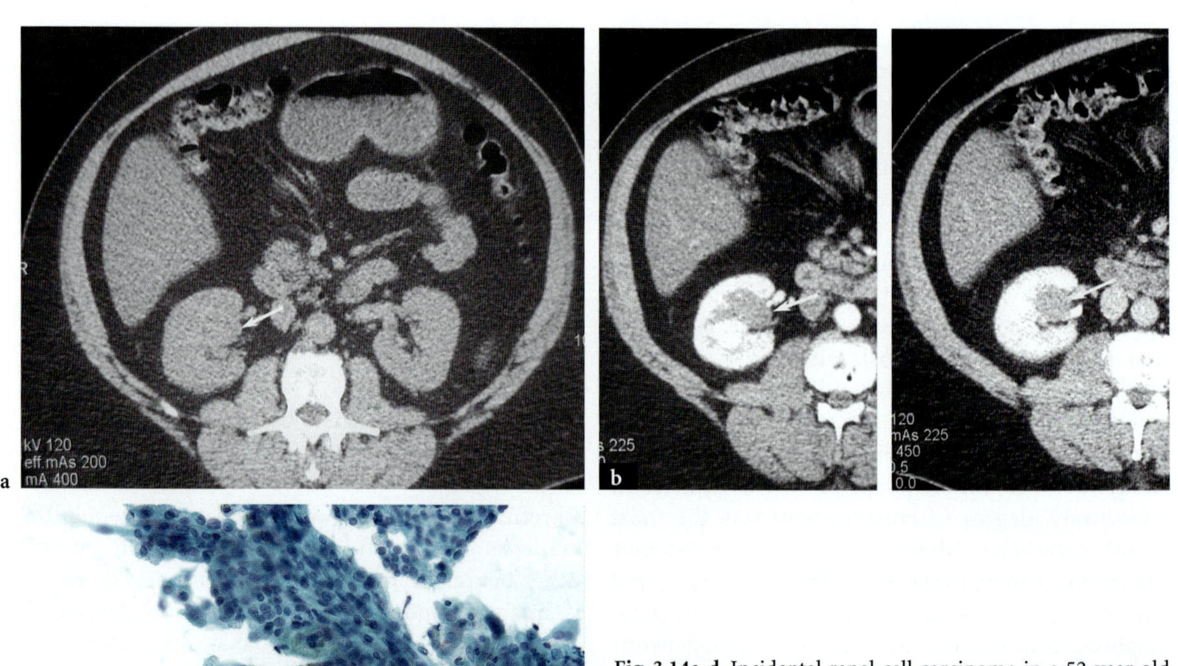

Fig. 3.14a-d. Incidental renal cell carcinoma in a 52-year-old man. **a** Axial unenhanced CT scan shows a subtle central soft tissue mass (*arrow*) in the right kidney. The ROI reading was 48 HU. **b** Axial contrast-enhanced CT scan in the AP shows that the mass (*arrow*) is not highly vascular. The ROI reading was 56 HU. **c** Axial contrast-enhanced CT scan in the EP shows some enhancement within the mass (*arrow*). The ROI reading was 60 HU. Because of the borderline enhancement, an ultrasound-guided percutaneous biopsy was performed. **d** Analysis of the fine-needle aspirate shows papillary renal cell carcinoma (Papanicolaou stain; original magnification, ×200). The patient underwent right nephrectomy.

from less than 1 cm to 15–20 cm. Although traditionally they have rarely been diagnosed before nephrectomy, preoperative diagnosis is desirable, as less aggressive surgery, such as enucleation or partial nephrectomy, is the preferred treatment. The CT appearance of a homogeneously enhancing large mass with a pseudo-capsule and a central scar should suggest the oncocytoma, since large RCC tend to enhance heterogeneously (Fig. 3.15). Small oncocytomas cannot be reliably distinguished from RCC with imaging (Fig. 3.16). With current improvements in cytopathological techniques, percutaneous biopsy can be useful in differentiating oncocytomas from RCC by demonstrating large eosinophilic epithelial cells with mitochondria rich cytoplasm, but there is significant overlap with renal cell cancer with oncocytic features (LIU and FANNING 2001).

3.6.1.2
Renal Angiomyolipoma

Angiomyolipomas are benign renal hamartomatous tumors composed of varying amounts of mature adipose tissue, smooth muscle, and abnormal blood vessels. Solitary angiomyolipomas are usually sporadic, whereas multiple lesions are part of the spectrum of renal abnormalities associated with tuberous sclerosis. Many of these tumors are small and detected serendipitously. On the other hand, large angiomyolipomas can hemorrhage and present acutely. In many cases a specific diagnosis can easily be established on CT by demonstrating even a small amount of fat within the lesion (Figs. 3.17, 3.18). Computed tomography can also detect intra- or perirenal blood as well as perinephric extension of angiomyolipomas (SHERMAN et al. 1981).

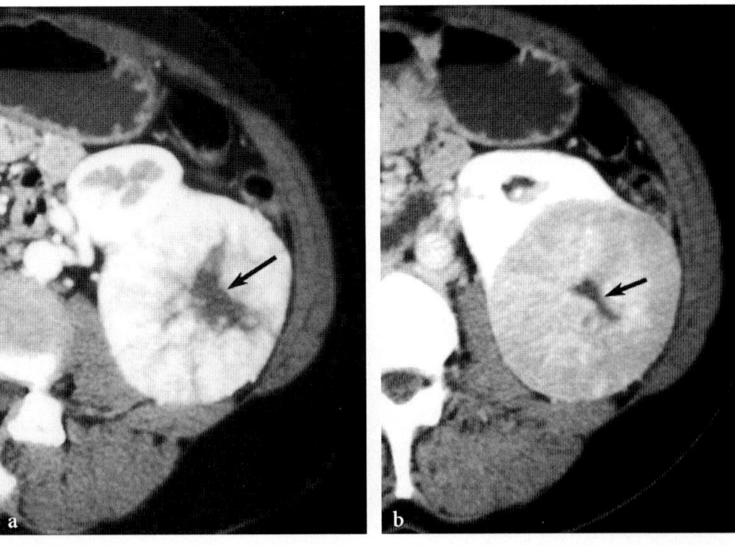

Fig. 3.15a,b. Incidental oncocytoma in a 45-year-old woman. **a** Axial contrast-enhanced CT scan in the AP shows a large hypervascular mass in the left kidney. Note that the tumor is enhancing homogeneously and has a central scar (*arrow*). **b** Axial contrast-enhanced CT scan in the VP shows that the mass central scar is well depicted (*arrow*). Partial left nephrectomy was performed and pathology revealed an oncocytoma.

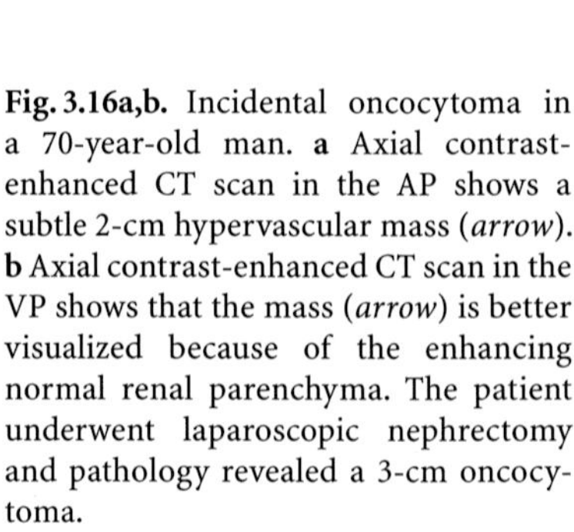
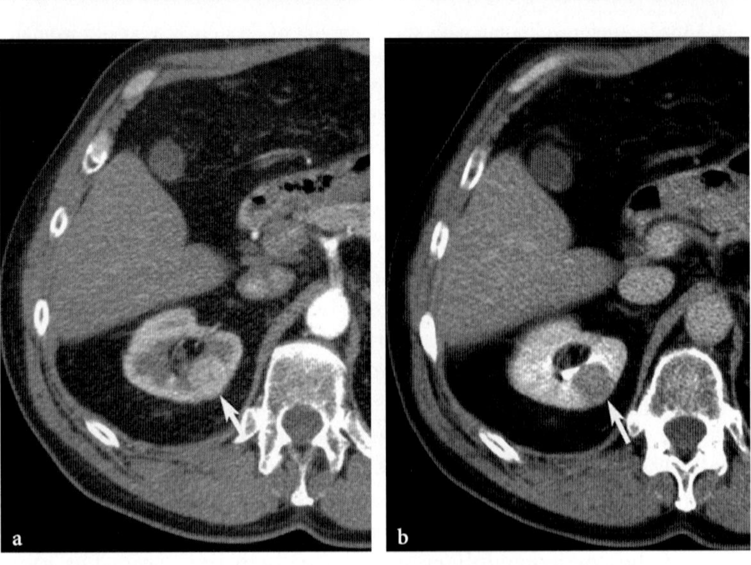

Fig. 3.16a,b. Incidental oncocytoma in a 70-year-old man. **a** Axial contrast-enhanced CT scan in the AP shows a subtle 2-cm hypervascular mass (*arrow*). **b** Axial contrast-enhanced CT scan in the VP shows that the mass (*arrow*) is better visualized because of the enhancing normal renal parenchyma. The patient underwent laparoscopic nephrectomy and pathology revealed a 3-cm oncocytoma.

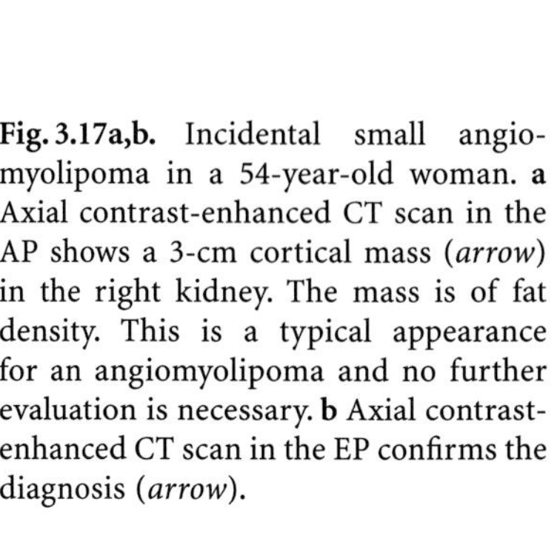
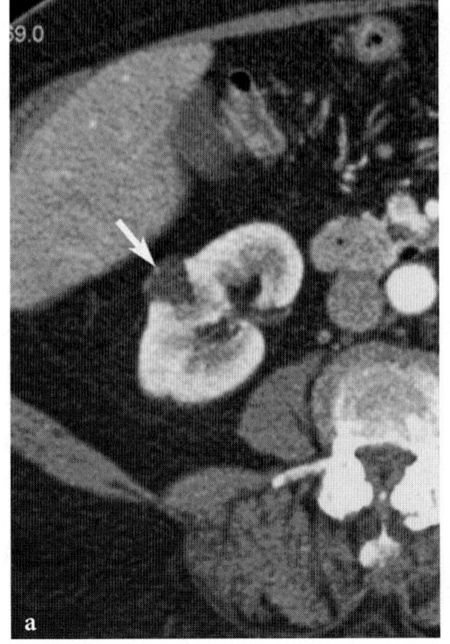
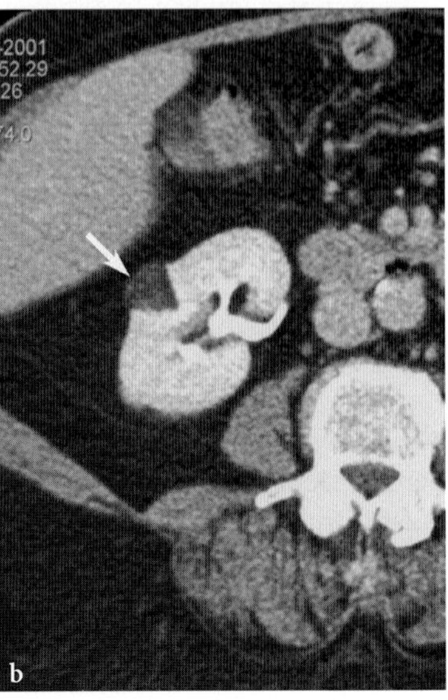

Fig. 3.17a,b. Incidental small angiomyolipoma in a 54-year-old woman. **a** Axial contrast-enhanced CT scan in the AP shows a 3-cm cortical mass (*arrow*) in the right kidney. The mass is of fat density. This is a typical appearance for an angiomyolipoma and no further evaluation is necessary. **b** Axial contrast-enhanced CT scan in the EP confirms the diagnosis (*arrow*).

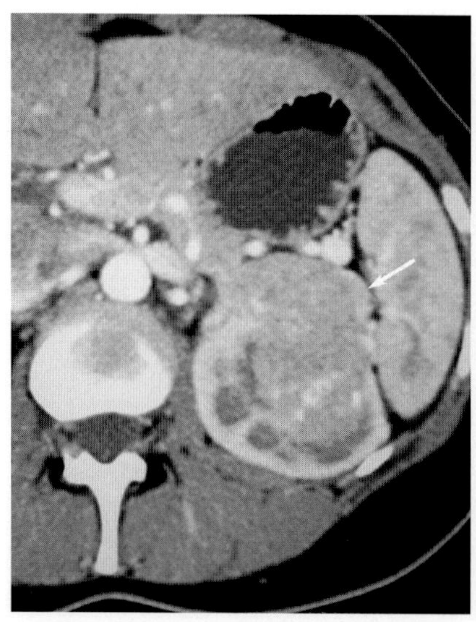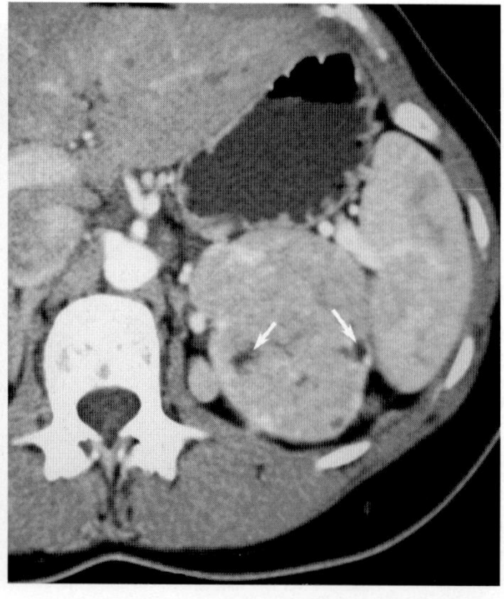

a · b

Fig. 3.18a,b. Angiomyolipoma with small amount of fat in a 37-year-old woman with history of left flank pain and previous bleed. **a** Axial contrast-enhanced CT scan in the AP shows a 6-cm vascular soft tissue mass in the left kidney (*arrow*). **b** Axial contrast-enhanced CT scan in the AP shows a small amount of fat (*arrows*) within the mass, indicating that this is most likely an angiomyolipoma. The patient underwent a successful partial left nephrectomy. The diagnosis of angiomyolipoma was confirmed at pathology.

Approximately 4.5% of angiomyolipomas contain only a minimal amount of fat that is below the detection threshold of CT (KIM et al. 2004), and they cannot be readily differentiated from RCC (SANT et al. 1984). The CT findings suggestive of angiomyolipomas with minimal fat include homogeneous high attenuation on pre-contrast scans, and homogeneous enhancement post-contrast scans (JINZAKI et al. 1997). KIM et al. (2004) suggest that prolonged lesion enhancement, defined as tumor attenuation values at least 20 HU higher in the excretory phase than in the corticomedullary phase, can help the differential diagnosis. In equivocal cases percutaneous biopsy is useful (SANT et al. 1990).

3.6.2
Malignant Renal Tumors Other Than Renal Cell Carcinoma

3.6.2.1
Intrarenal Transitional Cell Carcinoma

When transitional cell carcinoma spreads to the renal parenchyma, it presents as a centrally located infiltrating mass invading the renal sinus fat with poorly defined borders and lower enhancement than the normal renal parenchyma (Fig. 3.19; BREE et al. 1990; FUKUYA et al. 1994; IGARASHI et al. 1994). These tumors tend to be aggressive, with high-grade histology. Loco-regional and distant metastases are common and the prognosis is poor.

3.6.2.2
Renal Metastases and Lymphoma

Metastases are the most common malignant lesions found in the kidneys at autopsy (HIETALA and WAHLQVIST 1982). They reach the renal cortex via hematogenous spread and are generally asymptomatic. The most common primary cancers metastasizing to the kidneys include lung and breast cancers followed by melanoma and gastric carcinoma (BAILEY et al. 1998). In the oncological population, routine contrast CT images are usually obtained in the venous phase of enhancement. Renal metastases are easily diagnosed if multiple bilateral renal cortical lesions enhance less than the surrounding normal kidney; however, an increasing number of incidental small RCC are being detected on routine surveillance CT in patients with an extra-renal malignancy. In this population the finding of a solitary renal mass warrants image-guided biopsy to determine appropriate management.

The genitourinary tract is the most common location for spread of non-Hodgkin lymphoma, after the hematopoietic and reticuloendothelial system. A detailed discussion of the CT appearance of renal lymphoma is provided in Chapter 18.

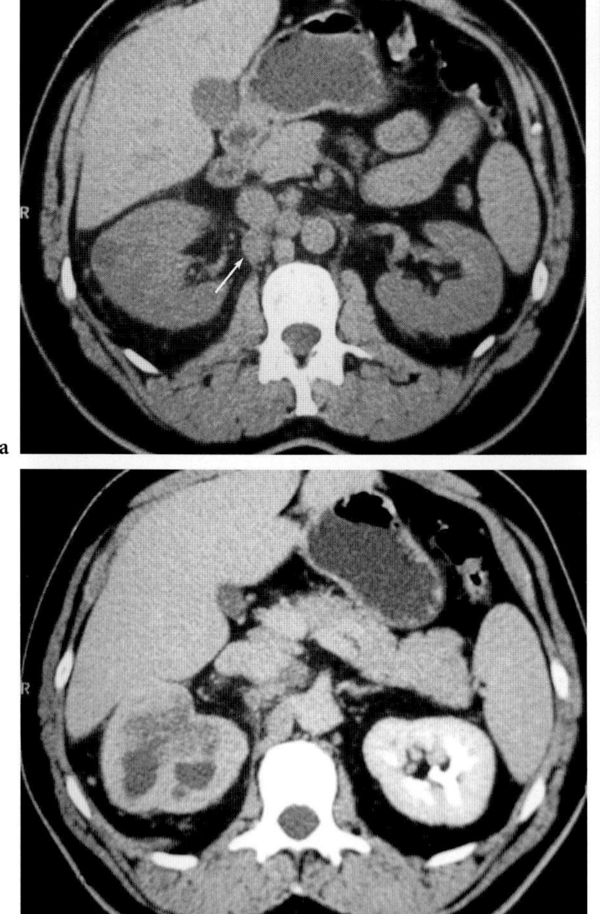

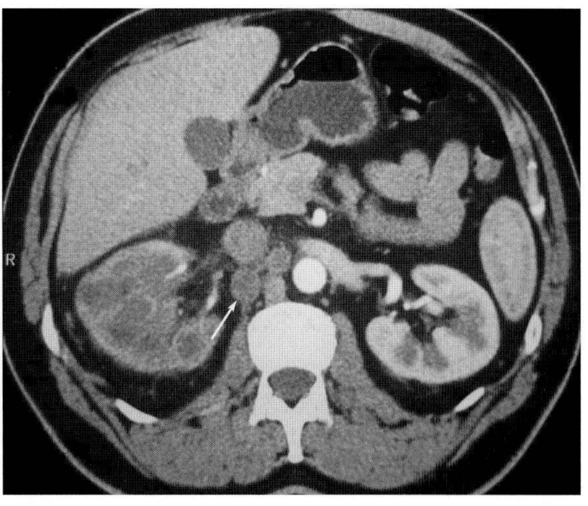

Fig. 3.19a-c. High-grade transitional cell carcinoma in a 45-year-old man with history of gross hematuria. **a** Axial unenhanced CT scan shows enlargement of the right kidney with soft tissue replacing the normal renal sinus fat. Note caval adenopathy (*arrow*). **b** Axial contrast-enhanced CT scan in the AP shows an infiltrating mass in the right kidney. Note delayed enhancement of this kidney and the caval adenopathy (*arrow*). **c** Axial contrast-enhanced CT scan in the EP shows delayed excretion in the right kidney. There is moderate hydronephrosis and soft tissue masses are infiltrating the collecting system. The diagnosis of high-grade transitional cell carcinoma was confirmed by ultrasound-guided biopsy. (With permission from Sheth et al. 2001)

3.7
Role of CT in Staging of Renal Cell Carcinoma

Accurate staging at the time of diagnosis is essential for determining prognosis and formulating a therapeutic plan. In 2004, multidetector CT remains the most widely available and single most effective modality for staging patients with RCC, with reported accuracy of 80–95% (CATALANO et al. 2003; HALLSCHEIDT et al. 2004; JOHNSON et al. 1987; SHETH et al. 2001).

Numerous studies have shown that the anatomic extent of the tumor at the time of diagnosis is the single most important factor in determining prognosis (DINNEY et al. 1992; THRASHER and PAULSON 1993). Disease-free survival is inversely correlated with increasing pathological stage, falling from 60 to 90% 5-year survival for patients with organ confined lesions to 5–10% for those with distant metastases.

The TNM classification, which defines the anatomic extent of the tumor more precisely, has gained wide acceptance and is progressively replacing the older Robson classification.

3.7.1
Tumors Confined Within the Renal Capsule

Patients with RCC confined to the kidney have the best prognosis with 5-year survival rates of 60–90% following nephrectomy (Fig. 3.20; THRASHER and PAULSON 1993). Many of these tumors are detected incidentally on cross-sectional imaging performed for unrelated indications. The recent modification of the TNM classification separating tumors 7 cm or less in size (stage T1) from lesions larger than 7 cm (stage T2) reflects the impact of tumor size on survival (RUSSO 2000).

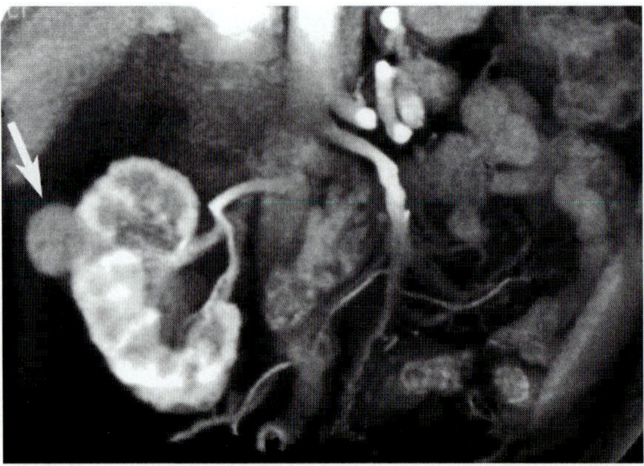

Fig. 3.20. Incidental renal cell carcinoma in a 62-year-old man. Coronal oblique plane 3D CT image in AP shows that the tumor measures 3 cm and is peripheral and exophytic (*arrow*). This is a stage T1 lesion. This tumor is in an ideal location for nephron-sparing surgery, which was performed successfully.

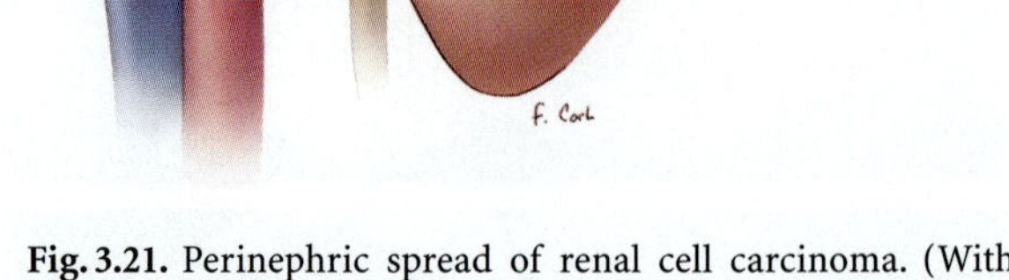

Fig. 3.21. Perinephric spread of renal cell carcinoma. (With permission from SHETH et al. 2001)

3.7.2
Perinephric Spread of Tumor

Under- and over-staging of perinephric invasion is the most common cause of staging errors on CT (CATALANO et al. 2003; JOHNSON et al. 1987; KOPKA et al. 1997). The presence of a pseudo-capsule suggests that the tumor is confined to the kidney (CATALANO et al. 2003). The most specific finding of stage T3a disease is the presence of an enhancing nodule in the perinephric space (Figs. 3.21, 3.22; JOHNSON et al. 1987). Tumor spread within the perinephric fat cannot always be reliably diagnosed, and differentiation between stage T2 and stage T3a tumors is problematic. Perinephric stranding does not reliably indicate tumor spread and is also found in about half of patients with localized T1 and T2 tumors. In these patients, perinephric stranding may be caused by edema, vascular engorgement of previous inflammation.

Diagnosis of perinephric extension has important prognostic as well as therapeutic implications, as T3a tumors are best treated with radical nephrectomy.

3.7.3
Imaging of the Ipsilateral Adrenal Gland

The incidence of adrenal metastases is low, reported as 4.3% in one large series (SAGALOWSKY et al. 1994). Evaluation of the adrenal gland is important for surgical management because the current trend is to spare the ipsilateral adrenal gland unless an abnor-

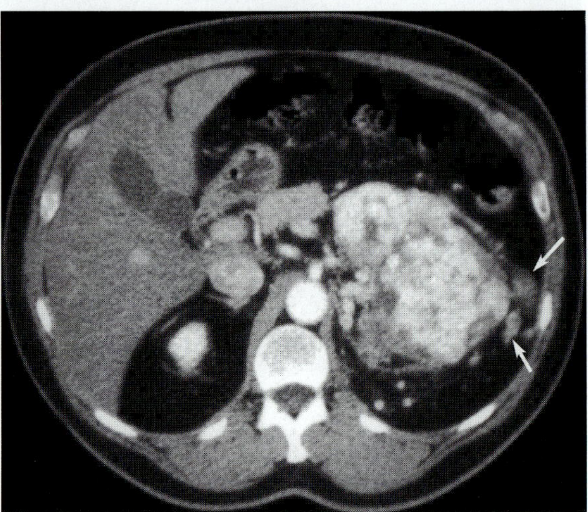

Fig. 3.22. Large renal cell carcinoma with perinephric tumor spread in a 65-year-old man with hematuria. Axial contrast-enhanced CT scan in the AP shows a large hypervascular mass in the left kidney. Several soft tissue nodules seen in the perinephric space indicate spread of tumor (*arrows*). The pathological stage of tumor was confirmed to be T3a at nephrectomy. (With permission from SHETH et al. 2001)

mality is suggested on CT. In one study of 157 patients with RCC who underwent radical nephrectomy, visualization of a normal adrenal gland on CT was associated with a 100% negative predictive value for tumor spread to the gland at pathology (SAGALOWSKY et al. 1994). By contrast, adrenal enlargement, displacement, or non-visualization were associated with malignant spread in 24% of cases, which indicates that adrenalectomy should be performed (RAMANI et al. 2003; SAGALOWSKY et al. 1994).

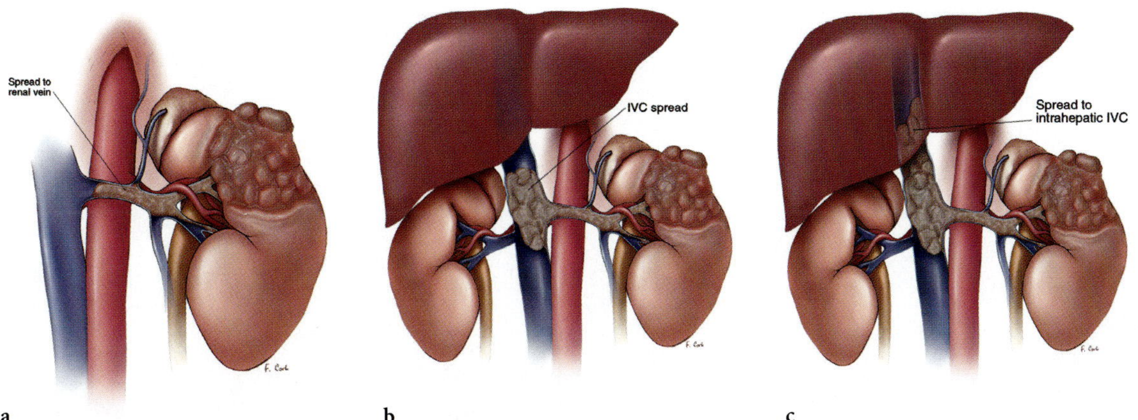

Fig. 3.23a-c. Venous spread of renal cell carcinoma. **a** Tumor spread limited to the renal vein (stage T3b). **b** Tumor spread into the inferior vena cava, infrahepatic (stage T3c). **c** Tumor spread into the inferior vena cava, hepatic (stage T3c). (With permission from SHETH et al. 2001)

3.7.4
Venous Spread of Tumor

Because RCC has a propensity to extend into the venous system, accurate preoperative evaluation of the renal vein and inferior vena cava is crucial. Extension of RCC limited to the renal vein (stage T3b) occurs in approximately 23% of patients and does not adversely affect the prognosis (Fig. 3.6; RUSSO 2000). Spread of the tumor into the inferior vena cava is found in 4–10% of patients and is more common with right-side lesions (KALLMAN et al. 1992). Patients with extensive IVC involvement and with nodal or distant metastases carry a relatively good prognosis with 5-year survival of 32–64%, provided that the thrombus is intraluminal, does not invade the vessel wall, and can be entirely resected (STAEHLER and BRKOVIC 2000). In these patients aggressive surgical resection with curative intent is justified (Fig. 3.24).

Helical CT has been shown to be highly accurate for diagnosing spread of RCC into the renal vein, with reported accuracy reaching 100% (CATALANO et al. 2003). The most specific sign of venous extension is the presence of a low-density filling defect within the vein (ZEMAN et al. 1988). An abrupt change in the caliber of the renal vein or the presence of a clot within collateral veins are helpful ancillary signs.

The CT appearance of the thrombus helps distinguish malignant from bland thrombus. Heterogeneous enhancement of the thrombus with contrast indicates neovascularity, and thus, tumor thrombus (Fig. 3.24). Direct continuity of the thrombus with the primary tumor suggests tumor thrombus.

If tumor spread is identified within the IVC, precise delineation of the superior extent of the thrombus is essential for the surgeon to plan the optimal surgical strategy for thrombectomy and minimize the risk of intraoperative tumor embolism (KALLMAN et al. 1992; STAEHLER and BRKOVIC 2000; SUGGS et al. 1991). The level of IVC involvement dictates the surgical approach. If the thrombus remains infrahepatic, it can be resected via an abdominal incision. If extension is detected to the level of the retrohepatic IVC, a right thoraco-abdominal approach allows access to the suprahepatic IVC.

3.7.5
Regional Lymph Node Metastases

The presence of regional lymph node metastases carries a poor prognosis with reported 5-year survival rates of 5–30% (Fig. 3.25; THRASHER and PAULSON 1993). The CT diagnosis of lymph node metastases relies on nodal enlargement above 1 cm short-axis diameter. This criterion was associated with a 4% false-negative rate in a series of 163 patients with RCC who underwent nephrectomy and regional lymph node dissection. This study also showed that in more than half of the patients, nodal enlargement was caused by benign inflammatory changes. This reactive nodal enlargement is often associated with extensive tumor necrosis or venous thrombosis and may represent a reactive immune response (RUSSO 2000; STUDER et al. 1990). Nodal enlargement demonstrated on CT should not disqualify patients for nephrec-

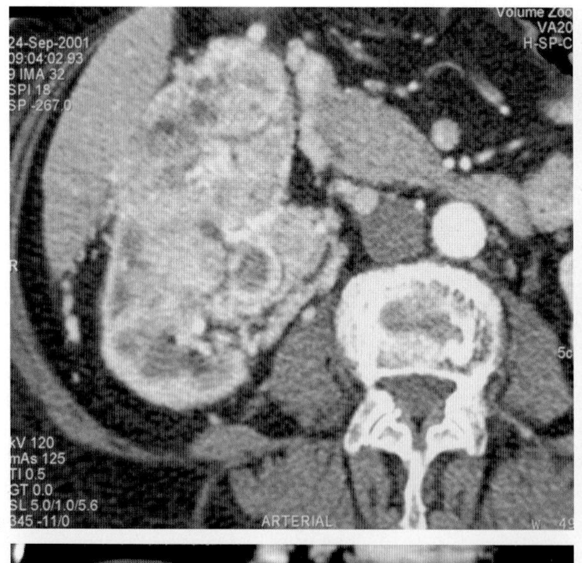

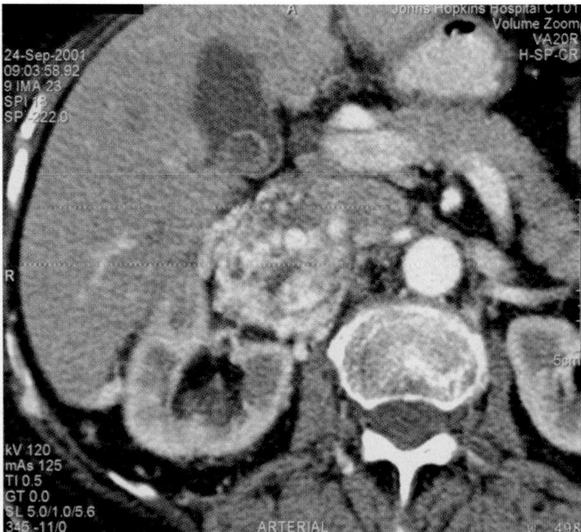

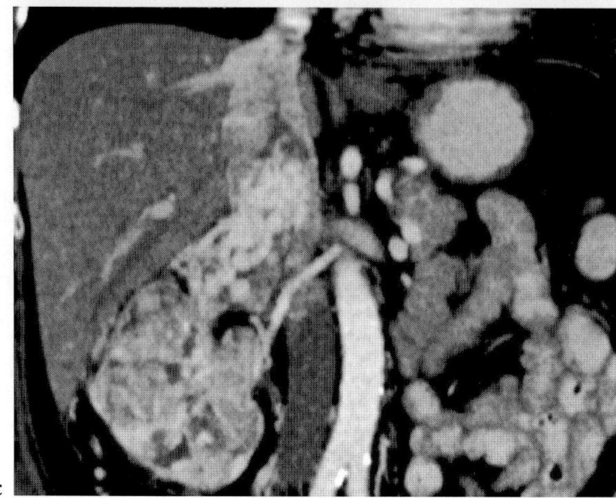

Fig. 3.24a-c. Renal cell carcinoma with extension into the inferior vena cava in a 72-year-old woman with hematuria. **a** Axial contrast-enhanced CT scan in the AP shows a large hypervascular mass in the right kidney. **b** Axial contrast-enhanced CT scan in the AP at the level of the renal veins shows that the right renal vein is enlarged and filled with an enhancing tumor thrombus. **c** Coronal 3D reconstruction CT image in the AP phase shows that the tumor thrombus extends into the hepatic inferior vena cava.

tomy unless metastatic spread is confirmed with fine-needle aspiration. The enhancement pattern within the node may also help differentiate reactive from malignant adenopathy: metastatic nodes may enhance, particularly if the primary tumor is very vascular (Fig. 3.25).

3.7.6
Local Extension and Distant Metastases

Direct extension of RCC outside Gerota's fascia into neighboring organs (stage T4a) is difficult to diagnose with certainty unless there is a demonstrable focal change in attenuation within the adjacent organ. Loss of tissue planes and irregular margins between the tumor and surrounding structures raise the possibility of direct infiltration, but can be seen in up to 15% of cases without surgically confirmed stage T4a disease (JOHNSON et al. 1987). Three-dimensional CT displays the tumor and its relationship to the adjacent organs in multiple planes and orientations and is very valuable in difficult cases to increase diagnostic confidence and help plan surgical resection (CATALANO et al. 2003; HALLSCHEIDT et al. 2004; SHETH et al. 2001).

Renal cell carcinoma metastasizes most frequently to the lungs and mediastinum, bones, and liver. Less common sites include the contralateral kidney, the adrenal gland, the brain, pancreas, mesentery, and abdominal wall (DINNEY et al. 1992; THRASHER and PAULSON 1993). Like the primary tumor, metastatic lesions tend to be hypervascular. The prognosis for these patients is dismal, with reported 5-year survival of 5–10%; however, patients with a solitary metastasis may benefit from aggressive management with nephrectomy and surgical removal of the metastatic lesion.

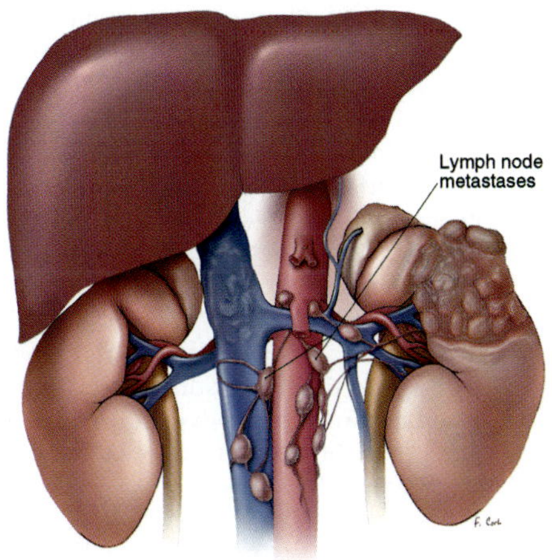

Fig. 3.25. Renal cell carcinoma with regional lymph node metastases. (With permission from SHETH et al. 2001)

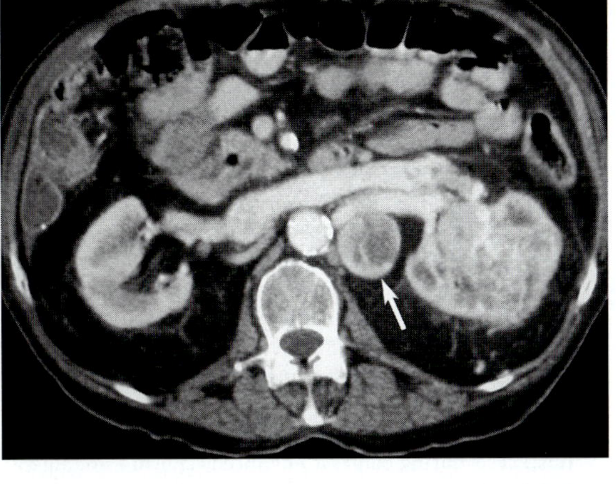

Fig. 3.26. Renal cell carcinoma with regional lymph node metastases in a 66-year-old man with hematuria. Axial contrast-enhanced CT scan in the AP shows hypervascular mass in the left kidney with hypervascular left para-aortic node (*arrow*).

3.8
Role of CT in Planning for Nephron-Sparing Surgery

In the past 20 years, the clinical presentation of RCC has evolved. The widespread use of cross-sectional imaging techniques has led to a dramatic increase in the number of incidentally discovered tumors. These asymptomatic tumors, which now comprise 25 to almost 50% of all surgically treated RCC, are generally confined to the renal capsule, relatively small in size (4–5 cm or less), and associated with an excellent prognosis following surgical removal.

These changes in the presentation of RCC have stimulated a growing trend towards nephron-sparing surgical techniques (NOVICK 1992; THRASHER et al. 1994). Nephron-sparing surgery entails complete excision of the renal tumor with a margin of at least 0.5 cm of normal renal tissue while preserving the largest amount of functioning renal parenchyma. It is the treatment of choice when radical nephrectomy would render the patient anephric with subsequent need for dialysis. Nephron-sparing surgery is also being increasingly advocated for the treatment of small RCC as current data show survival rates comparable to radical nephrectomy (HERR 1999).

Three-dimensional CT helps delineate the precise location of the renal mass, its relationship to the surface of the kidney, the collecting system, and the renal vessels. The arterial and venous anatomy of the kidney is depicted on the 3D CT angiogram (SMITH et al. 1999). The most suitable lesion for nephron-sparing surgery is small in diameter (<4 cm), polar, cortical, and far from the renal hilum and collecting system (Fig. 3.20).

3.9
Conclusion

With the advent of MDCT, the role of CT in the diagnosis and pre-surgical planning of RCC has been greatly expanded. Along with these technical improvements, new challenges facing the radiologist have emerged. These challenges include the adoption of scanning protocols designed to maximize diagnostic accuracy while at the same time minimizing radiation to the patient and image overload for the radiologist. Renal CT with multiple-phase image acquisitions as well as 3D reconstructions provides the clinician with all the information necessary for surgical planning.

References

Bailey JE, Roubidoux MA, Dunnick NR (1998) Secondary renal neoplasms. Abdom Imaging 23:266–274
Birnbaum BA, Jacobs JE, Ramchandani P (1996) Multiphasic renal CT: comparison of renal mass enhancement during the corticomedullary and nephrographic phases. Radiology 200:753–758

Bosniak MA (1986) The current radiological approach to renal cysts. Radiology 158:1–10

Bree RL, Schultz SR, Hayes R (1990) Large infiltrating renal transitional cell carcinomas: CT and ultrasound features. J Comput Assist Tomogr 14:381–385

Carrim ZI, Murchison JT (2003) The prevalence of simple renal and hepatic cysts detected by spiral computed tomography. Clin Radiol 58:626–629

Catalano C, Fraioli F, Laghi A, Napoli A, Pediconi F, Danti M, Nardis P, Passariello R (2003) High-resolution multidetector CT in the preoperative evaluation of patients with renal cell carcinoma. Am J Roentgenol 180:1271–1277

Cohan RH, Sherman LS, Korobkin M, Bass JC, Francis IR (1995) Renal masses: assessment of corticomedullary-phase and nephrographic-phase CT scans. Radiology 196:445–451

Coulam CH, Sheafor DH, Leder RA, Paulson EK, DeLong DM, Nelson RC (2000) Evaluation of pseudoenhancement of renal cysts during contrast-enhanced CT. Am J Roentgenol 174:493–498

Curry NS, Cochran ST, Bissada NK (2000) Cystic renal masses: accurate Bosniak classification requires adequate renal CT. Am J Roentgenol 175:339–342

Dinney CP, Awad SA, Gajewski JB, Belitsky P, Lannon SG, Mack FG, Millard OH (1992) Analysis of imaging modalities, staging systems, and prognostic indicators for renal cell carcinoma. Urology 39:122–129

Foley WD (2003) Renal MDCT. Eur J Radiol 45 (Suppl 1): S73–S78

Fukuya T, Honda H, Nakata H, Egashira K, Watanabe H, Naitou S, Kumazawa J, Masuda K (1994) Computed tomographic findings of invasive transitional cell carcinoma in the kidney. Radiat Med 12:6–10

Hallscheidt PJ, Bock M, Riedasch G, Zuna I, Schoenberg SO, Autschbach F, Soder M, Noeldge G (2004) Diagnostic accuracy of staging renal cell carcinomas using multidetector-row computed tomography and magnetic resonance imaging: a prospective study with histopathologic correlation. J Comput Assist Tomogr 28:333–339

Herr HW (1999) Partial nephrectomy for unilateral renal carcinoma and a normal contralateral kidney: 10-year follow-up. J Urol 161:33–35

Hietala SO, Wahlqvist L (1982) Metastatic tumors to the kidney. A postmortem, radiologic and clinical investigation. Acta Radiol Diagn (Stockh) 23:585–591

Hu H, He HD, Foley WD, Fox SH (2000) Four multidetector-row helical CT: image quality and volume coverage speed. Radiology 215:55–62

Igarashi T, Muakami S, Shichijo Y, Matsuzaki O, Isaka S, Shimazaki J (1994) Clinical and radiological aspects of infiltrating transitional cell carcinoma of the kidney. Urol Int 52:181–184

Jinzaki M, Tanimoto A, Narimatsu Y, Ohkuma K, Kurata T, Shinmoto H, Hiramatsu K, Mukai M, Murai M (1997) Angiomyolipoma: imaging findings in lesions with minimal fat. Radiology 205:497–502

Jinzaki M, Tanimoto A, Mukai M, Ikeda E, Kobayashi S, Yuasa Y, Narimatsu Y, Murai M (2000) Double-phase helical CT of small renal parenchymal neoplasms: correlation with pathologic findings and tumor angiogenesis. J Comput Assist Tomogr 24:835–842

Johnson CD, Dunnick NR, Cohan RH, Illescas FF (1987) Renal adenocarcinoma: CT staging of 100 tumors. Am J Roentgenol 148:59–63

Kallman DA, King BF, Hattery RR, Charboneau JW, Ehman RL, Guthman DA, Blute ML (1992) Renal vein and inferior vena cava tumor thrombus in renal cell carcinoma: CT, US, MRI and venacavography. J Comput Assist Tomogr 16:240–247

Kim JK, Kim TK, Ahn HJ, Kim CS, Kim KR, Cho KS (2002) Differentiation of subtypes of renal cell carcinoma on helical CT scans. Am J Roentgenol 178:1499–1506

Kim JK, Park SY, Shon JH, Cho KS (2004) Angiomyolipoma with minimal fat: differentiation from renal cell carcinoma at biphasic helical CT. Radiology 230:677–684

Kopka L, Fischer U, Zoeller G, Schmidt C, Ringert RH, Grabbe E (1997) Dual-phase helical CT of the kidney: value of the corticomedullary and nephrographic phase for evaluation of renal lesions and preoperative staging of renal cell carcinoma. Am J Roentgenol 169:1573–1578

Leslie JA, Prihoda T, Thompson IM (2003) Serendipitous renal cell carcinoma in the post-CT era: continued evidence in improved outcomes. Urol Oncol 21:39–44

Liu J, Fanning CV (2001) Can renal oncocytomas be distinguished from renal cell carcinoma on fine-needle aspiration specimens? A study of conventional smears in conjunction with ancillary studies. Cancer 93:390–397

Macari M, Bosniak MA (1999) Delayed CT to evaluate renal masses incidentally discovered at contrast-enhanced CT: demonstration of vascularity with deenhancement. Radiology 213:674–680

Neuzillet Y, Lechevallier E, Andre M, Daniel L, Coulange C (2004) Accuracy and clinical role of fine needle percutaneous biopsy with computerized tomography guidance of small (less than 4.0 cm) renal masses. J Urol 171:1802–1805

Novick AC (1992) The role of renal-sparing surgery for renal cell carcinoma. Semin Urol 10:12–15

Pickhardt PJ, Siegel CL, McLarney JK (2001) Collecting duct carcinoma of the kidney: Are imaging findings suggestive of the diagnosis? Am J Roentgenol 176:627–633

Ramani AP, Abreu SC, Desai MM, Steinberg AP, Ng C, Lin CH, Kaouk JH, Gill IS (2003) Laparoscopic upper pole partial nephrectomy with concomitant en bloc adrenalectomy. Urology 62:223–226

Richstone L, Scherr DS, Reuter VR, Snyder ME, Rabbani F, Kattan MW, Russo P (2004) Multifocal renal cortical tumors: frequency, associated clinicopathological features and impact on survival. J Urol 171:615–620

Rubin GD (2001) Techniques for performing multidetector-row computed tomographic angiography. Tech Vasc Interv Radiol 4:2–14

Russo P (2000) Renal cell carcinoma: presentation, staging, and surgical treatment. Semin Oncol 27:160–176

Sagalowsky AI, Kadesky KT, Ewalt DM, Kennedy TJ (1994) Factors influencing adrenal metastasis in renal cell carcinoma. J Urol 151:1181–1184

Sant GR, Heaney JA, Ucci AA Jr, Sarno RC, Meares EM Jr (1984) Computed tomographic findings in renal angiomyolipoma: an histologic correlation. Urology 24:293–296

Sant GR, Ayers DK, Bankoff MS, Mitcheson HD, Ucci AA Jr (1990) Fine needle aspiration biopsy in the diagnosis of renal angiomyolipoma. J Urol 143:999–1001

Sherman JL, Hartman DS, Friedman AC, Madewell JE, Davis CJ, Goldman SM (1981) Angiomyolipoma: computed tomographic–pathologic correlation of 17 cases. Am J Roentgenol 137:1221–1226

Sheth S, Scatarige JC, Horton KM, Corl FM, Fishman EK (2001)

Current concepts in the diagnosis and management of renal cell carcinoma: role of multidetector CT and three-dimensional CT. RadioGraphics 21S237–S254

Smith PA, Marshall FF, Corl FM, Fishman EK (1999) Planning nephron-sparing renal surgery using 3D helical CT angiography. J Comput Assist Tomogr 23:649–654

Staehler G, Brkovic D (2000) The role of radical surgery for renal cell carcinoma with extension into the vena cava. J Urol 163:1671–1675

Studer UE, Scherz S, Scheidegger J, Kraft R, Sonntag R, Ackermann D, Zingg EJ (1990) Enlargement of regional lymph nodes in renal cell carcinoma is often not due to metastases. J Urol 144:243–245

Suggs WD, Smith RB III, Dodson TF, Salam AA, Graham SD Jr (1991) Renal cell carcinoma with inferior vena caval involvement. J Vasc Surg 14:413-418

Sussman S, Cochran ST, Pagani JJ, McArdle C, Wong W, Austin R, Curry N, Kelly KM (1984) Hyperdense renal masses: a CT manifestation of hemorrhagic renal cysts. Radiology 150:207–211

Szolar DH, Kammerhuber F, Altziebler S, Tillich M, Breinl E, Fotter R, Schreyer HH (1997) Multiphasic helical CT of the kidney: increased conspicuity for detection and characterization of small (<3 cm) renal masses. Radiology 202:211–217

Thrasher JB, Paulson DF (1993) Prognostic factors in renal cancer. Urol Clin North Am 20:247–262

Thrasher JB, Robertson JE, Paulson DF (1994) Expanding indications for conservative renal surgery in renal cell carcinoma. Urology 43:160–168

Yuh BI, Cohan RH (1999) Different phases of renal enhancement: role in detecting and characterizing renal masses during helical CT. Am J Roentgenol 173:747–755

Yuh BI, Cohan RH, Francis IR, Korobkin M, Ellis JH (2000) Comparison of nephrographic with excretory phase helical computed tomography for detecting and characterizing renal masses. Can Assoc Radiol J 51:170–176

Zeman RK, Cronan JJ, Rosenfield AT, Lynch JH, Jaffe MH, Clark LR (1988) Renal cell carcinoma: dynamic thin-section CT assessment of vascular invasion and tumor vascularity. Radiology 167:393–396

4 Magnetic Resonance Imaging in Kidney Cancer

E. Scott Pretorius

CONTENTS

4.1
Introduction

Magnetic resonance (MR) imaging protocols for evaluation of patients with known or suspected renal malignancies have evolved with advancements in pulse sequences, surface coils, gradient magnets, and scanners. With improving MR imaging technology and increased radiologist experience, former limitations of relatively long imaging times and associated motion artifacts have largely been overcome. This has allowed renal diagnostic imagers to take fuller advantage of the many intrinsic advantages of MR imaging.

E. S. Pretorius, MD
Wallace T. Miller Sr. Chair of Radiologic Education, Residency Program Training Director, MRI Section, Department of Radiology, University of Pennsylvania Medical Center, 1 Silverstein, 3400 Spruce Street, Philadelphia, PA 19104, USA

The single greatest advantage of MR imaging over ultrasound (US) and computed tomography (CT) is that MR imaging generates the highest intrinsic soft tissue contrast of any cross-sectional imaging modality. Furthermore, whereas both US and CT have a single basis for generating tissue contrast, the ever-broadening array of MR imaging pulse sequences continues to expand our imaging armamentarium.

Like US, MR imaging is capable of directly imaging in any plane, although of course MR imaging does not suffer from the tissue-depth penetration limitations of US. The CT data acquisition remains limited to the axial plane, although reconstructed data from multidetector-row scanners can provide excellent resolution in interpolated planes. Although MR imaging's spatial resolution remains inferior to that of CT, in the vast majority of renal cases this limitation is more than compensated for by MR imaging's superior contrast and multiplanar capabilities.

Renal MR imaging is particularly useful for patients who should not receive iodine-based CT contrast agents, whether due to history of iodine allergy, renal insufficiency, or renal transplantation. All of the U.S. Food and Drug Administration-approved gadolinium-based chelates used for MR imaging have very favorable safety profiles relative to the intravenous iodine-based agents used for CT. True anaphylactic reaction to gadolinium chelates is extremely rare, and these agents may safely be used in patients with very limited renal function.

Optimal renal imaging with CT or MR imaging generally requires multiphasic data acquisition following intravenous contrast administration. Although radiation dose has become an issue with multiphasic CT examination, particularly in evaluation of children and women of childbearing age (Lockhart and Smith 2003), MR imaging, of course, employs no ionizing radiation and therefore multiphasic post-contrast data acquisition does not confer additional risk to the patient.

4.2
General Technical Considerations

Renal MR imaging examinations are best performed on high-field (1.0–1.5 T) systems, using a torso phased-array surface coil centered at the level of the kidneys to allow appropriately small fields of view (FOV) and to maximize the signal-to-noise ratio (SNR). A bellows may be placed around the patient's abdomen to permit the acquisition of respiratory-triggered images.

Use of low-field scanners for renal MR imaging examinations should, in general, be discouraged. Low-field scanners require very long imaging times to generate acceptable SNR, lack the gradient magnet speed and strength to acquire the thin slices required for adequate spatial resolution, and are incapable of imaging quickly enough to acquire truly dynamic post-contrast images. Although some patients and referring clinicians may specifically request the use of a low-field open scanner for a particular examination, it is incumbent upon the radiologist to fully disclose the limitations of renal MR imaging examinations performed on these systems.

Whole-body 3-T systems have recently become commercially available, and their role in renal MR imaging is likely to become prominent (Zhang et al. 2003; Norris 2003). They offer twice the SNR of 1.5-T scanners, which may obviate the need for use of surface coils. Furthermore, the increase in SNR afforded by 3-T systems is likely to expand the role of parallel imaging for renal MR imaging, thereby dramatically decreasing imaging times (McKenzie et al. 2004). Parallel imaging techniques, and partial parallel imaging techniques such as sensitivity encoding (van den Brink et al. 2003) and simultaneous acquisition of spatial harmonics (Bydder et al. 2002), allow fast imaging sequences to be accelerated by utilizing spatial information inherent in the geometry of the surface-coil array to generate missing lines of k-space (Heidemann et al. 2003). This effectively allows multiple lines of k-space to be generated for each phase-encoding step, decreasing imaging time; however, in parallel imaging, SNR decreases with increasing acceleration factor (Lin et al. 2004). A great advantage of 3-T scanners is that SNR lost to parallel imaging techniques could be compensated for by the higher SNR available at 3 T (due to increased spin polarization at the higher field strength), without compromising overall image quality. Limitations of 3-T renal imaging, however, include scanner cost and availability, as well as a probable increased incidence of severe patient claustrophobia due to the architecture of these scanners.

Intravenous contrast material is best administered with an MR-compatible power injector, to provide reliable and reproducible delivery of the gadolinium chelate. No difference in efficacy has been demonstrated among the FDA-approved extracellular gadolinium chelate contrast materials: gadopentetate dimeglumine (Magnevist, Berlex Laboratories, Wayne, N.J.), gadodiamide (Omniscan, Nycomed Amersham Imaging, Princeton, N.J.), and gadoteridol (Prohance, Bracco Diagnostics, Princeton, N.J.). For renal imaging, all three of these agents may be administered at a dose of 0.2 ml/kg. An injection rate of 2 ml/s is used, and the contrast material injection is followed with a saline flush of 20 ml.

As circulation times vary greatly among patients, the use of a fixed-time delay to imaging is not recommended. This is particularly important in avoiding venous contamination of arterial-phase images for optimal renal MR angiography (MRA) examinations. The routine use of automated bolus detection (Smartprep, GE Medical Systems, Milwaukee, Wis.) or "fluoroscopic" monitoring (Carebolus, Siemens Medical Systems, Erlangen Germany) provides high-quality reproducible MRA examinations.

4.3
Goals of Oncologic Renal MR Imaging Examinations

The MR imaging examinations of potential renal malignancies should be tailored to determine whether or not a renal mass is present, and, if present, whether the mass is benign or malignant. The MR imaging examinations can be used to stage renal malignancies and can serve as a guide to appropriate choice of therapy. Finally, MR imaging has an important role to play in follow-up imaging of patients who have had nephrectomy, partial nephrectomy, or percutaneous tumor ablation.

4.3.1
Renal Lesion Detection

Improved radiologic detection of renal masses by US, CT, and MR imaging has led to smaller average size of neoplasm at time of initial detection (Curry 2002), and most of these incidentally discovered renal cell carcinomas (RCC) are of low stage and tumor grade (TSUI et al. 2000). In prior decades, nearly all patients with RCC presented with hematuria or other genitourinary symptomatology. Presently, however, approximately 30% of all RCCs are incidentally identified on imaging studies performed for other purposes (BONO and LOVISOLO 1997).

Computed tomography with thin-section (5 mm or thinner), pre- and post-contrast images can characterize most renal neoplasms larger than 1 cm. Many renal masses detected on CT, however, will be found on enhanced studies performed for non-renal indications where pre-contrast images were not performed. As such, many of these masses will not be adequately characterized, as the degree of renal enhancement cannot be assessed. Further evaluation with dedicated renal CT or MR imaging may be required.

The ability of dedicated renal CT and gadolinium-enhanced MR imaging to detect and characterize renal lesions greater than 1 cm is similar, although MR imaging is superior in the detection of small polar lesions due its ability to image directly in non-axial planes (ROFSKY and BOSNIAK 1997). Magnetic

resonance imaging is the examination of choice for the characterization of renal masses in patients with limited renal function (creatinine >2.0 mg/dl), severe allergy to iodinated contrast, or for masses not adequately characterized by other imaging modalities. Neither CT nor MR imaging has been shown to be accurate in characterizing solid lesions smaller than 1 cm, although well-performed MR imaging is clearly capable of characterizing many of these lesions.

4.3.2
Renal Lesion Characterization

The goal of renal lesion characterization by CT or MR imaging, therefore, is to separate surgical lesions (RCC, cystic renal cell carcinoma, oncocytoma) from non-surgical lesions (cyst, hemorrhagic cyst, angiomyolipoma (AML), pseudotumor; Fig. 4.1). Some benign lesions, such as AML with minimal fat or renal leiomyomas, have imaging appearances

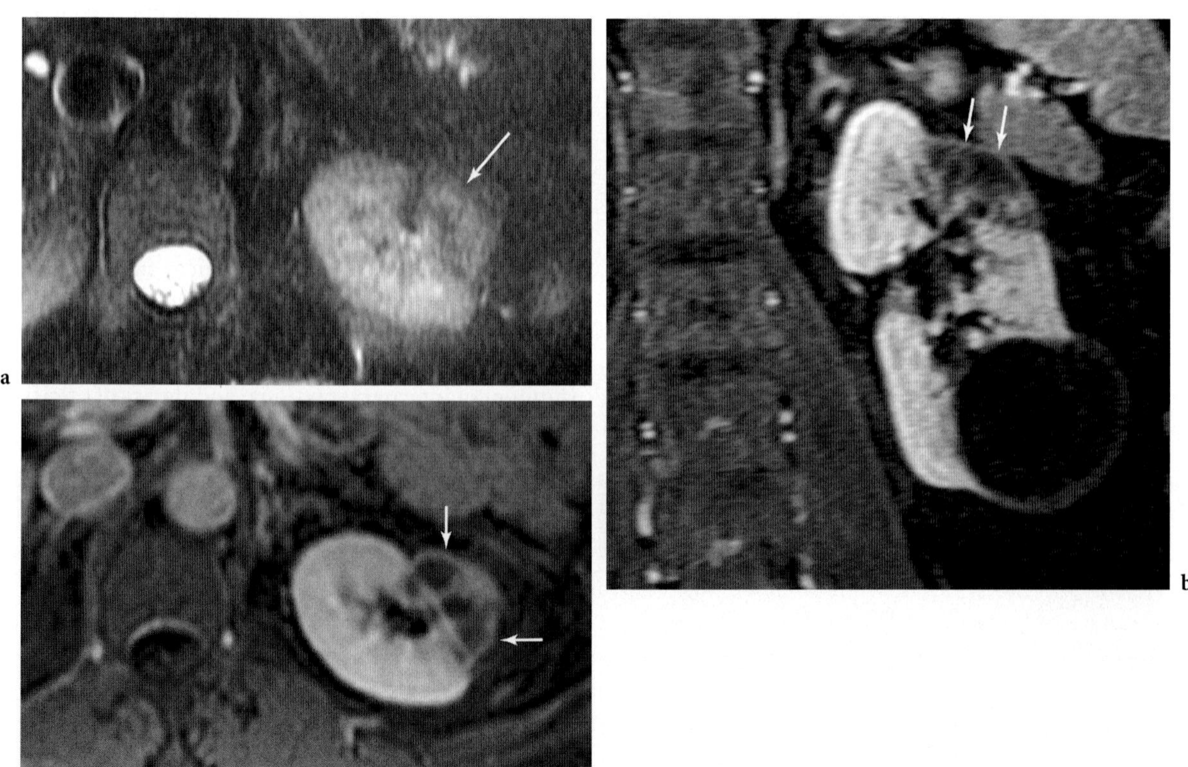

Fig. 4.1a-c. Flank pain and renal mass seen on US in a 46-year-old man. **a** Axial half-Fourier T2-weighted MR image (TR=not meaningful, TE=84 ms) demonstrates a possible mass (*arrow*) in the anterior interpolar region of the left kidney. **b** Coronal (TR=7.6 ms, TE=2.3 ms) and **c** axial (TR=195 ms, TE=1.4 ms) contrast-enhanced T1-weighted gradient-recalled-echo (GRE) MR images demonstrate very sharp, straight margins to the "mass," indicating that this is a vascular insult. There is preservation of capsular blood flow (*arrows*) in this region of infarct, which was due to embolic disease.

which may be indistinguishable from RCC on any imaging modality (ISRAEL and BOSNIAK 2003b).

Renal cell carcinoma has a highly variable appearance on MR imaging, due to the existence of multiple RCC histologies (SHINMOTO et al. 1998), and to variability in internal necrosis, hemorrhage (JOHN et al. 1997), and/or intratumoral lipid. On MR imaging, RCC most commonly appears hypointense or isointense to renal parenchyma on T1-weighted images, heterogeneously hyperintense on T2-weighted images, and enhances following gadolinium administration. Variability is the rule, however, and lesions may be primarily hyperintense, hypointense, or isointense to normal renal parenchyma on both T1- and T2-weighted images. Although RCCs enhance with intravenous gadolinium administration, they tend to enhance less than normal renal parenchyma, and are often most easily identified on post-contrast dynamic T1-weighted gradient-recalled-echo (GRE) images (YAMASHITA et al. 1995).

Clear cell RCCs, the most common subtype of RCC, may lose signal on opposed-phase gradient-echo images, due to the presence of microscopic lipid in some of these neoplasms (Fig. 4.2; OUTWATER et al. 1997). The presence of intracellular lipid in a renal lesion should therefore not by itself be used to make the diagnosis of AML. The presence of macroscopic lipid (Fig. 4.3) within a renal lesion, however, remains very specific for AML, although very rare RCCs which have undergone osseous metaplasia may contain fat (HELENON et al. 1997).

Approximately 10–15% of renal cell carcinomas display some cystic component (HARTMAN et al. 1986). As with CT, the architectural features and enhancement characteristics of non-simple cystic renal lesions are important in determining lesion management. The MR imaging features of cystic neoplasms that have been shown to be highly associated with malignancy include mural irregularity, mural nodules, increased mural thickness, and intense mural enhancement (BALCI et al. 1999).

Although the Bosniak classification system for cystic renal lesions was created for CT (BOSNIAK 1991), the morphologic features described in the various categories may be applied to MR imaging, with the limitation that calcifications are difficult to detect on MR imaging (ISRAEL and BOSNIAK 2004). Simple cysts are markedly T2 hyperintense, have a thin or imperceptible wall, display no internal architecture, and do not enhance (Fig. 4.4; NASCIMENTO et al. 2001). Lesions with a single thin septation or with fine mural calcification are probably benign (class II). Also in class II are small (<3 cm) CT "hyperdense" cysts, which contain internal protein or hemorrhage, and which therefore are hyperintense to normal renal parenchyma on T1-weighted images. These benign cysts do not enhance following contrast administration and have variable T2 signal intensity depending on their protein content. Subtraction imaging or direct region of interest (ROI) measurements on source images can be used to document lack of enhancement in these lesions. Cystic renal lesions with thicker septations, multiple septations or bulky calcifications are indeterminate, and should be excised (class III; Figs. 4.5, 4.6). Lesions with enhancing mural solid nodules (class IV) should be excised, and the majority of these lesions will be cystic RCCs (Fig. 4.7). Surgical cure rates for cystic RCC are very high (CORICA et al. 1999).

Category IIF lesions are lesions which are thought to be benign, but due to some internal complexity (number of internal septations, nodularity of calcification, T1-hyperintense cystic lesion >3 cm) require

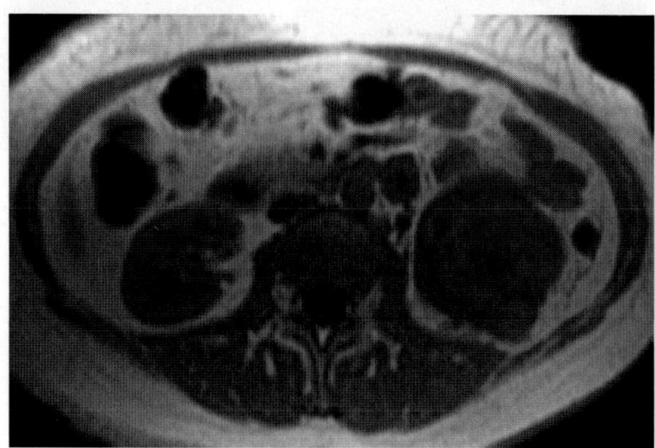
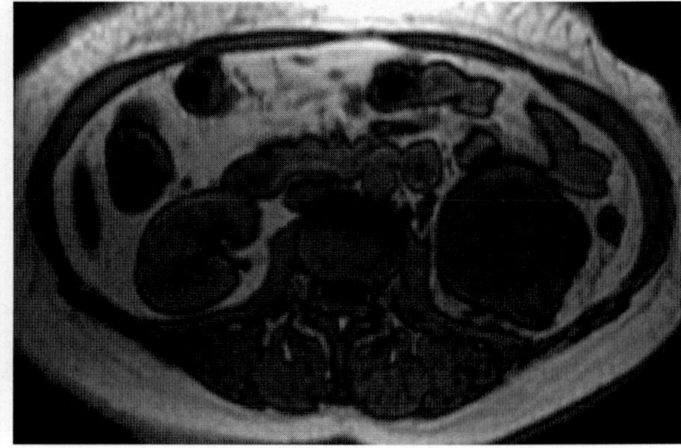

a   b

Fig. 4.2a,b. Hematuria and abdominal pain in a 54-year-old woman. Axial T1-weighted **a** in-phase (TR=185 ms, TE=4.2 ms) and **b** out-of-phase (TR=185 ms, TE=2.1 ms) GRE MR images demonstrate signal loss in this clear cell RCC of the left kidney due to the presence of intracytoplasmic lipid in the cells of the tumor.

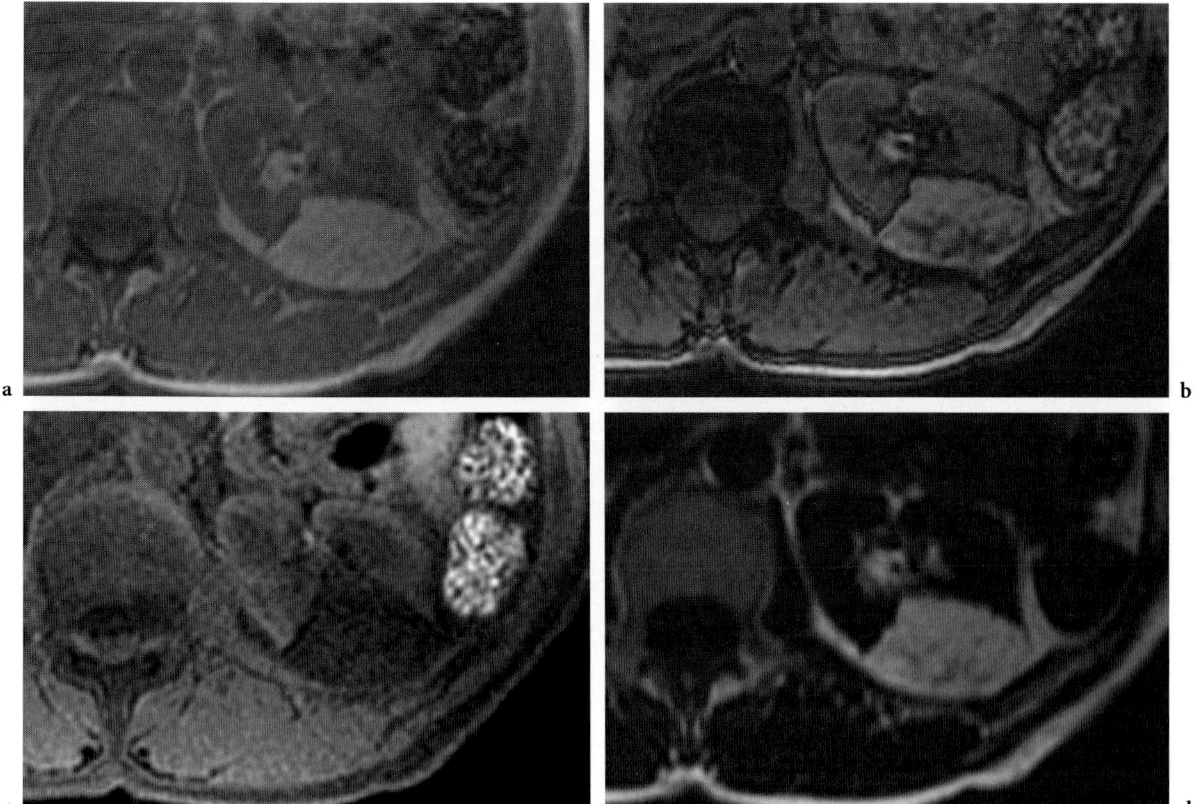

Fig. 4.3a-d. Renal angiomyolipoma in a 38-year-old woman. Axial T1-weighted gradient-echo MR images obtained **a** in phase (TR=275 ms, TE=4.6 ms), **b** out-of-phase (TR=275 ms, TE=2.3 ms), **c** with frequency-selective fat-suppression (TR=275 ms, TE=2.3 ms), and **d** with frequency-selective water saturation (TR=275 ms, TE=4.6 ms) demonstrate a benign left renal angiomyolipoma. Signal loss on the out-of-phase image relative to the in-phase image confirms the presence of both water and microscopic lipid. Signal intensity similar to that of the body wall fat on the fat-saturated and water-saturated images affirms the presence of macroscopic fat within the lesion, confirming the diagnosis of benign angiomyolipoma.

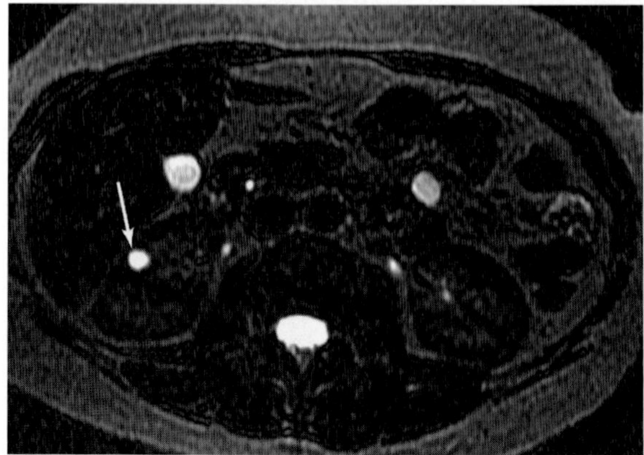

Fig. 4.4. Renal cyst in a 42-year-old woman. Axial heavily T2-weighted MR image (TR=not significant, TE=601 ms) demonstrates a thin-walled, fluid signal lesion (*arrow*) in the right kidney. This is a Bosniak I simple renal cyst.

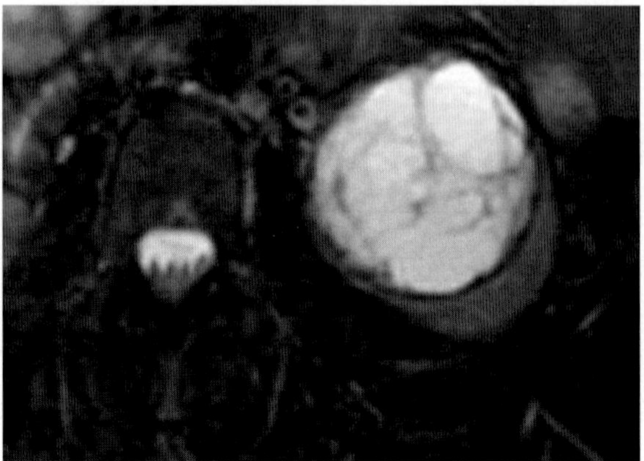

Fig. 4.5. Hematuria in a 42-year-old woman. Axial fat-suppressed respiratory-triggered fast-spin-echo T2-weighted MR image (TR=13043 ms, TE(eff)=120 ms) demonstrates a thickly septate, Bosniak III left renal lesion. This proved to be a cystic renal cell carcinoma.

follow-up at 6 and 12 months to determine stability (ISRAEL and BOSNIAK 2003a).

Most cystic neoplasms which require surgery will enhance greater than 20 Hounsfield units (HU) on CT, and enhancement of less than 12 HU is probably not significant in the absence of other lesion features suspicious for malignancy (SILVERMAN et al. 1994). Degree of CT enhancement is dependent on scanner software and calibration, and some helical-CT-rendering algorithms may erroneously increase post-contrast CT attenuation values in simple cysts adjacent to dense excreted iodine (MAKI et al. 1999). The absence of an absolute scale of intensity in MR imaging makes it difficult to quantify degree of enhancement, although an ROI increase of greater than 15% (nephrographic phase at 2–4 min compared with pre-contrast) is suspicious for malignancy (HO et al. 2002). Pre- and post-contrast MR images should always be obtained with identical imaging parameters, so that meaningful intensity comparisons can be made.

4.3.3
Staging of Renal Cell Carcinoma by MR Imaging

As RCC is relatively resistant to both radiotherapy and chemotherapy, surgical procedures have long been the mainstay of therapy (DEKERNION and MUKAME 1987). Accurate radiologic staging is critical in directing appropriate approach and resection for maximal disease control. Staging is also critical in determining prognosis, as tumor stage at time of diagnosis correlates directly with average survival. Renal cell carcinoma is most commonly staged using the Robson classification (ROBSON et al. 1969), although the TNM system may also be employed (Table 4.1; ERGEN et al. 2004).

Both CT and MR imaging have both been shown to be effective in staging RCC, with accuracies of approximately 90% reported for both modalities

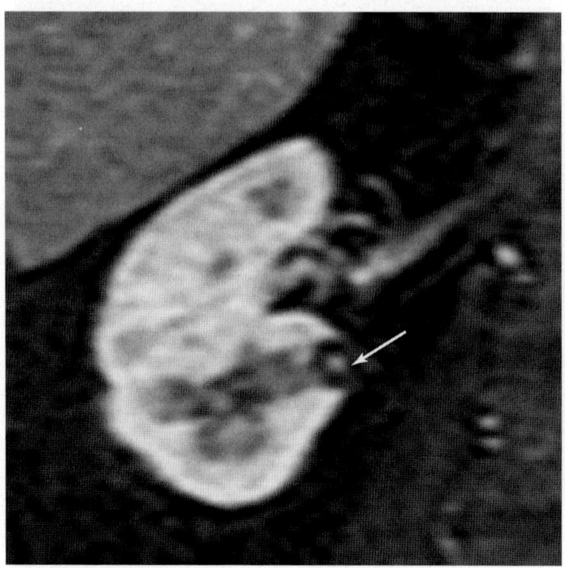

Fig. 4.6. Incidentally discovered cystic renal mass on CT in a 66-year-old woman. Coronal contrast-enhanced T1-weighted GRE MR image (TR=3.8 ms, TE=0.8 ms) demonstrates a thick internal septation (*arrow*) in this lesion, making this a Bosniak III lesion. Excision was advised, and this was a cystic RCC.

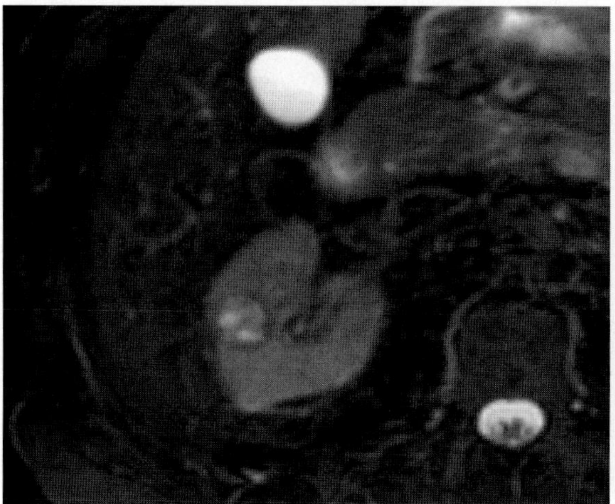

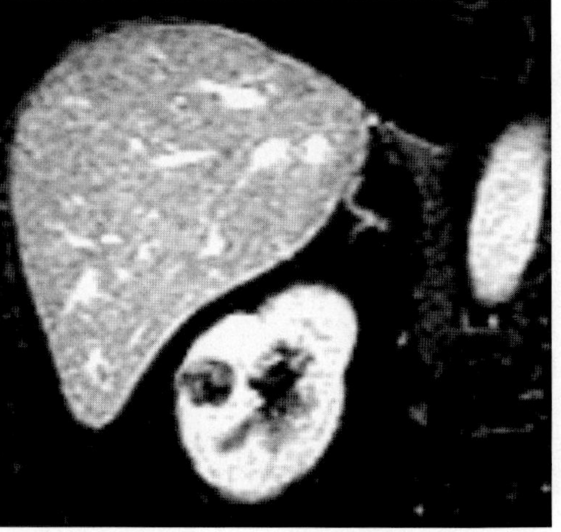

a   b

Fig. 4.7a,b. Hematuria in a 62-year-old man. **a** Axial fat-suppressed respiratory-triggered fast-spin-echo T2-weighted MR image (TR=12000 ms, TE=102 ms) demonstrates a cystic lesion with mural nodules in the right kidney. **b** Coronal 3D T1-weighted GRE MR image (TR=3.4 ms, TE=0.9 ms) demonstrates enhancement within the mural nodules. This is a Bosniak IV lesion, and was a cystic RCC.

Table 4.1. Staging of renal cell carcinoma

Robson stage	Description	TNM	TNM stage
I	Tumor confined to renal capsule		
	Small tumor (<2.5 cm)	T1	I
	Large tumor (>2.5 cm)	T2	II
II	Tumor spread to perinephric fat or adrenal	T3a	III
IIIA	Venous tumor thrombus		
	Renal vein thrombus only	T3b	III
	IVC thrombus	T3c	III
IIIB	Regional lymph node metastases	N1–N3	III/IV
IIIC	Venous tumor thrombus and regional nodes	T3b/c, N1–N3	III/IV
IVA	Direct invasion of adjacent organs outside Gerota's fascia	T4	IV
IVB	Distant metastases	M1	IV

(REZNEK 1996; ZAGORIA and BECHTOLD 1997). Magnetic resonance imaging appears to be superior for evaluation of tumor involvement of the perinephric fat, the renal vein, the inferior vena cava, and adjacent organs (PATEL et al. 1987). Ultrasound, although useful in screening for the presence of renal tumors, is limited in its ability to stage RCC because of difficulty in assessing retroperitoneal lymphadenopathy (BECHTOLD and ZAGORIA 1997). High accuracies for staging of advanced RCC have also been reported for fluorine-18 fluorodeoxyglucose (FDG) positron emission tomography (PET; RAMDAVE et al. 2001), although few such investigations have been performed.

Computed tomography cannot reliably differentiate Robson stage-I disease (tumor confined by the renal capsule) from Robson stage-II disease (tumor spread to the perinephric fat). This distinction has not historically been critical, as the perinephric fat would be routinely excised as part of a radical nephrectomy (CHOYKE 1997). If, however, partial nephrectomy is contemplated, it is desirable to know preoperatively if the perinephric fat is invaded by cancer, as this may affect the surgical approach (Fig. 4.8). One study has shown MR imaging to be slightly superior to CT in making this determination (FEIN et al 1987). In particular, the negative predictive value of MR imaging appears to be high; in one series, in 38 of 38 MR imaging cases (100%) in which the perinephric fat was thought to be uninvolved by tumor, this finding was confirmed at pathologic sectioning (Pretorius et al. 1999). This determination is best made on in-phase T1-weighted GRE images.

Fat-suppressed T2-weighted images are among the best MR images for detection of abdominal lymphadenopathy (Fig. 4.9). At present, MR imag-

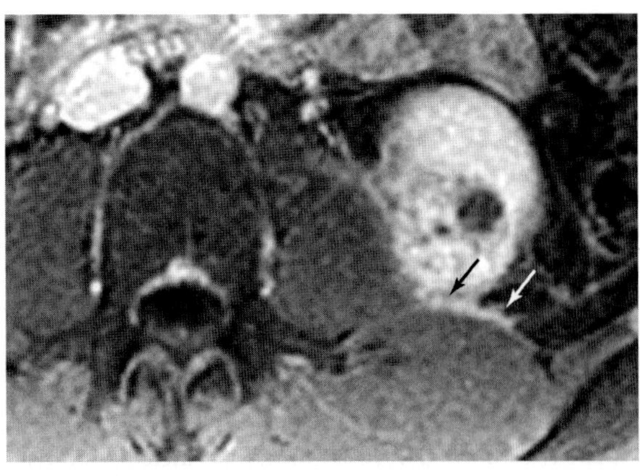

Fig. 4.8. Renal cell carcinoma invading perinephric fat in a 35-year-old man. Axial contrast-enhanced fat-suppressed gradient-echo T1-weighted MR image (TR=150 ms, TE=1.2 ms) demonstrates a left RCC. There is abnormal enhancement of the fat (*arrows*) posterior and medial to the kidney, adjacent to the left psoas muscle, representing tumor invasion of the perinephric fat.

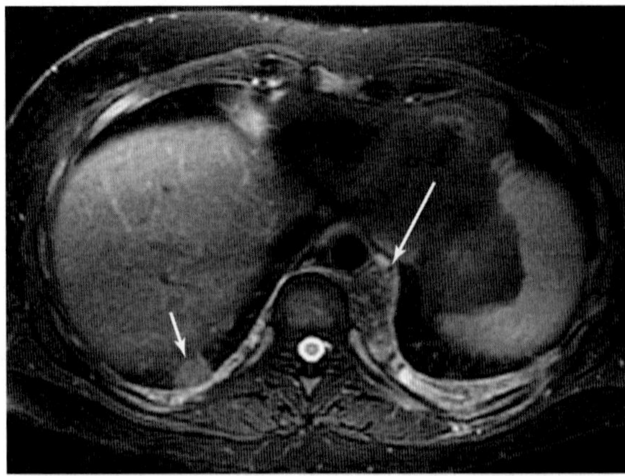

Fig. 4.9. Stage-IV RCC in a 55-year-old man. Axial fat-suppressed respiratory-triggered fast-spin-echo T2-weighted MR image (TR=5516 ms, TE(eff)=94.7 ms) demonstrates a large left retrocrural node (*long arrow*) and a right basilar pulmonary metastasis (*short arrow*) at time of presentation.

ing is limited to anatomical imaging for evaluation of tumor spread to lymph nodes, although MR imaging with iron-based agents have shown promise in differentiating malignant from hyperplastic nodes (ANZAL et al. 2003). Contrast-enhanced 3D MR venography (MRV) images can detect renal vein and inferior vena cava (IVC) thrombus, and MR imaging's direct multiplanar imaging capabilities make it superior to CT in determining whether adjacent organs are directly invaded by the RCC (HRICAK et al. 1988).

4.3.4
Therapy Planning

Radical nephrectomy, which involves resection of the entire kidney, the proximal ureter, and ipsilateral adrenal gland, was for many years the sole surgical therapy offered to patients with RCC (EL-GALLEY 2003). Recently, many studies have examined the efficacy of partial nephrectomy for select renal neoplasms, namely those that occur in solitary kidneys, synchronously in both kidneys, or in those patients with poor renal function. Reported rates of local tumor recurrence following radical nephrectomy are approximately 2% (ITANO et al. 2000). In one large series, local tumor recurrence from partial nephrectomy was approximately 3.2% (HAFEX et al. 1999), but overall patient survival has not differed significantly from that of patients with similar-stage disease who have undergone radical nephrectomy (D'ARMIENTO et al. 1997; LICHT et al. 1994; STEINBACH et al. 1995).

Many institutions now perform "elective" partial nephrectomy in patients with small renal neoplasms and normal contralateral kidneys, and studies have demonstrated no difference in patient 5- or 10-year survival (FERGANY et. al. 2000; GHAVAMIAN and ZINCKE 2001) or in patient quality of life (CLARK et al. 2001). Open partial nephrectomy may carry a slightly lower surgical complication rate than radical nephrectomy, although both procedures have relatively low morbidity and mortality (CORMAN et al. 2000).

Imaging parameters which suggest that a renal lesion can be successfully and completely removed by partial nephrectomy include: small (<4 cm) tumor size; peripheral location of the tumor; lack of invasion of the renal sinus fat, perinephric fat, and renal collecting system; presence of a pseudocapsule; lack of renal vein involvement; and absence of lymphadenopathy or distant metastases (PRETORIUS et al. 1999). Larger tumors and lesions that are locally invasive of the renal sinus fat (Fig. 4.10), renal collecting system, or perinephric fat may be removed by partial nephrectomy if there are compelling reasons (i.e., limited renal function, bilateral renal malignancies, or tumor in a solitary kidney). The presence of tumor thrombus or adjacent organ invasion excludes the possibility of a curative partial nephrectomy.

An evolving alternative to open surgery is laparoscopic partial nephrectomy (GUILLONNEAU et al. 2001). Although previously applied solely to benign disease, such as chronic pyelonephritis or calculus disease, the technique has now been advocated for use with small, indeterminate renal masses (HOLLENBECK and WOLF 2001). This is generally performed on lesions up to 2 cm and is associated with very low morbidity and mortality (JANETSCHEK et al. 1998). Laparoscopic access has also been used for tumor cryoablation, radiofrequency (RF) ablation, focused ultrasound, and microwave therapy (EDMUNDS et al. 2000; MURPHY and GILL 2001; NAITO et al. 1998; YOSHIMURA et al. 2001). Although technical procedural success has been reported, it remains to be seen whether these new therapies will match the high tumor cure rates achieved by open radical and partial nephrectomies (RASSWEILER et al. 2000).

Some institutions have performed MR-guided interventions on low-field, open MR imaging scan-

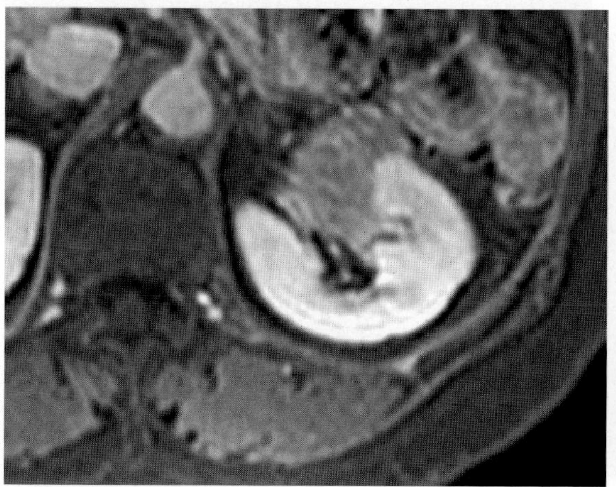
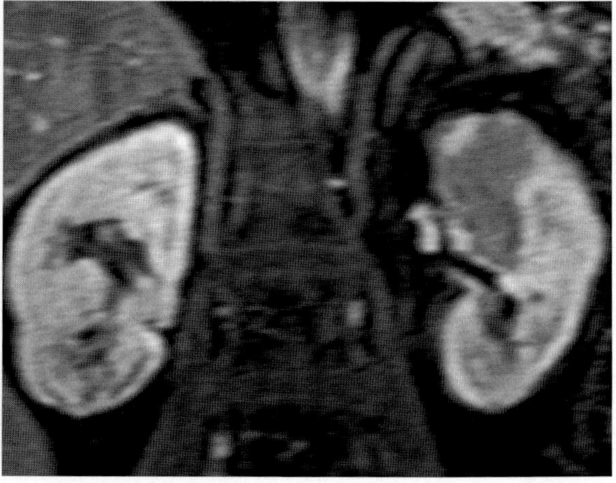

a   b

Fig. 4.10a,b. Renal mass in a 63-year-old woman with history of non-Hodgkin lymphoma. **a** Axial contrast-enhanced 2D T1-weighted GRE (TR=200 ms, TE=1.4 ms) and **b** coronal contrast-enhanced 3D T1-weighted GRE (TR=7.7 ms, TE=2.4 ms) MR images demonstrate a rounded mass of the left upper renal pole extending into the renal sinus fat. This was a renal recurrence of the patient's B-cell non-Hodgkin lymphoma.

ners (LEWIN et al. 1998; SEWELL et al. 2003), although CT guidance is more commonly used (HINSHAW and LEE 2004; ZAGORIA 2003). Among the advantages of combining real-time MR imaging with focused tumor ablation are the ability to confirm the presence of the RF electrode or cryoablation device within the tumor, and the ability to perform high-resolution, real-time imaging to confirm adequate tumor treatment. As availability of such open interventional scanners increases and image quality improves, the frequency of such procedures is likely to increase.

4.3.5
Post-Therapy Imaging

Authors differ in recommendations for imaging follow-up after surgical treatment for RCC, although recurrence rates are known to be related to the size, histologic grade, and stage of the primary neoplasm (BLUTE et al. 2000). In one retrospective study of 200 patients with RCC treated with radical or partial nephrectomy (Fig. 4.11), no patient with T1 neoplasm smaller than 4 cm had tumor recurrence at mean follow-up 47 months (GOFRIT et al. 2001), so patients with such tumors may not need routine imaging follow-up. Patients with larger tumors, high tumor grade, or advanced stage may be followed with semi-annual chest CT and with abdominal CT (GOFRIT et al. 2001) or MR imaging. Local tumor recurrence following complete resection is relatively rare (<2% at 5 years), but it carries a poor prognosis, with 28% survival at 5 years (Figs. 4.12, 4.13; ITANO et al. 2000).

Few studies have been performed on imaging following focal laparoscopic ablation of renal neoplasms. The MR imaging appearance of post-cryoablation has been reported, and most cryoablated lesions (95%) were isointense to hypointense to normal parenchyma on T2-weighted images, and a minority of lesions displayed a thin T2 hypointense rim. Serial imaging demonstrates interval decrease in size of the cryoablation site (REMER et al. 2000). The utility of MR imaging as follow-up imaging for RF ablation of solid renal tumors has also been established (Fig. 4.14; FARRELL et al. 2003).

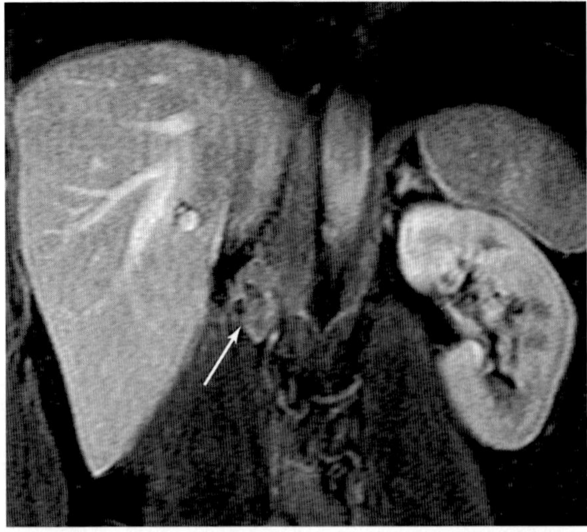

Fig. 4.12. Tumor recurrence in a 50-year-old man post-right nephrectomy. Coronal contrast-enhanced T1-weighted GRE MR image (TR=7 ms, TE=2.2 ms) demonstrates avidly enhancing nodal recurrence (*arrow*) posterior to the inferior vena cava.

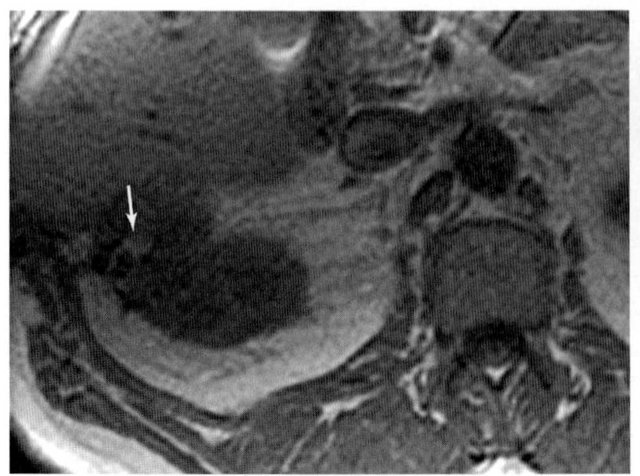

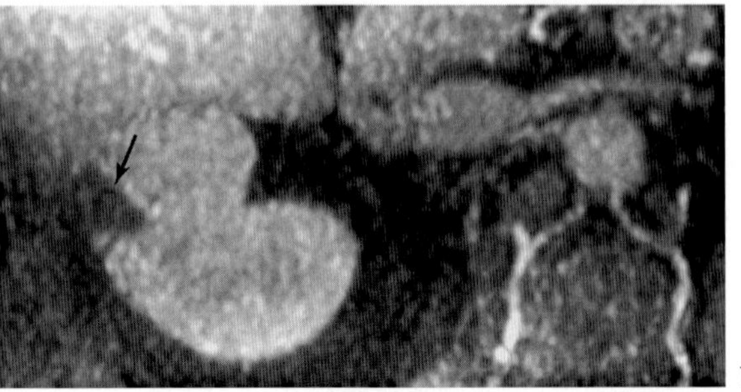

b

a

Fig. 4.11a,b. Follow-up MR imaging in a 62-year-old man with history of partial nephrectomy. Axial **a** in-phase (TR=160 ms, TE=4.7 ms) and **b** contrast-enhanced (TR=140 ms, TE=1.3 ms) T1-weighted GRE MR images demonstrate fat signal in the patient's partial nephrectomy defect (*arrow*). This is a common appearance, as fat is often used to fill the defect created by wedge resection.

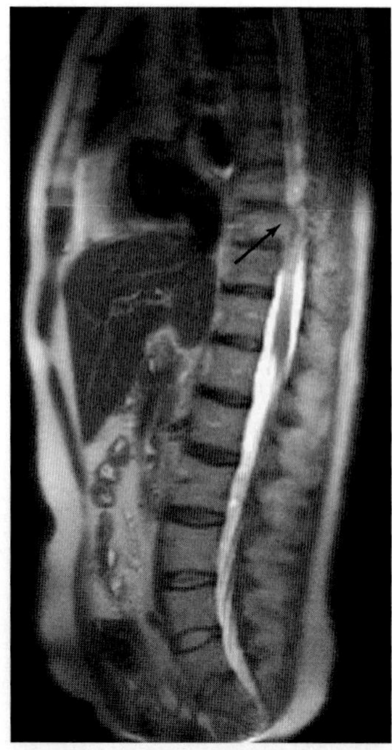

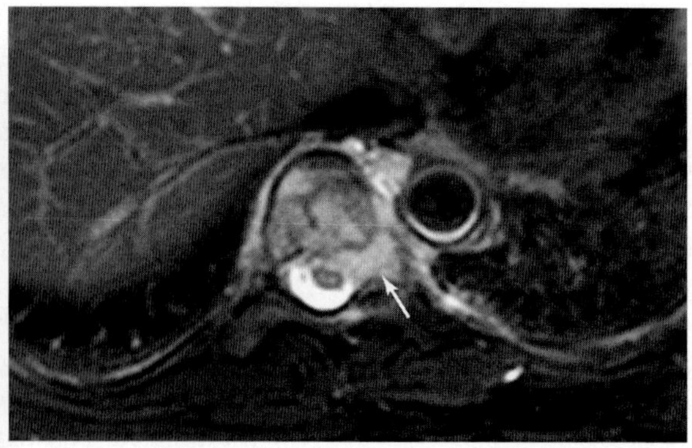

Fig. 4.13a,b. Osseous metastatic disease in a 44-year-old woman following partial nephrectomy. **a** Sagittal half-Fourier T2-weighted localizer (TR=not meaningful, TE=94 ms) MR image demonstrates osseous metastasis to T9 vertebral body with epidural extension (*arrow*). **b** Axial fat-suppressed respiratory triggered T2-weighted FSE MR image (TR=4754 ms, TE=90 ms) confirms this finding and shows the epidural involvement extending through the left neural foramen (*arrow*).

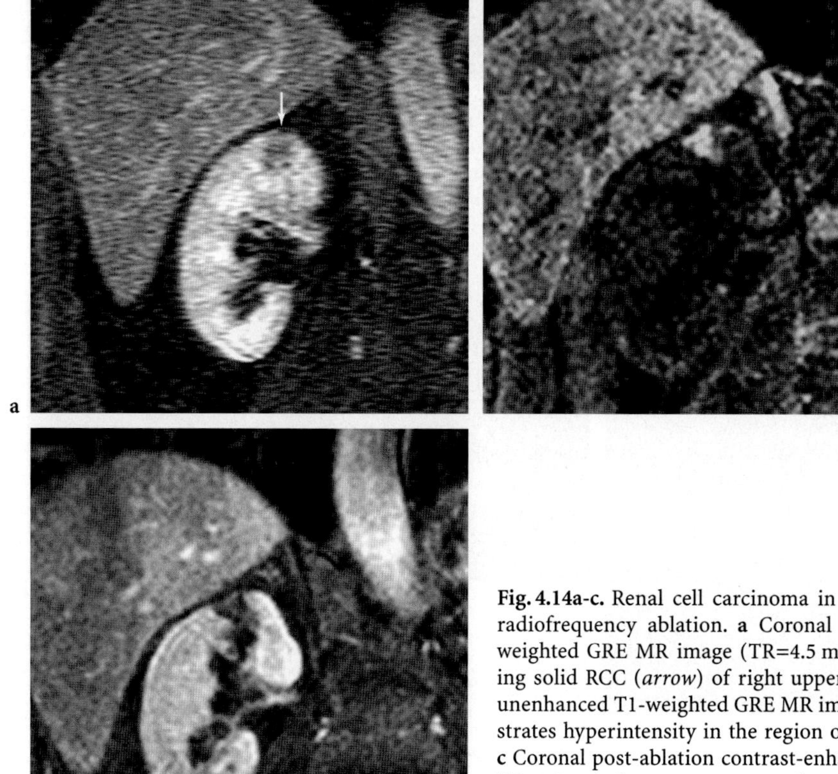

Fig. 4.14a-c. Renal cell carcinoma in a 56-year-old man before and after radiofrequency ablation. **a** Coronal pre-ablation contrast-enhanced T1-weighted GRE MR image (TR=4.5 ms, TE=2.0 ms) demonstrates enhancing solid RCC (*arrow*) of right upper renal pole. **b** Coronal post-ablation unenhanced T1-weighted GRE MR image (TR=4.7 ms, TE=1.8 ms) demonstrates hyperintensity in the region of ablation, representing hemorrhage. **c** Coronal post-ablation contrast-enhanced T1-weighted GRE (TR=4.7 ms, TE=1.8 ms) demonstrates no enhancement in this area, which was confirmed with region-of-interest placements. The absence of enhancing tissue confirms successful ablation.

4.4
Suggested MR Imaging Protocol

A suggested protocol for MR imaging of a potential renal mass is presented in Table 4.2.

4.4.1
Localizer Images

Localization may be performed in a breath-hold, with either a multiplanar 2D T1-weighted GRE sequence or with a half-Fourier single-shot T2-weighted sequence (Fig. 4.15). Either of these sequences can fulfill the purpose of localization, allowing selection of an appropriate center and field of view for the remainder of the examination. As the localizer sequence has the largest field of view of any sequence performed, however, there are some anatomic areas that are visualized on the localizer sequence only. As such, the T2-weighted sequence (single-shot fast spin echo (SSFSE), GE Medical Systems; half-Fourier acquisition single-shot turbo spin echo (HASTE), Siemens Medical Solutions) is preferred due to the superior tissue contrast of T2-weighted images. This allows characterization of pleural or pericardial effusions, as well as many findings in the bowel, bones, and pelvis.

It is not uncommon that the localizer sequence alone provide diagnostic information or reveal findings (e.g., solitary kidney, widespread metastatic disease) that may require modification of a standard renal protocol.

4.4.2
T1-Weighted Images

Chemical shift imaging with 2D, multishot in-phase and opposed-phase spoiled T1-weighted GRE images should be part of all abdominal MR imaging examinations (fast spoiled gradient-recalled (FSPGR), GE Medical Systems; fast low-angle shot (FLASH), Siemens Medical Solutions). If fat and water are present in the same voxel, loss of signal will be seen on the opposed-phase image relative to the in-phase images due to destructive interference of the fat and water signals. These sequences are used to detect the presence of intracytoplasmic lipid in hepatic steatosis, hepatic adenomas, hepatocellular carcinomas, and adrenal adenomas (OUTWATER et al. 1998). In the kidney, signal loss on chemical shift imaging is not specific for angiomyolipoma, as clear cell RCC may also contain intracytoplasmic lipid (Fig. 4.2; OUTWATER et al. 1998).

The TR of these 2D T1-weighted GRE images is adjusted based on the patient's ability to breath-hold, as it is desirable to image the entire kidney in a single breath-hold. At 1.5 T, the TE of the in-phase image will be 4.4 ms and the TE of the directly

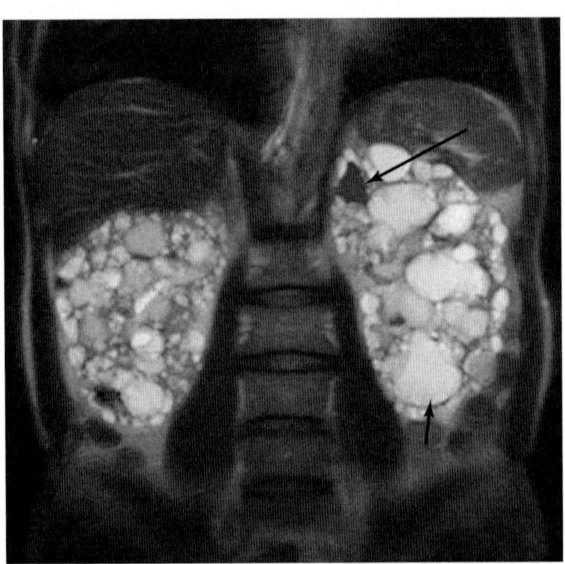

Fig. 4.15. Autosomal-dominant polycystic kidney disease in a 45-year-old man. Coronal half-Fourier T2-weighted localizer MR image (TR=not meaningful, TE=86 ms) reveals multiple simple (*short arrow*) and hemorrhagic (*long arrow*) cysts within greatly enlarged kidneys.

Table 4.2. Suggested protocol: renal mass on 1.5 T MR scanner. *FOV* field of view; *NA* not applicable

	Sequence	Plane	TR (ms)	TE (ms)	Flip angle (°)	FOV (cm)	Thickness (mm)	Skip (mm)
Localizer	T2 half-Fourier	Coronal/sagittal	NA	80–100	NA	40–48	8	2
Chemical shift	T1-GRE (in phase)	Axial	120–200	4.4	90	26–38	6	1
Chemical shift	T1-GRE (out of phase)	Axial	120–200	2.2	90	26–38	6	1
Respiratory triggered fat-suppressed T2	T2 FSE	Axial	4000–12,000	80–110(eff)	NA	26–38	7	1
Pre/post-contrast 3D	T1-GRE	Coronal	Minimum	Minimum	15	34	4 interpolated to 2	0
Delayed/post-contrast	T1-GRE	Axial	120–280	1.1–1.4	90	26–38	6	1

opposed phase image will be 2.2 ms. The software of some manufacturers employs sequences that are slightly off these values, but which nonetheless are capable of detecting signal loss on the opposed-phase image when fat and water protons are present in the same voxel. These sequences can be obtained simultaneously in a single breath-hold by acquiring two echoes per excitation and reconstructing the data as separate series. This technique is preferable to acquisition in two breath-holds, because it eliminates respiratory misregistration between the two sequences.

Renal angiomyolipomas are benign hamartomas which are composed of varying amounts of blood vessels, smooth muscle, and fat. They are common in patients with tuberous sclerosis (CASPER et al. 2002) but may also occur sporadically. As they are vascular lesions, AMLs may enhance avidly on CT and MR imaging and must be differentiated from RCCs. Angiomyolipomas may contain both intracytoplasmic lipid – detectable with chemical shift imaging – and macroscopic fat, which can be confirmed with use of frequency-selective fat-suppressed T1-weighted GRE and water-saturated T1-weighted GRE images (Fig. 4.3; Table 4.3). These are both breath-held sequences, and should be obtained while maintaining the TR of the original in-phase and opposed-phase T1-weighted GRE sequences. These sequences allow definitive detection and characterization of the macroscopic fat present in most angiomyolipomas. If present, macroscopic fat will follow the signal of the perinephric fat and the body-wall fat, becoming hypointense to renal parenchyma on the fat-suppressed T1-weighted GRE and remaining very hyperintense on the water-saturated T1-weighted GRE.

Some AMLs do not contain macroscopic fat. At present, these lesions cannot be reliably differentiated from RCC by diagnostic imaging (HOSOKAWA et al. 2002; JINZAKI et al. 1997). The renal leiomyoma, a rare benign lesion, is thought to represent an angiomyolipoma devoid of fat due to the increased incidence of leiomyomas in patients with tuberous sclerosis (STEINER et al. 1990; WAGNER et al. 1997).

For patients who cannot breath-hold, respiratory-triggered FSE T1-weighted imaging is an option for obtaining pre-contrast T1-weighted images. This technique is slower than T1-weighted GRE chemical shift imaging and provides less information, as the presence of microscopic lipid cannot be confirmed. This technique, therefore, is best reserved for sedated or ventilated patients.

4.4.3
T2-Weighted Images

For T2-weighted imaging, axial, fat-suppressed, respiratory-triggered FSE T2-weighted images offer excellent SNR and reasonable acquisition times. The FSE/TSE imaging is faster than conventional spin-echo imaging in that multiple-phase encodes are achieved in a single TR. The effective echo time of the sequence is determined by the TE of the phase encodes of the center of k-space, and this data dominates image contrast. Fat suppression is commonly applied to these sequences, as echo-train imaging results in higher signal intensity of fat than is routinely seen on conventional spin-echo T2-weighted images.

With respiratory triggering a bellows is placed around the patient's abdomen to monitor patient respiration. Acquisition of MR imaging data is performed at a fixed point in the respiratory cycle, minimizing respiratory-associated phase ghost artifacts. Although these images are generally excellent in quality, a detriment of this technique is that data can be collected in only a portion of the respiratory cycle, leading to relatively longer imaging times.

A promising alternative to respiratory triggering is navigator echo gating. This technique has been applied more in cardiac MR imaging than in abdominal imaging, but its potential for minimizing respiratory motion is well established (SODICKSON 2002). In navigator echo gating, targeted scans are used to establish the position of some anatomic object, such as the diaphragm, whose relationship to the organ of interest is predictable. Prior to each data acquisition, navigator echoes are generated by selectively exciting a column of tissue that traverses a high-contrast tissue interface, such as lung–diaphragm. Signal from this excitation is compared to a reference echo to establish the relative displacement of the navigator interface, and this data is used for

Table 4.3. Additional sequences: suspected angiomyolipoma on 1.5 T MR scanner

	Sequence	Plane	TR (ms)	TE (ms)	Flip angle (°)	FOV (cm)	Thickness (mm)	Skip (mm)
Fat suppression	T1-GRE	Axial	120–200	2.2	90	26–38	6	1
Water saturation	T1-GRE	Axial	120–200	4.4	90	26–38	6	1

respiratory gating of data acquired of the object of interest (FIRMIN and KEEGAN 2002). On most scanners, however, navigator echo gating is more challenging to optimize than respiratory triggering, and this has likely limited its use in routine imaging of the abdomen.

Although half-Fourier single-shot T2-weighted images (SSFSE, GE Medical Systems; HASTE, Siemens Medical Solutions) are adequate as localizer images, their SNR and contrast-to-noise ratio (CNR) relative to FSE/TSE T2-weighted images is too low to justify their routine use as the sole T2-weighted sequence of high-quality abdominal MR imaging. In half-Fourier imaging, just over one half of k-space is acquired in a single echo train, and k-space symmetry is used to infer the remainder of the non-acquired data. The result is a rapidly acquired image of low spatial resolution and relatively low contrast, which may render small or nearly T2-isointense renal malignancies undetectable (Fig. 4.16).

Half-Fourier imaging should not be the sole T2-weighted imaging sequence of a renal MR imaging examination; however, these sequences may serve as a useful adjunct to FSE/TSE T2-weighted images when employed as MR hydrography to evaluate the urothelium of a hydronephrotic, non-functioning kidney.

4.4.4
Pre- and Post-Contrast Imaging

The contrast-enhanced portion of the examination may be performed either as a 2D (FSPGR, GE Medical Systems; FLASH, Siemens Medical Solutions) or 3D (enhanced fast gradient-recalled echo (EFGRE), GE Medical Systems; volumetric interpolated breath-hold examination (VIBE), Siemens Medical Solutions) sequence (HEISS et al. 2000; ROFSKY et al. 1999). Three-dimensional images are greatly preferred, as they provide thinner sections, have no interscan gaps, suffer fewer partial-volume artifacts in evaluation of small lesions, and provide superior spatial resolution in the interpolated plane. The choice of 3D dynamic imaging allows renal MRA/MRV imaging to be performed at the same time that dynamically enhanced renal parenchyma data is acquired, although this commonly used approach requires some imaging compromises to be made. When primarily evaluating the renal parenchyma, a flip angle of 10–15° is used to minimize soft tissue saturation and optimize renal mass detection and characterization. If the study is for renal vascular evaluation, the flip angle is increased to 30–60° to optimize the contrast between enhanced vessels and

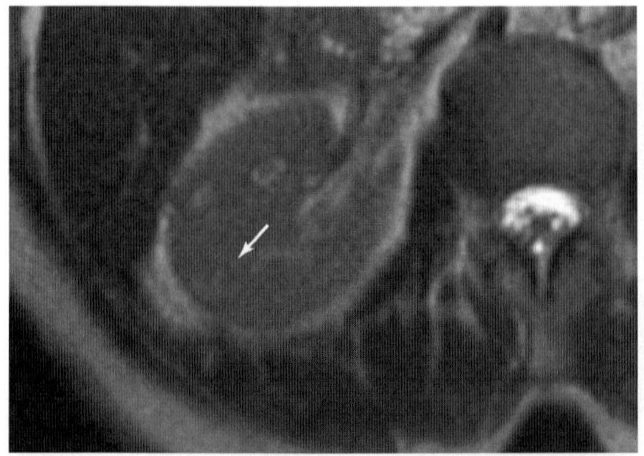

a

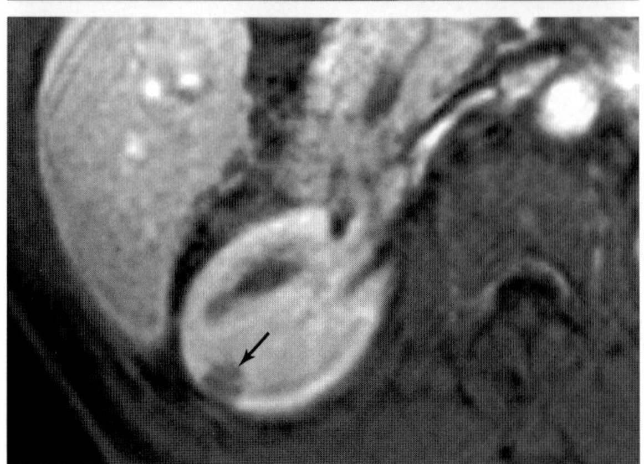

c

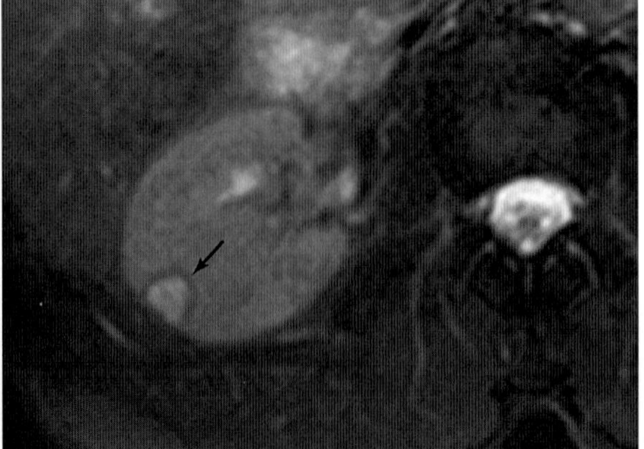

b

Fig. 4.16a-c. Renal cell carcinoma in a 74-year-old woman. **a** Axial half-Fourier T2-weighted MR image (TR=not meaningful, TE=91 ms) demonstrates an extremely subtle lesion (*arrow*) in the posterior aspect of the right interpolar kidney. This case illustrates why half-Fourier imaging, while adequate for localization purposes, should not be used as the sole T2-weighted sequence for abdominal imaging. **b** Axial fat-suppressed, respiratory triggered fast-spin-echo T2-weighted MR image (TR=5153 ms, TE=90 ms) at the same level as **a** clearly demonstrates this lesion (*arrow*). This sequence is superior to half-Fourier imaging in both contrast-to-noise and signal-to-noise ratio. **c** Axial contrast-enhanced fat-suppressed T1-weighted gradient-echo MR image (TR=4.7 ms, TE=1.8 ms) demonstrates internal lesion enhancement (*arrow*). This lesion, excised by partial nephrectomy, was an RCC.

the less-enhanced non-vascular soft tissues (ROFSKY et al. 1999). Field of view is also reduced in dedicated MRA examination, to increase spatial resolution.

For any contrast-enhanced MR imaging examination, a pre-contrast data set must be acquired. Its acquisition parameters must be identical to those of the post-contrast data sets so that potential lesion enhancement can be assessed. For renal parenchymal evaluation, images are acquired in both a corticomedullary phase and in a nephrographic phase. If the renal imaging is primarily for renal vascular evaluation, a renal arterial vascular phase may also be obtained, although use of a bolus timing technique is required to reliably capture this brief phase.

The coronal plane is generally chosen for the gadolinium-enhanced images as it allows dynamic evaluation of both kidneys, the renal vessels, and the inferior vena cava in the smallest number of slices or slabs. In general, though, for characterization of a known renal mass, one should choose the plane which best displays the mass. For exophytic anterior and posterior lesions, this may be the sagittal or axial plane. If the coronal plane is chosen, however, the patient's arms are elevated above the head to decrease phase-wrap artifact.

As dynamic 3D imaging of the kidneys necessarily may exclude portions of the liver, spleen, and other abdominal viscera to acquire the image within a reasonably short breath-hold, axial 2D delayed fat-saturated T1-weighted GRE images are obtained as the final sequence, imaging from the top of the hemidiaphragms to the iliac crests. This sequence provides full coverage of the contrast-enhanced abdominal viscera.

4.4.5
Subtraction Imaging

Subtraction imaging is a useful post-processing tool for interpretation of renal MR imaging. In subtraction imaging, each voxel of the pre-contrast data set is subtracted from a post-contrast data set. This may be performed by the technologist on the MR scanner, or by the radiologist on a workstation. Subtraction may be used to detect subtle enhancement in renal lesions (pre-contrast data set subtracted from nephrographic-phase data set); to improve the contrast-to-background ratio of MRA images (pre-contrast subtracted from arterial-phase data set); or to differentiate non-enhancing bland thrombus from enhancing tumor thrombus (precontrast subtracted

from MRV data set). One limitation of subtraction is respiratory misregistration between the pre-contrast and post-contrast data sets. This may result in "pseudoenhancement" of a renal lesion (Fig. 4.17). The presence of misregistration is identified by identifying a rim of hyperintensity around the kidneys and liver on the subtraction data set. If misregistration is severe, direct signal intensity measurements of the lesion in question on the pre- and post-contrast images must be performed to determine whether enhancement has occurred.

4.4.6
Functional Renal MR Imaging

Dynamic, multiphasic contrast-enhanced MR imaging can also be used as a form of functional renal imaging (HUANG et al. 2003; HUANG et al. 2004; TEH et al. 2003). This technique has been applied for quantification of renal cortical enhancement in patients with renal artery stenosis (GANDY et al. 2003), and in assessment of enhancement in RCC (CHOYKE et al. 2003). As tumor angiogenesis has become a recognized feature of renal and other malignancies, contrast-enhanced MR imaging has emerged as a modality capable of demonstrating tumor neovascularity, quantifying contrast agent wash-in/wash-out curves, and evaluating the effects of antiangiogenic therapies (which may not produce changes in lesion size; HAYES et al. 2002). Examinations tailored for functional MR imaging of renal cell carcinoma typically use slower injection rates (0.3 ml/s of 0.1 ml/kg gadolinium chelate) and 3D T1-weighted GRE imaging of the kidney is performed approximately every 30 s for 8–10 min.

4.4.7
MR Angiography

Three-dimensional arterial and venous-phase 3D data sets are post-processed to generate projection images of the renal arteries, renal veins, and inferior vena cava. As 3D volumetric sequences result in small, nearly isotropic voxels, maximum intensity projection (MIP) images of the renal arteries, renal veins, and inferior vena cava (IVC) may be generated in any plane. Axial and coronal projections are most commonly used, but oblique coronal or curved reformatted images are often optimal for display of renal vessel anatomy. Volume rendering of renal vessels may also be used.

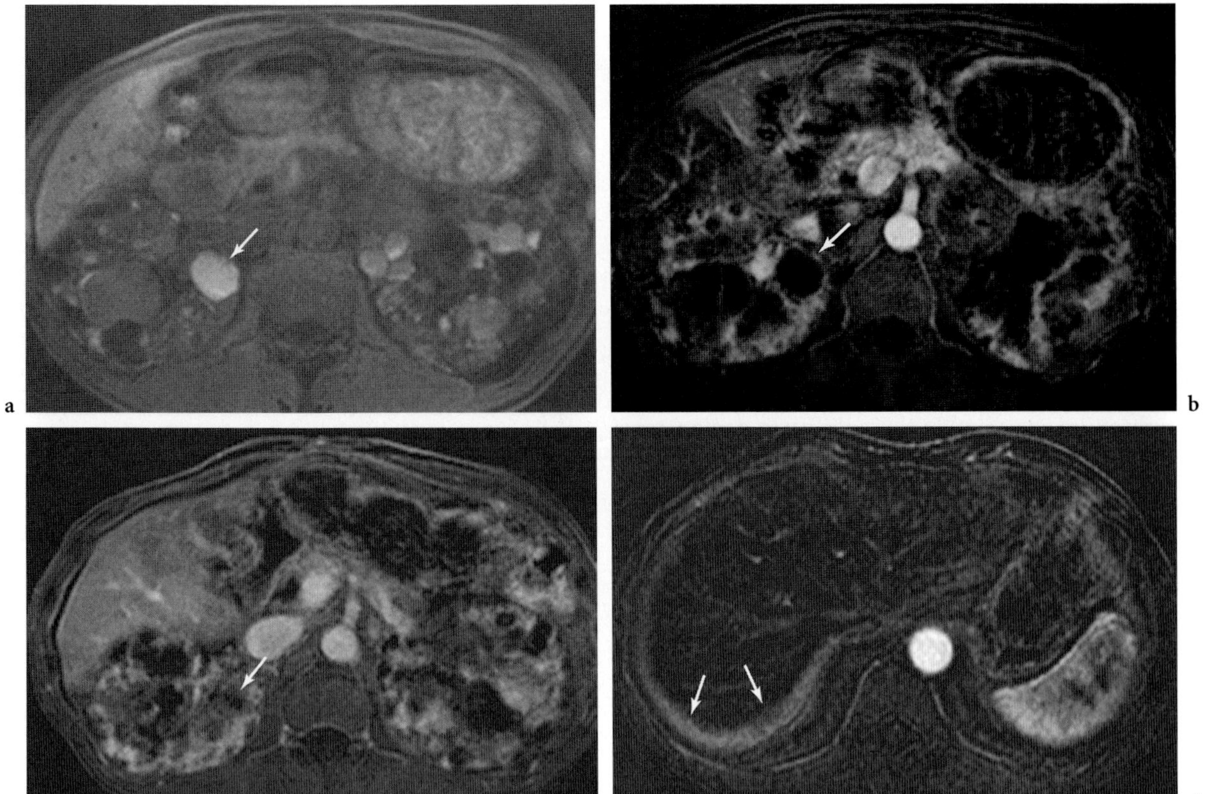

Fig. 4.17a-d. Autosomal-dominant polycystic kidney disease in a 45-year-old man. **a** Axial unenhanced fat-suppressed T1-weighted gradient-echo MR image (TR=3.8 ms, TE=0.9 ms) reveals many of the cysts to be hemorrhagic, including a large right posterior interpolar hemorrhagic cyst (*arrow*). As such, it can be difficult to determine if any of the cysts have internal enhancement. **b** Axial subtraction MR image reveals no internal enhancement in any of the cystic lesions. The right posterior interpolar lesion (*arrow*), in particular, does not enhance and is therefore a Bosniak II benign hemorrhagic cyst. **c** Axial subtraction image generated from a later contrast-enhanced acquisition. If contrast-enhanced images and unenhanced images are poorly registered due to differential breath-hold size, apparent enhancement in benign lesions (*arrow*) can result. **d** A more cranial axial MR image from the data set in c reveals a concentric bright band of misregistered enhancing tissue (*arrows*) around the liver. This confirms that this particular data set is poorly registered.

In MRA the order in which k-space is filled is an important consideration. Optimally, the central k-space data, which dominates the contrast of the image, should be acquired during the very brief time that gadolinium concentration is high in the renal arteries yet low in the renal veins. Use of a bolus timing technique is, of course, mandatory, but use of an elliptic–centric method of filling k-space (rather than traditional sequential filling) can effectively compress the time in which the critical central portion of k-space is filled (Fain et al. 2001; Wilman and Riederer 1997). This approach can be used to maximize contrast between the contrast-enhanced arteries and background.

The MRA/MRV constitutes an important part of the overall MR imaging evaluation of a renal malignancy, as several questions related to tumor staging and treatment strategy must be addressed (Kocak et al. 2001). The number and position of renal arteries, the number and morphology of renal veins, the presence/absence of tumor thrombus in the renal vein and IVC, and the status of the vasculature of the contralateral kidney should all be evaluated.

Magnetic resonance angiography has emerged as a powerful modality for imaging the renal arteries (Dong et al. 1999; Fain et al. 2001; Zhang and Prince 2004). Compared with conventional angiography, which is the traditional gold standard diagnostic examination, MRA is considerably less invasive and has the additional advantage of utilizing a non-nephrotoxic contrast agent that can be administered safely in patients with elevated creatinine. Both MRA and CT angiography (CTA) have been reported to be 100% sensitive for the detection of main renal arteries (Halpern et al. 2000; Rankin et al. 2001). Accessory renal arteries are common, however, occurring in approximately 29% of kidneys, and must be detected to allow proper surgical planning for radical nephrectomy (Fig. 4.18; NELSON et al. 1999).

Although early papers reported MRA to be inferior to conventional angiography for detection of accessory renal arteries (DEBATIN et al. 1993; MEYERS et al. 1995), MRA protocols have advanced (CARROLL and GRIST 2002) so that more recent investigations have found conventional angiography and dynamic, contrast-enhanced 3D MRA to be comparable (BUZZAS et al. 1997; LOW et al. 1998).

Computed tomography angiography and MRA are approximately equal in their ability to demonstrate accessory renal arteries, with sensitivities of greater than 90% reported for both modalities (RANKIN et al. 2001). Smaller (1–2 mm) accessory renal arteries are subject to higher rates of non-detection by imaging, as well as greater likelihood of interobserver disagreement. Both CTA and MRA examinations of renal donors have demonstrated high degrees of interobserver agreement for presence of accessory renal arteries and for the presence of early arterial bifurcations (HALPERN et al. 2000).

4.4.8
MR Venography

Although tumor thrombus may be suspected on conventional T1- and T2-weighted images, 3D contrast-enhanced sequences can be used to confirm the presence of renal vein or IVC thrombus (CHOYKE et al. 1997). Venous phase enhanced MR images have been reported to be 88–100% sensitive in detection of malignant tumor renal vein thrombus (CHOYKE et al. 1997; LAISSY et al. 2000). In the renal donor population, MRV has been shown to be superior to digital subtraction angiography in characterizing renal venous anatomy (GIESSING et al. 2003).

Renal cell carcinoma involves the IVC in 5–10% of cases (KEARNEY et al. 1981). In evaluation of the IVC, the second or third set of contrast-enhanced coronal images is ideal for detection and characterization of the extent of thrombus within the renal veins and IVC. Generally, tumor thrombus enhances while bland thrombus does not (Figs. 4.19, 4.20, 4.21; EILENBERG et al. 1990; NGUYEN et al. 1996); however, both types of thrombus are removed at time of surgery.

The sensitivity of MR imaging has been reported to be 90–100% for detection of IVC thrombus, which is superior to rates reported for CT (79%) and sonog-

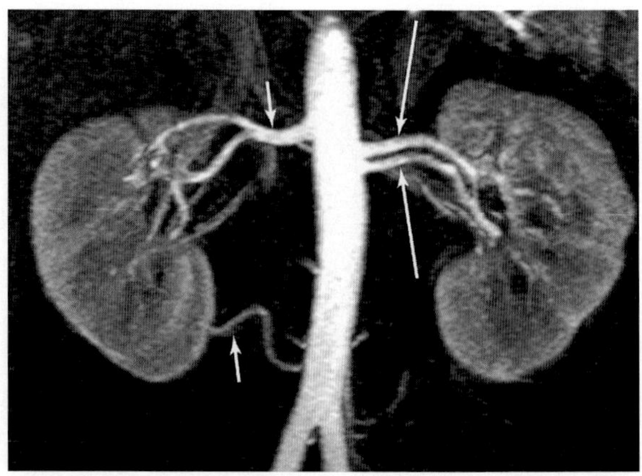

Fig. 4.18. Bilateral accessory renal arteries in a 47-year-old man. Maximum intensity projection (MIP) reformatted MR image of bolus-timed, arterial phase 3D T1-weighted GRE imaging of the kidneys (TR=3.8 ms, TE=0.9 ms) demonstrates two left renal arteries (*long arrows*) and two right renal arteries (*short arrows*).

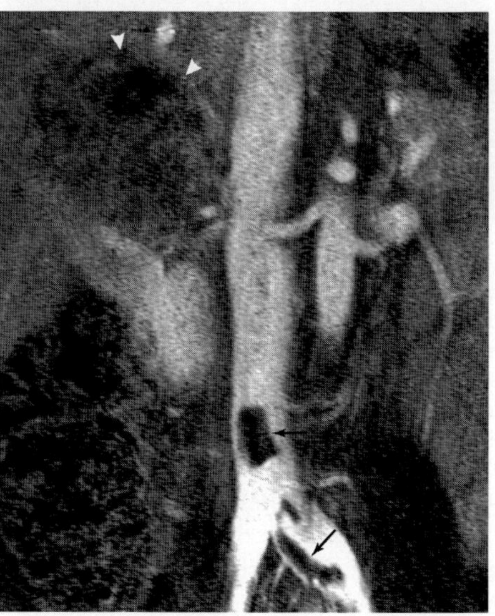

Fig. 4.19. Renal cell carcinoma in a 47-year-old woman. Coronal subtracted maximum intensity projection (MIP) image of contrast-enhanced MRV examination (TR=3.7 ms, TE=1.4 ms) demonstrates bland, non-enhancing, non-occlusive thrombus of the inferior vena cava and left common iliac vein (*arrows*). There is a large right-upper-pole-enhancing RCC (*arrowheads*).

raphy (68%; KALLMAN et al. 1992; ASLAM SOHAIB et al. 2002). The CT specificity for detection of IVC thrombus is limited by inflow artifact of unenhanced blood.

Magnetic resonance imaging is the modality of choice for the determination of the superior extent of IVC thrombus (ASLAM SOHAIB et al. 2002). The cephalad extent of tumor thrombus does not appear

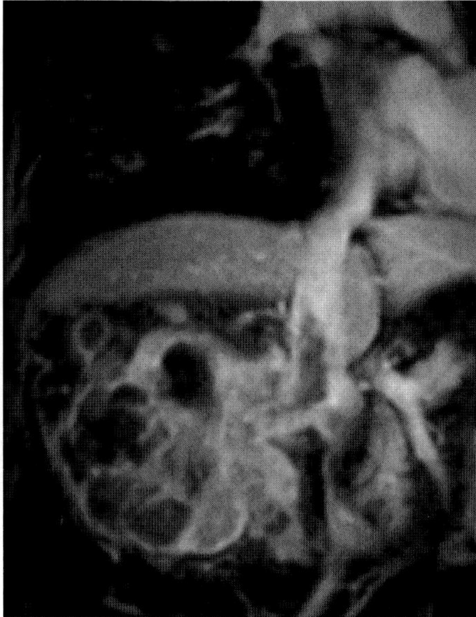

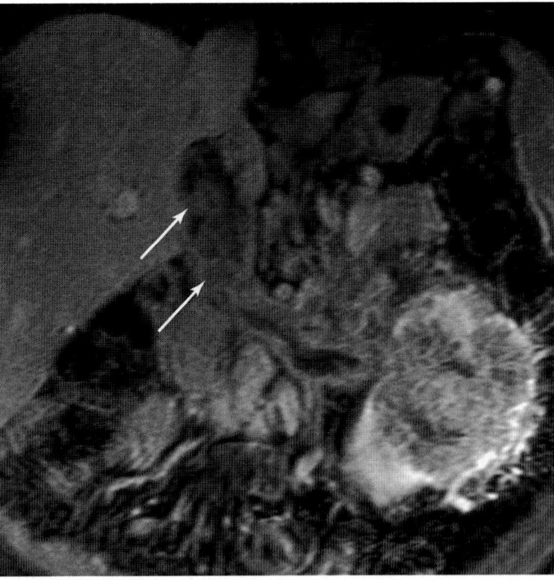

Fig. 4.20. Renal cell carcinoma in a 64-year-old man. Maximum intensity projection of coronal subtraction MRV (TR=4.7 ms, TE=1.6 ms) demonstrates avidly enhancing large right RCC with tumor thrombus in the right renal vein extending into the intrahepatic vena cava. No tumor thrombus above the diaphragm is seen.

Fig. 4.21. Left renal cell carcinoma in a 44-year-old man. Coronal contrast-enhanced fat-suppressed T1-weighted GRE MR image (TR=6.5 ms, TE=2.2 ms) demonstrates a large left renal cell carcinoma. There is thrombus in the left renal vein and inferior vena cava. Nodular regions of enhancement (*arrows*) indicate that this is malignant thrombus. The superior extent of the caval thrombosis into the intrahepatic cava, but not above the hepatic veins, is clearly delineated.

to affect expected survival (MONTIE et al. 1991) but has a significant impact on surgical approach (OTO et al. 1998). Level-I thrombus extends into the IVC, no more than 2 cm above the renal vein confluence with the IVC, and can be removed through either a standard flank approach or an anterior approach. Level II extends more than 2 cm above the renal veins, but remains inferior to the hepatic veins, and requires an anterior approach through bilateral subcostal transperitoneal or thoracoabdominal incisions (Fig. 4.20). Level-III thrombus involves the intrahepatic IVC but remains below the diaphragm (Fig. 4.21). The surgical approach for level-III thrombus is transperitoneal and thoracoabdominal similar to level-II thrombus, but may additionally require cardiac bypass and hypothermic circulatory arrest. Level-IV thrombus involves the supradiaphragmatic IVC or the right atrium. Excision of level-IV thrombus requires a median sternotomy, cardiac bypass, and hypothermic circulatory arrest, in addition to a transabdominal incision.

Renal vein anatomy is also assessed in candidates for radical nephrectomy. Normal variants such as the circum-aortic left renal vein (0.2–0.3%) and retro-aortic left renal vein (0.5–3%; Fig. 4.22) are readily demonstrable on MRV and should be reported as part of an overall MR imaging assessment of renal malignancy.

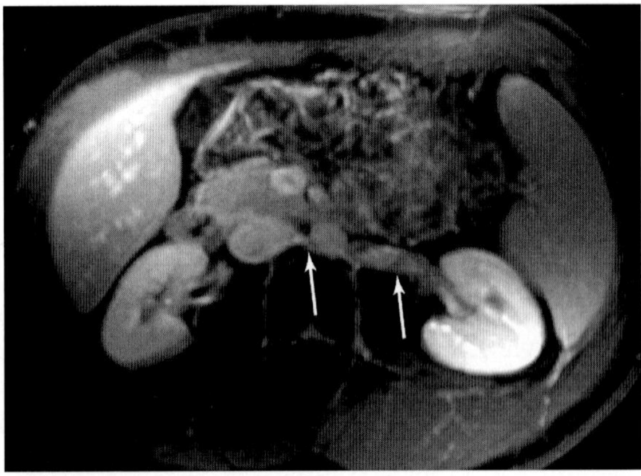

Fig. 4.22. Retro-aortic left renal vein in a 27-year-old man. Axial nephrographic phase contrast-enhanced fat-suppressed T1-weighted gradient echo MR image (TR=210 ms, TE=1.4 ms) demonstrates a retro-aortic left renal vein (*arrows*), a normal variant.

4.4.9
Flow-Related Vascular MR Imaging

Prior to development of contrast-enhanced breath-held MRA, time-of-flight imaging was a frequently used technique for evaluation of abdominal vasculature. Presently, however, time-of-flight renal vascular imaging is unnecessary if one is performing a contrast-enhanced study, as it has significant disadvantages relative to contrast-enhanced MRA; these include long imaging times, signal loss due to in-plane flow, severe motion artifacts, and an inability to demonstrate the distal portion of renal arteries (NELSON et al. (1999).

Phase-contrast MR imaging has been used to quantify flow in evaluation of renal artery stenosis (BINKERT et al. 2001). It is not used in renal vascular imaging in the oncologic setting, due to long imaging times and numerous artifacts.

4.4.10
MR Urography

Magnetic resonance urography is probably unnecessary as part of routine evaluation of a renal mass, although it can be very useful as part of the evaluation of suspected transitional cell carcinoma, for renal donor evaluation (HUSSAIN et al. 2003), for imaging of renal transplants, and for imaging in patients who cannot receive iodine-based contrast agents (Fig. 4.23; CHU et al. 2004; EL-DIASTY et al. 2003). For this examination, 10 mg of furosemide (American Regent Laboratories, Shirley, N.Y.) is injected with the gadolinium chelate (NOLTE-ERNSTING et al. 1998). Mild diuresis with furosemide both mildly dilates the renal collecting system to facilitate imaging, and simultaneously prevents excreted gadolinium chelate from a achieving high concentration, which could lead to T2* effect (Fig. 4.24; EL-DIASTY et al. 2003). Dynamic enhanced 3D images of the kidneys are acquired in arterial, venous, and nephrographic phases, and then the field of view is increased in the z plane to include the kidneys, ureters, and urinary bladder. Coronal 3D, breath-held, thin slab (2 mm interpolated to 1 mm) fat-suppressed T1-weighted GRE images are then acquired (3D EFGRE, GE Medical Systems; VIBE, Siemens Medical Solutions; Table 4.4). In situations where breath-hold imaging is not possible, respiratory-gated images can be acquired (ROHRSCHNEIDER et al. 2002).

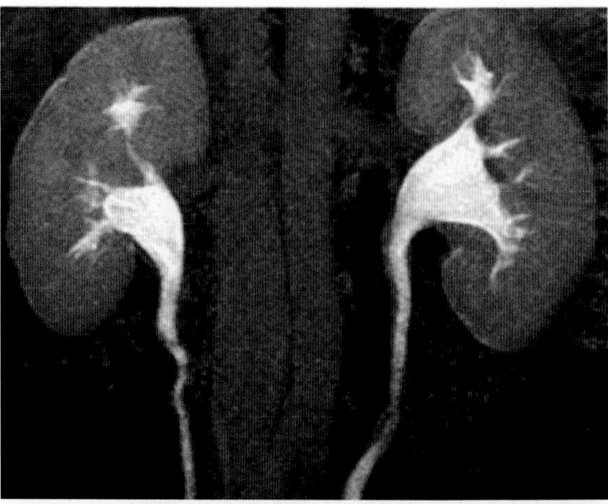

Fig. 4.23. Hematuria in a 39-year-old man. Coronal MIP reformatted MR image of 3D T1-weighted GRE excretory MR urogram (TR=5.5 ms, TE=1.1 ms) reveals normal collecting systems bilaterally.

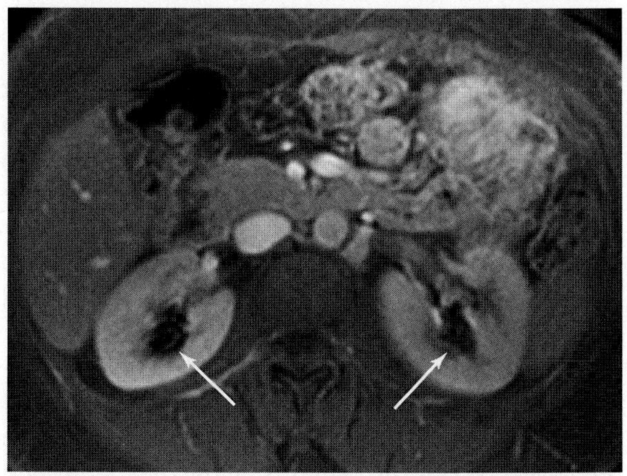

Fig. 4.24. Hematuria in a 42-year-old woman. Axial delayed contrast-enhanced fat-suppressed T1-weighted gradient-echo MR image (TR=150 ms, TE=1.4 ms) demonstrates markedly low hypointensity (*arrows*) within both renal collecting systems. This is the normal appearance of concentrated gadolinium chelate, and illustrates why furosemide is necessary to ensure excretion of a dilute and T1-hyperintense urine for T1-weighted excretory urography.

Table 4.4. Urothelial evaluation at 1.5 T MR scanner. *NA* not applicable

	Sequence	Plane	TR (ms)	TE (ms)	Flip angle(°)	FOV (cm)	Thickness (mm)	Matrix
Excretory MRU 3D	T1-GRE	Coronal	Minimum	Minimum	10	34	2 interpolated to 1	212/256
T2 Hydrography multislice	Half-Fourier T2	Coronal	NA	200	NA	36	5	256/256
T2 Hydrography thick slab	Half-Fourier T2	Coronal	NA	200	NA	36	70	256/256

Transitional cell carcinoma (TCC) is the second most common primary renal malignancy, although it is far more common in the urinary bladder than in the upper urinary tract. Between 30 and 75% of patients with upper tract TCC will have synchronous bladder tumors. Approximately 2–4% of patients with bladder TCC have synchronous upper tract disease (Fig. 4.25; Messing and Catalona 2000). Diagnosis of TCC, therefore, requires evaluation of the entire urothelium. Although MRU is capable of identifying large collecting system abnormalities (Huang et al. 1994), it remains inferior to conventional excretory urography in the detection of small calyceal abnormalities (Jung et al. 2000; Nolte-Ernsting et al. 1998).

Transitional cell carcinomas of the renal pelvis or renal collecting system are visualized on MRU or on T2-weighted images as filling defects, with or without proximal hydronephrosis (Fig. 4.26; Kanematsu et al. 1996). In contrast to calculi, TCC will enhance following the administration of gadolinium chelate (Wagner 1997), although tumors tend to enhance less than renal parenchyma. TCC is hypointense to urine on T2-weighted images. The MRU is known to be far inferior to unenhanced CT in detection of renal calculi, and the MRU identification of a non-enhancing filling defect in the renal collecting system is non-specific. Such a finding can represent stone, blood clot, gas bubble, or sloughed papilla (Kawashima et al. 2003).

A second option for collecting system evaluation in hydronephrotic or non-functioning kidneys is heavily T2-weighted MR hydrography (SSFSE, GE Medical Systems; HASTE, Siemens Medical Solutions; Figs. 4.27, 4.28, 4.29; (Table 4.4; Shokeir et al. 2004). These are heavily T2-weighted sequences identical to those used for MR cholangiopancreatography (MRCP) and, like MRCP, can be performed

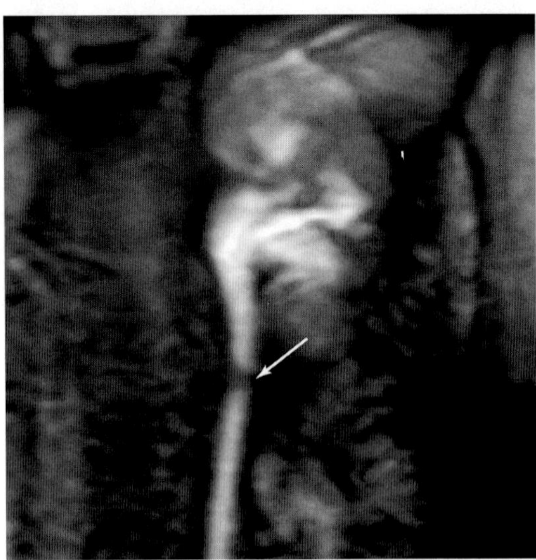

Fig. 4.26. Hematuria in a 66-year-old woman. Coronal T1-weighted gadolinium MRU (TR=6 ms, TE=0.8 ms) demonstrates a small, non-obstructing filling defect in the proximal left ureter (*arrow*). This was a transitional cell carcinoma.

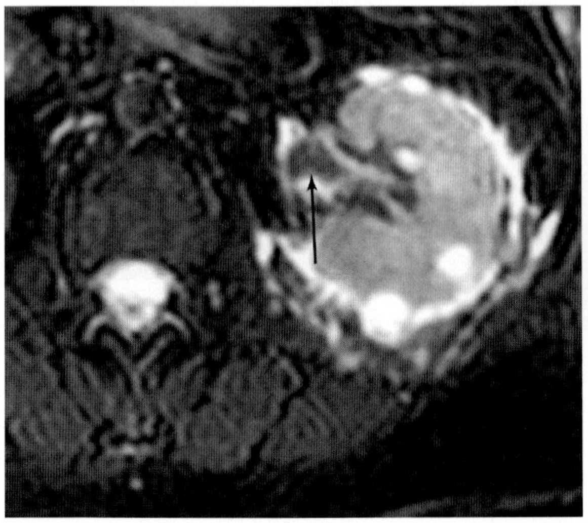

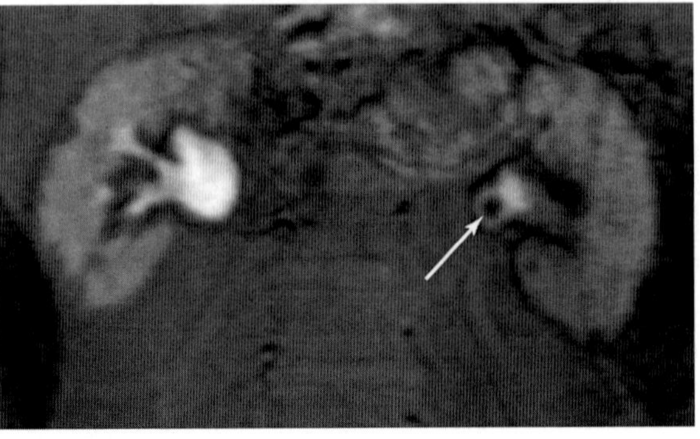

Fig. 4.25a,b. Transitional cell carcinoma of the left renal pelvis in an 82-year-old man. **a** Axial fat-suppressed respiratory-triggered fast-spin-echo T2-weighted MR image (TR=5700 ms, TE(eff)=106 ms) demonstrates a hypointense soft tissue mass (*arrow*) in the left renal pelvis. **b** Coronal T1-weighted gadolinium MRU (TR=5.5 ms, TE=1.2 ms) confirms the presence of a polypoid filling defect (*arrow*) in the left renal collecting system. The presence of enhancement within the lesion can be used to differentiate solid tumor masses from other potential causes of filling defects, including clot, stone, or air.

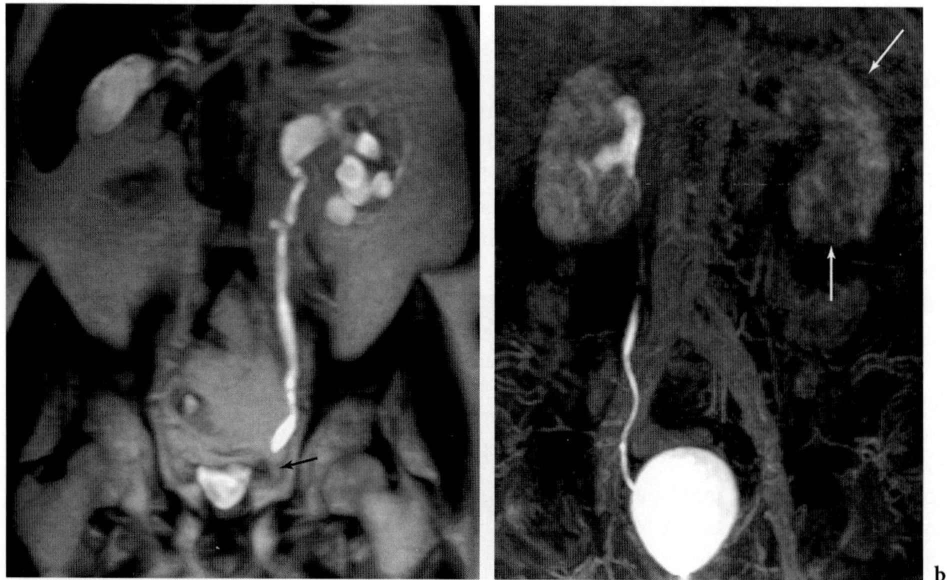

Fig. 4.27a,b. Obstructing transitional cell carcinoma at the left ureterovesical junction in a 67-year-old man. **a** Coronal half-Fourier T2-weighted MR image (TR=not significant, TE=92 ms) demonstrates left hydroureteronephrosis. There is a suggestion of a soft tissue mass (*arrow*) at the left ureterovesical junction (UVJ), which was confirmed on other images. No filling defect is seen in the visualized portion of the upper tract urothelium. **b** Coronal T1-weighted gadolinium MRU (TR=6.3 ms, TE=1.4 ms) demonstrates excretion from the functioning right kidney and a normal-caliber right ureter. The obstructed left kidney (*arrows*) is not functioning.

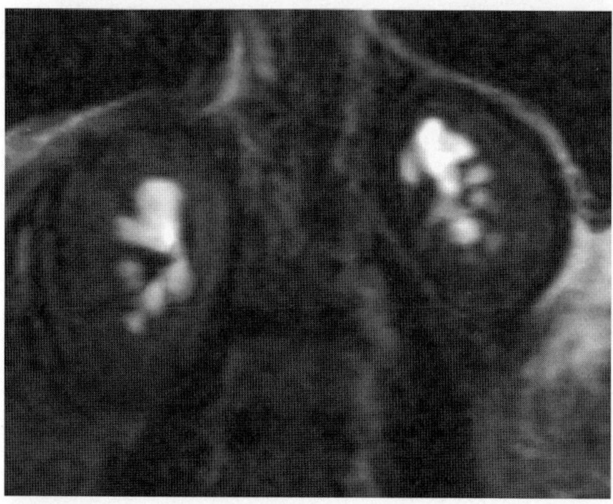

Fig. 4.28. Bilateral hydronephrosis in a 42-year-old woman. Coronal half-Fourier heavily T2-weighted MR hydrogram (TR=not meaningful, TE=431 ms) demonstrates fullness in both renal collecting systems. No calyceal or pelvic filling defect is present. In this case, hydronephrosis was due to compression from the patient's abnormal retroperitoneal soft tissue masses (not depicted), which were malignant histiocytes.

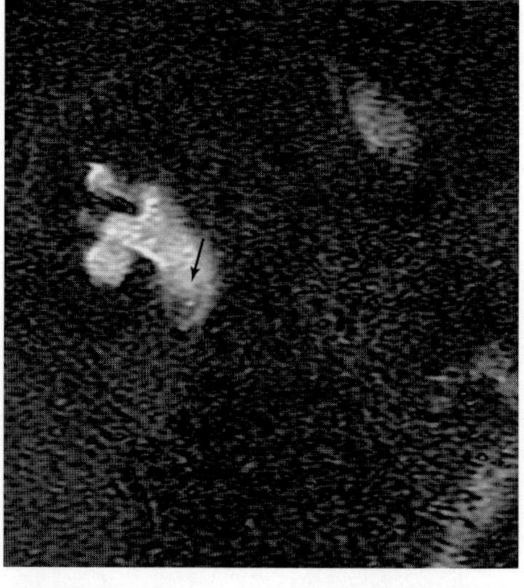

Fig. 4.29. Hematuria in a 56-year-old woman. Coronal half-Fourier heavily T2-weighted MR hydrogram (TR=not meaningful, TE=598 ms) demonstrates filling defect (*arrow*) in right renal pelvis resulting in hydronephrosis. This was obstructing transitional cell carcinoma.

as either multiple thin-section slices or as a single thick slab. Slices afford greater spatial information but, as single-shot half-Fourier images, have lower SNR (Fig. 4.29). These selected slices can then be viewed as an MIP projection to create a single image.

Thick-slab MRU creates a high SNR image, but high T2 signal intensity fluid in the bowel, the thecal sac, or in a dilated renal collecting system may obscure an urothelial tumor. These sequences can be useful in depicting an obstructed collecting system in a non-functioning kidney, but if renal function exists, 3D T1-weighted images of the excreted gadolinium are preferred for detection and characterization of small stones and urothelial tumors with MR imaging (NOLTE-ERNSTING et al. 2001).

4.5
Conclusion

Magnetic resonance imaging is a powerful and versatile tool for single-modality evaluation of potential renal malignancies. A well-planned and executed high-field MR imaging examination can simultaneously detect and characterize a renal neoplasm. Multiphasic post-contrast imaging can generate MRA/MRV/MRU data sets with which, after post-processing, the radiologist can characterize the renal vasculature and stage the tumor. Magnetic resonance imaging also has an important role to play in helping clinicians to select the proper therapy for a renal tumor and in evaluating the patient following therapy. Ongoing advances in MR imaging, including the development of new pulse sequences, the increased availability of whole-body 3-T scanners, and the growing practicality of parallel imaging techniques will likely expand the role of MR imaging in imaging patients with known or suspected renal malignancies.

References

Anzal Y, Piccoli CW, Outwater EK (2003) Evalution of neck and body metastases to nodes with Furumoxtran 10-enhanced MR Imaging: phase III safety and efficacy study. Radiology 228:777–788

Aslam Sohaib SA, Teh J, Nargund VH et al. (2002) Assessment of tumor invasion of the vena caval wall in renal cell carcinoma cases by magnetic resonance imaging. J Urol 167:1271–1275

Balci NC, Semelka RC, Patt RH et al. (1999) Complex renal cysts: findings on MR imaging. Am J Roentgenol 172:1495–1500

Bechtold RE, Zagoria RJ (1997) Imaging approach to staging of renal cell carcinoma. Urol Clin North Am 24:507–522

Binkert CA, Debatin JF, Schneider E et al. (2001) Can MR measurement of renal artery flow and renal volume predict the outcome of percutaneous transluminal renal angioplasty? Cardiovasc Intervent Radiol 24:233–239

Blute ML, Amling CL, Bryant SC et al. (2000) Management and extended outcome of patients with synchronous bilateral solid renal neoplasms in the absence of von Hippel-Lindau disease. Mayo Clin Proc 75:1020–1026

Bono AV, Lovisolo JA (1997) Renal cell carcinoma-diagnosis and treatment: state of the art. Eur Urol 31 (Suppl 1):47–55

Bosniak MA (1991) The small (≤3.0 cm) renal parenchymal tumor: detection, diagnosis, and controversies. Radiology 179:307–317

Buzzas GR, Shield CF III, Pay NT et al. (1997) Use of gadolinium-enhanced, ultrafast, three-dimensional, spoiled gradient-echo magnetic resonance angiography in the preoperative evaluation of living renal allograft donors. Transplantation 64:1734–1737

Bydder M, Larkman DJ, Hajnal JV (2002) Generalized SMASH imaging. Magn Reson Med 47:160–170

Carroll TJ, Grist TM (2002) Technical developments in MR angiography. Radiol Clin North Am 40:921–951

Casper KA, Donnelly LF, Chen B et al. (2002) Tuberous sclerosis complex: renal imaging findings. Radiology 225:451–456

Choyke PL (1997) Detection and staging of renal cancer. Magn Reson Imaging Clin North Am 5:29–47

Choyke PL, Walther MM, Wagner JR et al. (1997) Renal cancer: preoperative evaluation with dual-phase three-dimensional MR angiography. Radiology 205:767–771

Choyke PL, Dwyer AJ, Knopp MV (2003) Functional tumor imaging with dynamic contrast-enhanced magnetic resonance imaging. J Magn Reson Imaging 17:509–520

Chu WC, Lam WW, Chan KW et al. (2004) Dynamic gadolinium-enhanced magnetic resonance urography for assessing drainage in dilated pelvicalyceal systems with moderate renal function: preliminary results and comparison with diuresis renography. BJU Int 93:830–834

Clark PE, Schover LR, Uzzo RG et al. (2001) Quality of life and psychological adaptation after surgical treatment for localized renal cell carcinoma: impact of the amount of remaining renal tissue. Urology 57:252–256

Corica FA, Iczkowski KA, Cheng L et al. (1999) Cystic renal cell carcinoma is cured by resection: a study of 24 cases with long-term followup. J Urol 161:408–411

Corman JM, Penson DF, Hur K et al. (2000) Comparison of complications after radical and partial nephrectomy: results from the National Veterans Administration Surgical Quality Improvement Program. BJU Int 86:782–789

Curry NS (2002) Imaging the small renal mass. Abdom Imaging 27:629–636

D'Armiento M, Damiano R, Feleppa B (1997) Elective conservative surgery for renal carcinoma versus radical nephrectomy: a prospective study. Br J Urol 79:15–19

Debatin JF, Sostman HD, Knelson M et al. (1993) Renal magnetic resonance angiography in the preoperative detection of supernumerary renal arteries in potential kidney donors. Invest Radiol 28:882–889

DeKernion JB, Mukame E (1987) Selection of initial therapy for renal cell carcinoma. Cancer 60:539–546

Dong Q, Schoenberg SO, Carlos RC et al. (1999) Diagnosis of renal vascular disease with MR angiography. Radiographics 19:1535–1554

Edmunds TB Jr, Schulsinger DA, Durand DB et al. (2000) Acute histologic changes in human renal tumors after cryoablation. J Endourol 14:139–143

Eilenberg SS, Lee JKT, Brown JJ et al. (1990) Renal masses: evaluation with gradient-echo Gd-DTPA-enhanced dynamic MR imaging. Radiology 176:333–338

El-Diasty T, Mansour O, Farouk A (2003) Diuretic contrast-enhanced magnetic resonance urography versus intravenous urography for depiction of nondilated urinary tracts. Abdom Imaging 28:135–145

El-Galley R (2003) Surgical management of renal tumors. Radiol Clin North Am 41:1053–1065

Ergen FB, Hussain HK, Caoili EM et al. (2004) MRI for pre-operative staging of renal cell carcinoma using the 1997 TNM classification: comparison with surgical and pathologic staging. Am J Roentgenol 182:217–225

Fain SB, King BF, Breen JF et al. (2001) High spatial resolution contrast enhanced MR angiography of the renal arteries: a prospective comparisons with digital subtraction angiography. Radiology 218:481–490

Farrell MA, Charboneau WJ, DiMarco DS et al. (2003) Imaging-guided radiofrequency ablation of solid renal tumors. Am J Roentgenol 180:1509–1513

Fein AB, Lee JDT, Balfe DM et al. (1987) Diagnosis and staging of renal cell carcinoma. A comparison of MR imaging and CT. Am J Roentgenol 148:749–753

Fergany AF, Hafez KS, Novick AC (2000) Long-term results of nephron sparing surgery for localized renal cell carcinoma: 10-year follow-up. J Urol 163:442–445

Firmin D, Keegan J (2002) The use of navigator echoes in cardiovascular magnetic resonance and factors affecting their implementation. In: Manning WJ, Pennell DJ (eds) Cardiovascular magnetic resonance. Churchill Livingstone, Philadelphia, pp 186–195

Gandy SJ, Sudarshan TA, Sheppard DG et al. (2003) Dynamic MRI contrast enhancement of renal cortex: a functional assessment of renovascular disease in patients with renal artery stenosis. J Magn Reson Imaging 18:461–466

Ghavamian R, Zincke H (2001) Open surgical partial nephrectomy. Semin Urol Oncol 19:103–113

Giessing M, Kroencke TJ, Taupitz M et al. (2003) Gadolinium-enhanced three-dimensional magnetic resonance angiography versus conventional digital subtraction angiography: Which modality is superior in evaluating living kidney donors? Transplantation 76:1000–1002

Gofrit ON, Shapiro A, Kovalski N et al. (2001) Renal cell carcinoma: evaluation of the 1997 TNM system and recommendations for follow-up after surgery. Eur Urol 39:669–674

Guillonneau B, Bermudez H, Gholami S et al. (2001) Laparoscopic partial nephrectomy for renal tumor: single center experience comparison clamping and no clamping techniques of the renal vasculature. J Urol 169:483–486

Hafex KS, Fergany AF, Novick AC et al. (1999) Nephron sparing surgery for localized renal cell carcinoma: impact of tumor size on patient survival, tumor recurrence and TNM staging. J Urol 162:1930–1933

Halpern EJ, Mitchell DG, Wechsler RJ et al. (2000) Preoperative evaluation of living renal donors: comparison of CT angiography and MR angiography. Radiology 216:434–439

Hartman DS, Weatherby E III, Laskin WB et al. (1986) Cystic renal cell carcinoma. Urology 28:145–158

Hayes C, Padhani AR, Leach MO (2002) Assessing changes in tumor vascular function using dynamic contrast-enhanced magnetic resonance imaging. NMR Biomed 15:154–163

Heidemann RM, Ozsarlak O, Parizel PM et al. (2003) A brief review of parallel magnetic resonance imaging. Eur Radiol 13:2323–2337

Heiss SG, Shifrin RY, Sommer FG (2000) Contrast-enhanced three-dimensional fast spoiled gradient-echo renal MR imaging: evaluation of vascular and nonvascular disease. Radiographics 20:1341–1352

Helenon O, Merran S, Paraf F et al. (1997) Unusual fat-containing tumors of the kidney: a diagnostic dilemma. Radiographics 17:129–144

Hinshaw JL, Lee Jr FT (2004) Image-guided ablation of renal cell carcinoma. Magn Reson Imaging Clin North Am 12:429–448

Ho VB, Allen SF, Hood MN et al. (2002) Renal masses: quantitative assessment of enhancement with dynamic MR imaging. Radiology 224:695–700

Hollenbeck BK, Wolf JS Jr (2001) Laparoscopic partial nephrectomy. Semin Urol Oncol 19:123–132

Hosokawa Y, Kinouchi T, Sawai Y et al. (2002) Renal angiomyolipoma with minimal fat. Int J Clin Oncol 7:120–123

Hricak H, Thoeni RF, Carroll R (1988) Detection and staging of renal neoplasms a reassessment of MR imaging. Radiology 166: 643–649

Huang AJ, Lee VS, Rusinek H (2003) MR imaging of renal function. Radiol Clin North Am 41:1001–1017

Huang AJ, Lee VS, Rusinek H (2004) Functional renal MR imaging. Magn Reson Imaging Clin N Am 12:469-486

Huang CL, Liu GC, Sheu RS et al. (1994) Magnetic resonance imaging and computed tomography of transitional cell carcinoma of renal pelvis and ureter. Gaoxiong Yi Xue Ke Xue Za Zhi 10:194–202

Hussain SM, Kock MC, Ijzermans JN et al. (2003) MR imaging: a "one-stop shop" modality for preoperative evaluation of potential living kidney donors. Radiographics 23:505–520

Israel GM, Bosniak MA (2003a) Follow-up CT of moderately complex cystic lesions of the kidney (Bosniak category IIF). Am J Roentgenol 181:627–633

Israel GM, Bosniak MA (2003b) Renal imaging for diagnosis and staging of renal cell carcinoma. Urol Clin North Am 30:499–514

Israel GM, Bosniak MA (2004) MR imaging of cystic renal masses. Magn Reson Imaging Clin N Am 12:403–412

Itano NB, Blute ML, Spotts B et al. (2000) Outcome of isolated renal cell carcinoma fossa recurrence after nephrectomy. J Urol 164:322–325

Janetschek G, Daffner P, Peschel R et al. (1998) Laparoscopic nephron sparing surgery for small renal cell carcinoma. J Urol 159:1152–1155

Jinzaki M, Tanimoto A, Narimatsu Y et al. (1997) Angiomyolipoma: imaging findings in lesions with minimal fat. Radiology 205:497–502

John G, Semelka RC, Burdeny DA et al. (1997) Renal cell cancer: incidence of hemorrhage on MR images in patients with chronic renal insufficiency. J Magn Reson Imaging 7:157–160

Jung P, Brauers A, Nolte-Ernsting CA et al. (2000) Magnetic resonance urography enhanced by gadolinium and diuretics: a comparison with conventional urography in diagnosing the cause of ureteric obstruction. BJU Int 86:960–965

Kallman DA, King BF, Hattery RR et al. (1992) Renal vein and inferior vena cava thrombus in renal cell carcinoma: CT, US, MRI and venacavagraphy. J Comput Assist Tomogr 16:240–247

Kanematsu M, Hoshi H, Imaeda T et al. (1996) Renal pelvic and ureteral carcinoma with huge hydronephrosis: US, CT, and MR findings. Radiat Med 14:321–323

Kawashima A, Glockner JF, King Jr BF (2003) CT urography and MR urography. Radiol Clin N Am 41:945–961

Kearney GP, Waters RB, Klein LA et al. (1981) Results of IVC resection for renal cell carcinoma. J Urol 125:769–773

Kocak M, Sudakoff GS, Erickson S et al. (2001) Using MR angiography for surgical planning in pelvic kidney renal cell carcinoma. Am J Roentgenol 177:659–660

Laissy JP, Menegazzo D, Debray MP et al. (2000) Renal carcinoma: diagnosis of venous invasion with Gd-enhanced MR venography. Eur Radiol 10:1138–1143

Lewin JS, Connell CF, Duerk JL et al. (1998) Interactive MRI-guided radiofrequency interstitial thermal ablation of abdominal tumors: clinical trial for evaluation of safety and feasibility. J Magn Reson Imaging 8:40–47

Licht MR, Novick AC, Goormastic M (1994) Nephron-sparing surgery in incidental versus suspected renal cell carcinoma. J Urol 152:39–42

Lin FH, Kwong KK, Belliveau JW et al. (2004) Parallel imaging reconstruction using automatic regularization. Magn Reson Med 51:559–567

Lockhart ME, Smith JK (2003) Technical considerations in renal CT. Radiol Clin North Am 41:863–875

Low RN, Martinez AG, Steinberg SM et al. (1998) Potential renal transplant donors: evaluation with gadolinium-enhanced MR angiography and MR enhanced MR angiography. Am J Roentgenol 177:349–355

Maki DD, Birnbaum BA, Chakraborty DP et al. (1999) Renal cyst pseudo-enhancement: beam hardening effects on CT attenuation values. Radiology 213:468–472

McKenzie CA, Lim D, Ransil BJ et al. (2004) Shortening MR image acquisition time for volumetric interpolated breath-hold examination with a recently developed parallel imaging reconstruction technique: clinical feasibility. Radiology 230:589–594

Messing EM, Catalona W (2000) Urothelial tumors of the urinary tract. In: Walsh PC, Retik AB, Vaughan ED Jr, Wein AJ (eds) Campbell's urology, 7th edn. Saunders, Philadelphia, pp 2385–2387

Meyers SP, Talagala SL, Totterman S et al. (1995) Evaluation of the renal arteries in kidney donors: value of three-dimensional phase-contrast MR angiography with maximum-intensity-projection or surface rendering. Am J Roentgenol 164:117–121

Montie JE, Pontes JE, Novick AC et al. (1991) Resection of IVC tumor thrombi from renal cell carcinoma. Am Surg 57:56–61

Murphy DP, Gill IS (2001) Energy-based renal tumor ablation: a review. Semin Urol Oncol 19:133–140

Naito S, Nakashima M, Kimoto Y et al. (1998) Application of microwave tissue coagulator in partial nephrectomy for renal cell carcinoma. J Urol 159:960–962

Nascimento AB, Mitchell DG, Zhang XM et al. (2001) Rapid MR imaging detection of renal cysts: age-based standards. Radiology 221:628–632

Nelson HA, Gilfeather M, Holman JM et al. (1999) Gadolinium-enhanced breathhold three-dimensional time-of-flight renal MR angiography in the evaluation of potential renal donors. J Vasc Interv Radiol 10:175–181

Nguyen BD, Westra WH, Zerhouni EA (1996) Renal cell carcinoma and tumor thrombus neovascularity: MR demonstration with pathologic correlation. Abdom Imaging 21:269–271

Nolte-Ernsting CC, Bucker A, Adam GB et al. (1998) Gadolinium-enhanced excretory MR urography after low-dose diuretic injection: comparison with conventional excretory urography. Radiology 209:147–157

Nolte-Ernsting CC, Adam GB, Gunther RW (2001) MR urography: examination techniques and clinical applications. Eur Radiol 11:355–372

Norris DG (2003) High field human imaging. J Magn Reson Imaging 18:519–529

Oto A, Herts BR, Remer EM et al. (1998) Inferior vena cava tumor thrombus in renal cell carcinoma: staging by MR imaging and impact on surgical treatment. Am J Roentgenol 171:1619–1624

Outwater EK, Bhatia M, Siegelman ES et al. (1997) Lipid in renal clear cell carcinoma: detection on opposed-phase gradient-echo MR images. Radiology 205:103–107

Outwater EK, Blasbalg R, Siegelman ES et al. (1998) Detection of lipid in abdominal tissues with opposed-phase gradient-echo images at 1.5 T: techniques and diagnostic importance. Radiographics 18:1465–1480

Patel SK, Stack CM, Turner DA (1987) Magnetic resonance imaging in staging of renal cell carcinoma. Radiographics 7:703–728

Pretorius ES, Siegelman ES, Ramchandani P et al. (1999) Renal neoplasms amenable to partial nephrectomy: MR imaging. Radiology 212:28–34

Ramdave S, Thomas GW, Berlangieri SU et al. (2001) Clinical role of F-18 fluorodeoxyglucose positron emission tomography for detection and management of renal cell carcinoma. J Urol 166:825–830

Rankin SC, Jan W, Koffman CG (2001) Noninvasive imaging of living related kidney donors: evaluation with CT angiography and gadolinium-enhanced MR angiography. Am J Roentgenol 177:349–355

Rassweiler JJ, Abbou C, Janetschek G et al. (2000) Laparoscopic partial nephrectomy. The European experience. Urol Clin North Am 27:721–736

Remer EM, Weinberg EJ, Oto A (2000) MR imaging of the kidneys after laparoscopic cryoablation. Am J Roentgenol 174:635–640

Reznek RH (1996) Imaging in the staging of renal cell carcinoma. Eur Radiol 6:120–128

Robson CJ, Churchill BM, Anderson W (1969) The results of radical nephrectomy for renal cell carcinoma. J Urol 101:297–301

Rofsky NM, Bosniak MA (1997) MR imaging in the evaluation of small (≤3.0 cm) renal masses. Magn Reson Imaging Clin N Am 5:67–81

Rofsky NM, Lee VS, Laub G et al. (1999) Abdominal MR imaging with a volumetric interpolated breath-hold examination. Radiology 212:876–884

Rohrschneider WK, Haufwe S, Wiesel M et al. (2002) Functional and morphologic evaluation of congenital urinary tract dilation by using combined static-dynamic MR urography: findings in kidneys with a single collecting system. Radiology 224:683–694

Sewell PE, Howard JC, Shingleton WB et al. (2003) Interventional magnetic resonance image-guided percutaneous cryoablation of renal tumors. South Med J 96:708–710

Shinmoto H, Yuasa Y, Tanimoto A et al. (1998) Small renal cell carcinoma: MRI with pathologic correlation. J Magn Reson Imaging 8:690–694

Shokeir AA, El-Diasty T, Eassa W et al. (2004) Diagnosis of noncalcareous hydronephrosis: role of magnetic resonance urography and noncontrast computed tomography. Urology 63:225–229

Silverman SG, Lee BY, Seltzer SE et al. (1994) Small (< 3 cm) renal masses: correlation of spiral CT features and pathologic findings. Am J Roentgenol 163:597–605

Sodickson DK (2002) Clinical cardiovascular magnetic resonance imaging techniques. In: Manning WJ, Pennell DJ (eds) Cardiovascular magnetic resonance. Churchill Livingstone, Philadelphia. pp 18–30

Steinbach F, Stöckle M, Hohenfellner R (1995) Current controversies in nephron sparing surgery for renal cell carcinoma. World J Urol 13:163–165

Steiner MS, Quinlan D, Goldman SM et al. (1990) Leiomyomas of the kidney: presentation of 4 new cases and the role of computerized tomography. J Urol 143:994–998

Teh HS, Ang ES, Wong WC et al. (2003) MR renography using a dynamic gradient-echo sequence and low-dose gadopentetate dimeglumine as an alternative to radionuclide renography. Am J Roentgenol 181:441–450

Tsui KH, Shvarts O, Smith RB et al. (2000) Renal cell carcinoma: prognostic significance of incidentally detected tumors. J Urol 163:426–430

Van den Brink JS, Watanabe Y, Kuhl CK et al. (2003) Implications of SENSE MR in routine clinical practice. Eur J Radiol 46:3–27

Wagner BJ (1997) The kidney: radiologic–pathologic correlation. Magn Reson Imaging Clin N Am 5:13–28

Wagner BJ, Wong-You-Cheong JJ, Davis CJ Jr (1997) Adult renal hamartomas. Radiographics 17:155–169

Wilman AH, Riederer SJ (1997) Performance of an elliptical centric view order for signal enhancement and motion artifact suppression in breath-hold three-dimensional gradient echo imaging. Magn Reson Med 38:793–802

Yamashita Y, Miyazaki T, Hatanaka Y et al. (1995) Dynamic MRI of small renal cell carcinoma. J Comput Assist Tomogr 19:759–765

Yoshimura K, Okubo K, Ichioka K et al. (2001) Laparoscopic partial nephrectomy with a microwave tissue coagulator for small renal tumor. J Urol 165:1893–1896

Zagoria RJ (2003) Percutaneous image-guided radiofrequency ablation of renal malignancies. Radiol Clin North Am 41:1067–1075

Zagoria RJ, Bechtold RE (1997) The role of imaging in staging renal adenocarcinoma. Semin Ultrasound CT MR 18:91–99

Zhang H, Prince MR (2004) Renal MR angiography. Magn Reson Imaging Clin N Am 12:487–504

Zhang J, Pedrosa I, Rofsky NM (2003) MR techniques for renal imaging. Radiol Clin North Am 41:877–907

5 Angiography in Kidney Cancer

Jocelyn A. S. Brookes and Uday Patel

CONTENTS

5.1
Introduction

Modern renal arteriography has become much safer than in the past, with improved catheter design, radiographic contrast agents, and fluoroscopic equipment. Yet the indications for renal arteriography in the evaluation of renal masses have diminished. In the past, renal arteriography was a crucial component for the assessment of renal masses. Now most angiographic services perform few such studies. This is almost entirely due to advances in the cross-sectional imaging modalities, particularly multi-slice computed tomography (CT) and 3D volumetric imaging. In the modern era the role of

J. A. S. Brookes, MRCP, FRCR
Consultant Interventional Radiologist, Department of Radiology, The Middlesex Hospital, UCLH, Mortimer Street, London, W1T 3AA, UK
U. Patel, MRCP, FRCR
Consultant Interventional Radiologist, Department of Radiology, St. George's Hospital and Medical School, Blackshaw Road, London, SW17 0QT, UK

renal arteriography in the context of renal cancer is restricted to vascular mapping prior to therapeutic embolization or, rarely, surgery.

This chapter describes both the historical and modern role of renal arteriography in the assessment of renal cancer.

5.2
History of Angiography for the Assessment of Renal Masses

Radiographic contrast agents were first used experimentally in the 1920s and Dos Santos et al. (1929) reported the first successful angiogram. Through direct percutaneous puncture of the aorta an aortogram was performed. Good visualization was achieved, including the renal arteries and vasculature, but regular clinical use did not arrive until the 1950s. A large series from 1957 included one of the first large sample angiographic descriptions of renal cell carcinoma (Evans 1957). Of 126 angiographic diagnoses of renal cancers, 120 were proved to be correct on subsequent surgery. Subsequent reports, however, were less positive; finding that angiographic differentiation from simple renal cysts, benign renal masses such as angiomyolipoma, or inflammatory disease, for example, xanthogranulomatous pyelonephritis, were problematic. Nevertheless, in the sixth and seventh decades of the twentieth century renal angiography reached its climax in the assessment of renal cancer.

Improvements in angiographic technique and understanding of tumor pathology both led to the growth of renal angiography. Previously, angiographic diagnosis was thought to be technically difficult because it was subject to the morbidity of direct aortic puncture. Aortography also did not provide consistently good opacification of the renal vasculature, and some masses were intrinsically poorly vascular and impossible to separate from non-malignant renal diseases. Improved catheter designs, particularly the development of the Seldinger technique, and better radiographic methods, such as digital subtraction angiography, allowed more refined and consistent renal angiography. With this there was also progress in the theoretical groundings of renal angiography, with clearer definition and understanding of tumor vascularity (GAMMILL et al. 1976).

Analysis of tumor vascularity (or neo-vascularity) underlies the angiographic recognition of all malignancies, including renal cancer (Fig. 5.1). The development of new vessels appears crucial to the growth of malignant tissue and in particular tumor invasion. Existing vessels dilate and new vessels proliferate. Such neo-vessels are pathologically characterized by an absence of a complete smooth muscle. On angiography tumor vessels are described as irregular in outline, with a tortuous meandering course (Fig. 5.2) and random in distribution and branching pattern (Table 5.1). The irregularity of vessel walls may be extreme, forming vascular "lakes" or sinusoids. Abnormal venous communications may also be seen (LEVIN et al. 1976; LEVINE 1995). A separate, and equally important, development was improvement of the safety profile of contrast media (see below).

With these developments renal angiography became an important tool in the 1970s for the workup of renal masses, both for the diagnosis and staging of cancer. Accuracy rates of 75–95% (ELKIN 1990) for diagnosis were reported if small neo-vessels were carefully sought. Angiography (especially venography) was also used for staging, as there was no alternative prior to the advent of the cross-sectional modalities; however, smaller, or earlier-stage tumors, were still diagnostically difficult (Fig. 5.3), as were those cancers that were intrinsically less vascular, such as papillary cell cancers or cystic renal cell cancers (Fig. 5.4). Furthermore, some benign renal masses, e.g., angiomyolipoma, also depicted tumor neo-vascularity (Fig. 5.5). Pharmacoangiography was an attempt to further improve the sensitivity of renal angiography. Vascular dilators, such as glycerine trinitrate, were used to open up all renal vessels and conversely intra-renal injection of epinephrine (adrenaline) was used to selectively close "normal" renal arterioles, leaving the less responsive tumor neo-vessels open (ABRAHMS 1964).

These methods improved diagnostic accuracy, but the arrival of the cross-sectional modalities from the early 1980s onwards exposed the poor performance of renal angiography in the evalua-

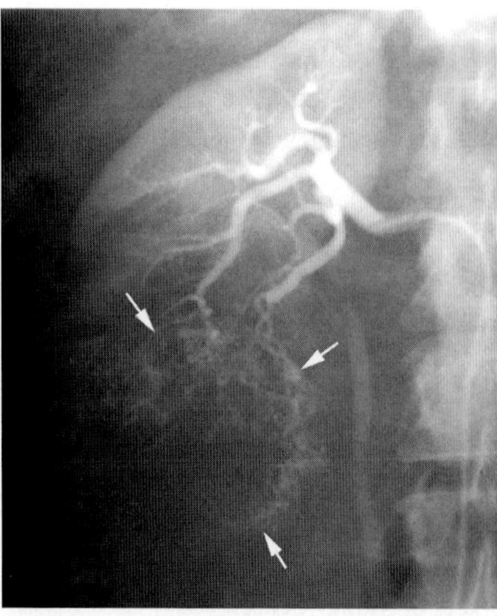

Fig. 5.1. Renal cell carcinoma in a 67-year-old man who presented with macroscopic hematuria. Anteroposterior selective right renal arteriography image demonstrates typical features of tumor vascularity, including large tortuous and meandering arteries and arterioles and numerous irregular branches (*arrows*), due to a lower pole renal cell carcinoma.

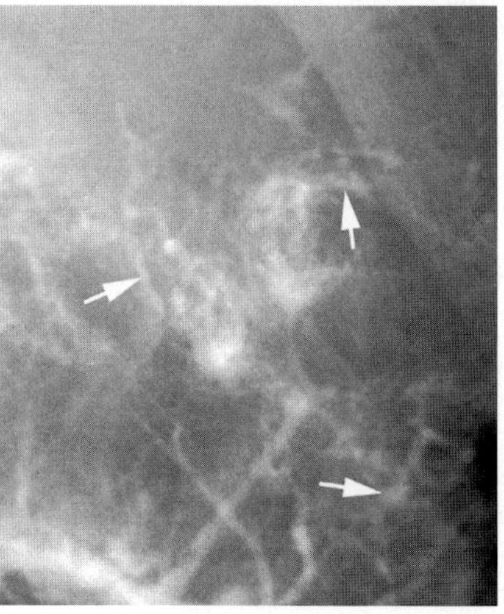

Fig. 5.2. Renal cell carcinoma diagnosed in a 43-year-old man. Anteroposterior magnified view from selective left renal arteriography shows the meandering, irregular features of tumor neovessels (*arrows*).

Table 5.1. Angiographic features of neovascularity

Tortuous arterioles
Meandering or wandering arterioles
Non-tapering arterioles
Irregular widening and narrowing of arterioles
Sinusoidal dilatation of arterioles or vascular "lakes"
Numerous irregular capillaries branching off arterioles
All of the above (but particularly the last) resulting in a tumor blush

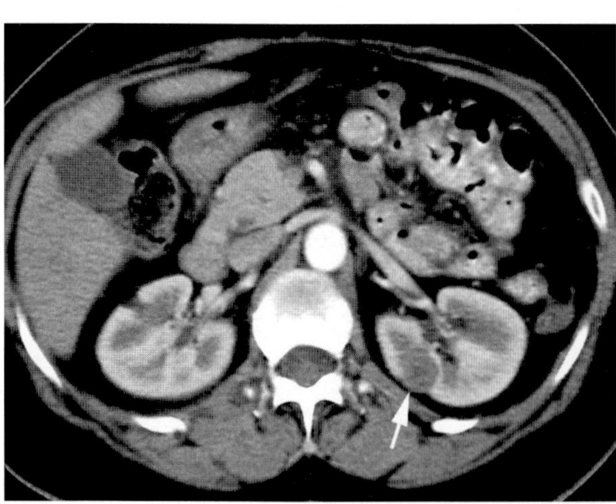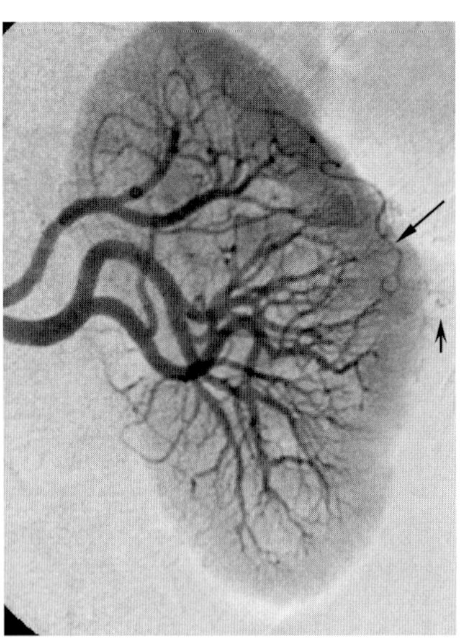

Fig. 5.3a,b. Small renal cell cancer in a 63-year-old woman. This was discovered incidentally on a routine renal ultrasound scan and later confirmed on CT. **a** Axial contrast-enhanced CT scan shows a small (12-mm) left renal mass (*arrow*). Although by CT criteria the mass was diagnosed as a renal tumor, angiography was carried out for pre-surgical vascular mapping. **b** Antero-posterior left angiography image shows hypertrophy of a capsular artery (*long arrow*), which is seen coursing along the renal capsule to supply the mass at the periphery, where a subtle increase in vascularity is seen (*short arrow*). This is a demonstration of how small renal masses are diagnostically difficult on angiography, yet well seen on CT. The superior diagnostic ability of US, CT, and MR imaging, particularly when faced with small renal masses, has displaced the diagnostic role of angiography.

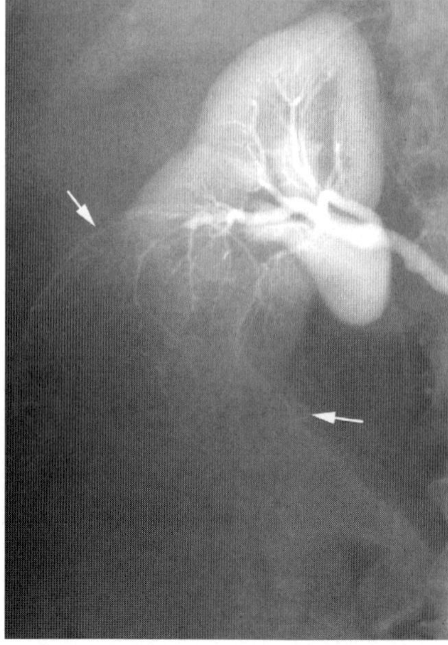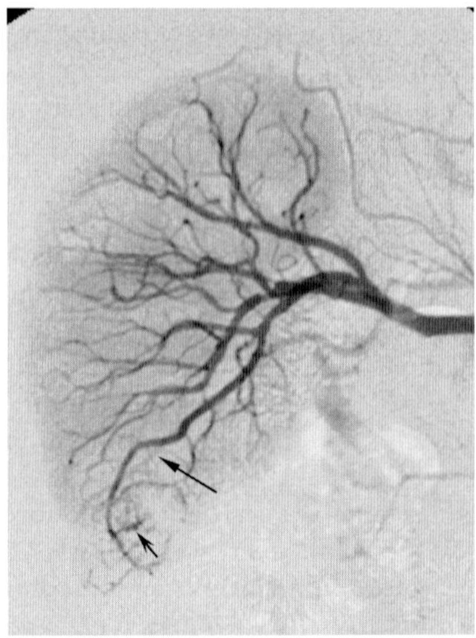

Fig. 5.4. Large cystic renal cell carcinoma arising from the lower pole in a 56-year-old woman. Anteroposterior right angiography image shows deviation of otherwise normal segmental branches (*arrows*) but does not demonstrate any convincing tumor vascularity. Arteriography performs poorly when faced with masses of intrinsically limited vascularity. Examples are cystic renal cell carcinoma or papillary renal cell carcinoma.

Fig. 5.5. Angiomyolipoma in a 69-year-old woman. Initial aortography (not shown) had demonstrated two right renal arteries. Selective renal arteriography was carried out after a catheter was advanced into the main renal artery. Anteroposterior right angiography image demonstrates subtly increased vascularity to the lower pole, with hypertrophy of a branch artery (*long arrow*) and tumor neo-vascularity (*short arrow*). This mass was an angiomyolipoma on histology and the angiogram was carried out prior to surgery. By angiographic criteria this mass is indistinguishable from renal cancer.

tion of renal masses. In the modern era renal angiography is now used very selectively. It retains a place in the evaluation of venous invasion, or in the occasional case with indeterminate or conflicting results from CT, MR imaging, and ultrasound. It may have some value in pre-operative vascular planning as explained below, but mainly it is now used as a prelude to embolization (briefly mentioned below and which is also further covered in Chap. 22).

5.3
Intravascular Contrast Media Used for the Assessment of Kidney Cancer

The fortuitous discovery of the safety and radiographic visibility of iodine led to the development of iodine-based compounds in the 1920s and 1930s. Since then, there have been further chemical refinements, but the fundamental structure of modern contrast media has remained constant: they are all benzene-based compounds with a variable amount of iodine atoms. All iodinated agents are also toxic to a lesser or greater degree. A major factor in contrast toxicity is osmolarity (ASPELIN et al. 2003). Early agents were hyperosmolar agents, but current agents are isoosmolar with high iodine content. This has improved morbidity and diagnostic visualization. Renal toxicity has decreased and patient acceptability is much better.

Yet, the important toxicity in clinical practice is still renal impairment, which is greater with selective intra-arterial injections. Pre-existing renal impairment (particularly a serum creatinine level of >200 mmol/l), diabetes mellitus, the use of renal toxic agents, such as non-steroidal anti-inflammatory agents, arterial disease, the use of ionic contrast media, and dehydration all enhance renal toxicity. Intravenous or oral hydration before and after contrast injection decreases the risk. Of other agents, the use of oral acetyl cysteine has been reported as useful (DERAY 2004; TEPEL and ZIDEK 2002), but further studies have not been confirmatory.

Apart from iodine compounds, the only other angiographic contrast agents used are carbon dioxide (Fig. 5.6; SANDHU et al. 2003) and gadolinium-based agents (KAUFMANN et al. 1999). Carbon dioxide is a negative contrast agent and requires more attention to technical details and special injectors but has the virtue of no renal toxicity and is less

viscous by a factor of 100 (Fig. 5.7). This low viscosity allows it to penetrate smaller arterioles, promising improved visualization of poorly vascular renal cancers, although in practice it has limitations (see below). Gadolinium agents have been used in some cases, although in approved doses it provides much poorer visualization as it has a lower atomic number than iodine. Experimentally, gadolinium agents are also renal toxic in animal studies, although there are insufficient data on this aspect in humans (THOMSEN et al. 2002).

5.4
Selective Renal Angiography

5.4.1
Preparation

The preparation of the patient commences with the first discussion of the decision to undergo angiography (which may be a prelude to therapeutic embolization) and where that fits in with the overall clinical management plan (MOLINE 2000). Signed consent is obtained in the non-operative environment. Blood screens for hematology, "group and

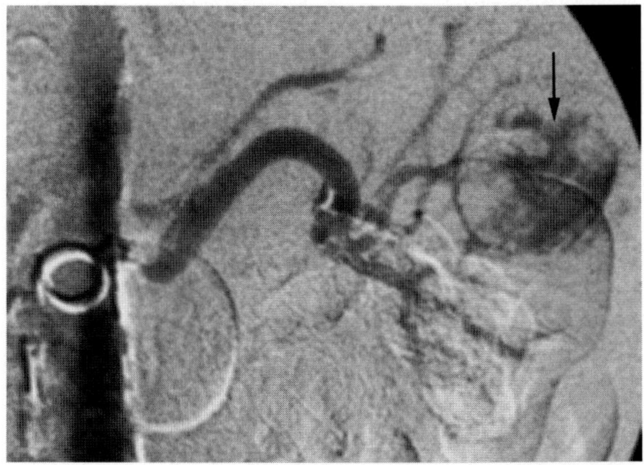

Fig. 5.6. Renal cell carcinoma in a 73-year-old man. Anteroposterior left carbon dioxide (CO_2) angiography image clearly shows the mass in the upper pole (*arrow*) of the kidney which was not visible on conventional contrast injection. As CO_2 is much less viscous than iodinated contrast media, it can penetrate small vessels much better. In practice, this advantage is negated by the peripheral break-up of the CO_2 bolus with degradation of image quality, and many small renal masses are not visible on iodinated or CO_2 arteriography. This inability to angiographically visualize all renal masses limits the use of renal arteriography in the modern era. Nevertheless, it can occasionally be useful.

Fig. 5.7a,b. Stage-III renal cell carcinoma in a 59-year-old man. On CT scan, the right renal vein was thought to be involved, but it was not clear if the inferior vena cava also had tumor thrombus. Magnetic resonance imaging could not be performed because the patient was claustrophobic. **a** Anteroposterior cavography image with iodinated contrast media shows patent inferior vena cava but neither renal vein is seen (*arrow* points to the renal vein ostium). **b** Carbon-dioxide (CO_2) cavography image shows that CO_2 better delineates the extent of right renal vein involvement (*short arrow*), and the tumor is seen to just project into the inferior vena cava (*long arrow*). This was confirmed at operation.

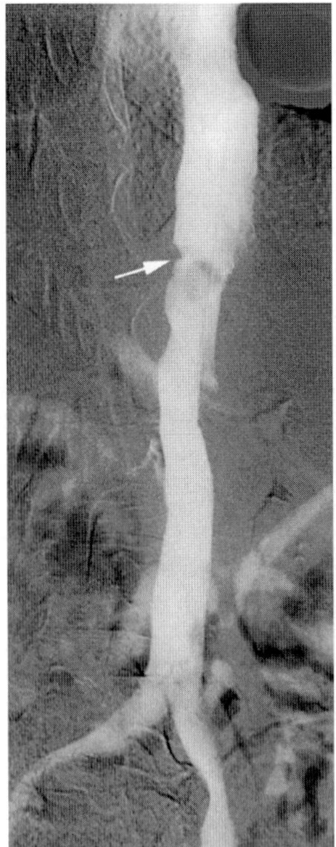

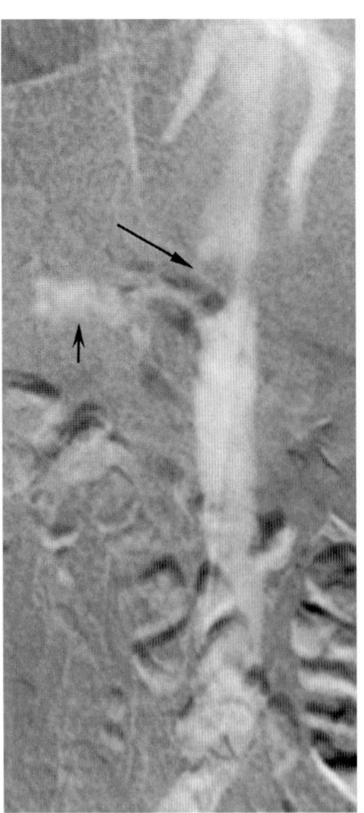

a   b

save," blood chemistry, and coagulation profile are taken. Hydration of the kidneys is the best protection against contrast media nephrotoxicity (see above), but in cases of pre-existing renal failure, there is evidence to suggest a useful role for N-acetyl cysteine, taken orally in two separate doses (600 mg) over the 12 h before the procedure (DERAY 2004; TEPEL and ZIDEK 2002). Light fluid meals are allowed on the day of the procedure, but the patient should be kept "nil by mouth" for 2 h beforehand especially if sedation is planned. Nausea is a common consequence of renal embolization, although it is now rarely seen with modern contrast agents after simple angiography, and an empty stomach is required. An intravenous saline drip should be established to preserve good hydration during this period and to preserve good venous access for sedation. On arrival in the endovascular suite, the patient is checked and cardiovascular monitoring is established.

Light sedo-analgesia (e.g., Midazolam 2–3 mg intravenously and an opiate, such as Fentanyl 50-100 µg intravenously) is commonly used (BARIS et al. 2001). Although for many patients reassurance, constant information, and the soothing voices of well-trained and caring staff provide sufficient anxiolysis (HAGEN et al. 2003), some patients will be irritable and unable to lie still due, for instance, to

flank pain which occurs very soon after successful embolization. In these cases the help of an anesthetist should be sought to provide deeper conscious sedation.

5.4.2
Technique

The right (or left) common femoral artery is punctured (with or without ultrasound guidance) approximately 2 cm inferior to the inguinal ligament, over the femoral head. A hemostatic sheath of 4- or 5-F gauge is inserted, and a 4-F femoro-visceral "cobra"-shaped single-end-hole catheter is advanced over a 0.035-inch hydrophilic wire to the renal artery. The left renal artery is usually at a less acute angle to the aorta than the right. For definitive angiography, a pump injection rate of 20 ml of contrast injected at 5 ml/s is used initially. Hand injections of 10 ml are then sufficient to guide further selective catheterization in the context of therapeutic embolization or vascular mapping. For vascular mapping, first all the renal arteries arising from the aorta are individually identified and injected. Next the anterior and posterior divisions of the main renal artery are injected, to define whether the tumor has a unidivisional supply or not. Further selective injections may be required to define the tumor-supplying segmental branches. It is important to avoid vascular spasm during selective angiographic mapping, and glyceryl trinitrate or an alternative vasodilator should be used as necessary. Well-mapped tumor supply is then evaluated for planning surgery or embolization.

Digital subtraction angiographic (DSA) imaging is continued through to the venous phase and repeated in anteroposterior and right anterior oblique planes. Rotational angiography is better, if available, to obtain all possible oblique planes of view with one dose of contrast and one radiation exposure (SEYMOUR et al. 2001). Newer endovascular angiography suites provide single-acquisition rotational 3D angiography, which can provide interactive 3D models for assistance in reaching awkward, super-selective destinations (HAGEN et al. 2003).

For studying the inferior vena cava (IVC), it is preferable to carry out a separate venous puncture rather than depend on the venous opacification after an arterial injection. The right (or left) femoral vein is punctured under ultrasound guidance, or blindly using anatomical markings, and a 4- to 5-F pigtail catheter is advanced over a guidewire till it rests in the lower IVC. Iodinated contrast is than injected using a pump. A volume of 40 ml pumped at 15 ml/s provides adequate visualization. Visualization is further improved if the study is carried out under Valsalva maneuver.

5.4.3
Renal Embolization

Having established an angiographic roadmap of the renal vascular tree, embolization can then be undertaken if clinically indicated. The prerequisite of embolization of active bleeding sites or prophylactic embolization of potential bleeding sites is to obtain a stable catheter foothold as close to the target as possible so as to control the entire target circulation while causing the least "collateral damage" to benign tissue.

Stability of the catheter is essential to allow safe extrusion of the embolic material, be it alcohol, thrombogenic coils, PVA particles, microspheres, Gelfoam pledgets or cyanoacrylate glue. With the use of hydrophilic-coated 4-F catheters it is rarely necessary to resort to coaxially delivered microcatheters to reach even the most distally situated target vessel. Great care with wire positioning is necessary to avoid inadvertent renal perforation,

the catastrophic effects of which may only manifest after the withdrawal of the catheter and wire at the end of the procedure.

As in all situations of acute unstable arterial bleeding, the effective embolization of the bleeding site results in near instantaneous recovery of the monitored hemodynamic parameters.

Where the embolization is prophylactic or palliative, the first response to embolization may be the onset of ischemic pain in the flanks. This should be anticipated in the sedative cocktail (see above) and titrated against the patient response as necessary. As mentioned above, in the acute situation or with a fragile patient, the assistance of an anesthetist to optimize sedation and analgesia is good practice.

5.4.4
Finishing the Procedure

Having obtained angiographic images on completion of the procedure, the catheter and wire are withdrawn. The sheath is removed and manual pressure is applied proximal to the puncture site for 15 min. If, however, the patient is irritable, unstable, obtunded, or due for transfer to theatre, any one of several arterial closure devices can be used to seal the puncture site and avoid predictable hematoma, pseudoaneurysm, and the rare but real complication of exsanguination. Closure devices are broadly of three designs: thrombin plugs; arterial wall staple; or arterial wall suture. The latter design carries the advantage of permitting instant re-puncture, if necessary, whereas the others require 3 months before re-puncture can be attempted (JONES and McCUTCHEON 2004; VAITKUS 2002).

5.4.5
Aftercare

The patient is required to remain flat in bed for 4 h following manual hemostasis or 30 min after a closure device has been placed. Most patients requiring embolization in the context of renal cancer require close clinical monitoring following the procedure, in particular to manage discomfort and pain. Infarction of large volumes of tissue may cause pain, nausea, mild pyrexia, and mild elevation of the white count. This is known as the "post-embolization syndrome" and may persist for up to 3 days after the procedure.

5.5
Angiography in the Evaluation and Management of Renal Masses

5.5.1
Historical Applications

Up till the introduction of the cross-sectional modalities renal masses mostly presented with symptoms. Symptoms were either directly related to the renal tumor, such as hematuria or a palpable loin/abdominal mass (LEVINE 1995), or originated from metastasis such as bone pain or fracture. In other cases a renal cancer was suspected on non-specific systemic symptoms. Consequently, most renal cancers were diagnosed late and at a higher clinical stage. For example, in reviews from the early 1980s only around 10% renal cell cancers were detected at a pre-symptomatic stage (RITCHIE and CHILSHOLM 1983), but in more recent studies around 40% were incidentally detected (ZAGORIA 2000).

Before the advent of cross-sectional imaging, preoperative diagnosis began with an intravenous urography (IVU). The signs of renal cancer on an IVU are those of mass effect with distortion of the renal outline or the calyces, signs that may also be mimicked by any other renal mass including the much more common simple renal cyst (Fig. 5.8). As these signs are non-specific, further investigation is necessary, and the only available next test in the past was renal angiography (Table 5.2). The arteriographic signs of renal cancer are described above (Table 5.1), and for symptomatic masses diagnostic accuracy was believed to be high. Older reviews report figures as high as 95% (ELKIN 1990; EVANS 1957). In one study 78% of renal cancers were seen on angiography (WATSON et al. 1968), and a later study reported an even better accuracy of 90% (LANG et al. 1972), but these data are based on observational and not controlled studies. Figure 5.9 demonstrates the typical angiographic appearances of renal carcinoma; these are little different from those seen with other renal masses such as angiomyolipoma, or other benign conditions such as renal inflammation. Furthermore, not all masses are angiographically visible: Fig. 5.3 shows a smaller renal cancer, and despite a selective angiogram, neovascularity is not seen. The appearances are indistinguishable from those of a renal cyst (Fig. 5.10; USON 1963).

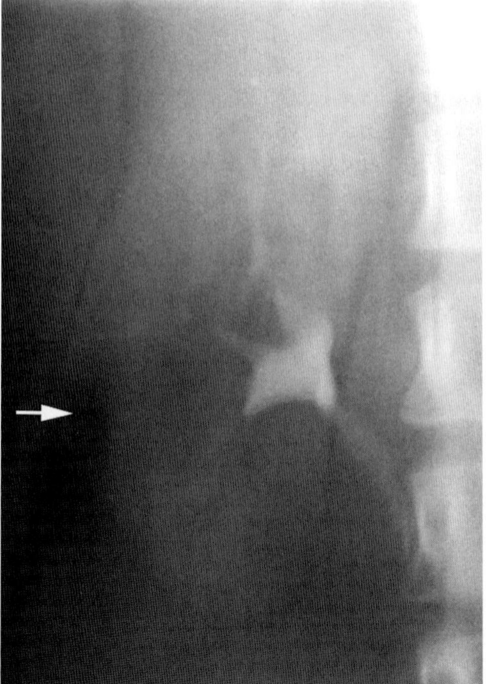
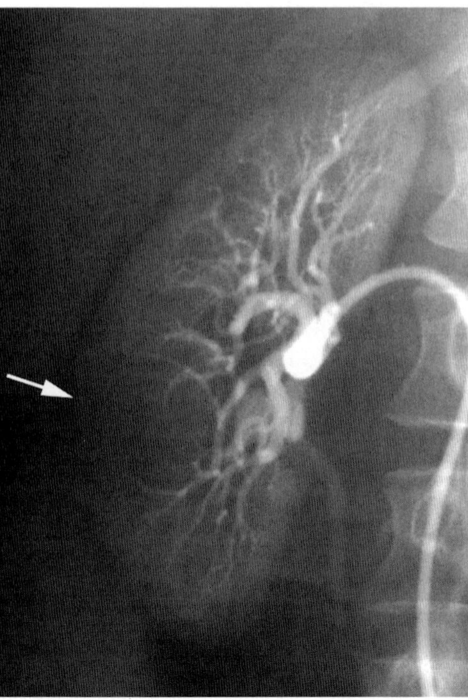

Fig. 5.8a,b. Small renal mass in a 44-year-old man who presented with hematuria. **a** Anteroposterior plain tomographic view from intravenous urography shows the right calyces are splayed by the small renal mass (*arrow*). **b** Corresponding anteroposterior renal angiography image shows splaying of renal arteries (*arrow*) and no evidence of neovascularity. This mass proved to be a simple cyst.

Table 5.2. Value of angiographic assessment in kidney cancer

	Comments
Diagnosis of renal cancer	75–95% accuracy in old series, but accuracy is around 47–61% in modern series as smaller renal masses are more common now
Staging of renal cancer	68–100% in old series; in modern series 36–40%, when compared with CT. Venography still has a limited role
Assessment of renal masses that are intermediate on current CT or MR imaging	Accuracy only 16% in modern series

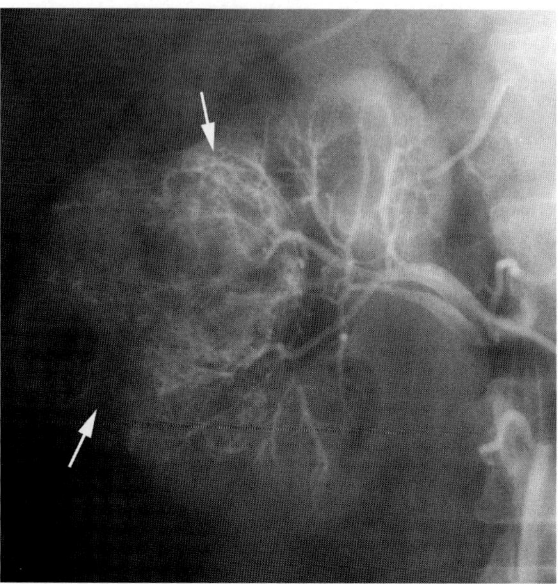

Fig. 5.9. Renal cell cancer in a 57-year-old man. Anteroposterior right angiography image demonstrates typical angiographic features (*arrows*) of renal cell cancer including large tortuous and meandering arteries and arterioles associated with numerous irregular branches.

These limitations of renal angiography become more pressing still with smaller renal masses, the type that form the bulk of contemporary clinical practice, when over half of renal masses are asymptomatic or incidental presentations (LEVINE 1995). In one study only 16% of indeterminate renal cancers were identified on angiography (BALFE et al. 1982). Smaller renal masses are particularly difficult to demonstrate angiographically. Only about half (47%) of renal cancers <3 cm were visualized in one study (YAMASHITA et al. 1992). In another study neovascularity was seen in 8 of 13 (61%) small renal cancers, and the use of carbon dioxide injection better demonstrated neo-vessels in only 1 of 13 tumors (SANDHU et al. 2003); thus, in the modern era renal angiography has a very limited role in the diagnosis of renal cancers, but does have some value

in pre-surgical planning for nephron-sparing surgery, although modern CT and MR imaging are also challenging this role.

Angiography was also used in the past for preoperative staging of renal cancer. The size of the cancer could be measured and invasion of adjacent structures or lymph nodes could be assessed. Regarding venous invasion, either a selective intravenous venography was carried out or delayed images from a selective renal arteriography could be used to image the renal veins and the cava, although less well; however, renal arteriography for staging is relatively insensitive. Although in one report (WEYMAN et al. 1980) angiographic accuracy for staging was 68% for perinephric extension, 79% for renal vein invasion and 100% for caval involvement this study would have involved much larger and more advanced tumors than seen in current practice. These figures would not be reproducible now, and others have reported much poorer accuracies of 40% (DAS et al. 1977) and 36% (BRACKEN and JONSSON 1979). Angiography has now no primary place in the staging of renal cancer either, although the occasional intravenous cavography (Fig. 5.7) is still performed if cross-sectional modalities are non-diagnostic.

Table 5.3. Current indications for renal angiography in kidney cancer

Diagnosis and staging (including cavography)
Therapeutic embolization for post-biopsy bleeding complications

Adjunctive management
  Surgical planning/preparation
  Prophylactic embolization pre-surgery to reduce vascularity (including inferior vena cava tumor thrombus)

Therapeutic embolization
  For post-surgical bleeding complications
  For actively bleeding tumors
  Palliative embolization for unresectable tumors

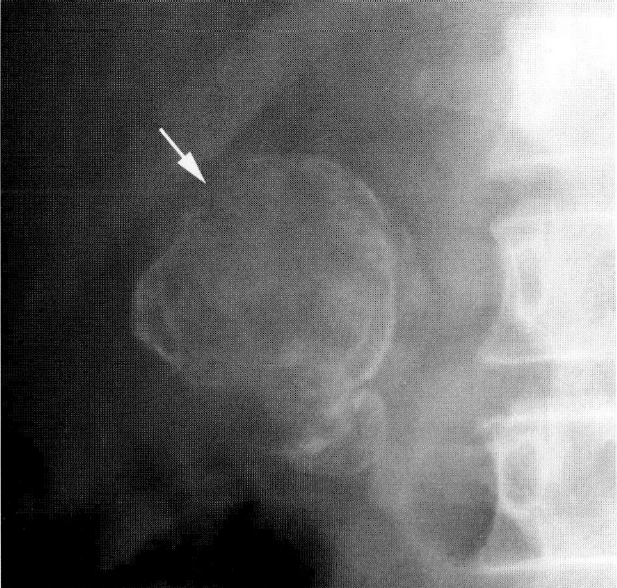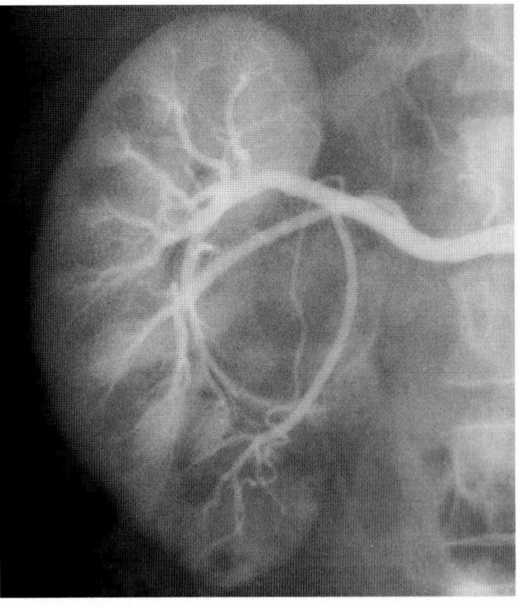

a

b

Fig. 5.10a,b. Calcified renal cell cancer in a 61-year-old woman who presented in 1982. **a** Anteroposterior plain film shows a calcified right renal mass (*arrow*). **b** Corresponding anteroposterior renal angiography image does not demonstrate any features of neovascularity. Computed tomography was not available. On percutaneous biopsy and subsequent histological examination of the nephrectomy specimen this mass proved to be a calcified renal cell cancer.

5.5.2
Current Applications

The current indications for traditional renal angiography are very limited (Table 5.3) and should become less so with the rapid advances in CT and MR angiography. The diagnostic focus has long ago shifted to the non-invasive modalities of ultrasound, CT, and MR imaging (see above). Although there are limited instances where angiography may contribute to diagnosis and staging, it is of secondary importance and presently rarely performed. The main role of renal angiography in the management of renal tumors is chiefly for pre-planning prior to therapeutic embolization, but the occasional case may require vascular planning prior to surgery. Although there are no modern series comparing cavography vs CT or MR imaging, the occasional patient may require cavography to confirm the extent of suspected venous tumor thrombus, particularly its caudal extent (McClennan and Deyoe 1994). In our experience, knowledge of the renal arterial anatomy aids vascular control during partial nephrectomy (Sandhu et al. 2003); however, the limitation, as also discussed above, is that tumor neovascularity of small tumors is poorly seen. In our experience only about half demonstrate clear

tumoral vessels, even with selective injections (Fig. 5.11).

Nevertheless, the likely dominant tumor supply can be predicted from any observed mass effect. From this information the surgeon can be informed of which divisional or segmental branches supply the tumor, and these can be selectively identified and clamped during the operation to reduce intra-operative bleeding. The method used for such angiographic mapping is shown in Fig. 5.12. In patients with suspected abnormal renal anatomy, e.g., renal cell cancer in a horseshoe kidney or pelvic kidney, arteriography will define accessory renal arteries if CT or MR angiography have been inconclusive.

Angiography and embolization is a vital service to support diagnostic renal parenchymal biopsy (Whittier and Korbet 2004). The majority of renal cell cancers are diagnosed accurately on imaging criteria alone, but occasionally core biopsy may be required. The risks associated with performing a percutaneous renal biopsy have substantially decreased in the past two decades because of technical advances in the method; however, significant bleeding complications still occur in 1–2% of cases (Manno et al. 2004). Many post-biopsy hemorrhages can be managed conservatively, as the tough renal capsule contains the hemorrhage, but if there

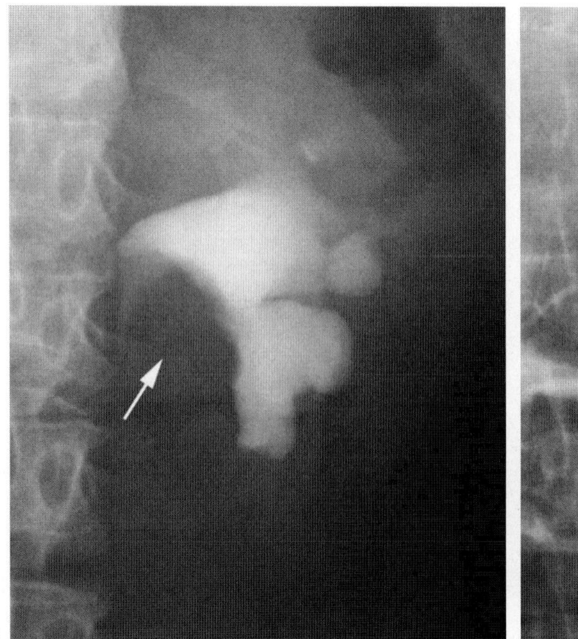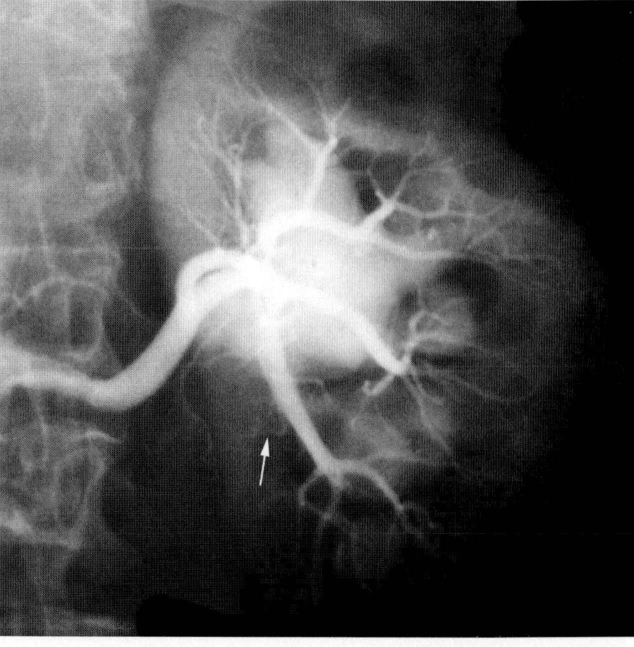

Fig. 5.11a,b. Transitional cell cancer in a 71-year-old man. **a** Anteroposterior intravenous urography image shows that a mass effect (*arrow*) is seen affecting the left renal pelvis resulting in hydronephrosis. **b** Anteroposterior angiography image shows subtle neovascularity (*arrow*). On pathology this mass proved to be a transitional cell cancer of the renal pelvis.

is evidence of a large, continuing renal hemorrhage, than selective renal arteriography as a prelude to embolization should not be delayed.

The place of angiography for surgical planning has now been mostly superseded by MR imaging and CT, particularly with the advances in 3D volumetric rendering (UEDA et al. 2004), but in the context of large and complex renal tumors the literature shows that complete pre-operative renal artery embolization facilitates the excision of large hypervascular vein-invading renal cell carcinomas. In one study patients who underwent pre-operative embolization required less blood transfusion volume (250 vs 800 ml), even though embolized tumors were larger (BAKAL et al. 1993). The authors further concluded that embolization has to be technically meticulous to confer most benefit, underlying the importance of thorough pre-operative angiographic mapping for planning of embolization.

There is also some evidence to suggest that complete pre-operative embolization offers a survival advantage. In a recent study the 5- and 10-year survival rate after embolization was 62 and 47%, respectively, compared with 35 and 23% in those not embolized (ZIELINSKI et al. 2000). The optimal delay between embolization and operation on meta-analysis, is 1 day. The embolization material of choice is chiefly but not exclusively ethanol (KALMAN and VARENHORST 1999, LIN et al. 2003). Angiographic embolization also has a role for the treatment of post-surgical bleeding complications after nephron-sparing surgery (partial nephrectomy or tumor enucleation). Such bleeding may be catastrophic, related to arteriovenous fistulas, and can be controlled by selective arterial embolization (ROY et al. 1999).

Renal embolization offers a minimally invasive means of renal ablation as a primary palliative procedure. In this context it is indicated to control pain, hematuria, IVC obstruction, and paraneoplastic syndromes. Due to the large volume of tissue infarction, an evanescent post-embolization syndrome is common (FICHTNER et al. 2003). Even in the presence of distant metastases, there is evidence to suggest a survival advantage derived from aggressive embolization (ONISHI et al. 2001).

5.6
Conclusion

From occupying a central role in the evaluation of kidney cancer, renal arteriography has been relegated to a problem-solving secondary role in the

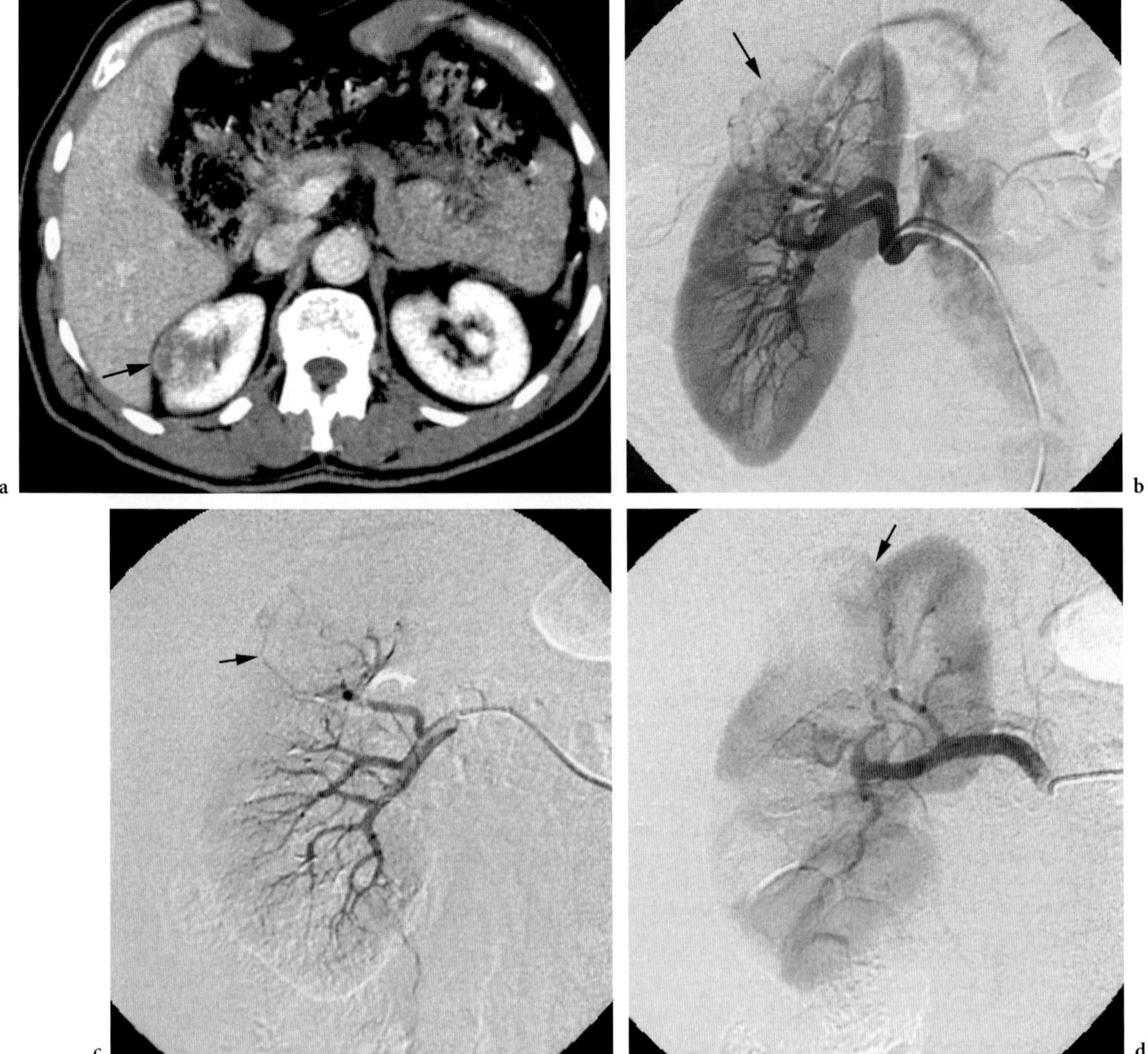

Fig. 5.12a-d. Cystic renal cell cancer in a 63-year-old woman. **a** Axial contrast-enhanced CT scan shows a cystic renal cell cancer close to the right collecting system (*arrow*). Partial nephrectomy was planned. **b** Anteroposterior angiography image shows that the kidney (and tumor, *arrow*) is supplied by a single main renal artery. Super-selective angiography images into the **c** anterior and **d** posterior division branches show that both divisions supply the tumor (*arrows*). Intra-operative vascular control would require clamping of the main renal artery or both divisions. This montage demonstrates the use of selective renal angiography for surgical planning. The knowledge that the tumor is supplied by just one artery can help the surgeon plan vascular control of the renal mass prior to partial nephrectomy.

modern era. This is partly due to the changing presentation of renal tumors; most are now identified at an early stage, and renal arteriography is insensitive when compared with the cross-sectional modalities for evaluation of small renal masses. Arteriography is now seldom used for diagnosis. For staging it may help in the occasional case with indeterminate findings regarding venous involvement on CT and MR imaging. It may have some utility for pre-operative surgical planning, but mostly it is now used for planning of therapeutic or palliative tumor embolization.

References

Abrahms HL (1964) The response of neoplastic renal vessels to epinephrine in man. Radiology 82:217–223

Aspelin P, Aubry P, Fransson S-G, Strasser R, Wilenbrock R, Berg KJ (2003) Nephrotoxic effects in high-risk patients undergoing angiography. N Engl J Med 348:491–499

Bakal CW, Cynamon J, Lakritz PS, Sprayregen S (1993) Value of preoperative renal artery embolization in reducing blood transfusion requirements during nephrectomy for renal cell carcinoma. J Vasc Interv Radiol 4:727–731

Balfe DM, McClennan BL, Stanley RJ, Weyman PJ, Sagel SS (1982) Evaluation of renal masses considered indeterminate on computerised tomography. Radiology 142:421–428

Baris S, Karakaya D, Aykent R, Kirdar K, Sagkan O, Tur A (2001) Comparison of midazolam with or without fentanyl for conscious sedation and hemodynamics in coronary angiography. Can J Cardiol 17:277–281

Bracken B, Jonsson K (1979) How accurate is angiographic staging of renal carcinoma? Urology 14:96–99

Das G, Chisholm GD, Sherwood T (1977) Can angiography stage renal carcinoma? Br J Urol 49:611–614

Deray G (2004) Value of N-acetylcysteine to prevent nephrotoxicity from iodinated contrast agents. J Radiol 85:725–727

Dos Santos R, Lamas A, Caldas JP (1929) Arteriography of the aorta and the abdominal blood vessels. Bull Mem Soc Nat Chir 55:587–601

Elkin M (1990) Stages in the growth of uroradiology. Radiology 175:297–306

Evans AT (1957) Renal cancer: translumber arteriography for its recognition. Radiology 69:657–662

Fichtner J, Swoboda A, Hutschenreiter G, Neuerburg J (2003) Percutaneous embolization of the kidney: indications and clinical results. Aktuelle Urol 34:475–477

Gammill SL, Shipkey FH, Himmelfarb EH, Parvey LS, Rabinowitz JG (1976) Roentgenology–pathology correlative study of neovascularity. Am J Roentegenol 126:376–385

Hagen G, Wadstrom J, Magnusson A (2003) 3D rotational angiography of transplanted kidneys. Acta Radiol 44:193–198

Jones T, McCutcheon H (2004) A meta-analysis of percutaneous vascular closure devices after diagnostic catheterization and percutaneous coronary intervention. J Invasive Cardiol 16:243–246

Kalman D, Varenhorst E (1999) The role of arterial embolization in renal cell carcinoma. Scand J Urol Nephrol 33:162–170

Kaufmann JA, Geller SC, Bazari H, Waltman AC (1999) Gadolinium based contrast agents as an alternative at vena cavography in patients with renal insufficiency: early experiences. Radiology 212:280–284

Lang EK, Johnson B, Chance HL, Enright JR, Fontenot R, Trichel BE, Martin EC (1972) Assessment of avascular renal masses: the use of nephrotomography, arteriography, cyst puncture, double contrast study and histochemical and histopathologic examination of the aspirate. South Med J 65:1–10

Levin DC, Gordon D, Kinkhabwala M, Becker JA (1976) Reticular neovascularity in malignant and inflammatory renal masses. Radiology 120:61–68

Levine E (1995) Renal cell carcinoma: clinical aspects, imaging diagnosis and staging. Semin Roentgenol 30:128–148

Lin PH, Terramani TT, Bush RL, Keane TE, Moore RG, Lumsden AB (2003) Concomitant intraoperative renal artery embolization and resection of complex renal carcinoma. J Vasc Surg 38:446–450

Manno C, Strippoli GF, Arnesano L, Bonifati C, Campobasso N, Gesualdo L, Schena FP (2004) Predictors of bleeding complications in percutaneous ultrasound-guided renal biopsy. Kidney Int 66:1570–1577

McClennan BL, Deyoe LA (1994) The imaging evaluation of renal cell carcinoma: diagnosis and staging. Radiol Clin North Am 32:55–69

Moline LR (2000) Patient psychologic preparation for invasive procedures: an integrative review. J Vasc Nurs 18:117–122

Onishi T, Oishi Y, Suzuki Y, Asano K (2001) Prognostic evaluation of transcatheter arterial embolization for unresectable renal cell carcinoma with distant metastasis. BJU Int 87:312–315

Ritchie AW, Chisholm GD (1983) The natural history of renal carcinoma. Semin Oncol 10:390–400

Roy C, Tuchmann C, Morel M, Saussine C, Jacqmin D, Tongio J (1999) Is there still a place for angiography in the management of renal mass lesions? Eur Radiol 9:329–335

Sandhu C, Belli AM, Patel U (2003) Demonstration of renal arterial anatomy and tumor neovascularity for vascular mapping of renal cell carcinoma: the value of CO2 angiography. Br J Radiol 76:89–93

Seymour HR, Matson MB, Belli AM, Morgan R, Kyriou J, Patel U (2001) Rotational digital subtraction angiography of the renal arteries: technique and evaluation in the study of native and transplant renal arteries Br J Radiol 74:134–141

Tepel M, Zidek W (2002) Acetylcysteine and contrast media nephropathy. Curr Opin Nephrol Hypertens 11:503–506

Thomsen HS, Almen T, Morcos SK (2002) Gadolinium containing contrast media for radiographic examinations: a position paper. Eur Radiol 12:2600–2605

Ueda T, Tobe T, Yamamoto S, Motoori K, Murakami Y, Igarashi T, Ito H (2004) Selective intra-arterial three-dimensional computed tomography angiography for pre-operative evaluation of nephron-sparing surgery. J Comput Assist Tomogr 28:496–504

Uson AC, Melicow MM, Lattimer JK (1963) Is renal arteriography a reliable test in the differential diagnosis between renal cysts and neoplasms? J Urol 89:554–559

Vaitkus PT (2002) Effectiveness of mechanical compression devices in attaining hemostasis after femoral sheath removal. Am J Crit Care 11:155–162

Watson RC, Fleming RJ, Evans JA (1968) Arteriography in the diagnosis of renal cell carcinoma: review of 100 cases. Radiology 91:888–897

Weyman PJ, McClennan BL, Stanley RJ, Levitt RG, Sagel SS (1980) Comparison of computed tomography and angiography in the evaluation of renal cell carcinoma. Radiology 137:417–424

Whittier WL, Korbet SM (2004) Renal biopsy: update. Curr Opin Nephrol Hypertens 13:661–665

Yamashita Y, Takahashi M, Watanabe O, Yoshimatsu S, Ueno S, Ishimaru S, Kan M, Takano S, Ninomiya M (1992) Small renal cell carcinoma: pathologic and radiologic correlation. Radiology 184:493–498

Zagoria RJ (2000) Imaging of small renal masses. A medical success story. Am J Roentgenol 175:945–955

Zielinski H, Szmigielski S, Petrovich Z (2000) Comparison of preoperative embolization followed by radical nephrectomy with radical nephrectomy alone for renal cell carcinoma Am J Clin Oncol 23:6–12

6 PET and PET/CT in Kidney Cancer

Christiaan Schiepers

CONTENTS

6.1
Introduction

Renal cell carcinoma (RCC) is not a common disease, having an incidence of about 3% of all cancers. In the U.S. 35,710 new cases were diagnosed in 2004, and 12,480 are expected to die from their disease. There is a gender difference with more men affected than women. The male-to-female ratio is 1.620 for incidence and 1.707 for mortality. Advanced renal cell cancer carries a poor prognosis (Jemal et al. 2004). New treatment strategies, such as immunotherapy, are being employed in an attempt to delay the progression of disease but remain controversial (Figlin et al. 1999). Non-invasive tests for diagnosing, staging, and monitoring the course of disease are desirable.

Various imaging modalities, such as radiography, computed tomography (CT), magnetic resonance (MR) imaging, ultrasound (US), and positron emission tomography (PET), are available for diagnosis and staging of RCC. PET is based on imaging of biochemical processes in vivo, and creates tomographic cuts similar to CT and MR imaging. PET is unique because it supplies an image representing the metabolic activity of the underlying tissue processes. PET has been in existence since the 1960s, and gained clinical acceptance in the mid 1990s.

Considerable effort has been invested in improving preoperative staging by using tomographic imaging. Anatomic modalities are excellent for detecting neoplasms but fail to reliably distinguish between benign and malignant tumors. Metabolic imaging using the glucose analogue ^{18}F-fluorodeoxy-glucose (FDG) is currently used for staging of a variety of malignancies. The first well-established application of PET was the characterization of solitary pulmonary nodules or chest masses (Coleman 2002; Wahl 1999), yielding high sensitivity and specificity (Gould et al. 2001), and staging of the mediastinum in lung cancer (Dwamena et al. 1999). PET using FDG is reimbursed by the Centers for Medicare and Medicaid for lung, breast, colorectal, head and neck, thyroid, and esophageal cancer, lymphoma, and melanoma. PET using FDG for RCC is not an approved imaging procedure.

The introduction of dual-modality imaging, by combining a CT and PET scanner into one gantry, has further enhanced the clinical armamentarium (Townsend and Cherry 2001). Again, lung cancer was the first neoplasm to be studied in detail and the use of PET/CT in staging and restaging has been established (Lardinois et al. 2003).

The basics of PET are beyond the scope of this chapter. Phelps (2004) provides a standard text for the interested reader and Valk (2003) edited a book focused on the clinical applications.

At present, it is appropriate to speak of correlative imaging, in which all imaging modalities have their specific contribution, and are not seen as competitive modalities. Diagnostic schemes or algorithms for an efficient diagnostic work-up are available for

C. Schiepers, MD, PhD
Professor, Department of Molecular and Medical Pharmacology; Professor, Department of Radiological Sciences, David Geffen School of Medicine at UCLA, 10833 Le Conte Avenue, AR-144 CHS, Los Angeles, CA 90095-6942, USA

common cancers such as lung, breast, and colorectal, but have not been established for renal cell cancer.

6.2
Methods

To perform PET or PET/CT imaging, the following are essential:
1. Injection of the radiopharmaceutical FDG for PET (contrast for CT if requested)
2. Dedicated scanners for the detection of low-energy (CT) and high-energy (PET) photons
3. Computers and monitors with hardware and software for image acquisition, processing, and display

For a description of CT acquisition and processing the reader is referred to Chap. 3. Herein the specifics of PET imaging using FDG are discussed. The clinical protocol used at the University of California at Los Angeles (UCLA) for PET/CT is briefly reviewed.

6.2.1
Uptake Mechanism

The best-known PET radiopharmaceutical for oncological applications is the glucose analogue 2-^{18}F-fluoro-2-deoxy-D-glucose. The ability to non-invasively image glucose utilization is important, since high rates of glycolysis are found in many malignant tumor cells (Warburg 1956; Warburg et al. 1924). Malignant cells also have increased glucose transporters and upregulated hexokinase enzymes. The uptake of FDG varies greatly for different tumor types; however, a high uptake is usually associated with a high number of viable tumor cells and high expression of glucose transporter 1 (GLUT-1). Lung cancer has among the highest expressions of GLUT-1, and therefore is readily detectable, whereas renal cell cancers show the opposite trend (Brown and Wahl 1993; Miyauchi et al. 1996; Wahl 1996).

Increased FDG uptake is by no means specific for neoplasms. Inflammatory processes also have increased uptake, and false-positive results have been reported for tuberculosis, fungal infections, sarcoidosis, non-specific granulomas, suture granulomas, benign fibrous mesotheliomas, acute postoperative changes, radiation changes, abscesses, pancreatitis, and fractures. Kubota et al. (1991,

1992, 1993) studied the uptake of FDG in macrophages and granulation tissue as well as in tumors.

6.2.2
Acquisition

The whole-body imaging mode was introduced in the late 1980s by UCLA and subsequently became the standard for PET imaging in oncology (Dahlbom et al. 1992; Hoh et al. 1993; Hoh et al. 1997). Multiple acquisitions are performed sequentially to encompass the patient's body. The intuitive advantage of this technique is that many cancers are systemic diseases requiring imaging of the entire body. PET images are tomographic and permit full 3D review in the axial, coronal, and sagittal planes. This is the favorite mode of searching for disease outside the limited primary field of view, which is still the standard in CT imaging.

As the photons pass through the tissues, varying degrees of attenuation will affect the final number that reaches the detectors and can be used for imaging. This attenuation effect is corrected for by acquiring a transmission scan, and by calculating the regional attenuation factors. The transmission scan has to be performed separately from the emission scan, and is a lengthy procedure due to the low-photon flux of a positron source. In a PET/CT scanner, the CT images are used to generate the attenuation map. Since the photon flux in CT is an order of 3 to 4 higher than in PET, this takes only a fraction of the transmission scan, e.g., 30–90 s vs 12–30 min. With the current multislice-CT systems, whole-body CT can be acquired in approximately 30 s.

The spatial resolution of a modern CT or MR imaging system is better than that of a PET system; however, this is not the only determining factor in detecting abnormalities. The difference in metabolic activity of the lesion and its surroundings (target-to-background ratio) or the "contrast resolution" helps to find disease; thus, metabolically very active lesions of 3–4 mm have been detected with FDG-PET.

6.2.3
Quantification

Dynamic imaging and biological tracer detection enables PET to measure the tissue concentrations of radiotracer, and to assess the kinetics of physiologic and biochemical processes in vivo. In this respect,

PET is similar to autoradiography. A numerical value or index, representing the local tracer concentration or tracer accumulation rate in a tumor, may characterize that tumor. In addition, serial imaging allows measurement of changes induced by therapy. Dynamic PET imaging and kinetic modeling is still a research tool and not used clinically (PHELPS 2004).

Clinical studies can be analyzed semi-quantitatively by using the standardized uptake value (SUV; KEYES 1995; ZASADNY and WAHL 1993). The SUV is the ratio of the measured radioactivity concentration in a lesion to the estimated body tracer concentration, assuming a uniform distribution. It is generally assumed that tumors achieve a plateau concentration around 1–2 h, at the time of image acquisition. Standardization of the SUV is necessary to compare results between different equipment and between institutions. This SUV parameter offers a more objective way of reporting metabolic activity than visual interpretation. The SUV technique works well for most tumors. Quantification appears especially relevant for monitoring of therapy, i.e., to guide treatment protocols or initiate change of treatment regimen.

6.2.4
Patient Preparation and Diagnostic Protocol

Patients are studied in a prolonged fasting state to produce low insulin levels and induce low rates of glucose utilization of normal tissues, e.g., the normal muscular tissues including the myocardium. Malignant tissues are less dependent on hormone regulation, and thus will have higher uptake when compared with the surrounding normal tissues.

A dose of 250–500 MBq (7–15 mCi) of FDG is the usual adult dose administered intravenously. After an uptake period of about 1 h, the patient is asked to void and is positioned in the scanner. In general, images are acquired for 2–5 min duration per bed position and reconstructed using available software. Scans are usually from the pelvis to head, taking advantage of the low bladder uptake (after voiding) at the beginning of acquisition.

A separate transmission scan is performed either with a PET source (^{68}Ge) or derived from the CT map. If CT attenuation factors are used in PET imaging, they need to be scaled to 511 keV, the photon energy of annihilation radiation.

Since FDG is filtered but not reabsorbed by the glomerulus, high FDG activity may be present in the urinary tract. Interventions to clear the excreted tracer for better evaluation of the surrounding tissues are usually not necessary. The currently used iterative reconstructions are no longer hampered by streak artifacts, which were common with older techniques such as filtered back projection. High uptake is sometimes seen in the bowel, and some have proposed anti-peristalsis and anti-motility drugs to overcome this problem. Many institutions utilize mild sedatives for patient comfort during the relatively lengthy acquisition of an emission plus transmission PET. In addition, muscle and brown fat uptake can be decreased significantly with benzodiazepines. For a PET/CT system, muscles and brown fat can be easily distinguished on the CT part of the study, and no longer pose a problem for the image interpretation (COHADE et al. 2003b).

For PET/CT, UCLA uses a protocol that comprises one CT acquisition of the torso, i.e.. from the base of the skull to the mid-thigh level, followed by a PET scan of the same area. Figure 6.1 shows a representative normal PET/CT study. Currently, we have a dual-slice CT that provides images of diagnostic quality with the following settings: 130 kVp; 80 mAs; pitch 1; and reconstruction slice thickness 5 mm. The helical CT takes about 80 s to image the upper body. Oral contrast is given if indicated for the delineation of the bowel. Nine hundred milliliters of oral contrast (Ready-Cat) with 2% barium sulfate, but without glucose, is given orally over 75 min before the acquisition starts. Intravenous contrast is non-ionic (Omnipaque), and a volume of 100–130 ml at a rate of 1.5 ml/s is administered. The intravenous contrast may cause regions of high attenuation that lead to typical CT-based attenuation artifacts and pseudo-FDG uptake (Fig. 6.2). The FDG dose is 0.19 mCi/kg (7.0 MBq/kg) with a maximum of 15 mCi (555 MBq). The uptake interval between tracer administration and start of acquisition is 1 h. The patient rests comfortably in a chair with armrests, in a dimly lit room without radio or television to minimize brain stimulation. The patient is covered under blankets to prevent shivering and activation of brown adipose tissue (Figs. 6.2, 6.3). Just before acquisition, the bladder is emptied. Our PET scanner has fast detectors (LSO lutetium-ortho-silicate) allowing for imaging of 1–4 min per bed position to accumulate the necessary counts. Body weight determines the imaging time, <75 kg, 1 min/bed, <100 kg, 2 min/bed, etc. The overall PET acquisition takes 6–26 min. With this setup, a standard whole-body PET/CT can be completed within 45 min.

With dual-modality imaging, FDG in the outflow tract can easily be distinguished on the CT images.

The axial cuts in Fig. 6.1 show activity in the renal pelvis bilaterally. A patient with an abnormal left outflow tract is shown in Fig. 6.4 and FDG in the renal pelvis and ureter can easily be differentiated from uptake in soft tissues.

6.3
Objective

From an oncologist's point of view, imaging needs to be focused on diagnosis, grading, and staging of tumors. Tumor grade in general does not correlate well with FDG uptake. There is not enough data to propose PET as a prognostic imaging modality in the routine clinical environment, including RCC. On the other hand, PET appears exquisitely equipped to stage newly detected disease or to signal relapse of disease. If PET discloses unexpected or occult lesions, high-resolution imaging with CT or MR imaging of the suspicious areas is indicated to delineate the structural involvement.

As has been pointed out by VALK (1996), the reference standard in comparing modalities is imperfect, because full validation of findings with biopsy

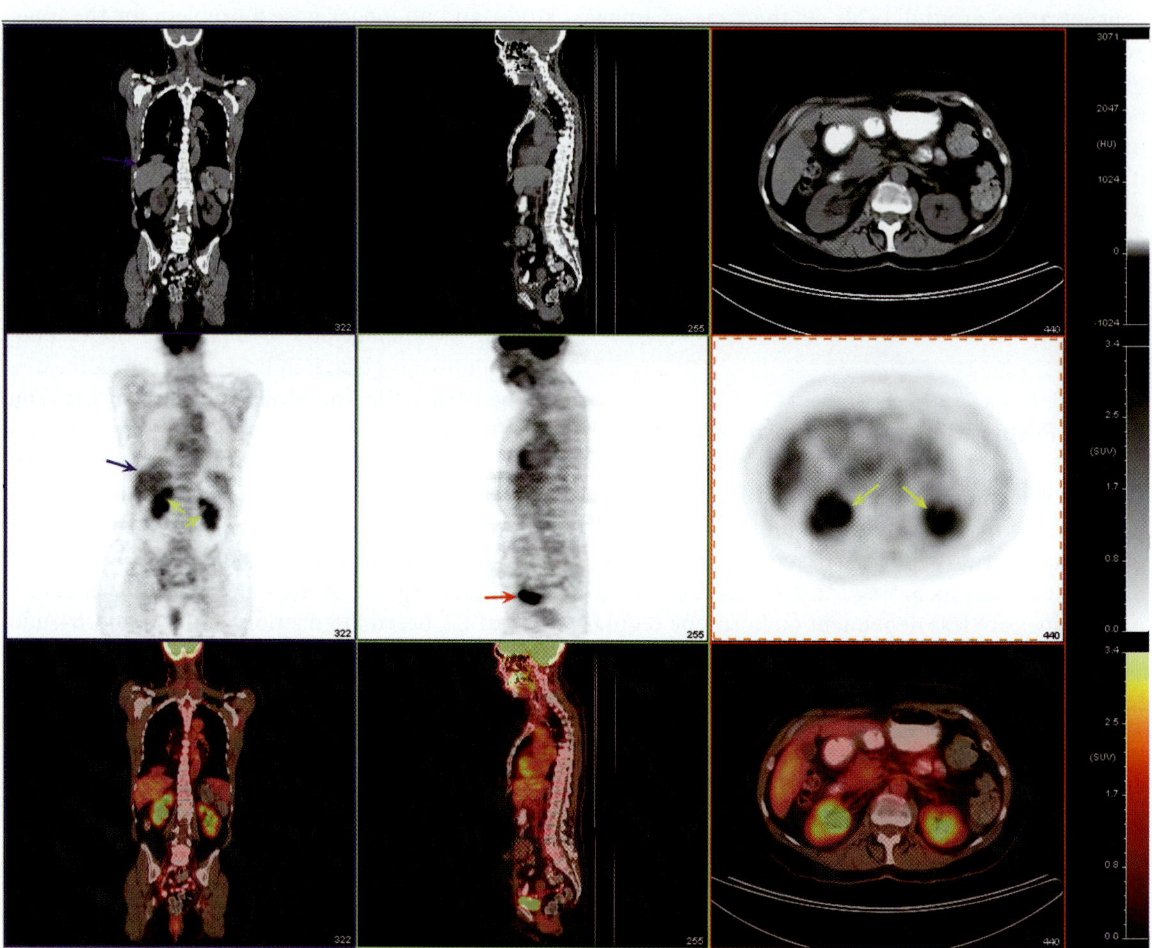

Fig. 6.1. Normal PET/CT scan in a 69-year-old woman. Coronal (*left column*) and axial cuts (*right column*) are displayed at the level of the kidneys. In the middle column the midline sagittal cuts are presented. The *top row* shows the CT slices in the kidney soft tissue window. The *middle row* shows the corresponding PET planes. The bottom row demonstrates the fused images, CT in black and white with PET superimposed in color. Note the window settings on the *right intensity bars*, the top in Hounsfield units (HU), the middle in standardized uptake value (SUV), and the bottom color bar also in SUV. The kidneys have mild uptake, whereas the hot spots are related to excreted FDG in the renal calyces and pelvis (*yellow arrows*). Note the "hot" bladder on the sagittal plane (*red arrow*). The uptake in the brain is high, because this organ uses glucose exclusively for its metabolism. Note the "double dome" of the liver, due to breathing at the time of the passage through the CT gantry. This causes attenuation correction artifacts in the dome of the liver on PET (*blue arrow*). Oral contrast can be seen in the bowel. No intravenous contrast was administered for this study.

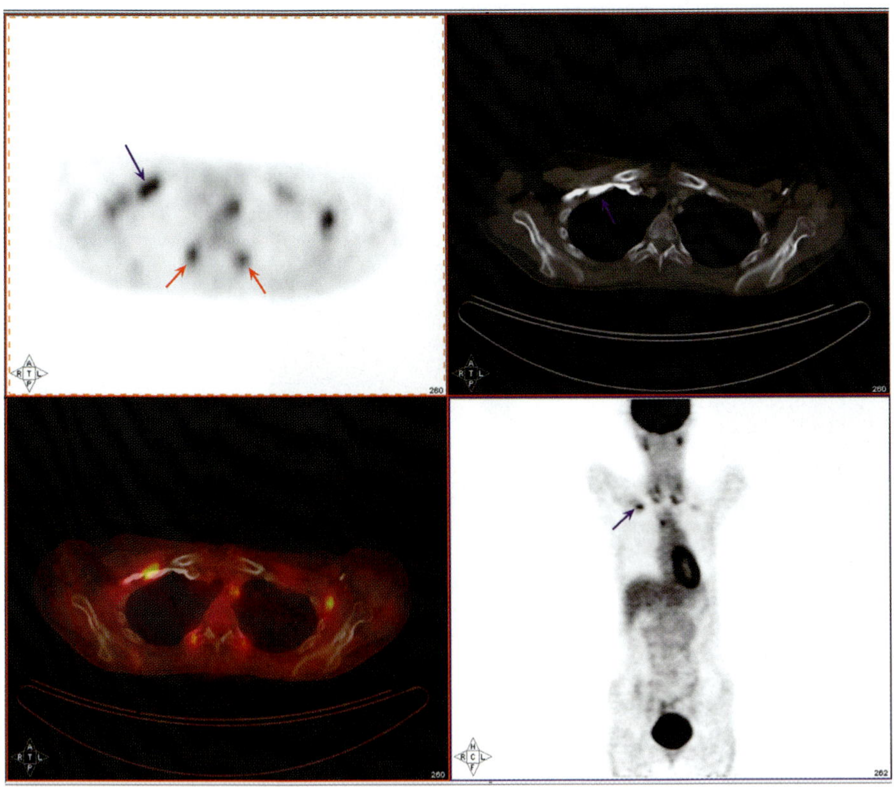

Fig. 6.2. Pseudo-FDG uptake in the right infra-clavicular region, related to incorrect attenuation correction in a 28-year-old woman. At the time of the CT scan, a high concentration of contrast is present (*blue arrow, right upper quadrant*), generating high-attenuation coefficients in this region. At the time of PET acquisition, contrast is no longer present in the initial high concentration. Since the CT is used for attenuation correction, the generated attenuation coefficients are too high (assuming contrast) and overcorrect the voxels, leading to an "apparent" increase or pseudo-FDG uptake (*left upper quadrant*). The CT scan (*right upper quadrant*), here presented in the bone window, clearly shows the contrast. Note the paraspinal muscle uptake (*red arrows*), as the CT scan does not reveal any bone abnormalities. *The left lower quadrant* shows the fused axial image, and the *right lower quadrant* the coronal PET slice at the level of the right subclavian vein.

and histology is not feasible; thus, there are no truly double-blind studies available comparing the performance of PET to conventional imaging in the majority of cancers. In the typical clinical context, on the other hand, it is not meaningful to evaluate the assumed "separate" contribution of each imaging modality. The purpose of imaging is to supply the diagnosis, which will prompt the surgical, medical, or radiation oncologist to watch and wait, or to administer a treatment regimen.

6.4
Clinical Experience

Over the past decade, few studies have been reported on the use of FDG-PET in RCC. In a review from Germany, Hofer et al. (2001) concluded that FDG-

PET offers no significant benefits over conventional imaging modalities. A review from the UK in 2003 concluded that RCC is FDG avid and visible (Hain and Maisey 2003). The FDG-positive patients had higher tumor grades than FDG-negative patients.

6.4.1
Diagnosis

In the study by Bachor et al. (1996) 29 patients with solid renal masses were scanned prior to surgery. PET using FDG was true positive in 20 of 26 histologically confirmed RCCs, and was false negative in 6 patients. In 3 patients with benign lesions (angiomyolipoma, pericytoma, and pheochromocytoma), false-positive results were obtained. In another 3 patients, FDG PET detected regional lymph node metastases, suggesting a role in staging of RCC.

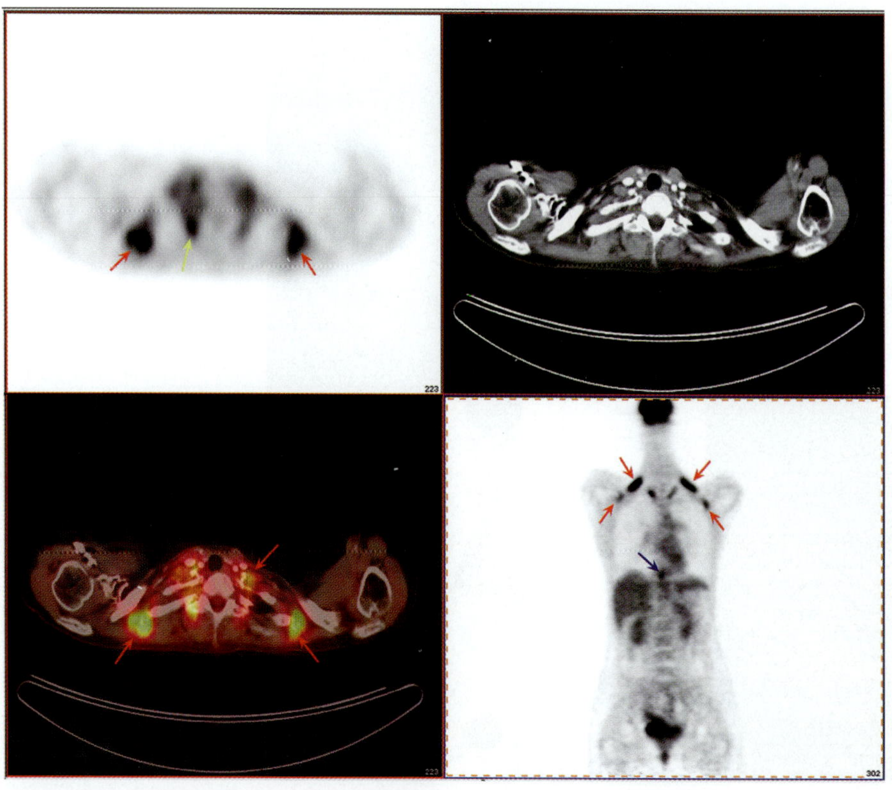

Fig. 6.3. Normal variants in a slender and tense 28-year-old woman. Increased FDG uptake (*left upper quadrant*: PET slice; *left lower quadrant*: PET/CT fused image) in brown adipose tissue (*red arrows*) corresponding to regions with fat density HU on corresponding CT (*right upper quadrant*). Increased uptake in muscle (*yellow arrow*). Coronal PET slice (*right lower quadrant*) shows activity in the midline (*blue arrow*) which corresponds to the lower gastro-esophageal junction, and is commonly seen. Increased uptake in muscles and brown adipose tissue is commonly seen in young patients, and more in women. (See Cohade et al. 2003b)

Goldberg et al. (1997) performed 26 FDG-PET studies in 21 patients. They evaluated the ability of FDG-PET to characterize solid renal masses (10 patients) and indeterminate renal cysts (11 patients) as malignant or benign. PET correctly classified solid lesions as malignant in 9 of 10 histologically confirmed tumors (6 RCC, 3 lymphoma). One patient with bilateral RCC was false negative. PET correctly classified indeterminate renal cysts as benign in 7 of 8 patients confirmed by surgery or needle aspiration. PET was false negative in one patient with a 4-mm papillary neoplasm. The authors suggested that a positive FDG-PET scan in the appropriate clinical setting might obviate the need for cyst aspiration in indeterminate renal masses.

Montravers et al. (2000) performed FDG-PET in 13 patients with renal masses who subsequently had nephrectomy or surgical resection. PET correctly characterized eight of nine malignant tumors, was false positive in 1 patient with renal tuberculosis, and was true negative in 3 patients with benign masses (one angiomyolipoma, two renal cysts), and false negative in 1 patient with a 3-cm RCC.

These early studies with a limited number of patients revealed that FDG-PET had a high positive predictive value, suggesting its utility for non-invasive characterization of indeterminate renal masses in patients in whom surgical resection or biopsy is not feasible.

Kang et al. (2004) reported a large retrospective study with 99 scans in 66 patients. The sensitivity for primary RCC was 60%, and the specificity 100%.

Fig. 6.4a,b. Incidental finding of a mega-ureter of the left kidney in a 73-year-old woman with newly diagnosed lymphoproliferative disorder. The urine in the renal pelvis and ureter contains excreted FDG, which shows up as hot spots on PET slices (*top rows*). The CT scans show the dilated pelvis and dilated ureter in these coronal cuts (*bottom rows*). Panel **a** has the more anterior cuts with bladder and distal ureter, whereas panel **b** has the more posterior cuts with the kidneys.

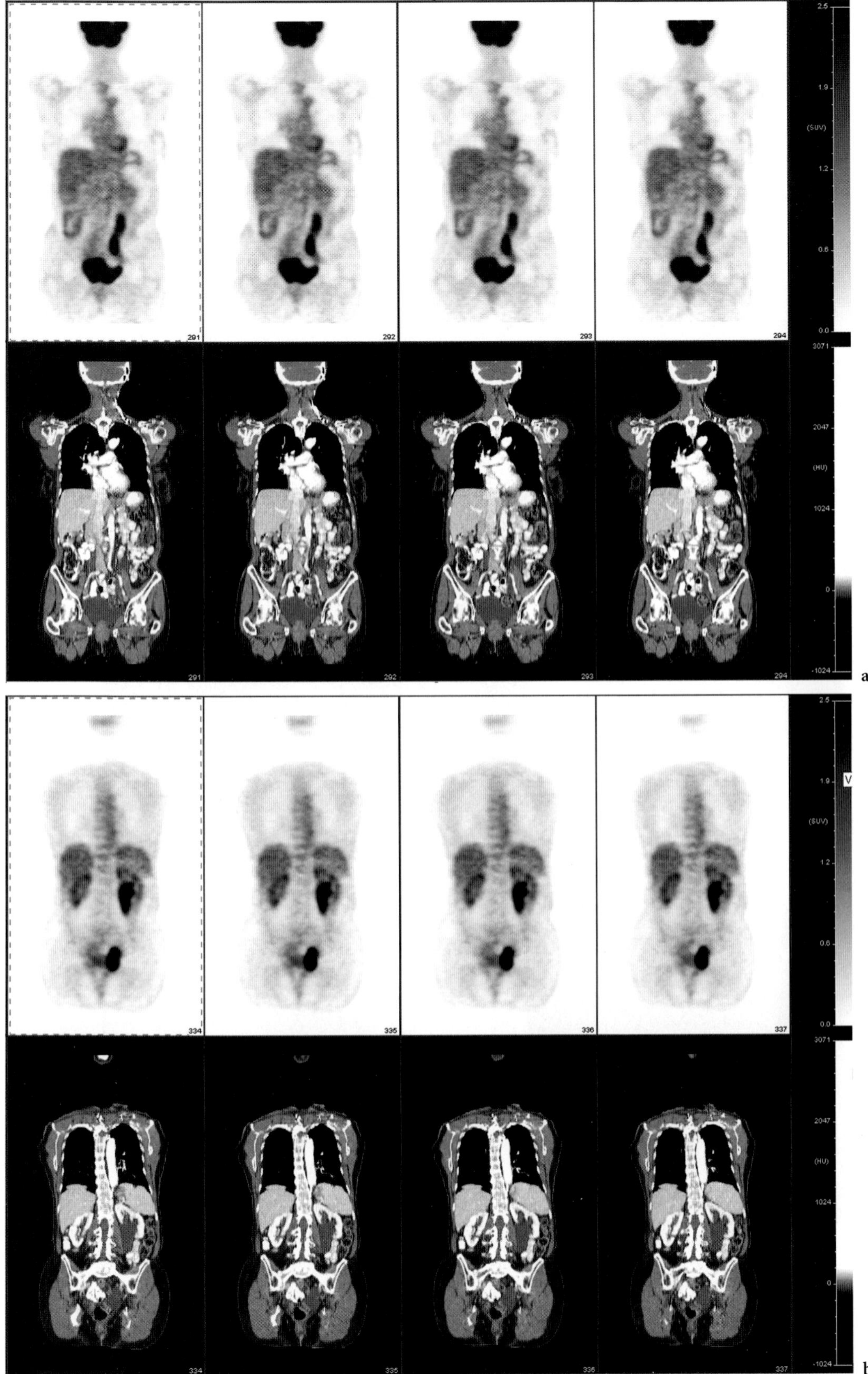

The authors concluded that PET with FDG is limited due to the low sensitivity.

To investigate why RCC patients had negative FDG-PET scans, WAHL compared several biological characteristics (BROWN and WAHL 1993; MIYAUCHI and WAHL 1996; WAHL 1996). They demonstrated that patients with positive scans at the primary tumor site had higher tumor grades and higher GLUT-1 expression than patients with negative PET scans. Since GLUT-1 is the key transporter for FDG, with low expression in RCC, most renal cancers are missed (MIYAUCHI et al. 1996). MIYAUCHI et al. (1996) compared several biological characteristics of renal tumors in relation to glycolysis. They studied 11 patients with newly diagnosed RCC and compared FDG uptake to the expression of glucose transporters, tumor size, and tumor grade. They

concluded that renal cancers that are well visualized by FDG-PET tended to have higher tumor grades and higher GLUT-1 expression, compared with poorly visualized RCC. MIYAKITA et al. (2002) also studied the correlation between GLUT-1 immunoreactivity and FDG positivity. They found no correlation and concluded that FDG-PET may not be a useful tool for RCC. An example of a false-negative RCC is given in Fig. 6.5.

6.4.2
Staging

KOCHER et al. (1994) performed pre-surgical staging with FDG-PET in 10 patients with renal cancer and found that PET predicted the presence or absence

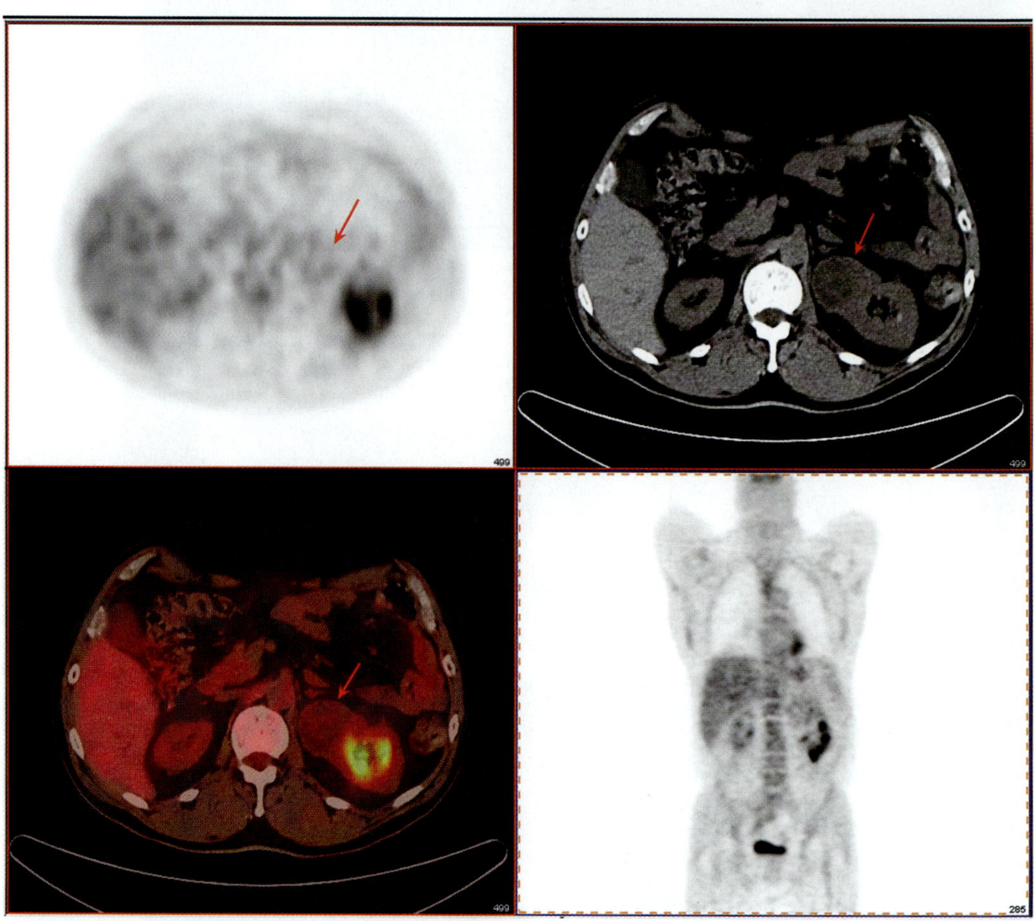

Fig. 6.5. Kidney mass in a 55-year-old man who was diagnosed with large B-cell lymphoma 2 years previously, and was in complete remission after chemotherapy and radiation therapy. Axial CT scan (*right upper quadrant*) shows the mass of the upper pole of the left kidney. The corresponding PET image (*left upper quadrant*) shows normal uptake, suggestive of a benign lesion (*arrow*). Subsequent biopsy revealed a renal cell carcinoma. This case shows that some renal cell carcinomas have normal metabolism, and are therefore not detected with FDG-PET. The *left lower quadrant* shows the fused axial image, and the *right lower quadrant* shows the coronal PET slice at the level of the kidneys.

of lymph node metastases in all cases (3 positive, 7 negative). Bachor et al. (1996) reported that FDG-PET correctly identified regional lymph node metastases in 3 of 26 patients. Finally, Montravers et al. (2000) reported that PET correctly staged 11 of 12 patients (4 true positive, 7 true negative). The sites of positive PET findings were in the bone, lung, and lymph nodes.

An Australian study investigated the effect of staging on patient management (Ramdave et al. 2001). The authors concluded that PET had an accuracy similar to CT (94%) and changed patient management in 40% of patients.

Safaei et al. (2002), from our institution, assessed the utility of FDG-PET for restaging 36 patients with advanced RCC. In this retrospective study, the additional value of whole-body PET to conventional imaging (CT, MR imaging, US, radiography, and bone scintigraphy) was demonstrated. The patient-based analysis demonstrated that FDG-PET correctly classified the clinical stage in 32 of 36 patients (89%) and was incorrect in 4 patients (11%). The lesion-based analysis showed that metabolic imaging correctly classified 21 of 25 lesions (81%), subsequently verified by surgical biopsy. PET was true positive in 14, true negative in 7, false positive in 1, and false negative in 3 lesions. This resulted in a sensitivity of 82%, specificity of 88%, and accuracy of 81% for lesion detection. Typical examples for restaging and characterization of lesions in RCC are given in Figs. 6.6–6.8.

More recently, Majhail et al. reported on the evaluation of distant metastases in 24 patients with RCC (Majhail et al. 2003). The sensitivity was 64%, the

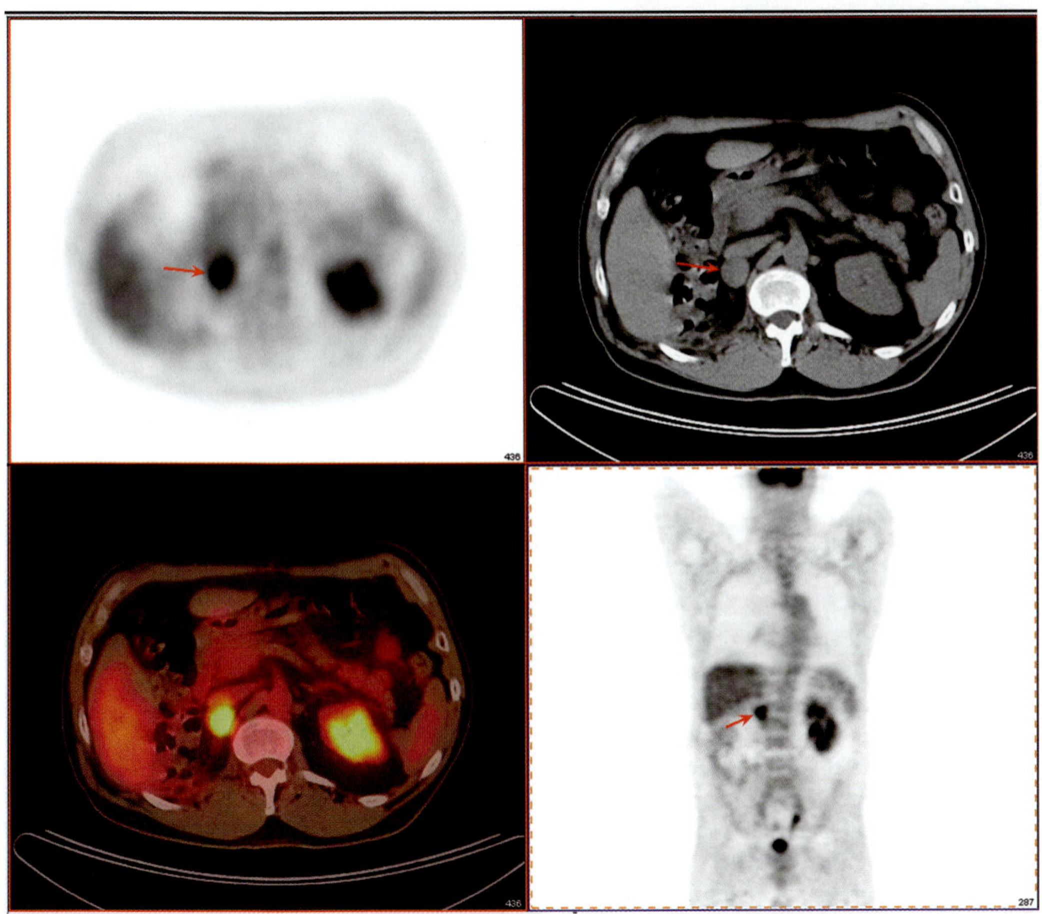

Fig. 6.6. Recurrent renal cell carcinoma in a 60-year-old man with a metastasis near the surgical site. This patient was diagnosed with right papillary renal cell cancer 3 years previously. He had right nephrectomy, lymphadenectomy, and chemotherapy. Recent outside CT showed a suspicious retro-caval lymph node. Axial CT scan (*right upper quadrant*) shows a node anterior to the right nephrectomy site (*arrow*), which is hypermetabolic on PET (*arrow, left upper quadrant*) confirming recurrence. The *left lower quadrant* shows the fused axial image, and the *right lower quadrant* shows the coronal PET slice at the level of the kidneys.

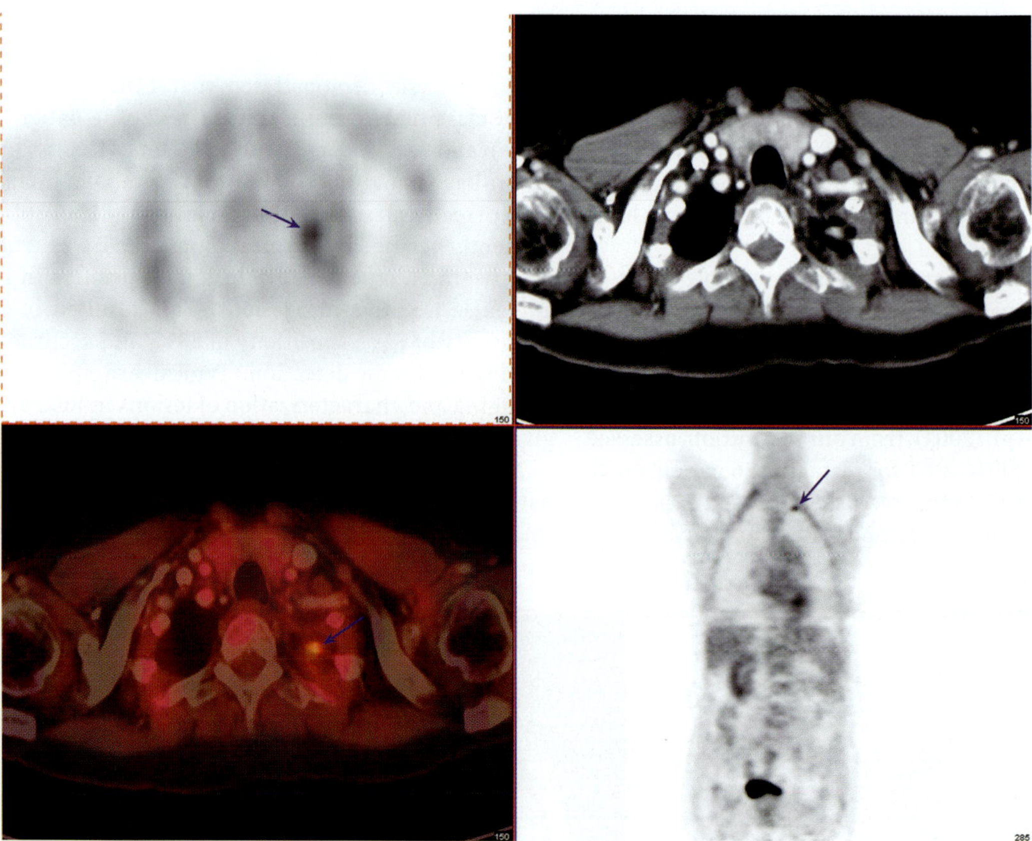

Fig. 6.7. Renal cell carcinoma in a 72-year-old man 7 years after left nephrectomy. Axial contrast-enhanced CT scan (*right upper panel*) shows new nodule in the left lung apex (*arrow*), which is hypermetabolic on PET (*left upper panel*). The *left lower panel* shows the axial PET/CT fusion image. The *right lower panel* is a coronal PET cut with the apical lesion (*arrow*) and only the right kidney visible.

specificity 100%, and the positive predictive value 100%. Interestingly, they found that the false-negative results were all related to lesions less than 1 cm in size. Similar results were published by JADVAR et al. (2003), demonstrating a modest accuracy for restaging of RCC. In 25 patients they found a sensitivity of 71%, specificity of 75%, and accuracy of 72%. With a negative predictive value of 33% and a positive predictive value of 94%, these authors concluded that a negative study does not exclude disease, whereas a positive study is suspicious for malignancy. KANG et al. (2004) arrived at the same conclusion by finding a sensitivity of 75% and specificity of 100% for lymph node metastasis from RCC.

The general opinion is that PET using FDG suffers from limited sensitivity in RCC (Fig. 6.5). This is partially related to the low glucose utilization of renal tumors (low GLUT-1 expression). The fact that small lesions (<1 cm) are missed is in part related to the spatial resolution of the PET systems used and, therefore, not specific for RCC.

6.4.3
Outlook

Therapy monitoring is an approved indication in the US for the common cancers. There are no studies on RCC in this domain. The significance of FDG uptake relative to the prognostic outcome is unknown. In

Fig. 6.8a,b. Metastatic renal cell carcinoma in a 60-year-old woman 7 years after nephrectomy. The patient had finished interleukin therapy (IL-2) 8 months previously. Recent CT scan revealed mediastinal lymphadenopathy, hilar lymphadenopathy, lung nodules in the thorax, as well as an ileocecal mass and a pancreatic head mass in the abdomen. FDG-PET scan is performed for characterization of lesions. Additional distant metastases from renal cell carcinoma were seen in unexpected locations. **a** A lesion in the left anterior cardiophrenic space (*red arrow*). **b** Lymph node in the abdomen (*red arrow*). Note the extensive involvement in the upper mediastinum, right hilum, and left aortopulmonary window seen on coronal PET slice (*blue arrows, right lower panel*).

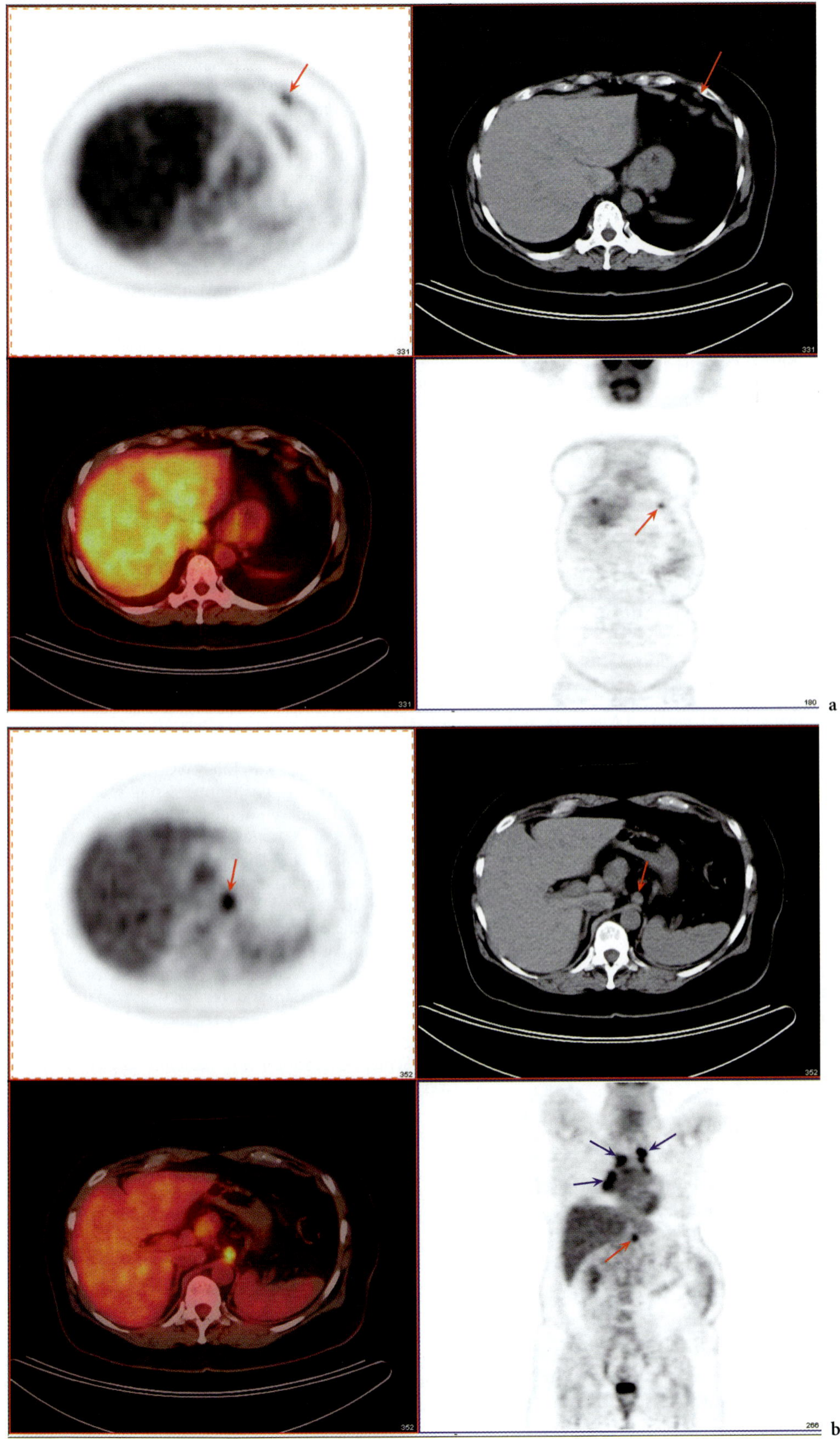

our institution, Hoh et al. (1998) investigated the utility of the FDG-PET imaging technology in RCC in a limited series.

In addition to the biological characteristics of renal malignancies, the normal renal excretion of FDG results in residual parenchymal activity as well as pooling of excreted tracer in the pelvicalyceal system. This excreted FDG limits the ability of metabolic imaging alone in diagnosis. As stated previously, small lesions may be below the spatial resolution of existing PET scanners (approximately 5 mm). Currently, PET/CT is en vogue and the superiority of dual-modality imaging over PET alone and CT alone has been demonstrated for lung cancer (Lardinois et al. 2003) and colorectal cancer (Cohade et al 2003a; Schiepers 2003). To date, there are no series reporting on the accuracy of PET/CT in RCC. The co-registration of PET to CT may solve interpretation problems related to excreted FDG in the urine and outflow tract (Fig. 6.4). In Fig. 6.6, an example of a positive PET/CT in recurrent RCC is given, and in Fig. 6.7, an occult metastasis was discovered in the left lung apex.

As recently outlined by Wahl (2004), imaging of abdominal and pelvic cancer in the future will be almost exclusively done by PET/CT. This is based on the experience of the Johns Hopkins PET Center, where over 2700 studies were performed in a 2-year period.

6.5
Conclusion

Renal cell carcinoma comprises about 3% of all malignancies. FDG has a modest affinity for RCC related to a lower expression of GLUT-1 than other cancers. Metabolic imaging using FDG and PET has a modest accuracy for primary lesions and local recurrence. The data for staging and restaging of RCC is similar: low sensitivity and high specificity. Possible interpretation problems related to the excreted FDG can be overcome by fusion of anatomic and metabolic images (PET/CT). Newer-generation scanners have improved spatial resolution, which will reduce false negatives. To date, there are no series available about the utility of this emerging dual-modality imaging technique in RCC. The modality is also suitable for therapy monitoring, but again there is insufficient data to assess the contribution of PET or PET/CT.

References

Bachor R, Kotzerke J, Gottfried HW, Brandle E, Reske SN, Hautmann R (1996) Positron emission tomography in diagnosis of renal cell carcinoma. Urologe A 35:146–150

Brown RS, Wahl RL (1993) Overexpression of Glut-1 glucose transporter in human breast cancer. An immunohistochemical study. Cancer 72:2979–2985

Cohade C, Osman M, Leal J, Wahl RL (2003a) Direct comparison of (18)F-FDG PET and PET/CT in patients with colorectal carcinoma. J Nucl Med 44:1797–1803

Cohade C, Osman M, Pannu HK, Wahl RL (2003b) Uptake in supraclavicular area fat ("USA-Fat"): description on 18F-FDG PET/CT. J Nucl Med 44:170–176

Coleman RE (2002) Value of FDG-PET scanning in management of lung cancer. Lancet 359:1361–1362

Dahlbom M, Hoffman EJ, Hoh CK, Schiepers C, Rosenqvist G, Hawkins RA, Phelps ME (1992) Whole-body positron emission tomography. 1. Methods and performance characteristics. J Nucl Med 33:1191–1199

Dwamena BA, Sonnad SS, Angobaldo JO, Wahl RL (1999) Metastases from non-small cell lung cancer: mediastinal staging in the 1990s: meta-analytic comparison of PET and CT. Radiology 213:530–536

Figlin RA, Thompson JA, Bukowski RM, Vogelzang NJ, Novick AC, Lange P, Steinberg GD, Belldegrun AS (1999) Multicenter, randomized, phase III trial of CD8(+) tumor-infiltrating lymphocytes in combination with recombinant interleukin-2 in metastatic renal cell carcinoma. J Clin Oncol 17:2521–2529

Goldberg MA, Mayo-Smith WW, Papanicolaou N, Fischman AJ, Lee MJ (1997) FDG PET characterization of renal masses: preliminary experience. Clin Radiol 52:510–515

Gould MK, Maclean CC, Kuschner WG, Rydzak CE, Owens DK (2001) Accuracy of positron emission tomography for diagnosis of pulmonary nodules and mass lesions: a meta-analysis. J Am Med Assoc 285:914–924

Hain SF, Maisey MN (2003) Positron emission tomography for urological tumours. BJU Int 92:159–164

Hofer C, Kubler H, Hartung R, Breul J, Avril N (2001) Diagnosis and monitoring of urological tumors using positron emission tomography. Eur Urol 40:481–487

Hoh CK, Hawkins RA, Glaspy JA, Dahlbom M, Tse NY, Hoffman EJ et al. (1993) Cancer detection with whole-body PET using 2-[F-18]fluoro-2-deoxy-D-glucose. J Comput Assist Tomogr 17:582–589

Hoh CK, Schiepers C, Seltzer MA, Gambhir SS, Silverman DH, Czernin J, Maddahi J, Phelps ME (1997) PET in oncology: Will it replace the other modalities? Semin Nucl Med 272:94–106

Hoh CK, Seltzer MA, Franklin J, deKernion JB, Phelps ME, Belldegrun A (1998) Positron emission tomography in urological oncology. J Urol 159:347–356

Jadvar H, Kherbache HM, Pinski JK, Conti PS (2003) Diagnostic role of [F-18]-FDG positron emission tomography in restaging renal cell carcinoma. Clin Nephrol 60:395–400

Jemal A, Tiwari RC, Murray T, Ghafoor A, Samuels A, Ward E, Feuer EJ, Thun MJ; American Cancer Society (2004) Cancer statistics, 2004. CA Cancer J Clin 54:8–29

Kang DE, White RL Jr, Zuger JH, Sasser HC, Teigland CM (2004) Clinical use of fluorodeoxyglucose F 18 positron emission tomography for detection of renal cell carcinoma. J Urol 171:1806–1809

Keyes JW Jr (1995) SUV: standard uptake or silly useless value? J Nucl Med 36:1836–1839

Kocher F, Grimmel S, Hautmann R (1994) Positron emission tomography. Introduction of a new procedure in diagnosis of urologic tumors and initial clinical results. J Nucl Med 35:223P

Kubota K, Ishiwata K, Kubota R, Yamada S, Tada M, Sato T, Ido T (1991) Tracer feasibility for monitoring tumor radiotherapy: a quadruple tracer study with fluorine-18-fluorodeoxyglucose or fluorine-18-fluorodeoxyuridine, L-[methyl-14C]methionine, [6-3H]thymidine, and gallium-67. J Nucl Med 32:2118–2123

Kubota K, Kubota R, Yamada S (1993) FDG accumulation in tumor tissue. J Nucl Med 34:419–421

Kubota R, Yamada S, Kubota K, Ishiwata K, Tamahashi N, Ido T (1992) Intratumoral distribution of fluorine-18-fluorodeoxyglucose in vivo: high accumulation in macrophages and granulation tissues studied by microautoradiography. J Nucl Med 33:1972–1980

Lardinois D, Weder W, Hany TF, Kamel EM, Korom S, Seifert B, Schulthess GK von, Steinert HC (2003) Staging of non-small-cell lung cancer with integrated positron-emission tomography and computed tomography. N Engl J Med 348:2500–2507

Majhail NS, Urbain JL, Albani JM, Kanvinde MH, Rice TW, Novick AC, Mekhail TM, Olencki TE, Elson P, Bukowski RM (2003) F-18 fluorodeoxyglucose positron emission tomography in the evaluation of distant metastases from renal cell carcinoma. J Clin Oncol 21:3995–4000

Miyakita H, Tokunaga M, Onda H, Usui Y, Kinoshita H, Kawamura N, Yasuda S (2002) Significance of 18F-fluorodeoxyglucose positron emission tomography (FDG-PET) for detection of renal cell carcinoma and immunohistochemical glucose transporter 1 (GLUT-1) expression in the cancer. Int J Urol 9:15–18

Miyauchi T, Wahl RL (1996) Regional 2-[18F]fluoro-2-deoxy-D-glucose uptake varies in normal lung. Eur J Nucl Med 23:517-523

Miyauchi T, Brown R, Grossman H, Wojno K (1996) Correlation between visualization of primary renal cancer by FDG-PET. J Nucl Med 37 (Suppl):64P

Montravers F, Grahek D, Kerrou K, Younsi N, Beco V de, Talbot JN (2002) Sensitivity of FDG CDET (2D dual-head coincidence gamma camera) for the detection of occult or doubtful recurrences of colorectal cancer. Histopathological correlation. Clin Positron Imaging 3:169

Phelps ME (ed) (2004) PET: molecular imaging and its biological applications. Springer, Berlin Heidelberg New York

Ramdave S, Thomas GW, Berlangieri SU, Bolton DM, Davis I, Danguy HT, Macgregor D, Scott AM (2001) Clinical role of F-18 fluorodeoxyglucose positron emission tomography for detection and management of renal cell carcinoma. J Urol 166:825–830

Safaei A, Figlin R, Hoh CK, Silverman DH, Seltzer M, Phelps ME, Czernin J (2002) The usefulness of F-18 deoxyglucose whole-body positron emission tomography (PET) for restaging of renal cell cancer. Clin Nephrol 57:56–62

Schiepers C (2003) PET/CT in colorectal cancer. J Nucl Med 44:1804–1805

Townsend DW, Cherry SR (2001) Combining anatomy and function: the path to true image fusion. Eur Radiol 11:1968–1974

Valk PE (1996) Sense and sensitivity: issues in technology assessment. J Nucl Med 37:1436–1437

Valk P (ed) (2003) Positron emission tomography: basic science and clinical practice. Springer, Berlin Heidelberg New York

Wahl RL (1996) Targeting glucose transporters for tumor imaging: "sweet" idea, "sour" result. J Nucl Med 37:1038–1041

Wahl RL (1999) Positron emission tomography in cancer patient management. Cancer J Sci Am 5:205–207

Wahl RL (2004) Why nearly all PET of abdominal and pelvic cancers will be performed as PET/CT. J Nucl Med 45 (Suppl 1):82S–95S

Warburg O (1956) On the origin of cancer cells. Science 123:309–314

Warburg O, Posener K, Negelein E (1924) The metabolism of cancer cells. Biochem Zeitschr 152:129–169

Zasadny KR, Wahl RL (1993) Standardized uptake values of normal tissues at PET with 2-[fluorine-18]-fluoro-2-deoxy-D-glucose: variations with body weight and a method for correction. Radiology 189:847–850

7 Renal Cell Carcinoma

David W. Barker and Ronald J. Zagoria

CONTENTS

7.1
Introduction

With a variety of imaging modalities in his or her armamentarium, the genitourinary radiologist plays an important role in the detection and management of patients with renal cell carcinoma (RCC). Appropriate and cost-effective use of these modalities, proper recognition of specific benign and malignant radiological features, and the keenness to "pick up" the sometimes subtle finding of an incidental renal mass on a study ordered for another purpose are all required skills.

7.2
General Discussion

7.2.1
Incidence

Renal cell carcinoma, also known as renal adenocarcinoma, Grawitz tumor, hypernephroma, and renal clear cell carcinoma, is the most common neoplasm of the kidney, accounting for 90–95% of all renal tumors (Landis et al. 1999). The incidence of RCC has been rising steadily over the past 50 years (Chow et al. 1999), and approximately 30,000 new cases are now diagnosed in the United States annually (American Cancer Society 1996). Renal cell carcinoma accounts for 3% of all adult malignancies, and it is the sixth leading cause of cancer death (Greenlee et al. 2000).

7.2.2
Histology

Renal cell carcinoma arises from renal tubular epithelium and usually develops in the cortex of the kidney. Based on morphological and molecular characterization, there are four subtypes of RCC (in decreasing frequency): clear cell; papillary; chromophobe; and collecting duct (Eble et al. 2004). The clear cell subtype, also known as conventional RCC, comprises 75–85% of all RCCs and is characterized by its lipid and glycogen-rich cytoplasm. Papillary RCC, also known as the chromophilic subtype, tends to be multifocal and bilateral. It generally has a better prognosis than the clear cell tumors. Chro-

D. W. Barker, MD
Senior Radiologist, Tennessee Cancer Specialists, PLLC, Medical Director, LifeCare Partners, LLC, 1450 Dowell Springs Boulevard, Suite 230, Knoxville, TN 37909, USA
R. J. Zagoria, MD, FACR
Professor of Radiology, Section Head of Abdominal Imaging, Vice-Chairman for Clinical Affairs, Department of Radiology, Wake Forest University School of Medicine, Medical Center Boulevard, Winston-Salem, NC 27157, USA

mophobic RCC arises from the cortical collecting duct and is characterized by its large polygonal cells with pale reticular cytoplasm. It also has a better prognosis than clear cell RCC. Finally, the collecting duct subtype arises from the medullary collecting duct, tends to affect younger patients, and often has an aggressive clinical course.

7.2.3
Risk Factors

Renal cell carcinoma typically presents in the sixth and seventh decades of life and is more common in males (two- to threefold increased risk). Risk factors also include cigarette smoking, which doubles risk, obesity, and heavy analgesic use. Diseases associated with RCC are tuberous sclerosis and von Hippel-Lindau disease. Finally, there is increased risk with renal dialysis and with immunosuppression for renal transplants.

7.2.4
Clinical Presentation

Because of its protean and often nonspecific clinical manifestations, RCC is sometimes referred to as the "great imitator" by clinicians. Most common presentations are hematuria (50–60%), pain (40%), and a palpable abdominal or flank mass (30–40%), with the entire triad present in only about 10–20% of patients (MOTZER et al. 1996). Patients may also present with a variety of paraneoplastic syndromes, including hypercalcemia, hypertension, erythrocytosis, hyperglycemia, cachexia, anemia, and Stauffer syndrome (nonmetastatic hepatic dysfunction).

7.2.5
Classification

Renal cell carcinoma can be staged with either the Robson or TNM classifications. The Robson classification is the most widely used in imaging literature (Table 7.1; ERGEN et al. 2004).

More recently, the American Joint Committee on Cancer (AJCC) and the "Union Internationale Contre le Cancer" (UICC) have devised a TNM-based system for RCC (GUINAN et al. 1997). The TNM classification describes the loco-regional extent of disease in greater detail and is more accurate than the Robson classification at predicting survival by stage (Tables 7.2, 7.3).

Table 7.1. Robson renal cell carcinoma classification

Stage I: confined to kidney
Stage II: through renal capsule but confined to Gerota's fascia
Stage IIIA: involvement of renal vein or IVC
Stage IIIB: involvement of local lymph nodes
Stage IIIC: involvement of vessel(s) and nodes
Stage IV: spread to local organs or distant metastases

7.2.6
Therapy

The mainstay of therapy for localized disease is surgery. Radical nephrectomy is the procedure of choice and classically includes resection of the kidney along with all contents within Gerota's fascia including perinephric fat, regional lymph nodes, and the ipsilateral adrenal gland. Nephron-sparing surgery may be an option for patients with small tumors (DEKERNION 1987). The role of radical nephrectomy in patients with metastatic disease is controversial. Adjuvant radiotherapy does not improve survival, but may be used for palliation in patients who are not surgical candidates.

Despite numerous clinical trials, RCC has proven resistant to all forms of chemotherapy. A review by YAGODA et al. (1995), of over 80 phase-II trials published between 1983 and 1993 testing various cytotoxic agents, showed an overall response rate of only 6%.

Biological agents are another consideration. The observation of occasional spontaneous remissions, the presence of lymphocytes within RCCs, and the results of early clinical trials have prompted the investigation of such agents. Specifically, use of high-dose IL-2 in patients with metastatic RCC showed a 19% response rate (FISHER et al. 2000), though complete and durable response was achieved in only 5% of patients.

7.2.7
New Trends in Detection

"Look and you will find it. What is unsought will go undetected." – Sophocles

Renal cell carcinoma is often identified incidentally. In the past, approximately 10% of RCCs were diagnosed incidentally. Now, with the widespread use of cross-sectional imaging techniques including ultrasound, CT, and MR imaging, this percentage is approximately 36% (LESLIE et al. 2003).

Incidental RCCs are typically smaller and of a lower stage and lower grade. These smaller tumors

Table 7.2. The TNM classification

Primary tumor (T)	Regional lymph nodes (N)[a]	Distant metastasis (M)
TX: primary tumor cannot be assessed	NX: regional lymph nodes cannot be assessed	MX: distant metastasis cannot be assessed
T0: no evidence of primary tumor	N0: no regional lymph node metastasis	M0: no distant metastasis
T1: tumor 7 cm or less in greatest dimension limited to the kidney	N1: metastasis in a single regional lymph node	M1: distant metastasis
T2: tumor more than 7 cm in greatest dimension limited to the kidney	N2: metastasis in more than one regional lymph node	
T3: tumor extends into major veins or invades adrenal gland or perinephric tissues but not beyond Gerota's fascia		
T3a: tumor invades adrenal gland or perinephric tissues but not beyond Gerota's fascia		
T3b: tumor grossly extends into the renal vein(s) or vena cava below the diaphragm		
T3c: tumor grossly extends into the renal vein(s) or vena cava above the diaphragm		
T4: tumor invades beyond Gerota's fascia		

[a]Laterality does not affect the N classification

Table 7.3. American Joint Committee on Cancer stage groupings

Stage I	T1, N0, M0
Stage II	T2, N0, M0
Stage III	T1, N1, M0
	T2, N1, M0
	T3a, N0, M0
	T3a, N1, M0
	T3b, N0, M0
	T3b, N1, M0
	T3c, N0, M0
	T3c, N1, M0
Stage IV	T4, N0, M0
	T4, N1, M0
	Any T, N2, M0
	Any T, any N, M1

are usually less biologically aggressive and have a generally slow but variable rate of growth. Bosniak et al. (1995) followed 40 tumors 3.5 cm in diameter or smaller and reported a growth rate of 0.1–1 cm/year (mean 0.36 cm/year).

Not surprisingly, patients with incidentally discovered RCCs have a more favorable prognosis than patients who present with urological symptoms attributable to the tumor. Sweeney et al. (1996) showed a 5-year survival rate of 85% for incidental tumors vs 53% for patients with symptomatic lesions. The overall 5-year survival rate for renal cancer has increased from 45% (1970–1973) to 61% (1989–1996; Landis et al. 1998; Greenlee et al. 2001). This has occurred despite no significant progress in therapy. Lead-time and length biases may play some role in

the apparent survival benefits, but the data strongly suggest improved outcomes due to earlier diagnosis; therefore, it appears that progress has been substantial with regard to survival for patients with RCC. Much of this improvement can be attributed to early radiological diagnosis of renal malignancies that in turn has resulted in a higher proportion of tumors that can be cured with surgical resection. For this reason the detection and accurate diagnosis of renal masses are important tasks for radiologists.

7.3
Imaging Modalities

Because of its improved sensitivity and specificity over other imaging modalities, such as intravenous urography and ultrasound (US), contrast-enhanced CT has emerged as the procedure of choice for detecting RCC. Both CT and MR imaging are useful for staging and restaging. In the future, other modalities, such as PET, may also play a significant role.

7.3.1
Plain Radiographs

Occasionally, RCC may be found on an abdominal radiograph, usually appearing as an expansile ball-shaped mass extending from the kidney. Calcifications may also be detected, with approximately 15%

of RCCs containing calcifications that are visible on abdominal radiographs. Gross calcification within any renal mass is worrisome for RCC. Prior to the refinement of cross-sectional imaging, a urology rule-of-thumb was "a calcified renal mass is a surgical renal mass."

Patterns of calcification include thin peripheral rim calcification, irregular central calcification, or a combination of both. Eighty percent of masses on conventional radiography with thin, peripheral rim calcification are benign cysts, and 20% are malignancies, typically cystic RCC. At the opposite end of the spectrum, renal masses that contain central, irregular calcification (Fig. 7.1) are likely to be malignant. Eighty-seven percent of these lesions are RCCs, and the remaining 13% are cysts complicated by previous infection or hemorrhage. Masses that contain both thin, peripheral calcification, and focal, central calcification have a 50% chance of being malignant. Taking all of these variables into account, 60% of renal masses that contain calcium that is visible on an abdominal radiograph, regardless of the calcification pattern, are RCCs (BRACKEN 1987). Other renal masses that frequently contain calcium are focal xanthogranulomatous pyelonephritis, chronic perirenal hematomas, hemangiomas, aneurysms, and vascular malformations. Cross-sectional imaging allows distinction between benign and malignant calcified renal masses in most patients.

Other plain radiograph findings that may be important are skeletal abnormalities. Renal cell carcinoma often spreads hematogenously to the skeleton, causing lytic skeletal lesions. These lesions sometimes grow slowly and lead to bubbly lesions that focally expand the bone. They can mimic other types of bone lesions, including primary bone neoplasms and myeloma. Finally, patients with tuberous sclerosis, a disease associated with RCC, can have multiple osteomas, which predominate in the skull and spine.

7.3.2
Intravenous Urography

Intravenous urography (IVU) can be performed as follows:
1. Before injection of contrast material, a preliminary radiograph of the abdomen is always obtained.
2. Using bolus technique, 100 ml of 30 mg% contrast material is administered over 30–60 s.
3. One-minute coned radiograph of both kidneys or nephrotomogram.
4. Five-minute coned radiograph of both kidneys. Apply abdominal compression.
5. Ten-minute coned radiograph of both kidneys with abdominal compression, then release compression.
6. Fifteen-minute abdominopelvic plain radiographs, frontal and both obliques.
7. Postvoid abdominopelvic plain radiograph.

It is important to carefully analyze the scout radiograph, particularly for abnormal calcifica-

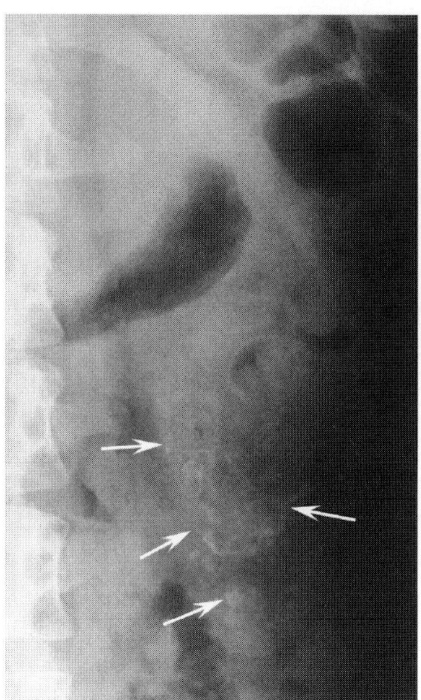

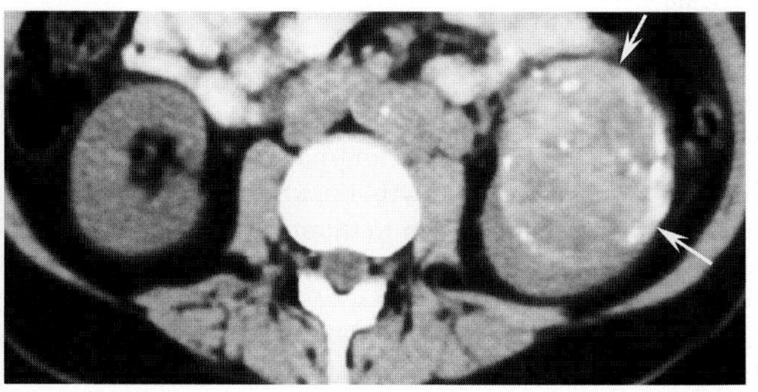

Fig. 7.1a,b. Calcifications in RCC in a 56-year-old woman. a Anteroposterior cone down radiograph of left upper quadrant demonstrates irregular calcifications (*arrows*) extending from, and projecting over, the lower pole of the left kidney. This pattern is very worrisome for RCC. b Axial unenhanced CT scan of same patient demonstrates large, solid RCC (*arrows*) of left kidney. Mass contains numerous calcifications corresponding to those seen on abdominal radiograph.

tions. Renal cell carcinoma is typically expansile and appears as a focal bulge extending from the kidney, displacing normal renal structures (Fig. 7.2). Such contour abnormalities are optimally detected with nephrotomography performed during the nephrogram phase of the IVU. Large masses lead to calyceal splaying, stretching, and draping. Occasionally, an RCC grows predominantly outward and no detectable mass effect is exerted on the calyceal system. Furthermore, RCCs that extend either exclusively anteriorly or posteriorly from the kidney are very difficult to detect with IVU, since the mass contour is obscured by superimposed normal kidney.

Other IVU signs of RCC include notching of the renal pelvis or the ureter, obstruction or invasion of the collecting system, and diminished or absent renal function. Notching results from enlargement of ureteric and renal pelvic vessels, which are recruited to feed or drain an RCC, the majority of which are hypervascular. Focal or diffuse hydronephrosis usually occurs with a large RCC and is due to compression of major calyces, the renal pelvis, or the upper ureter. Less commonly, an RCC grows by infiltration rather than by expansion. In these cases, malignant stricturing of the collecting system may occur secondary to encasement and invasion of the urothelium. Renal cell carcinoma has a predilection for venous extension, which may result in decreased or absent renal function. In fact, the finding of globally decreased function in a kidney with a renal mass is nearly diagnostic of RCC. Less commonly, diminished or absent renal function can result from high-grade ureteral obstruction caused by the RCC compressing the adjacent ureter or from diffuse parenchymal replacement by tumor.

Excretory urography lacks sufficient specificity to accurately characterize renal masses as benign or malignant; therefore, every renal mass detected with or suggested by excretory urography must be imaged with another technique. The most cost-effective approach is to go directly to renal US. With this technique approximately 80% of detected renal masses are characterized as simple cysts, thus ending their diagnostic evaluation (EINSTEIN et al. 1995). The remaining 20% of renal masses require further study with CT or MR imaging.

7.3.3
Ultrasound

The US features of RCC are typical but not diagnostic. Most RCCs appear as expansile, solitary renal masses. They may be hypoechoic, isoechoic, or hyperechoic in comparison with the renal parenchyma, with larger lesions developing heterogeneous echo patterns and internal cystic areas. Most small RCCs are slightly hyperechoic (Fig. 7.3), but approximately one-third are markedly hyperechoic (Fig. 7.4; FORMAN et al. 1993) and may mimic a benign angiomyolipoma (AML; Fig. 7.5). In distinguishing the two, the ultrasound findings of an anechoic perimeter or internal cystic areas strongly favor RCC, though CT or MR imaging is required for

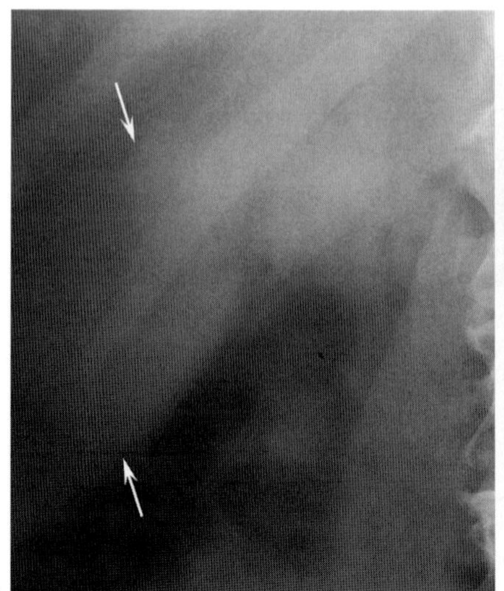
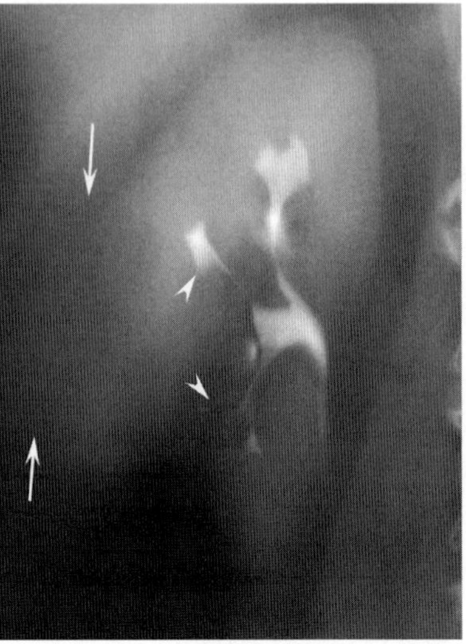

a   b

Fig. 7.2a,b. Renal mass in a 49-year-old woman. **a** Anteroposterior scout abdominal radiograph shows contour abnormality (*arrows*) along lateral aspect of right kidney. **b** Anteroposterior nephrotomogram shows mass (*arrows*) with splaying of collecting system (*arrowheads*).

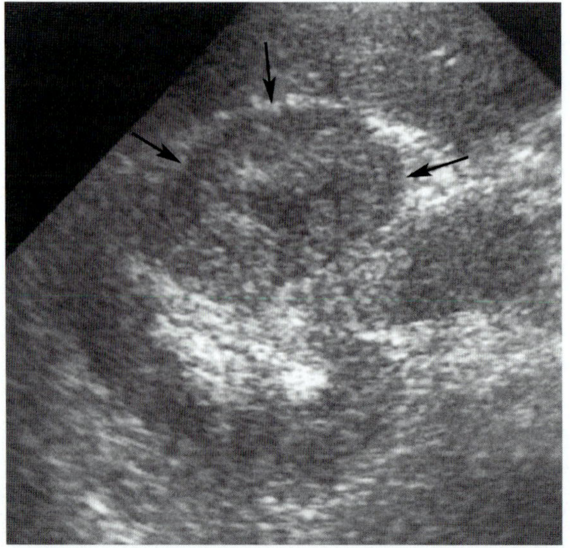

Fig. 7.3. Renal cell carcinoma in a 55-year-old man. Axial US image demonstrates expansile right renal mass (*arrows*). This mass is slightly hyperechoic and heterogeneous compared with normal renal parenchyma. These features are typical of most RCC.

further characterization (YAMASHITA et al. 1993). Both CT and MR imaging are exquisitely sensitive for the detection of intratumoral fat, the presence of which is highly suggestive of AML (Fig. 7.5; TAKAHASHI et al. 1993) and excludes an RCC except in the rare case that the tumor has grown to engulf normal renal sinus or perirenal fat.

Another interesting US feature is the capacity to demonstrate the internal architecture of renal tumors better than other imaging techniques. Some renal masses appear cystic or homogeneous with CT and MR imaging. Ultrasound examination of these lesions may demonstrate complex internal components with septations, fronds of solid tissue lining the periphery of the mass, or other evidence of malignancy; therefore, US may be used as an adjunctive test when CT findings are equivocal. In particular, US may be useful when CT findings suggest a cystic lesion not clearly a simple cyst but not obviously malignant (Fig. 7.6).

An infiltrating RCC may cause only subtle US abnormalities or none at all, but may lead to second-

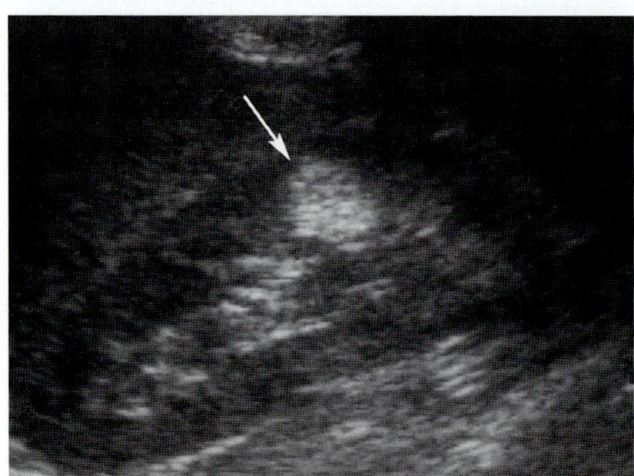

a

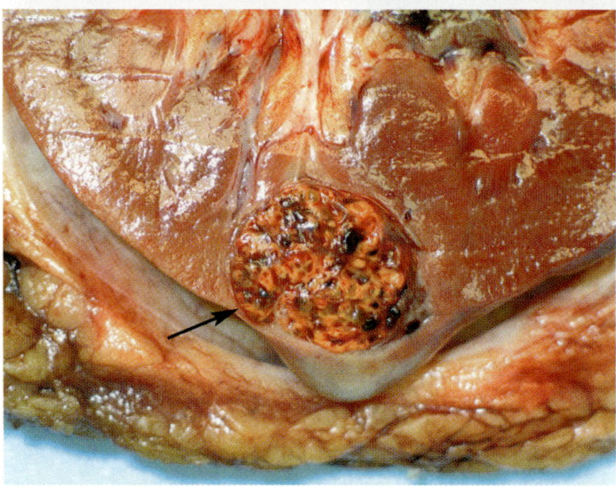

c

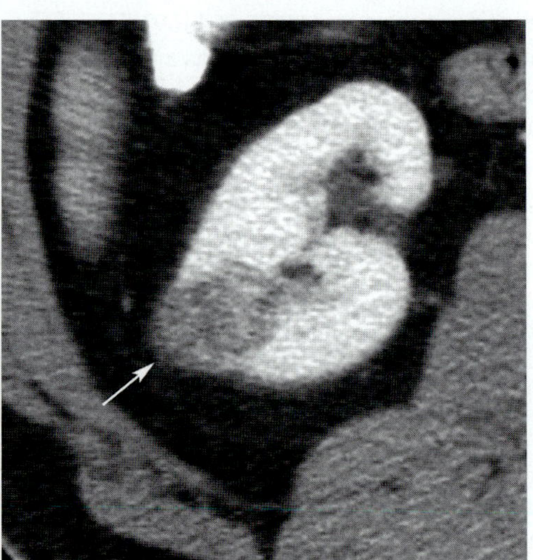

b

Fig. 7.4a–c. Renal cell carcinoma in a 66-year-old woman. **a** Longitudinal US image reveals markedly hyperechoic renal cell carcinoma (*arrow*) indistinguishable from angiomyolipoma. **b** Axial contrast-enhanced CT scan reveals solid enhancing lesion (*arrow*) with no detectable fat. **c** Pathology specimen shows yellow-orange mass (*arrow*) with spongy consistency and areas of hemorrhage. Final diagnosis was conventional RCC.

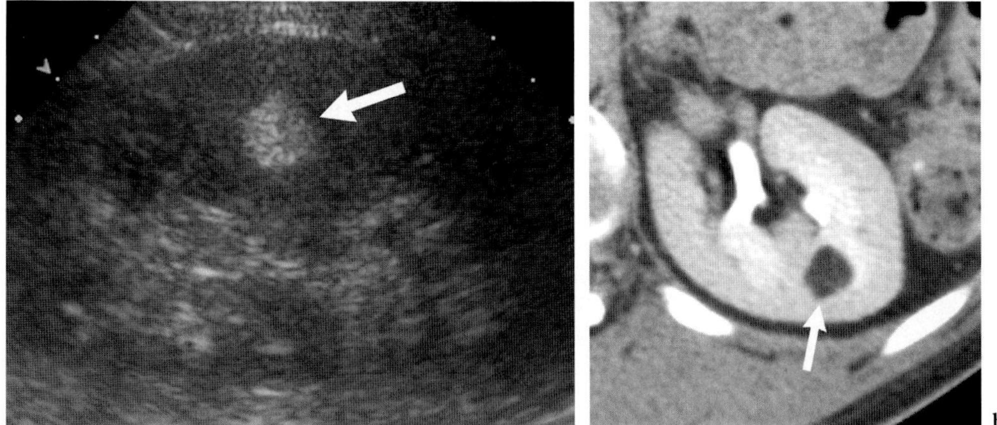

Fig. 7.5a,b. Angiomyolipoma in a 41-year-old woman. **a** Longitudinal ultrasound image shows small hyperechoic lesion (*arrow*) within renal parenchyma typical of angiomyolipoma. **b** Axial contrast-enhanced CT scan reveals fat density within lesion, confirming diagnosis (*arrow*).

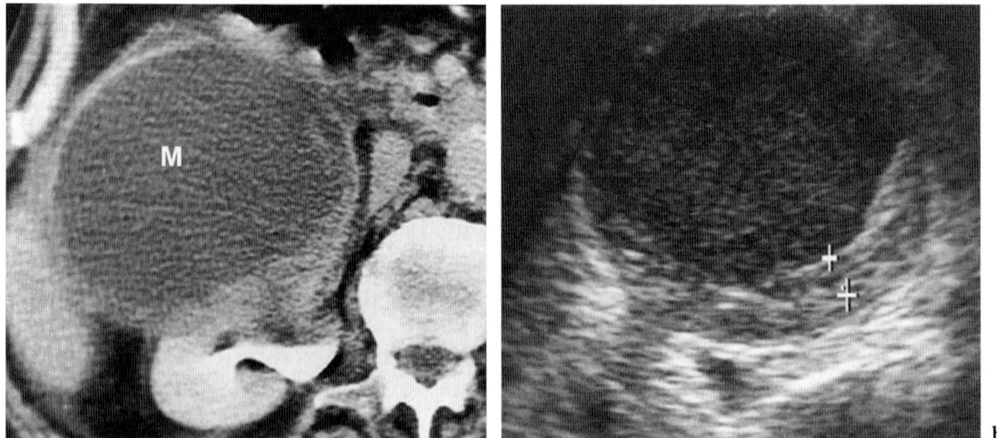

Fig. 7.6a,b. Papillary RCC in a 44-year-old man. **a** Axial contrast-enhanced CT scan demonstrates renal mass (*M*). Most of mass appears cystic. **b** Axial US image through right kidney in this patient better demonstrates thick rind of solid tissue. The cystic component contains many low-level echoes and this component of mass is not simply cystic.

ary abnormalities, including hydronephrosis and vascular encasement with diminished Doppler flow to the area of involvement. Alteration of the normal central sinus echo complex may also be seen.

Ultrasound is less accurate than either CT or MR imaging for staging RCC. Ultrasound should not be used as the sole modality for staging RCC, but it may be a helpful adjunct to other imaging techniques. The major limitations of US in staging RCC are the inability to image the renal vein and the subhepatic inferior vena cava reliably, and limited detection of abdominal lymphadenopathy. For staging, it is used mainly as an adjunct examination when tumor extension into the inferior vena cava is detected with CT but the exact superior extent of the tumor thrombus cannot be determined with CT. In these cases, US is highly accurate (95%) in determining whether tumor thrombus extends into the intrahepatic inferior vena cava (Fig. 7.7; GUPTA et al. 2004). This portion of the inferior vena cava can be visualized with US in 100% of cases, and tumor thrombus in this region is identifiable whenever present. Although this area can also be evaluated with either MR imaging or venography, US is the most cost-effective technique to resolve this isolated staging problem.

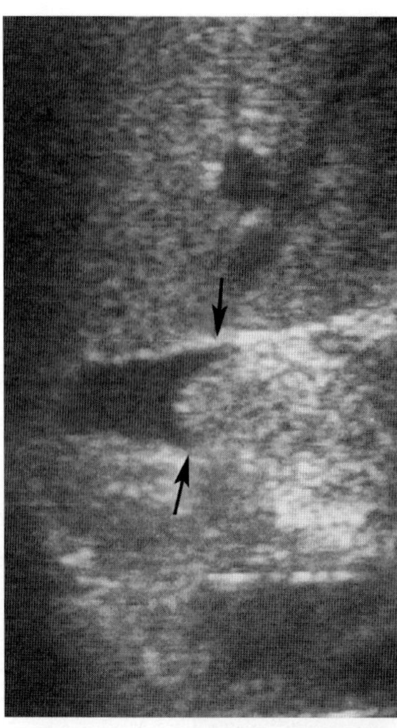

Fig. 7.7. Tumor extension into the inferior vena cava in a 66-year-old man. Longitudinal transabdominal US image demonstrates upper extent of a RCC (*arrows*) within intrahepatic inferior vena cava.

7.3.4
Angiography

Renal angiography, once a basic element in the diagnosis of renal masses (WATSON et al. 1968), is now of little value. Angiography has traditionally been reserved for mapping vascular supply to the kidney harboring a renal mass when a partial nephrectomy is contemplated. Since noninvasive techniques, such as CT or MR angiography, can be used to derive similar information, these techniques have largely replaced catheter angiography for this indication at most centers.

Renal arteriography in concert with embolization may be useful in the treatment of some RCCs. Tumor embolization can reduce intraoperative blood loss, or can diminish symptoms in patients considered inoperable. In rare cases, angiography may be useful to distinguish among various renal masses. In particular, angiography may be an alternative to open biopsy in the evaluation of infiltrating renal neoplasms, the differential diagnosis for which includes urothelial neoplasm, inflammatory lesion, infarct, or infiltrating RCC. Each of these entities, except RCC, is nearly always hypovascular or avascular; therefore, an infiltrating renal mass that is hyper-

vascular strongly suggests an infiltrating RCC. This finding is important as RCC is traditionally treated with nephrectomy, whereas transitional cell carcinoma is treated with nephroureterectomy, and many other infiltrating lesions are treated medically.

7.3.5
Cross-Sectional Imaging

7.3.5.1
Protocols

Conventional renal CT can be performed as follows:
1. Oral contrast (dilute Gastrografin or barium) is utilized.
2. Intravenous contrast is utilized with injection of 125 ml of 30 mg% contrast medium at a rate of 2–4 ml/s.
3. Evaluation should include contiguous 2.5-mm sections through the kidneys with unenhanced and contrast-enhanced sequences. Five-millimeter sections can be used elsewhere in the abdomen/pelvis.
4. The kidneys should be scanned during the corticomedullary phase (70 s) and the tubular/nephrographic phase (120 s).
5. A CT angiogram can also be obtained obviating the need for later catheter angiography for surgical planning. This requires initial scanning during the arterial phase (25 s).

Magnetic resonance imaging of the kidney can be performed as follows:
1. Unenhanced and contrast-enhanced T1-weighted spin-echo or gradient-echo images in the axial and coronal planes are recommended. An image section thickness of 5–7 mm is recommended. Prior to contrast administration and immediately afterward, breath-hold 3D fast spoiled gradient-echo images, with 4 mm or less section thickness, should be obtained. The torso phased-array coil is used routinely to image the kidneys.
2. Fast spin-echo T2-weighted images of the kidneys in the axial or coronal plane are obtained. These images are usually supplemented with a heavy T2-weighted sequence such as single-shot fast spin-echo (SSFSE, General Electric) or half-Fourier acquisition single-shot turbo spin echo (HASTE, Siemens).
3. The liver, adrenal glands, and upper retroperitoneum should also be evaluated routinely.

4. Flow-compensated T1-weighted spoiled gradient-echo images are used to evaluate patency of the renal veins and inferior vena cava. This pulse sequence can be implemented alone or as a component of MR venography.

7.3.5.2
Diagnosis

With CT or MR imaging alone, RCC can be diagnosed with better than 95% accuracy (BECHTOLD and ZAGORIA 1997). In our own experience with CT, 94% of RCCs are detected as expansile masses, whereas the remaining 6% grow by infiltration without significant disruption of the reniform shape of the involved kidney (GASH et al. 1992). The precontrast density of RCC compared with the background renal parenchyma can be hypodense, isodense, or hyperdense. Hyperdensity presumably results from acute hemorrhage, calcium, or proteinaceous debris within the tumor. Almost half of RCCs display a transient hyperdense blush during bolus contrast material injection (Fig. 7.8).

Note that the above CT protocol calls for imaging both during the corticomedullary phase (which also corresponds to the portal venous phase of liver enhancement) and the tubular phase of renal enhancement. Dual-phase imaging is important because during the corticomedullary phase, where renal parenchymal enhancement predominates in the cortex, there is decreased conspicuity of hypervascular cortical tumors and similar decreased conspicuity of hypovascular medullary tumors. The optimal phase for renal mass detection with helical CT is during the tubular phase (ZAGORIA et al. 1990). Again, this typically occurs about 120 s after the initiation of intravenous contrast material injection. Virtually all renal tumors appear less dense than enhanced renal parenchyma during this phase of enhancement.

Tumor homogeneity, distinctness of the RCC–kidney interface, and the shape and sharpness of the tumor margins are largely dependent on tumor size. The RCCs less than 5 cm in diameter are usually homogeneous masses with a distinct mass–kidney interface and smooth, sharp margins (Fig. 7.9). These features are rare in large RCCs, which usually display malignant findings, including central necrosis as a result of inadequate vascular supply, marginal lobulation reflecting differential growth rates within the tumor, infiltration of surrounding tissues including the renal collecting system (Fig. 7.10), and

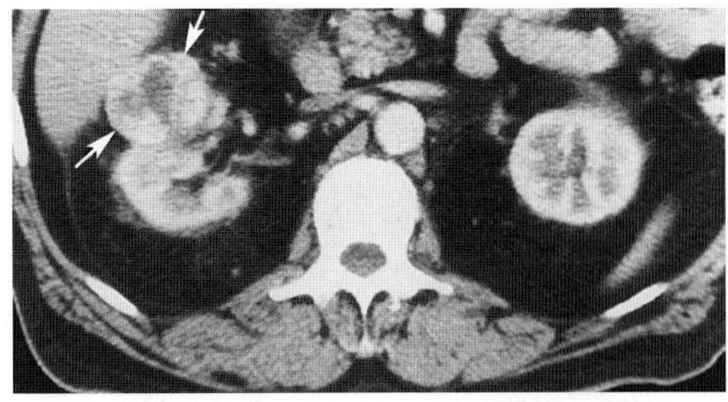

Fig. 7.8. Transient hyperdense blush in a 68-year-old man with RCC. Axial CT scan taken during a bolus injection of intravenous contrast material demonstrates expansile right renal mass (*arrows*). This mass enhances slightly greater than does normal renal parenchyma. This feature is commonly seen with hypervascular RRC.

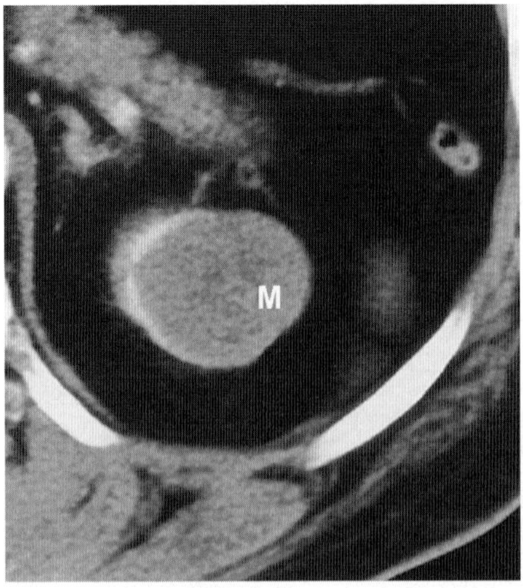

Fig. 7.9. Small RCC in a 58-year-old man. Axial contrast-enhanced CT scan demonstrates homogenous renal mass (*M*) which has a distinct interface with normal enhancing renal parenchyma. This feature is typically seen with small RCC. The 4-cm mass was proven to be RCC.

production of an indistinct mass–kidney interface (Fig. 7.11). Calcifications are visible by CT in 31% of RCCs (ZAGORIA et al. 1990) and are more common in papillary (32%) and chromophobe (38%) RCCs than in conventional RCC (11%; KIM et al. 2002).

Thus far, the major role of MR imaging in RCC evaluation lies in staging of cases deemed indeterminate after CT evaluation or in imaging patients in whom obtaining optimal CT scans is impossible. The MR imaging characteristics of RCC are similar to those described for CT. With gadolinium injection, as with iodinated contrast material injection for CT, RCCs enhance and become conspicuous within the renal parenchyma. A recent study showed that

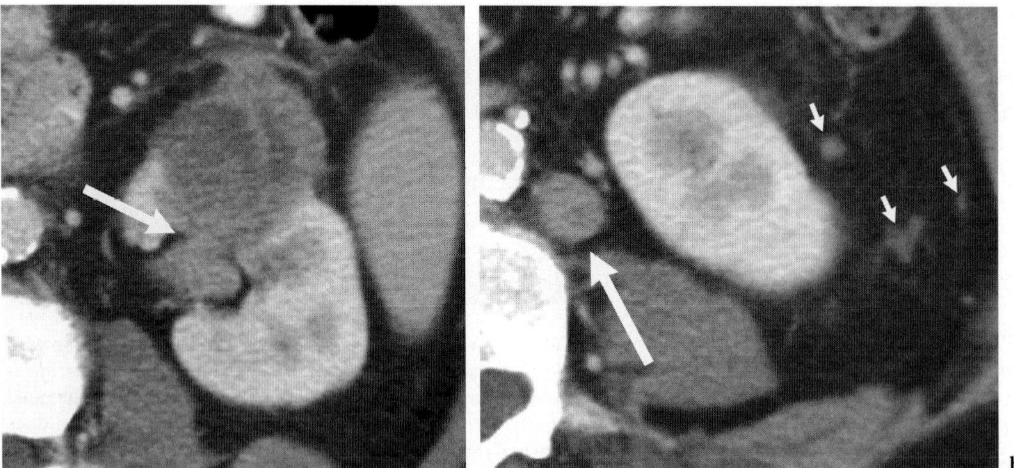

Fig. 7.10a,b. Renal cell carcinoma in a 57-year-old man. **a** Axial contrast-enhanced CT image shows large exophytic solid mass with invasion into renal collecting system (*arrow*). **b** Axial CT scan at different level shows enlarged para-aortic lymph node (*large arrow*) and small perinephric nodules (*small arrows*), both suspicious for malignant involvement.

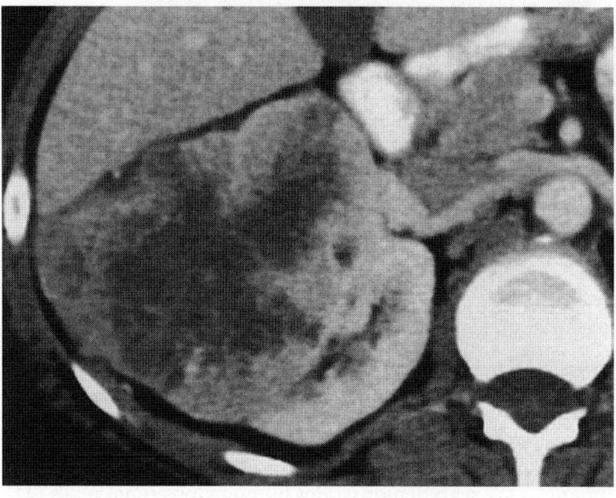

Fig. 7.11. Large RCC in a 61-year-old woman. Axial contrast-enhanced CT scan shows a large right RCC demonstrating features typical of larger RCC. Heterogeneity with central necrosis, irregular margins, and indistinct interface with normal kidney are all demonstrated in this renal mass.

enhancement of a renal mass of greater than 15% on scans made 3–5 min after gadolinium injection is strongly suggestive of a malignancy (Ho et al. 2002). This measurement of enhancement is predicated on the fact that all imaging parameters are set exactly the same before and after gadolinium injection. Gadolinium injection also improves the imaging quality of MR renal angiograms, if they are obtained early after bolus injection. Magnetic resonance imaging is particularly useful for the diagnosis of RCC in patients for whom iodinated intravascular contrast media present a significant health risk, such as patients with a history of a major adverse reaction or those with renal insufficiency. Although gadolinium is more nephrotoxic than iodinated contrast materials on a milliliter-to-milliliter basis, at the smaller doses required for MR imaging it is safe in patients with renal insufficiency.

Infiltrating RCCs, an uncommon subtype, do not substantially alter the reniform shape of the kidney, and these lesions often have homogeneous internal architecture (Fig. 7.12). They are detectable mainly because of their hypodensity compared with surrounding parenchyma on contrast-enhanced CT or MR imaging. Without the use of other diagnostic modalities, such as angiography or biopsy, these tumors may be indistinguishable from invasive urothelial malignancies.

Renal cell carcinomas sometimes appear cystic, and about 22% of proven RCCs are predominantly cystic (ZAGORIA et al. 1990); these are discussed in section 7.4.1.

7.3.5.3
Staging

Once RCC is suspected, staging is critical for appropriate treatment planning. It is often impossible to differentiate between stage I and stage II RCC with CT and MR imaging. Although this distinction does affect prognosis, it traditionally does not affect management, since radical nephrectomy is the treatment of choice in either case. More recently, a growing number of surgeons are treating early-stage

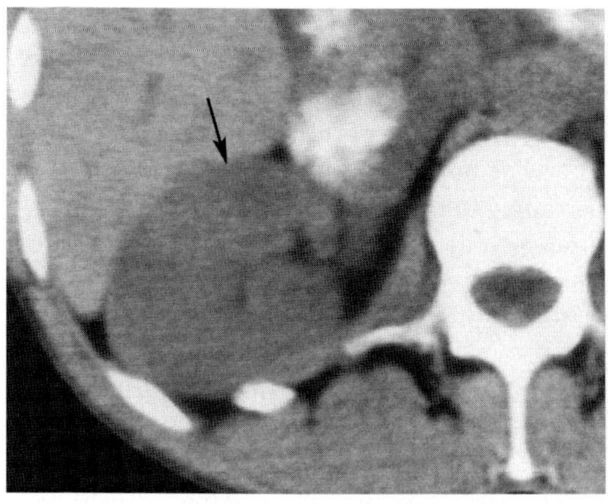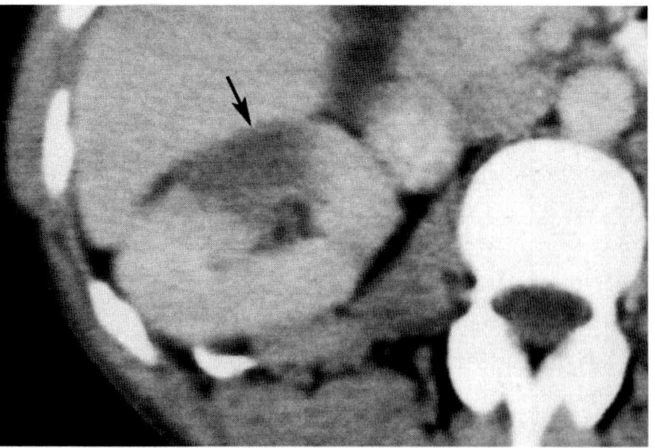

Fig. 7.12a,b. Typical CT appearance of infiltrating renal mass in a 69-year-old man. **a** Axial unenhanced CT scan shows infiltrating mass in the right kidney (*arrow*) which is barely discernable as a subtle hypodense area. **b** Axial contrast-enhanced CT scan shows a readily identifiable geographic area of decreased enhancement (*arrow*). Typical of infiltrating lesions, this RCC does not grossly affect bean shape of kidney.

RCC with partial nephrectomy or tumorectomy (LJUNGBERG 2004). Results indicate that partial nephrectomy is as effective a treatment for both stage I and stage II RCC as radical nephrectomy. When partial nephrectomy is being considered, it is important to scrutinize the ipsilateral adrenal gland for evidence of tumor involvement. When present, this form of stage II RCC will necessitate adrenalectomy in conjunction with tumor removal; otherwise, the adrenal gland is spared.

Some signs have been considered suggestive of extracapsular (stage II) tumor spread. These signs include visualization of the following features in the perinephric space: fat obliteration; collateral vessels; stranding or cobwebbing; fascial thickening; and discrete soft tissue masses. Obliteration of perinephric fat and visualization of perinephric collateral vessels are not reliable signs of stage II disease, and their significance for staging is minimal. Fat obliteration indicates only mass effect, not invasion, in the perinephric space, and collateral vessels form in response to tumor angiogenesis factor, but do not indicate extension of tumor. Likewise, perinephric stranding should not be considered a sign of extracapsular tumor spread. Perinephric stranding results from thickening of perinephric septa by edema, inflammation, or vascular congestion. Although fascial thickening is in fact often due to direct tumor spread, it may also occur as a result of reactive edema or hyperemia. The most reliable imaging sign of RCC spread to the perinephric space is the presence of a discrete perinephric soft tissue mass. The presence of a focal perinephric mass larger than 1 cm in diameter is strongly indicative

of stage II RCC; however, this finding is seen in less than half of patients with stage II disease. To date, reliable differentiation between stage I and stage II disease remains in the domain of the pathologist.

With MR imaging, as with CT, no reliable criteria have been established for differentiating between stage I and stage II RCC. Because they are multiplanar, MR images can be helpful in determining the presence of adjacent organ invasion when this remains unclear after CT and US. Sagittal and coronal images are usually definitive in excluding the presence of direct adjacent organ invasion when a fat plane exists between the RCC and that organ. Altered signal characteristics within adjacent organs must be interpreted with care when they are the sole abnormality, as signal changes in compressed segments of liver, for example resulting from congestion and edema, may mimic changes of direct invasion.

Often the most difficult imaging task with CT is accurate evaluation of tumor extension into the renal vein. After power-injected contrast material administration, thin (5 mm or less) CT slices made through the level of the renal vein will yield 95% accuracy in detecting renal vein thrombus complicating RCC (WELCH and LEROY 1997). Secondary signs of renal vein involvement are unreliable. Renal vein enlargement and displacement are not accurate indicators of venous invasion, as the renal vein is often enlarged simply due to the high flow of blood from a hypervascular RCC. Venous displacement may reflect distortion of its normal course from a bulky renal tumor or displacement from extrinsic nodal disease. The normal left renal vein may have an abrupt caliber change as it crosses between the

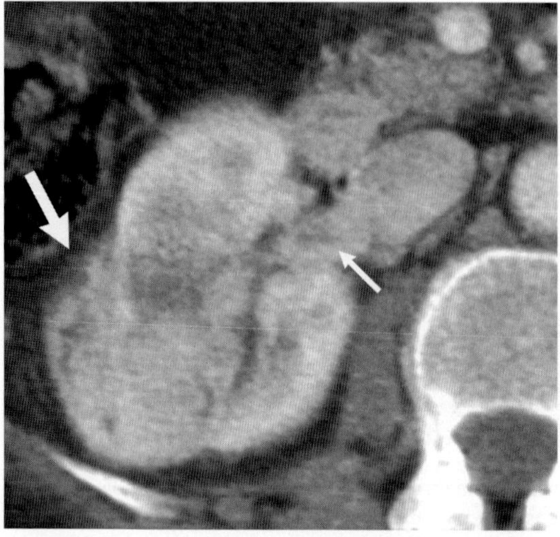

Fig. 7.13. Tumor extension into renal vein in a 54-year-old woman with RCC. Axial contrast-enhanced CT scan shows solid mass (*large arrow*) and filling defect (*small arrow*) in the renal vein compatible with tumor extension.

superior mesenteric artery and aorta; elsewhere such changes usually indicate the presence of tumor thrombus. The most reliable sign of tumor invasion is direct visualization of the hypodense thrombus in an otherwise opacified vein (Fig. 7.13). These criteria also apply to the diagnosis of tumor thrombus in the inferior vena cava.

The degree of venous tumor extension is also accurately depicted with multiplanar MR imaging (Fig. 7.14). Venous extension of tumor thrombus is well demonstrated with standard spin-echo T1-weighted images, on which flowing blood appears black because of signal void, with relative increased signal of the tumor thrombus. Alternatively, low-flip-angle gradient-echo scans enhance the signal of flowing blood. The resulting "bright-blood" images are similar in appearance to inferior vena cavograms and renal vein phlebography; thrombus appears as a hypointense filling defect surrounded by the hyperintensity of flowing blood. Tumor extension at or

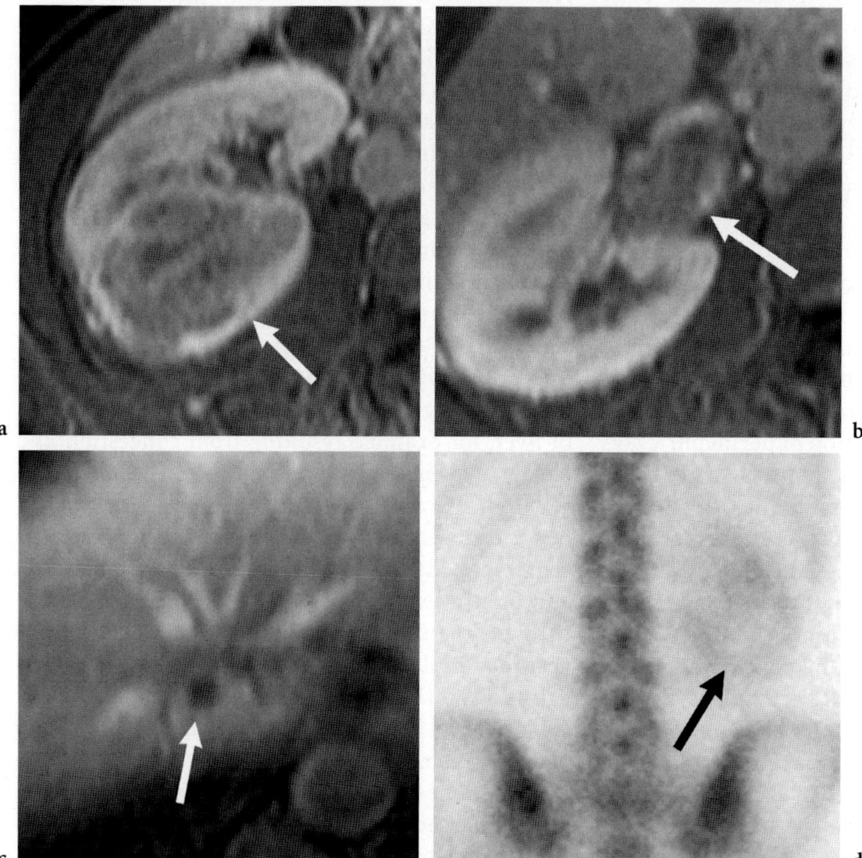

Fig. 7.14a-d. Venous involvement in a 72-year-old man with RCC. Axial contrast-enhanced fat-suppressed T1-weighted MR images show **a** RCC (*arrow*), **b** extension of tumor into renal vein (*arrow*), and **c** extension within inferior vena cava to level of hepatic veins (*arrow*). **d** Staging bone scan (posterior view) incidentally shows the right renal mass as an area of photopenia (*arrow*). The left kidney was surgically absent.

above the level of the hepatic veins dictates the surgical approach. If the tumor does not extend beyond hepatic inflow, an abdominal approach may be used for tumor excision and thrombectomy. Extension above this level necessitates an intrathoracic approach, and requires intraoperative cardiopulmonary bypass.

Clotted blood, also known as bland thrombus, may develop in veins adjacent to tumor thrombus, and the appearance may suggest more extensive tumor thrombus than is actually present. Both CT and MR imaging can be used to differentiate bland thrombus from tumor thrombus only when neovascularity (Fig. 7.15) or substantial contrast enhancement is detectable within the tumor thrombus (Fig. 7.16).

Both CT and MR imaging are very effective in detecting retroperitoneal lymphadenopathy. Nodes 1.5 cm or larger in short axis are pathologically enlarged and therefore suggestive of lymphatic metastases. This criterion assures accurate detection of most nodal metastases. Unfortunately, malignant lymphadenopathy cannot be differentiated from lymph node enlargement due to reactive

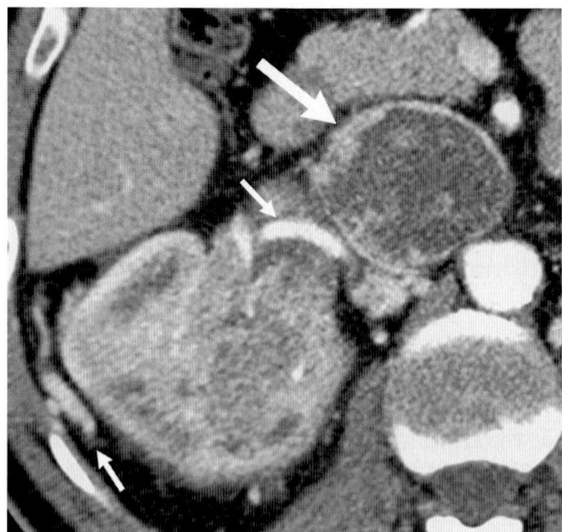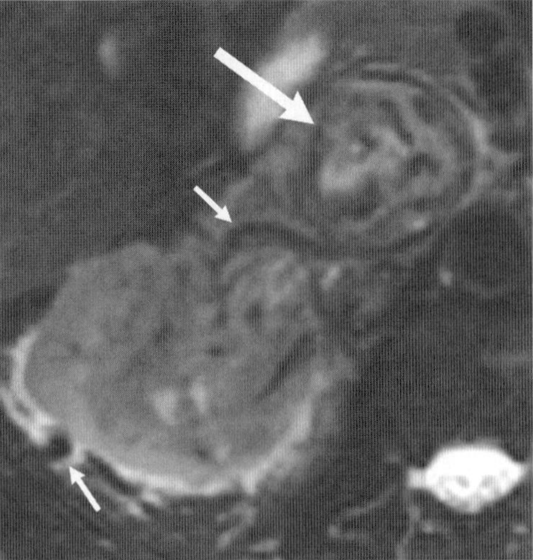

Fig. 7.15a,b. Neovascularity within tumor thrombus in a 54-year-old man with RCC. **a** Axial contrast-enhanced CT scan shows tumor thrombus extending into renal vein and distended inferior vena cava (*large arrow*). Tumor neovascularity in tumor thrombus and perinephric vessel enlargement are also noted (*small arrows*). **b** Axial T2-weighted MR image again shows the inferior vena cava thrombus (*large arrow*). Thrombus neovascularity and perinephric vessel enlargement are identified as flow voids (*small arrows*).

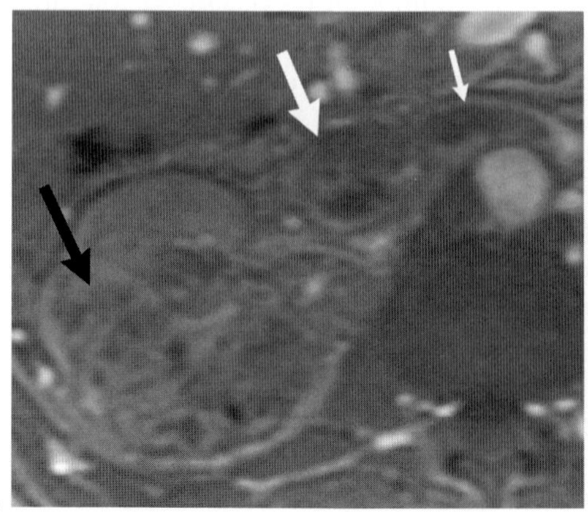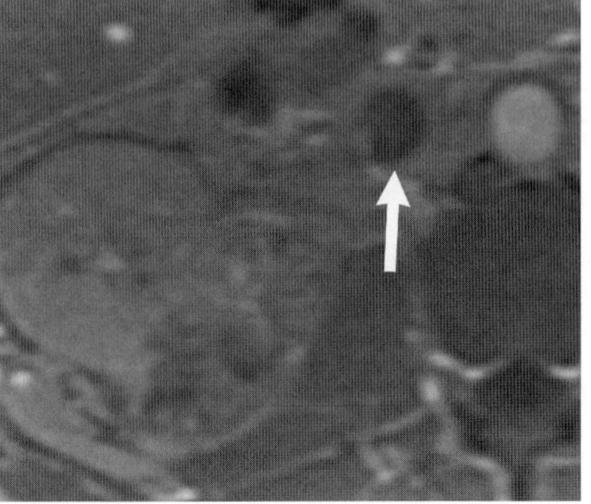

Fig. 7.16a,b. Bland thrombus and tumor thrombus in a 39-year-old man with RCC. Axial delayed contrast-enhanced fat-suppressed T1-weighted MR images show **a** renal mass (*black arrow*), enhancing tumor thrombus within inferior vena cava (*large white arrow*), and non-enhancing filling defect within left renal vein (*small white arrow*) compatible with bland thrombus. **b** Similar bland thrombus is identified in more inferior aspect of the inferior vena cava (*arrow*).

hyperplasia. Reactive hyperplasia in regional nodes is more commonly seen with RCCs complicated by tumor necrosis and venous extension. Also, nodes in the 1- to 1.5-cm range, particularly if they are more numerous than expected, are considered indeterminate but suspicious for spread of malignant disease. Occasionally, normal-sized nodes (<1 cm) harbor microscopic tumor foci.

Distant metastases to liver and bone are generally easy to identify with CT or MR imaging. Organ-appropriate window settings of scans should be done in all cases to maximize the CT visualization of metastatic deposits. Since RCC metastases are often hypervascular, making them difficult to detect in the enhanced liver, CT images of the liver during the hepatic arterial phase of liver enhancement are helpful in identifying many of these lesions. With MR imaging, metastatic deposits in the liver can be readily detected and distinguished from benign hemangiomas and cysts. Metastases to the spleen can be very difficult to identify because of the MR imaging characteristics of the spleen, which can mask focal tumors. Finally, MR imaging may be more sensitive than CT in the detection of unsuspected bony metastases because of its exquisite bone marrow imaging capability.

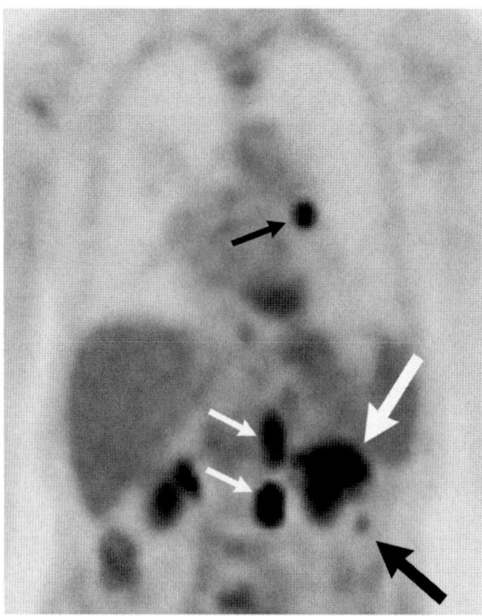

Fig. 7.17. Metastatic survey in a 61-year-old man with RCC. Coronal FDG-PET image shows increased radiotracer uptake in large left renal mass (*large white arrow*), perinephric focus (*large black arrow*), para-aortic lymph nodes (*small white arrows*), and left hilar lymph node (*small black arrow*). all compatible with metastatic disease.

7.3.6
PET Imaging

Oncological PET imaging with F-18 deoxyglucose (FDG) is predicated on the increased glucose utilization exhibited by tumor cells. Regarding the diagnosis of primary lesions, FDG-PET is limited by physiological radiotracer uptake in the kidney as well as by overall modest uptake within the tumor itself. Regarding staging and restaging, the overall sensitivity of FDG-PET (64–71%) in the detection of metastatic foci is limited (MAJHAIL et al. 2003; JADVAR et al. 2003). FDG-PET may play a complementary role in the restaging of RCC patients related to superior specificity and positive predictive value compared with conventional imaging (Fig. 7.17; KANG et al. 2004).

7.4
Additional Considerations

7.4.1
Cystic Renal Cell Carcinoma

Cystic renal masses have been studied extensively with CT and US. The Bosniak classification system is useful for categorizing these lesions as to their etiology and serving as a guide for treatment (BOSNIAK 1997). It is summarized as follows:

1. Class I lesions are simple cysts. Findings that are diagnostic of a simple renal cyst include a water-density mass that does not enhance and has an imperceptible or barely perceptible peripheral margin. Ultrasound findings include an anechoic lesion with thin walls and increased through-sound transmission (Fig. 7.18).

2. Class II lesions have thin septation(s) (Fig. 7.19), thin peripheral calcifications, are non-enhancing hyperdense cysts, or have features typical of infected cysts. With CT, one can be reasonably confident that these class II lesions are benign; however, they do merit follow-up CT scanning in 6–12 months to exclude progression. Septations and hyperdense internal material are thought to develop after cyst infection or hemorrhage, which leads to the development of fibrinous internal septa, dystrophic calcifications in the wall of the cyst, or internal proteinaceous material reflected by hyperdensity on unenhanced CT scans. The hyperdense cysts are the most problematic for radiologists. These lesions appear to be of higher

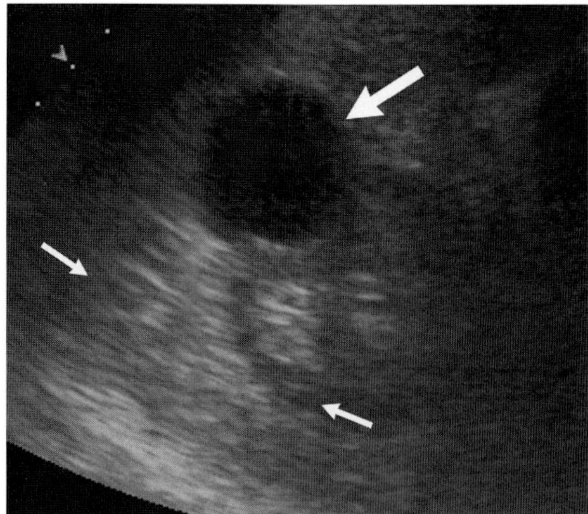

Fig. 7.18. Bosniak I lesion in a 37-year-old woman. Axial US image shows anechoic lesion (*large arrow*) with thin walls and evidence of increased through-sound transmission (*small arrows*) confirming simple cyst.

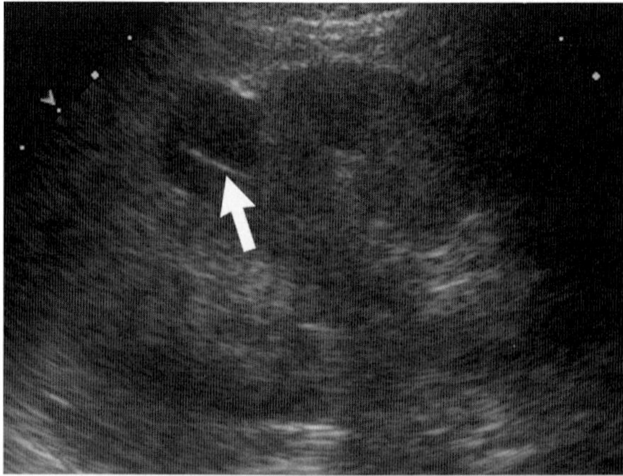

Fig. 7.19. Bosniak II lesion in a 40-year-old woman. Longitudinal US image shows cyst with single thin septation (*arrow*).

density than the kidney on unenhanced CT. With contrast infusion, they appear hypodense to the enhanced renal parenchyma, and there is no interval enhancement of these lesions with contrast material injection. Management of these lesions is somewhat controversial. Although the lack of enhancement seems to indicate that these are benign lesions, some researchers believe that US of these lesions is helpful in confirming that they are benign, albeit complicated, cysts. Unfortunately, these lesions often contain internal echoes when imaged with US. In such cases, follow-up imaging or even surgical extirpation may be nec-

essary. Since the overwhelming majority of these lesions are benign, follow-up CT seems to be the more prudent approach. If these lesions contain enhancing components, they are not class II lesions, but rather class IV lesions, and surgical removal is indicated.

3. Class III lesions have more complex imaging characteristics, including dense, thick calcifications, numerous septa or multiple locules, septal nodularity, or solid components that do not enhance. Approximately one-half of these lesions are cystic RCCs; the remainder are benign lesions such as cysts complicated by infection or hemorrhage, or the benign tumor known as multilocular cystic nephroma. There is no reliable way to distinguish among these lesions without surgery. Since many of them are benign, renal-sparing surgery can be considered for these patients, but surgical excision is generally recommended for complex cystic masses. Magnetic resonance imaging may be helpful in evaluating cystic lesions that are equivocal by US and CT (Fig. 7.20).

4. Class IV lesions are always considered malignant. The major criterion of a class IV lesion is an area of enhancing solid tissue. With cystic neoplasms, this tissue often is at the periphery, and enhancement may be subtle (Fig. 7.21). Careful comparison of the margins of the cystic mass between the unenhanced and the contrast-enhanced CT scan may reveal an area of enhancement. If so, the lesion should be presumed to be RCC and surgery is indicated.

As stated previously, approximately 20% of RCCs are predominantly cystic on CT or MR imaging. Three-quarters of these are solid RCCs that have undergone central liquefaction necrosis. With growth, these lesions tend to outstrip their blood supply, and central areas become ischemic and necrotic. The remaining lesions are truly cystic RCCs. This subgroup usually has a papillary cellular growth pattern, which has been associated with a decreased rate of metastases and better prognosis than other forms of RCC. Papillary RCCs are also often multifocal and may be familial. These tumors tend to be slow-growing masses with fronds of tissue protruding centrally from the margins. Fluid may be a large component of these masses. They are usually hypovascular, even after attaining a large size. Although these lesions may have subtle features indicating their true nature on CT, US often better demonstrates the complex internal architecture (Fig. 7.6) typical of a papillary RCC.

Cysts may be associated with renal malignancies in other ways. Since renal cysts are quite common,

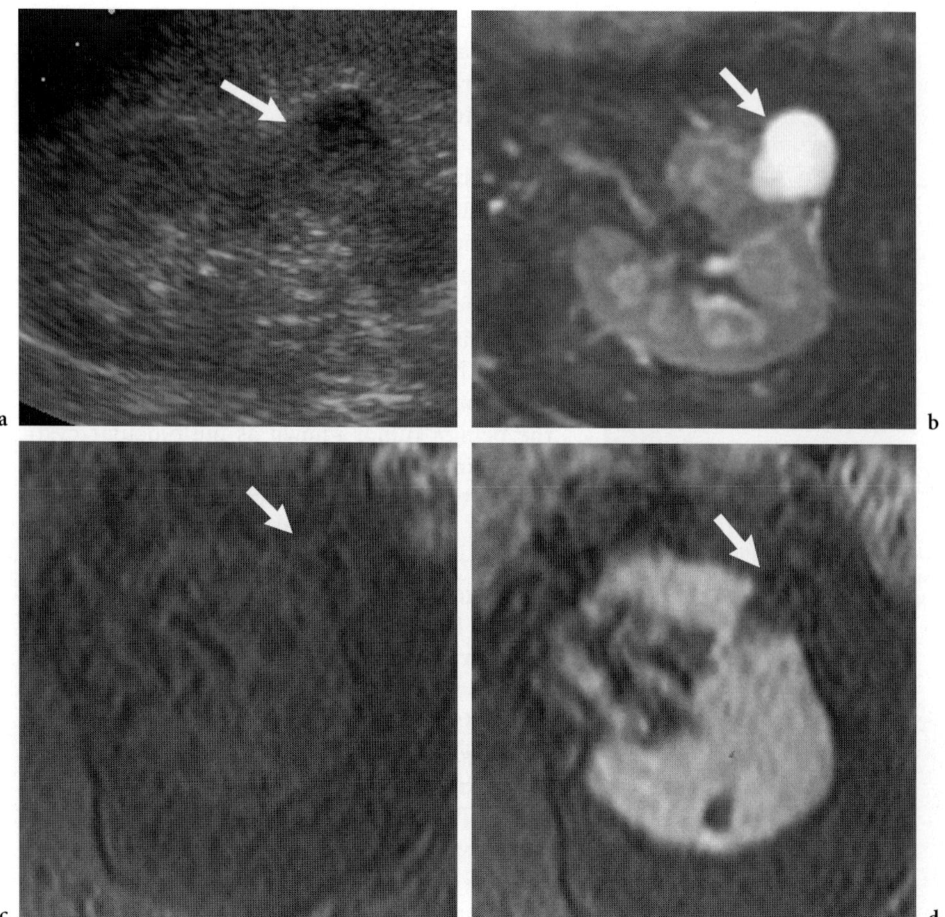

Fig. 7.20a-d. Cystic lesion in a 44-year-old man. **a** Longitudinal US image shows exophytic cystic lesion with ill-defined margins and questionable solid component (*arrow*). **b–d** Axial MR images show the lesion (*arrow*) to be homogeneous and hyperintense on T2-weighted image (**b**) and hypointense on unenhanced fat-suppressed T1-weighted image (**c**). There is no evidence of enhancement on contrast-enhanced fat-suppressed T1-weighted image (**d**). These findings are compatible with benign lesion.

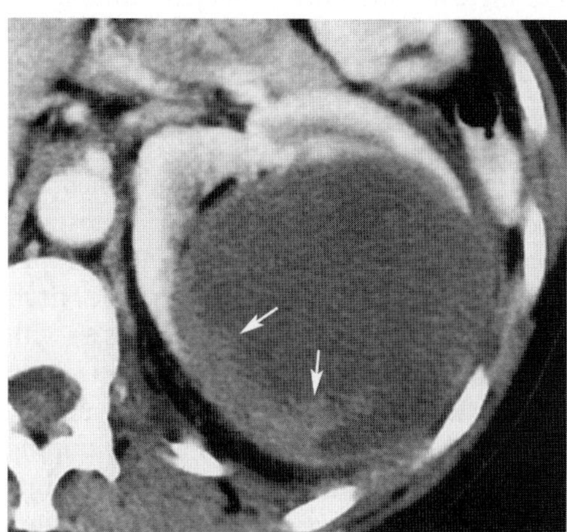

Fig. 7.21. Suspicious cystic renal mass in a 58-year-old man. Axial CT scan of this papillary RCC demonstrates solid tissue with subtle peripheral enhancement (*arrows*). Enhancing tissue in a cystic renal mass strongly suggests a malignant tumor.

cysts and tumors may occur in the same kidney and yet be causally unrelated. A renal tumor may occur adjacent to a solitary or dominant cyst. This pattern of abnormalities is likely related and occurs because the neoplasm obstructs renal tubules and causes dilatation and cyst formation. Since recognition of these cysts may lead to detection of the nearby renal tumor, these focal, solitary cysts are sometimes referred to as "sentinel" cysts. Some conditions cause formation of both renal cysts and renal neoplasms. This category includes von Hippel-Lindau disease (CHOYKE et al. 1990; JENNINGS and GAINES 1988), tuberous sclerosis (SEIDENWURM and BARKOVICH 1992), and long-term dialysis (SIEGEL et al. 1988). Finally, the rarest cyst–renal neoplasm association is the formation of an RCC in the wall of a preexisting simple renal cyst. Once sizable, these neoplasms can be detected with US, CT, or MR imaging as a solid nodule originating in the wall of cyst. The solid component of such a mass usually enhances with contrast material injection, and these tumors are managed identically to other RCCs.

7.4.2
Differential Diagnosis of Renal Masses

Several entities may mimic RCC; these include complex cysts, AML, abscess, metastases, oncocytoma, multilocular cystic nephroma (MLCN), and focal

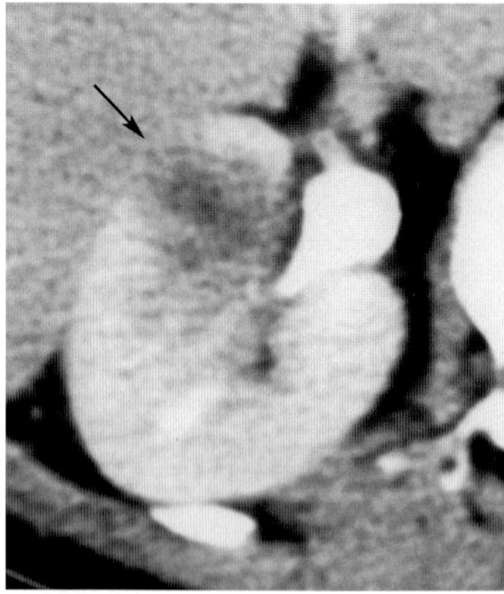

Fig. 7.22. Renal abscess in a 59-year-old woman. Axial contrast-enhanced CT scan shows hypodense lesion (*arrow*) with ill-defined margins in the right kidney. Distinction from RCC was made based on clinical presentation and follow-up.

xanthogranulomatous pyelonephritis (XGP). Complex cysts and AML are discussed in section 7.4.1 and section 7.3.3, respectively.

Renal abscesses usually result from inadequate treatment of pyelonephritis, which leads to central liquefaction and formation of a discrete intrarenal lesion. Abscesses, when visible, appear as thick-walled cystic masses on IVU or US. With CT, abscesses appear as rounded, well-defined, low-density masses with central liquefaction (Fig. 7.22). Distinction from RCC is based on clinical presentation. Rarely, patients present with a true renal abscess but have an underlying RCC. In these cases, the necrotic tumor center becomes secondarily infected. Follow-up renal imaging studies of patients with renal abscess, after resolution of their symptoms, are necessary to exclude an occult RCC.

Occasionally, a solitary renal metastasis or solitary focus of renal lymphoma may occur. In a patient with known extrarenal malignancy, percutaneous biopsy or surgical biopsy is usually necessary to distinguish RCC from a solitary metastasis. Primary sources that account for most renal metastases include carcinoma of the breast, lung, gastrointestinal tract, or malignant melanoma. Also, lymphoma commonly spreads to the kidneys, but true primary renal lymphoma is extremely rare.

Oncocytomas are benign renal tumors, comprising 5% of resected renal masses (SCHATZ and LIEBER 2003), and having no metastatic potential. Unfortunately, preoperative diagnosis is often impossible since imaging characteristics of these lesions substantially overlap with those of RCC (Fig. 7.23). In addition, biopsy is of little value, since

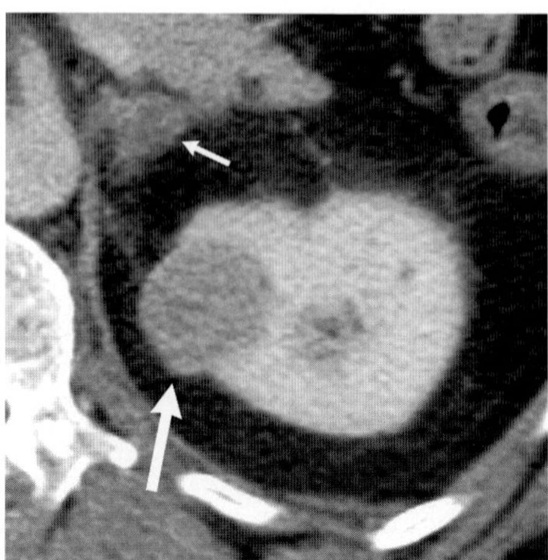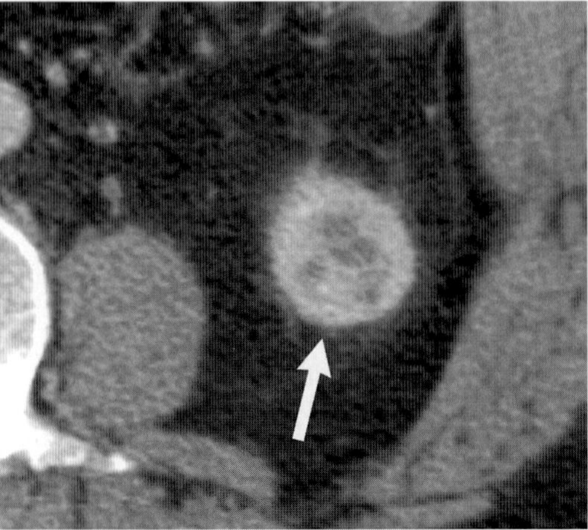

a   b

Fig. 7.23a,b. Oncocytoma and RCC in a 44-year-old man. **a** Axial contrast-enhanced CT scan shows solid enhancing mass (*large arrow*) in the left mid-kidney and suspicious para-aortic lymph node (*small arrow*). This mass was proved to be RCC. **b** Axial contrast-enhanced CT scan caudad to **a** shows a second solid enhancing left kidney lesion (*arrow*) which proved to be oncocytoma.

some RCCs contain benign-appearing oncocytic elements that are indistinguishable from an oncocytoma. On IVU, oncocytomas are often large at initial detection and have very smooth margins. The US findings are nonspecific. Oncocytomas are usually isoechoic to the kidney, with well-demarcated margins. (Fig. 7.24) A central scar, typical of oncocytoma, may be visible with US. With CT or MR imaging, these lesions appear well circumscribed and have homogeneous enhancement patterns. Often the appearance of a pseudocapsule is seen at the periphery of the mass. The pseudocapsule is formed from renal parenchyma compressed around the edge of the mass. The above mentioned central stellate scar may also be detectable with CT (Fig. 7.25) or MR imaging. Although this scar is typical of oncocytoma, it is not diagnostic, and RCC may have an identical appearance. Angiography may be obtained prior to attempting renal-sparing surgery. The typical angiographic pattern of an oncocytoma is one of a "spoke wheel" with circumferential vessels at the periphery of the lesions and feeding vessels penetrating to the avascular central scar. These tumors lack the bizarre tumor vascularity often seen with RCC. A renal mass with these features may be an oncocytoma, but renal cell carcinoma can have identical imaging findings; thus, a renal mass with some, or all, of these features should be considered a "surgical" renal mass. At best, the presence of some of these imaging features may suggest the possibility of an oncocytoma and may prompt an attempted renal-sparing approach to the tumor. At the time of surgery, histological assessment of the entire lesion can confirm the

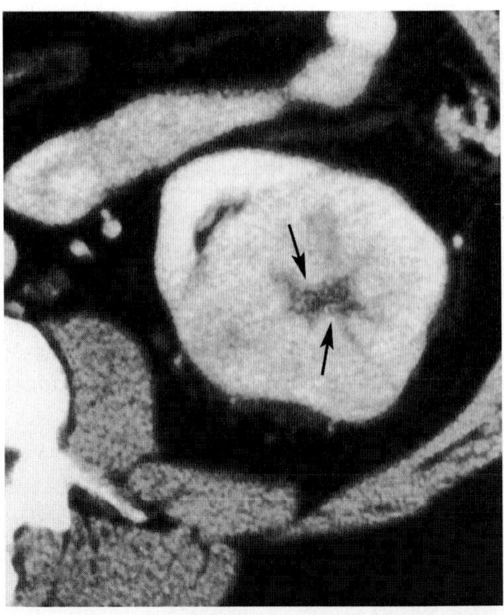

Fig. 7.25. Oncocytoma in a 55-year-old man. Axial contrast-enhanced CT scan demonstrates homogenous renal mass with central stellate scar (*arrows*). Although this mass was an oncocytoma, there is considerable overlap of these imaging features with RCC.

diagnosis of oncocytoma. If malignant elements indicating an RCC are found, partial or radical nephrectomy can be completed.

With CT or MR imaging, MLCNs are well-defined masses with visible septations (Fig. 7.26). Internal hemorrhage is characteristically absent in these benign tumors. They are hypovascular or avascular. Like oncocytomas, these tumors have characteristic features, none of which, however, distinguish them reliably from RCC; therefore, at best, one can sug-

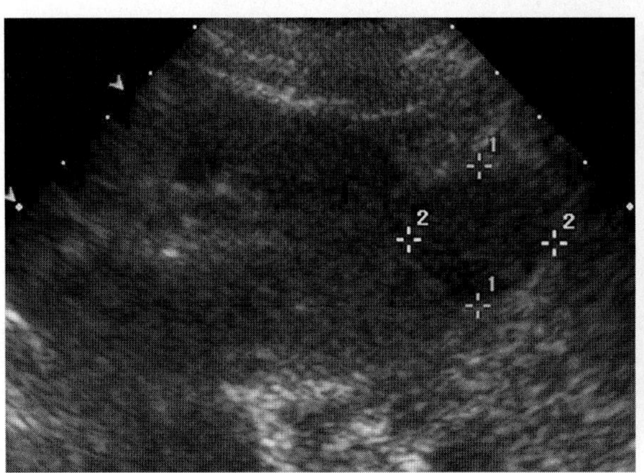
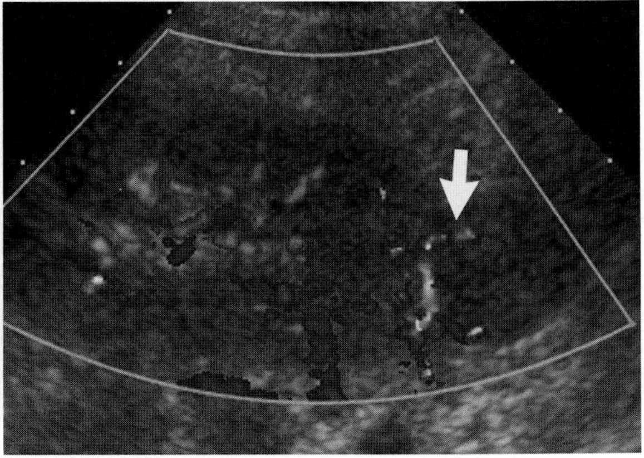

Fig. 7.24a,b. Oncocytoma in a 54-year-old woman. a Longitudinal US image shows solid lesion with homogeneous echo texture. b Longitudinal color Doppler image shows vessel extending from kidney into lesion (*arrow*).

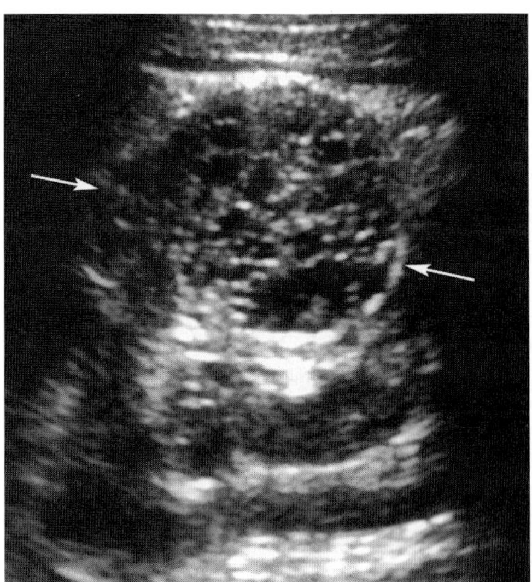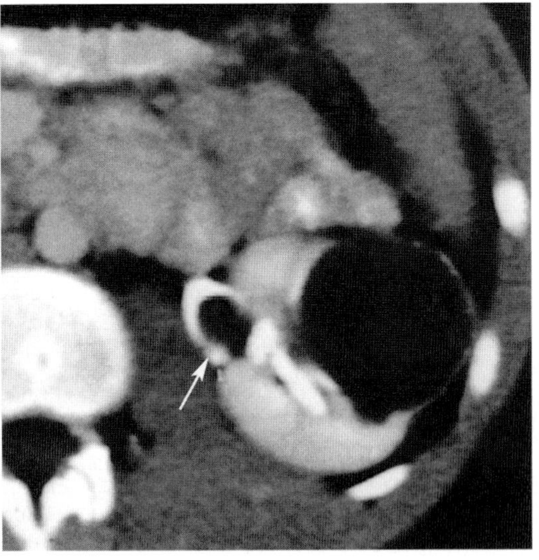

Fig. 7.26a,b. Multilocular cystic nephroma in a 42-year-old woman. **a** Oblique US image of a renal mass (*arrows*) demonstrates numerous cystic locules with interposed septa. **b** Axial contrast-enhanced CT scan of this same mass demonstrates features typical of a multilocular cystic nephroma. This cystic mass is well circumscribed with thin septations. Centrally it is seen to herniate (*arrow*) into the renal pelvis.

gest the diagnosis preoperatively, so that renal-sparing surgery can be attempted in some cases.

Tumefactive or focal XGP results from a focal area of renal inflammation often associated with stone disease. No imaging characteristics are diagnostic of focal XGP. With IVU, a hypofunctioning focal mass is evident. With US, this mass may have increased echogenicity due to the innumerable lipid-laden macrophages that make up the mass. On CT, focal XGP appears as a nonspecific solid or cystic renal mass (Fig. 7.27), often in association with a renal calculus. Typical history may suggest the diagnosis of focal XGP preoperatively. These lesions are irreversible and are best treated with renal-sparing surgery.

7.4.3
Spontaneous Perirenal Hemorrhage

Nontraumatic spontaneous renal, subcapsular, or perirenal hemorrhage (SPH; Fig. 7.28) is an unusual presentation of RCC, causing patients to seek medical evaluation. Of all SPHs, up to 55% are due to underlying RCCs (ZHANG et al. 2002). Unfortunately, extensive hemorrhage often obscures the underlying tumor, making it undetectable with CT or MR imaging. In these cases, if a renal mass is not detected when SPH is initially diagnosed, a renal arteriogram should be acquired to detect evidence of a vasculitis or vascular lesion; if none is detected, CT or MR

imaging should be repeated in 1 month to search again for a renal mass while the hemorrhage is resolving. Follow-up CT or MR imaging should be repeated if no lesion is detected. If a benign mass, such as an AML, which is commonly associated with SPH, is detected, it can be treated nonsurgically or with renal-sparing surgery. Detection of an RCC usually

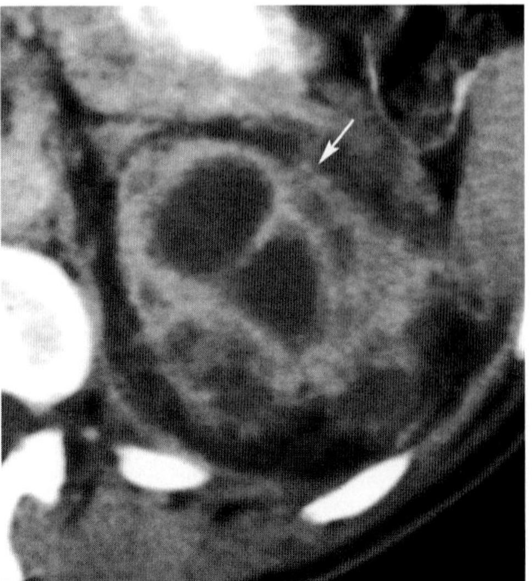

Fig. 7.27. Focal xanthogranulomatous pyelonephritis in a 50-year-old man. Axial contrast-enhanced CT scan shows multicystic ill-defined mass (*arrow*) upper pole left kidney. Renal cell carcinoma could have similar appearance.

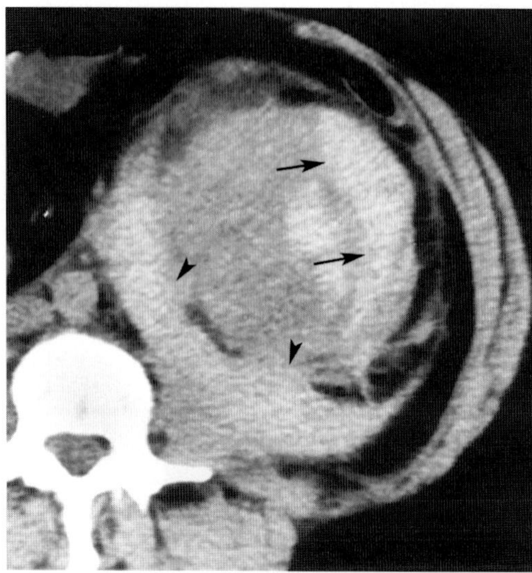

Fig. 7.28. Spontaneous perirenal hemorrhage in a 69-year-old man with RCC. Axial unenhanced CT scan demonstrates subcapsular (*arrows*) and perirenal (*arrowheads*) hyperdense fluid. This is typical of acute hemorrhage and suggests underlying pathology in that kidney. Further scanning demonstrated a solid renal mass with features typical of RCC in this kidney.

leads to nephrectomy. This approach to SPH helps to minimize nephrectomy for benign diseases.

7.5
Conclusion

Because a significant percentage of RCCs are discovered incidentally on an imaging study ordered for another purpose, the radiologist must remain vigilant. Once a suspected mass is identified, US is a cost-effective means to further characterize those lesions that are statistically most likely to be simple cysts. Solid or complex cystic lesions are best characterized by CT or MR imaging. These cross-sectional modalities are also indispensable in the staging and restaging of suspected RCC lesions, although other modalities, such as PET, may play a complementary role.

References

American Cancer Society (1996) Cancer facts and figures – 1996. American Cancer Society, Atlanta

Bechtold RE, Zagoria RJ (1997) Imaging approach to staging of renal cell carcinoma. Urol Clin North Am 24:507–522

Bosniak MA, Birnbaum BA, Krinsky GA et al. (1995) Small renal parenchymal neoplasms: further observations on growth. Radiology 197:589–597

Bosniak MA (1997) The use of the Bosniak classification system for renal cysts and cystic tumors. J Urol 157:1852–1853

Bracken RB (1987) Renal carcinoma: clinical aspects and therapy. Semin Roentgenol 22:241–247

Chow WH, Devsa SS, Warren JL et al. (1999) Rising incidence of renal cell cancer in the United States. J Am Med Assoc 281:1628–1631

Choyke PL, Filling-Katz MR, Shawker TH et al. (1990) Von Hippel-Lindau disease: radiologic screening for visceral manifestations. Radiology 174:815–820

Eble JN, Sauter G, Epstein JI et al. (eds) (2004) Tumors of the kidney. In: WHO classification of tumours: tumours of the urinary system and male genital organs. IARC Press, Lyon, France

Einstein DM, Herts BR, Weaver R et al. (1995) Evaluation of renal masses detected by excretory urography: cost-effectiveness of sonography versus CT. Am J Roentgenol 164:371–375

Ergen FB, Hussain HK, Caoili EM (2004) MRI for preoperative staging of renal cell carcinoma using the 1997 TNM classification: comparison with surgical and pathologic staging. Am J Roentgenol 182:217–225

Fisher RI, Rosenberg SA, Fyfe G (2000) Long-term survival update for high-dose recombinant interleukin-2 in patients with renal cell carcinoma. Cancer J Sci Am 6 (Suppl 1):55–57

Forman HP, Middleton WD, Melson GL et al. (1993) Hyperechoic renal cell carcinomas: increase in detection at US. Radiology 188:431–434

Gash JR, Zagoria RJ, Dyer RB (1992) Imaging features of infiltrating renal lesions. Crit Rev Diagn Imaging 33:293–310

Greenlee RT, Murray T, Bolden S, Wingo PA (2000) Cancer statistics, 2000. CA Cancer J Clin 50:7–33

Greenlee RT, Hill-Harmon MB, Murray T, Thun M (2001) Cancer statistics, 2001. CA Cancer J Clin 51:15–36

Guinan P, Sobin LH, Algaba F (1997) TNM staging of renal cell carcinoma: Workgroup no. 3 (Union International Contre le Cancer UICC) and the American Joint Committee on Cancer (AJCC). Cancer 80:992–993

Gupta NP, Ansari MS, Khaitan A et al. (2004) Impact of imaging and thrombus level in management of renal cell carcinoma extending to veins. Urol Int 72:129–134

Ho VB, Allen SF, Hood MN et al. (2002) Renal masses: quantitative assessment of enhancement with dynamic MR imaging. Radiology 224:695–700

Jadvar H, Kherbache HM, Pinski JK et al. (2003) Diagnostic role of [F-18]-FDG positron emission tomography in restaging renal cell carcinoma. Clin Nephrol 60:395–400

Jennings CM, Gaines PA (1988) The abdominal manifestation of von Hippel-Lindau disease and a radiological screening protocol for an affected family. Clin Radiol 39:363–367

Kang DE, White RL Jr, Zuger JH et al. (2004) Clinical use of fluorodeoxyglucose F 18 positron emission tomography for detection of renal cell carcinoma. J Urol 171:1806–1809

deKernion JB (1987) Management of renal adenocarcinoma. In: deKernion JB, Paulson DF (eds) Genitourinary cancer management. Lea and Febiger, Philadelphia, pp 187–217

Kim JK, Kim TK, Ahn HJ et al. (2002) Differentiation of subtypes of renal cell carcinoma on helical CT scans. Am J Roentgenol 178:1499–1506

Landis SH, Murray T, Bolden S, Wingo PA (1998) Cancer statistics, 1998. CA Cancer J Clin 48:6–29

Landis SH, Murray T, Bolden S, Wingo PA (1999) Cancer statistics, 1999. CA Cancer J Clin 49:8–31

Leslie JA, Prihoda T, Thompson IM (2003) Serendipitous renal cell carcinoma in the post-CT era: continued evidence in improved outcomes. Urol Oncol 21:39–44

Ljungberg B (2004) Nephron-sparing-surgery strategies for partial nephrectomy in renal cell carcinoma. Scand J Surg 93:126–131

Majhail NS, Urbain J, Albani JM et al. (2003) F-18 fluorodeoxyglucose positron emission tomography in the evaluation of distant metastases from renal cell carcinoma. J Clin Oncol 21:3995–4000

Motzer RJ, Bander NH, Nanus DM (1996) Renal cell carcinoma. N Engl J Med 335:865–875

Schatz SM, Lieber MM (2003) Update on oncocytoma. Curr Urol Rep 4:30–35

Seidenwurm DJ, Barkovich AJ (1992) Understanding tuberous sclerosis. Radiology 183:23–24

Siegel SC, Sandler MA, Alpern MB et al. (1988) CT of renal cell carcinoma in patients on chronic hemodialysis. Am J Roentgenol 150:583–585

Sweeney JP, Thornhill JA, Graiger R et al. (1996) Incidentally detected renal cell carcinoma: pathological features, survival trends and implications for treatment. Br J Urol 78:351

Takahashi K, Honda M, Okubo RS et al. (1993) CT pixel mapping in the diagnosis of small angiomyolipomas of the kidneys. J Comput Assist Tomogr 17:98–101

Watson RC, Fleming RJ, Evans JA (1968) Arteriography in the diagnosis of renal carcinoma: review of 100 cases. Radiology 91:888–897

Welch TJ, LeRoy AJ (1997) Helical and electron beam CT scanning in the evaluation of renal vein involvement in patients with renal cell carcinoma. J Comput Assist Tomogr 21:467–471

Yagoda A, Abi-Rached B, Petrylak D (1995) Chemotherapy for advanced renal-cell carcinoma: 1983–1993. Semin Oncol 22:42–60

Yamashita Y, Ueno S, Makita O et al. (1993) Hyperechoic renal tumors: anechoic rim and intratumoral cysts in US differentiation of renal cell carcinoma from angiomyolipoma. Radiology 188:179–182

Zagoria RJ, Wolfman NT, Karstaedt N et al. (1990) CT features of renal cell carcinoma with emphasis on relation to tumor size. Invest Radiol 25:261–266

Zhang JQ, Fielding JR, Zou KH (2002) Etiology of spontaneous perirenal hemorrhage: a meta-analysis. J Urol 167:1593–1596

8 Transitional Cell Carcinoma

Ronan F. Browne and William C. Torreggiani

CONTENTS

8.1
Introduction

Transitional cell carcinoma (TCC) of the urothelium is the second most common urological tumor after prostate carcinoma (Herranz-Amo et al. 1999), and usually presents with hematuria. Although these tumors are most commonly encountered in the urinary bladder, up to 5% are found in the upper urinary tract. The evaluation of hematuria, however, also requires assessment of the renal parenchyma for masses and the urinary tract for calculi. In addition, the urothelium must be examined in its entirety because of the multicentric nature of TCC. Conventional imaging modalities, such as

R. F. Browne, MD
Fellow in Abdominal Imaging, Abdominal Division, Department of Radiology, Vancouver General Hospital, 899 West 12th Avenue, Vancouver V5Z 1M9, British Columbia, Canada
W. C. Torreggiani, MD
Consultant Radiologist, Department of Radiology, Adelaide and Meath Hospital, Tallaght, Dublin 24, Ireland

intravenous urography (IVU), retrograde pyelography (RP), and ultrasound (US), still play a key role in diagnosis in combination with cystoscopy and endourological techniques. Recently, the technique of multiphasic computed tomographic urography (CTU) has evolved as an alternative method of assessing patients with hematuria, offering superior detection of urinary calculi and renal parenchymal masses, and in some studies, improved detection of urothelial lesions. Because surrounding structures can also be assessed, CTU is rapidly becoming the definitive study for these patients, potentially shortening the duration of diagnostic evaluation. Magnetic resonance (MR) imaging, including the newer techniques of MR angiography (MRA) and MR urography (MRU), is also being used, particularly in patients who cannot tolerate iodinated contrast, and in whom multiplanar, vascular, and collecting system imaging is required.

Although there are pathological and imaging features common to TCC occurring anywhere in the urinary tract, certain findings are more typical of tumors of the upper urinary tract. Synchronous or metachronous tumor of either ipsilateral or contralateral collecting system is common, necessitating vigilant urological and radiological follow-up. This chapter reviews the characteristic imaging features of renal TCC and outlines the role of imaging in diagnosis, pre-operative staging, and follow-up.

8.2
Incidence

Transitional cell carcinoma of the kidney arises from the urothelium of the renal pelvis or calices overlying the renal parenchyma, and is the most common urothelial malignancy of the urinary tract (Scolieri et al. 2000). Five percent of urothelial tumors arise in the kidney or ureters, accounting for approximately 10% of upper-tract neoplasm

(HALL et al. 1998; KIRKALI and TUZEL 2003). Renal TCC most frequently arises in the extrarenal part of the pelvis, followed by the infundibulocalyceal region.

Distribution is equal between left and right kidneys, with 2–4% occurring bilaterally. Twenty-five percent of upper-tract tumors occur in the ureter, and only 25% of these are found in the upper third (KIRKALI and TUZEL 2003)

8.3
Etiology

Renal TCC typically occurs in the sixth and seventh decades of life, with men affected three times more often than women. Besides increasing age and male gender, the most important risk factor is smoking, with smokers two to three times more likely to develop renal TCC than non-smokers (KIRKALI and TUZEL 2003). Chemical carcinogens (aniline, benzidine, aromatic amine, azo dyes), cyclophosphamide therapy, and heavy caffeine consumption are also associated with TCC, and all predispose to synchronous and metachronous tumor development (KIRKALI and TUZEL 2003). These substances are metabolized and excreted in the urine as carcinogenic substances that act locally on the urothelium. Because urine is in contact with mucosa in the bladder reservoir for a longer time and because the surface area of the bladder is larger than other parts of the urinary tract, bladder carcinomas are 30–50 times more common than tumors of the upper tract (WONG-YOU-CHEONG et al. 1998). Stasis of urine and structural abnormalities, such as horseshoe kidneys which predispose to stasis, are therefore also associated with increased prevalence. Renal TCC is very common in families affected with "Balkan endemic nephropathy." Familial metabolic abnormalities in these patients lead to tubulointerstitial nephritis, renal failure, carcinogenic glomerular–tubular toxins and multiple tumors (KIRKALI and TUZEL 2003). Analgesic abuse, particularly long-term use of phenacetin, produces capillosclerosis and predisposes to a highly invasive type of TCC that preferentially involves the renal pelvis (LEE et al. 1997). Human papilloma virus and hereditary non-polyposis colon cancer have also been suggested as risk factors for renal TCC, and the incidence is also significantly higher in areas where endemic "blackfoot disease" is seen (KIRKALI and TUZEL 2003).

8.4
Presentation

Patients with renal TCC typically present with hematuria, which may be frank or microscopic. Up to a third of patients with ureteric lesions may present with flank pain or acute renal colic. The gradual expansion of the ureteral lumen around these slow-growing tumors, however, makes these symptoms, which are more commonly associated with calculi, less likely than may be expected. Occasionally, tumors may be discovered incidentally during radiological investigations performed for unrelated symptomatology. Tumor spread occurs by mucosal extension or local, hematogenous, or lymphatic invasion. Occasionally, patients may present with distant metastases usually to the liver, bone, and lungs (CHAN et al. 2002).

8.5
Pathophysiology

Approximately 80% of TCC is low-stage, superficial, papillary neoplasm with a broad base and frond-like morphologic structure (BARENTSZ et al. 1996). These tumors are usually small at time of diagnosis, grow slowly, and follow a relatively benign course (URBAN et al. 1997a).

Pedunculated or diffusely infiltrating tumor accounts for approximately 20% of TCC and tends to behave more aggressively and be more advanced at diagnosis (BUCKLEY et al. 1996). Infiltrating tumors are characterized by thickening and induration of the renal pelvic wall, often with invasion into the renal parenchyma. This infiltrative growth pattern, however, preserves renal contour and differs from renal cell carcinomas (RCC), which are largely expansile.

Synchronous bilateral TCC has been reported to occur in 1–2% of cases of renal lesions. Eleven to 13% of patients with upper-tract TCC subsequently develop metachronous upper-tract tumor (WONG-YOU-CHEONG et al. 1998). Furthermore, up to 50% of patients initially presenting with upper-tract TCC develop metachronous tumor in the bladder, typically developing within 2 years of surgical treatment and seen more commonly with ureteral than renal tumors (KEELEY et al. 1997; KIRKALI and TUZEL 2003). On the other hand, 2% of patients with bladder TCC have synchronous upper-tract tumor at time of evaluation (HERRANZ-AMO et al. 1999). In patients with bladder cancer, metachronous upper-tract disease occurs in up to 6%, invariably seen in patients with cystoscopic evidence of recurrent bladder tumor, typically occurring within 3 years and carrying a relatively poor prognosis (Hession et al. 1999; Kirkali and Tuzel 2003). The incidence is higher with multifocal or high-grade tumor, distal ureteric involvement, or vesicoureteral reflux (Kirkali and Tuzel 2003; Wong-You-Cheong et al. 1998).

8.6
Diagnosis

The standard work-up of patients with hematuria as recommended by the American Urological Association consists of urinalysis and cytology, cystoscopy, and IVU (Grossfeld et al. 2001; O'Malley et al. 2003). The initial diagnosis of TCC is usually made on the basis of urine cytology and diagnostic yield is improved with selective lavage and collection, and brush biopsies performed at cystoscopy or retrograde ureteropyelography; however, these techniques are invasive and technically demanding. The limitations of IVU in assessing the renal parenchyma usually requires the supplemental use of US, CT, or MR imaging to evaluate the kidneys for masses (Gray Sears et al. 2002; Kawashima et al. 2003; Maher et al. 2004). Furthermore, additional imaging is also

often required to clarify indeterminate findings on IVU. Computed tomographic urography offers the potential to diagnose calculi, urothelial tumors, and renal parenchymal tumors as a single investigation, although further studies are required before it becomes the standard first-line investigation for hematuria. Cystoscopy remains the gold standard for the diagnosis and follow-up of carcinoma of the bladder, and is therefore performed in all patients presenting with hematuria in whom tumor is suspected (Lang et al. 2003; O'Malley et al. 2003).

8.6.1
Intravenous Urography

The diagnosis of renal TCC is most frequently made on IVU in patients undergoing investigation for hematuria or flank pain. Intravenous urography remains the non-invasive method of choice for imaging the detailed anatomy of the pelvicalyceal system and ureters (Kawashima et al. 2003; O'Malley et al. 2003; Scolieri et al. 2000; Yousem et al. 1988), although this is likely to change as CTU becomes more refined and accepted as a primary diagnostic investigation. The appearances of renal lesions on IVU are well described. Calcification may be visualized on preliminary radiographs but is uncommon, occurring in 2–7% of tumors, and, when present, may mimic urinary tract calculi (Fig. 8.1;

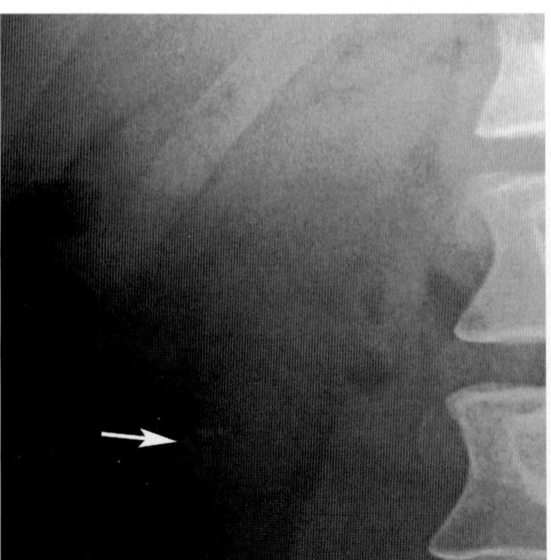
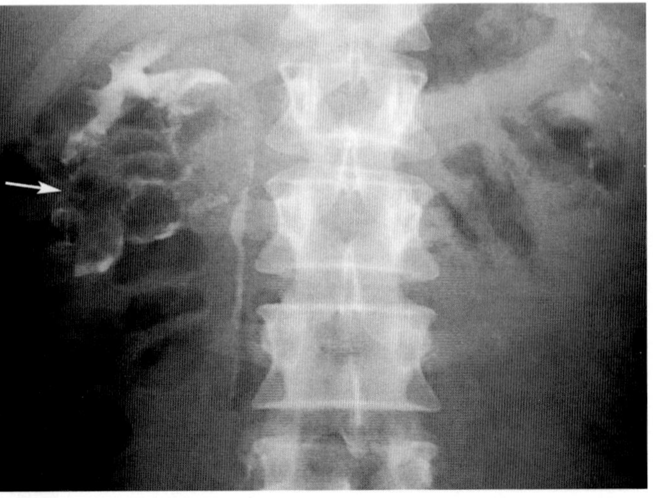

a   b

Fig. 8.1a,b. Transitional cell carcinoma of the renal pelvis in a 65-year-old man. **a** Oblique intravenous urography (IVU) scout film reveals microscopic calcification (*arrow*) overlying the lower pole of the right kidney, subsequently shown to represent transitional cell carcinoma. **b** Anteroposterior IVU 15-min film reveals a large stippled filling defect involving the collecting system of the right kidney. Calcification in the periphery is again noted and discerned from contrast by reference to the scout film (*arrow*).

WONG-YOU-CHEONG et al. 1998). Renal enlargement is seen only with very large tumors. On IVU renal TCC usually manifests as a filling defect within the contrast-enhanced renal collecting system. Filling defects may be single or multiple and smooth, irregular (Fig. 8.2), or stippled. The stipple sign refers to tracking of contrast into the interstices of a papillary lesion (Fig. 8.1b; KIRKALI and TUZEL 2003; WONG-YOU-CHEONG ct al. 1998). This sign, however, may also be seen with blood clot and fungus balls, and should be interpreted with caution. Stricture-like lesions of the pelvicalyceal system may be evident and, if multiple, may mimic renal tuberculosis. Filling defects within dilated calices may occur secondary to tumor obstruction of the infundibulum, and may lead to calyceal amputation (Fig. 8.3). Tumor-filled, distended calices have been called "oncocalices/phantom calices" which fail to opacify with contrast. It is important to remember that longstanding tumor obstruction of the uretero-pelvic junction or ureter may lead to generalized hydronephrosis and poor excretion. In this case alternative imaging modalities are often required for diagnosis. This is a major disadvantage of IVU when compared with CTU, which allows assessment of non-functioning kidneys. Because pelvicalyceal filling defects may be non-specific and urinary obstruction may obscure distal synchronous ureteric tumors, RP is often required to clarify the diagnosis.

8.6.2
Retrograde Pyelography

Retrograde pyelography is usually performed during cystoscopy or to further characterize abnormalities detected on IVU, in inadequately excreting kidneys, or in cases of contrast allergy. Retrograde pyelography, although invasive, can confirm the radiological diagnosis while also facilitating ureterorenoscopy with biopsy/brushings and cytological examination of localized urine collection. As with IVU, renal TCC typically appears as an intraluminal filling defect, which may be smooth, irregular, or stippled (Figs. 8.4–8.6). Opacification of a tumor-involved calyx may show irregular papillary or nodular mucosa (Figs. 8.7, 8.8). If TCC involves an infundibulum, then an "amputated" calyx may be seen with/without focal hydronephrosis and "oncocalyx" (Fig. 8.9). If renal lesions extend into the upper ureter, ureteric fixation may occur secondary to diffuse mural infiltration.

8.6.3
Ultrasound

At present, renal US is frequently used for patients with hematuria to assess for renal parenchymal masses. Ultrasound, however, is not as sensitive as

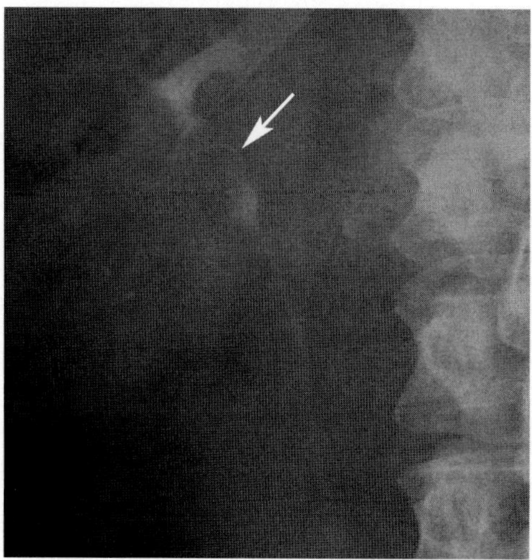

Fig. 8.2. Transitional cell carcinoma of the renal pelvis in a 60-year-old man with painless hematuria. Oblique IVU 15-min film demonstrates a large irregular filling defect (*arrow*) involving the right renal pelvis and extending into the lower-pole calyceal system due to transitional cell carcinoma.

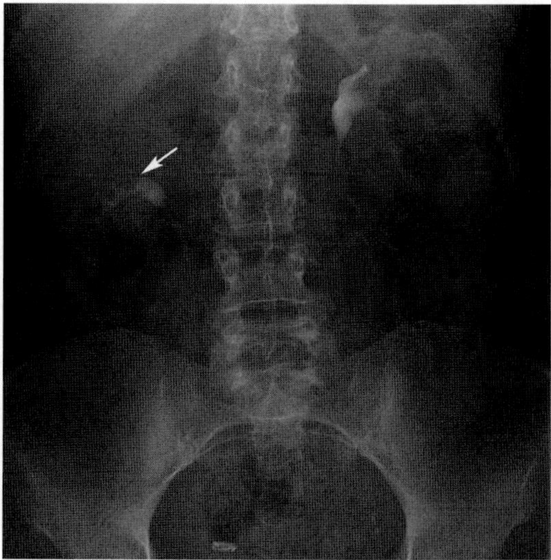

Fig. 8.3. Transitional cell carcinoma of the upper-pole collecting system in a 58-year-old woman. Anteroposterior IVU 15-min film shows amputation of the upper-pole calyx secondary to transitional cell carcinoma (*arrow*).

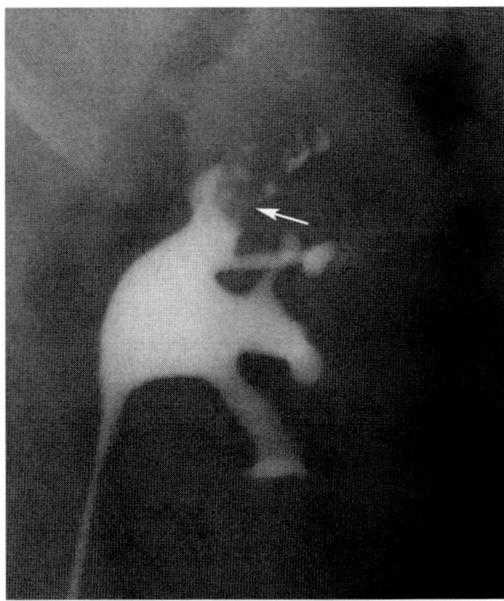

Fig. 8.4. Transitional cell carcinoma of the upper pole in a 70-year-old man. Anteroposterior retrograde pyelography (RP) view shows distortion and an irregular filling defect involving the left upper-pole calyx (*arrow*).

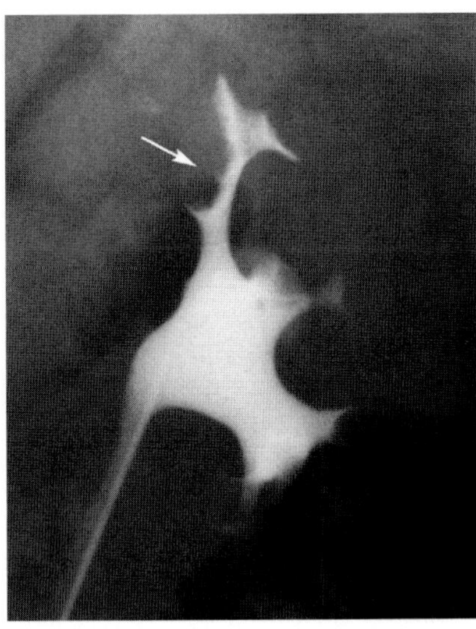

Fig. 8.5. Transitional cell carcinoma of the upper pole of left kidney in a 67-year-old man. Anteroposterior RP view shows a large, irregular filling defect involving the upper-pole calyx (*arrow*).

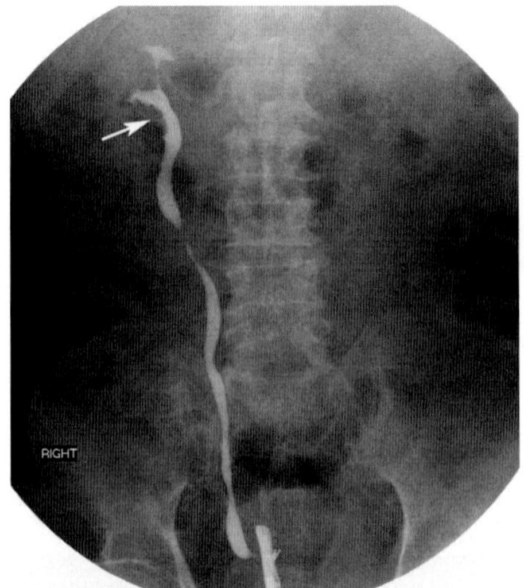

Fig. 8.6. Transitional cell carcinoma of the lower pole of right kidney in a 70-year-old man. Anteroposterior RP view shows a large, irregular mass arising from and distorting the lower-pole collecting system (*arrow*).

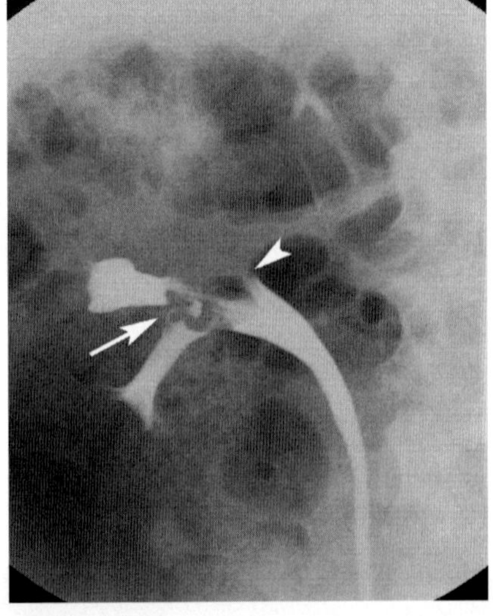

Fig. 8.7. Transitional cell carcinoma in a 72-year-old man. Anteroposterior RP view shows an irregular, papillary filling defect of the lower/mid-pole calyces due to transitional cell carcinoma (*arrow*). Complete amputation of the upper pole calyx is seen (*arrowhead*).

CT in identifying or characterizing renal masses (GRAY SEARS et al. 2002; JOFFE et al. 2003; KIM and CHO 2003; PERLMAN et al. 1996), and as CTU emerges as an initial imaging investigation of hematuria, US will also likely play only a limited diagnostic role in the future. Ultrasound can be useful in patients with renal impairment or iodinated contrast allergy, although MR imaging is becoming established as the investigation of choice in these

patients. Ultrasound can also assess the degree of hydronephrosis and guide interventional procedures in the setting of acute obstruction. The US features of renal pelvic TCC are non-specific, but usual appearances are of a central soft tissue mass in the echogenic renal sinus, with or without hydronephrosis (Figs. 8.10–8.12). Infundibular tumors may cause focal hydronephrosis (Fig. 8.13). Transitional cell carcinoma is usually iso- or hypoechoic relative

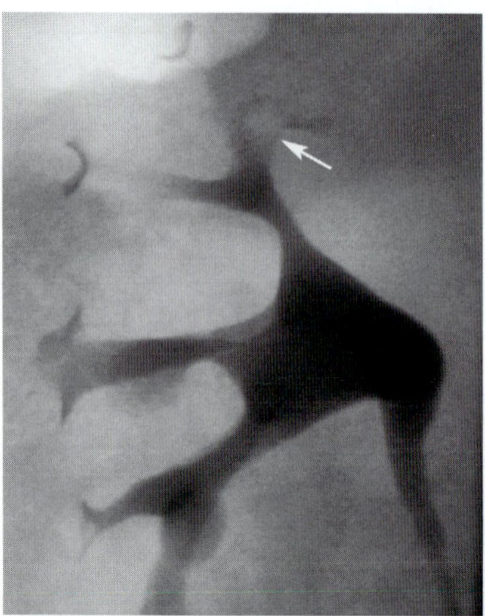

Fig. 8.8. Transitional cell carcinoma in a 61-year-old woman. Anteroposterior RP view shows a diffuse infiltrating transitional cell carcinoma involving the right upper-pole calyx with nodular irregularity of the involved mucosa (*arrow*).

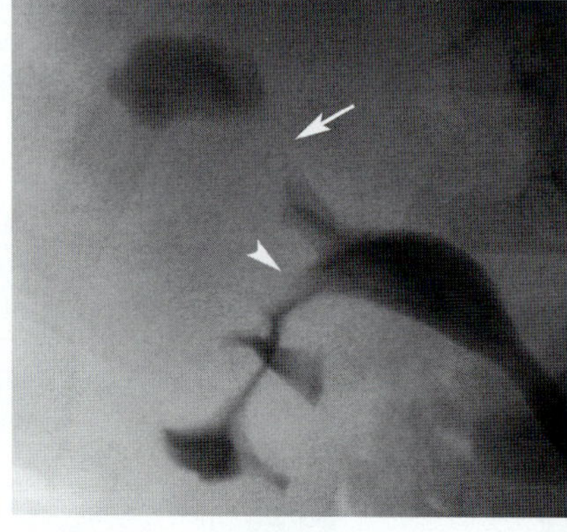

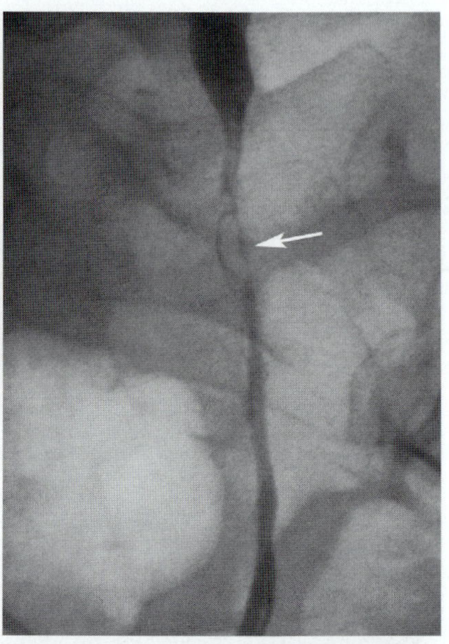

Fig. 8.9a,b. Multifocal transitional cell carcinoma in an 83-year-old woman. **a** Anteroposterior RP view of the right kidney demonstrates amputation of the interpolar calyx (*arrowhead*) and stricture of the upper pole infundibulum (*arrow*) with local upper-pole hydronephrosis and "oncocalyx" due to multifocal transitional cell carcinoma. **b** Anteroposterior RP view of the left ureter shows diffuse infiltration of the lower ureter with mural irregularity, intraluminal filling defects (*arrow*) and proximal dilatation.

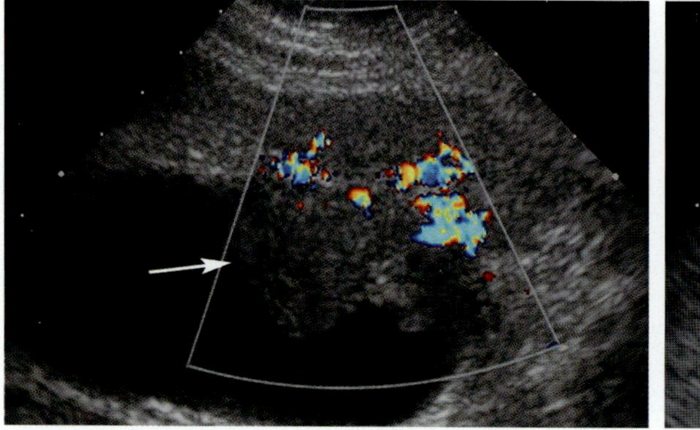

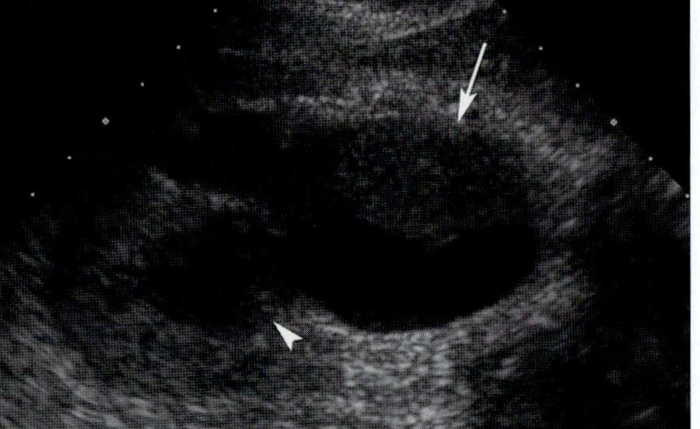

Fig. 8.10a,b. Transitional cell carcinoma in a 62-year-old man with gross hematuria. **a** Longitudinal Doppler US image shows gross hydronephrosis of the right kidney secondary to a large transitional cell carcinoma (*arrow*) arising from the anterior aspect of the renal pelvis. Note the moderate Doppler flow within the lesion. **b** Longitudinal US image again shows transitional cell carcinoma (*arrow*), with further tumor identified within the mid-pole calyx (*arrowhead*).

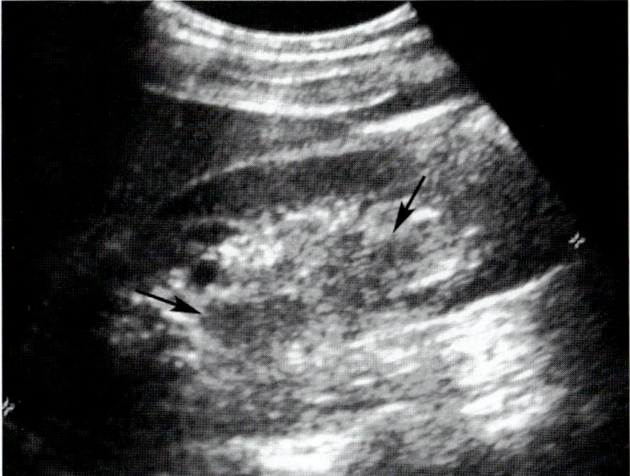

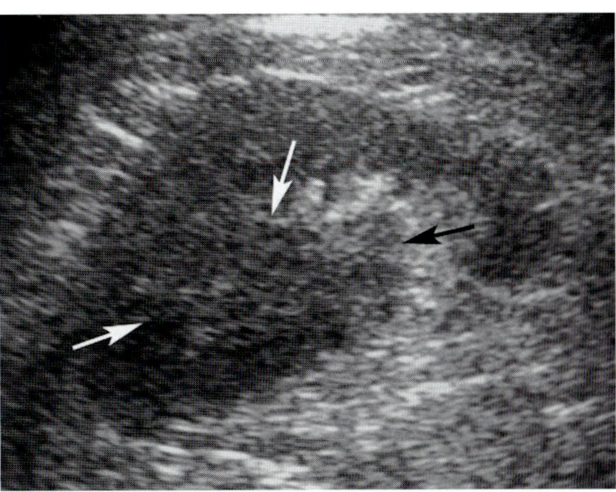

Fig. 8.11. Transitional cell carcinoma of renal pelvis in a 58-year-old woman. Longitudinal US image shows large mass (*arrows*) in the echoic right renal sinus. The tumor itself is isoechoic to renal parenchyma.

Fig. 8.12. Transitional cell carcinoma of left kidney in a 67-year-old woman. Longitudinal US image shows large lesion, isoechoic to renal parenchyma (*arrows*). The renal sinus fat is obliterated in the upper pole suggestive of parenchymal invasion.

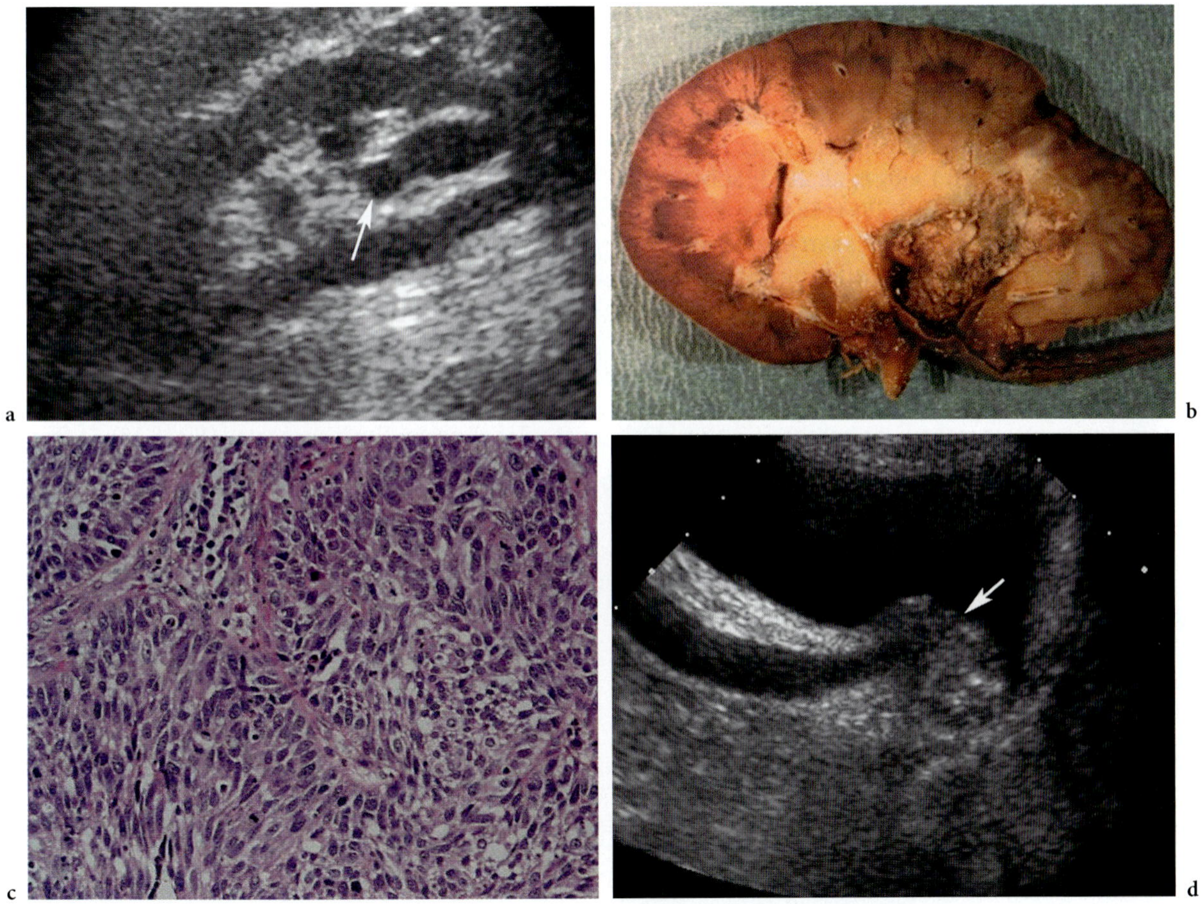

Fig. 8.13a-d. Multifocal transitional cell carcinoma in a 78-year-old man. **a** Longitudinal US image shows focal mid- and lower-pole hydronephrosis (*arrow*) secondary to transitional cell carcinoma. **b** Gross pathological section shows tumor in the renal pelvis with extension to involve the lower-pole calyx. **c** Microscopic pathological section of tumor (hematoxylin and eosin stain; original magnification, ×100). **d** Longitudinal US image of the contralateral vesicoureteric junction demonstrates transitional cell carcinoma (*arrow*) with proximal hydroureter.

to surrounding renal parenchyma, but occasionally high-grade TCC may show areas of mixed echogenicity (Fig. 8.14). Ultrasound can sometimes help differentiate tumor from radiolucent calculi, which appear more echogenic and cause a greater degree of acoustic shadowing. Although lesions may extend into the renal cortex and cause focal contour distortion, typically TCC is infiltrative and does not distort the renal contour. Recent developments in high-resolution endoluminal US performed during ureterorenoscopy have shown promise in the evaluation of renal TCC, offering potential advantages over other imaging techniques, and may assume a more prominent role in future diagnosis (HADAS-HALPERN et al. 1999).

8.6.4
Computed Tomography

Computed tomography is well established in the preoperative staging and assessment of upper-tract TCC. Computed tomography is more sensitive than either US or IVU in the detection of small renal mass lesions and urinary tract calculi (CAOILI et al. 2002; FIELDING et al. 1999; LANG et al. 2003; SCOLIERI et al. 2000; SILVERMAN et al. 1994; SZOLAR et al. 1997; TAWFIEK and BAGLEY 1997; WARSHAUER et al. 1988). The recent advent of CTU, offering single breath-hold coverage of the entire urinary tract, improved resolution and the ability to capture multiple phases of contrast, offers improved diagnostic potential over IVU and US in the assessment of patients with hematuria due to calculi or tumor (CAOILI et al.

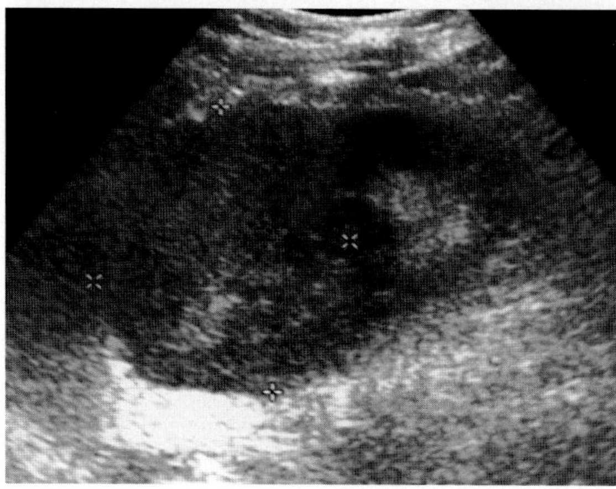

Fig. 8.14. Transitional cell carcinoma of the right upper pole in a 63-year-old woman. Longitudinal US image shows large mixed echoic lesion with obvious parenchymal invasion and distortion.

2002; CORRIE and THOMPSON 1987; GRAY SEARS et al. 2002; LANG et al. 2003; MAHER et al. 2004). Recent studies have also shown higher detection rates for upper- and lower-tract urothelial malignancies by CTU over IVU (KAWASHIMA et al. 2003; MCCARTHY and COWAN 2002; NEWHOUSE et al. 2000). Although the American College of Radiology still recommends IVU in the investigation of hematuria, as CTU becomes more prevalent it is likely to become the investigation of choice, as the urothelium, renal parenchyma, and perirenal tissues can be assessed at a single examination. Typically, CTU consists of a multiphasic helical CT protocol comprising four sequences:

1. A pre-enhancement helical CT scan from the upper pole of the kidney to the lower edge of the symphysis, to exclude urinary tract calculi.
2. A late arterial, early corticomedullary phase helical CT scan of the kidney and lower pelvis, beginning 15–25 s after infusion of 150 ml of nonionic contrast medium, to evaluate for vascular abnormalities.
3. A nephrographic phase helical CT scan of the kidney, 80–140 s after contrast infusion, to assess renal parenchyma.
4. An excretory phase helical CT scan from the upper pole of the kidney to the symphysis pubis 4–8 min after contrast infusion, to detect urothelial disease.

In the interest of decreasing radiation exposure and time of examination, many protocols omit the late arterial, early corticomedullary phase scan, unless a vascular abnormality is suspected (Fig. 8.15). In fact, some authors advocate a two-phase protocol where a nephropyelographic phase scan is performed if the initial non-contrast phase does not demonstrate a satisfactory cause for the patient's hematuria. This involves two contrast infusions with a delay of 10–15 min between them, allowing assessment of the renal parenchyma in the nephrographic phase and the entire collecting system in the pyelographic phase simultaneously. Saline is infused after the first bolus to distend the ureters. Other authors have utilized abdominal compression, prone scanning, and diuretics to obtain optimum distension and opacification (JOFFE et al. 2003; KAWASHIMA et al. 2003; MAHER et al. 2004). Oral contrast is omitted to facilitate three-dimensional (3D) reformats, which typically include thick- and thin-slab coronal and sagittal maximum intensity projections (MIPs) for kidneys, ureters, and bladder, although other 3D reconstruction techniques can be used. These pro-

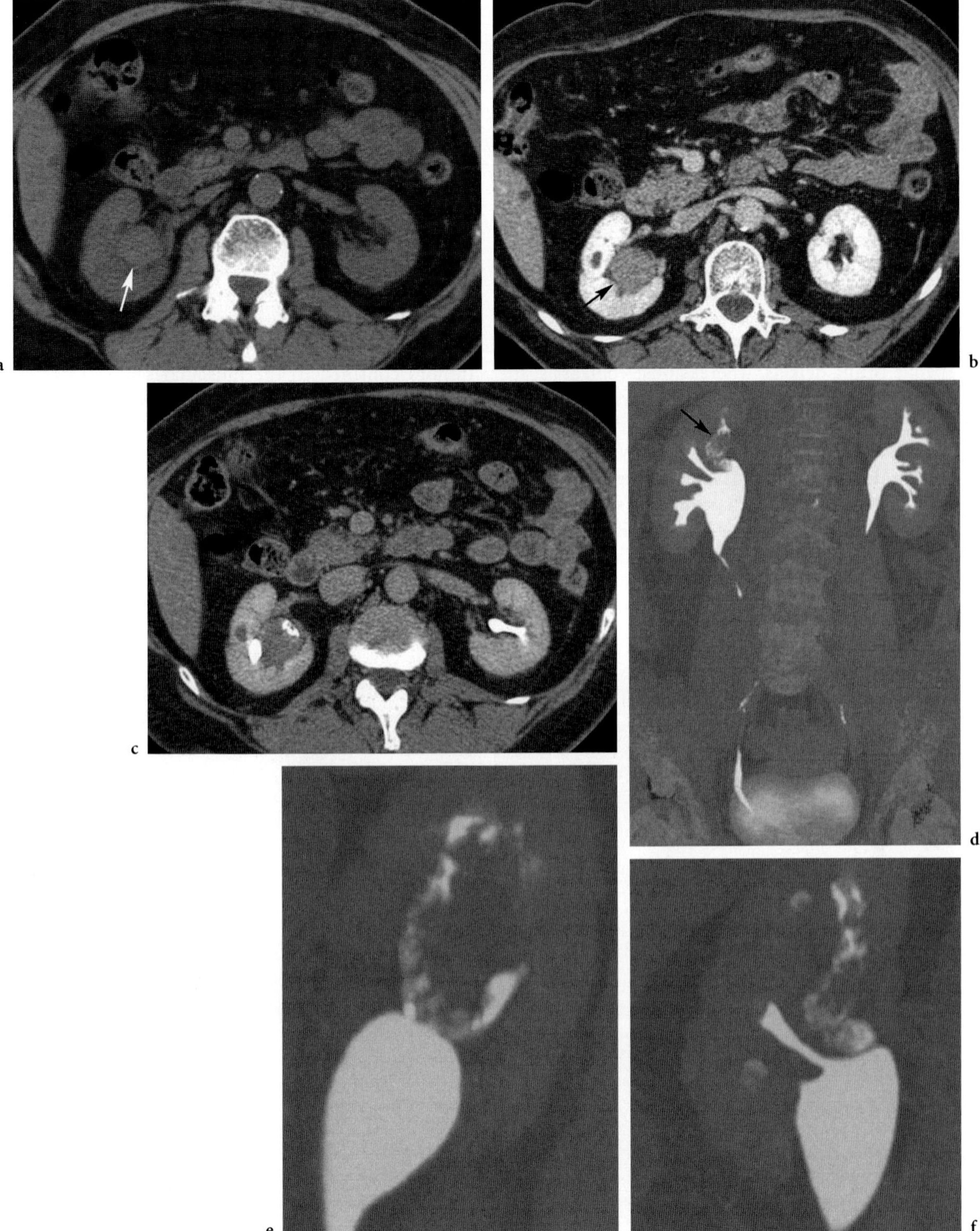

Fig. 8.15a-f. Upper-pole transitional cell carcinoma on CT urography in a 59-year-old man. **a** Axial pre-enhancement CT scan shows mass (*arrow*) in the right upper-pole calyx slightly hyperdense relative to the renal parenchyma. **b** Axial nephrographic phase-contrast-enhanced CT scan demonstrates characteristic early enhancement of the mass (*arrow*) which is less than surrounding renal parenchyma. **c** Axial excretory phase-contrast-enhanced CT scan confirms tumor within the upper-pole calyx with surrounding excreted contrast medium. **d** Coronal maximum intensity projection (MIP) reformatted image displaying the upper pole tumor (*arrow*) in IVU format. **e** Sagittal and **f** coronal MIP reformatted images further demonstrate the lesion.

vide urologists with a familiar imaging format while still demonstrating small filling defects, although most radiologists diagnose primarily from the axial images, using the planar images to confirm or better display an abnormality. Coronal reconstructions in particular demonstrate the longitudinal extent of a lesion and assess for multicentric tumor (Fig. 8.15d). Viewing the opacified system at wider window settings, such as bone windows, can aid in identifying and differentiating subtle lesions. Unlike IVU, imaging is not dependent on a functioning kidney and the tract distal to a lesion can be evaluated. Pre-contrast scans are necessary to obtain accurate density values and differentiate tumor from other non-opaque filling defects, whereas post-contrast scans aid in confirming lesion location and extent. On pre-contrast imaging TCC is typically hyperdense (5–30 HU) to urine and renal parenchyma (Fig. 8.16) but less dense than other pelvic filling defects such as clot (40–80 HU), papillary necrosis (20–40 HU), or calculus (>100 HU). Calcified TCC may occasionally be difficult to distinguish from calculi, in which case enhancement of the non-calcified portions of the tumor should be sought.

Short-interval follow-up is occasionally required to differentiate between clot and tumor (McNicholas et al. 1998; Urban et al. 1997a). Post-contrast early enhancement and de-enhancement, although more typical of RCC, is also seen with TCC (Garant et al. 1998). Computed tomographic urography may also reveal other causes of hematuria such as calculi, papillary necrosis, inflammatory lesions, or infarcts. Renal TCC is characteristically seen as a filling defect in the excretory phase, which expands centrifugally with compression of the renal sinus fat (Figs. 8.17–8.19). Other appearances include pelvicalyceal irregularity, focal or diffuse mural thickening, oncocalyx, and focally obstructed calices. Early tumors confined to the muscularis are separated from the renal parenchyma, either by renal sinus fat or excreted contrast, and have normal-appearing peripelvic fat. Advanced TCC extends into the renal parenchyma in an infiltrating pattern which distorts normal architecture (Fig. 8.20). Reniform shape is typically preserved, however, unlike RCC (Fig. 8.21). Renal cell carcinoma, being hypervascular, also tends to enhance more, although the two tumors often cannot be differentiated. Transitional

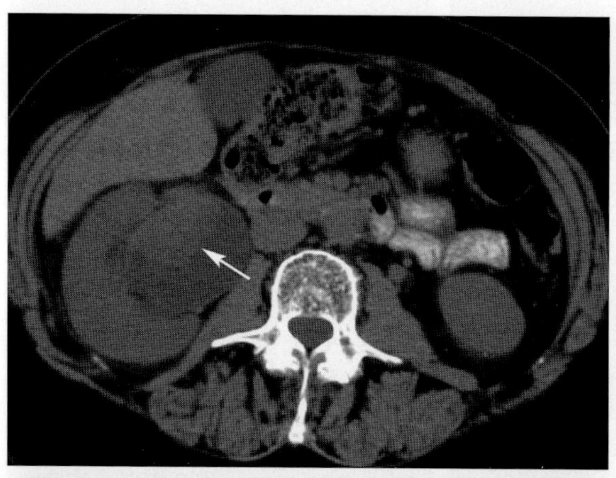

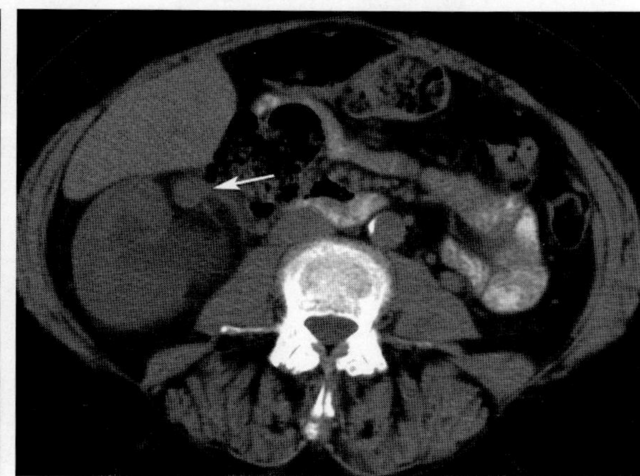

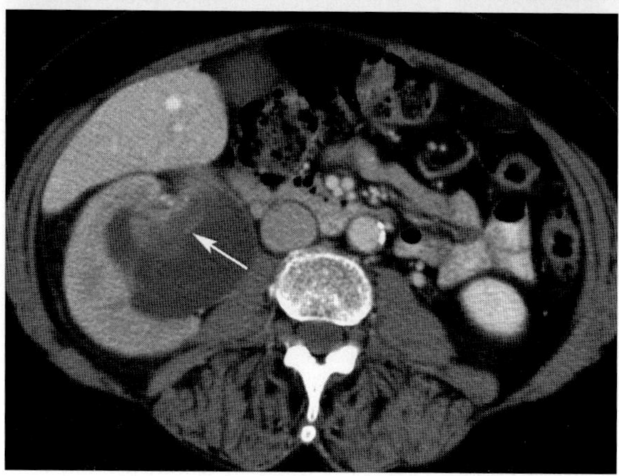

Fig. 8.16a-c. Transitional cell carcinoma arising from the anterior wall of right renal pelvis in a 68-year-old woman. a Axial pre-enhancement CT scan shows hyperdense tumor (*arrow*) with surrounding hypodense urine in an obstructed kidney. b Axial pre-enhancement CT scan at a slightly lower level shows extension of tumor into the upper ureter (*arrow*) causing obstruction. c Axial nephrographic phase contrast-enhanced CT scan shows enhancement of tumor within the obstructed pelvis (*arrow*).

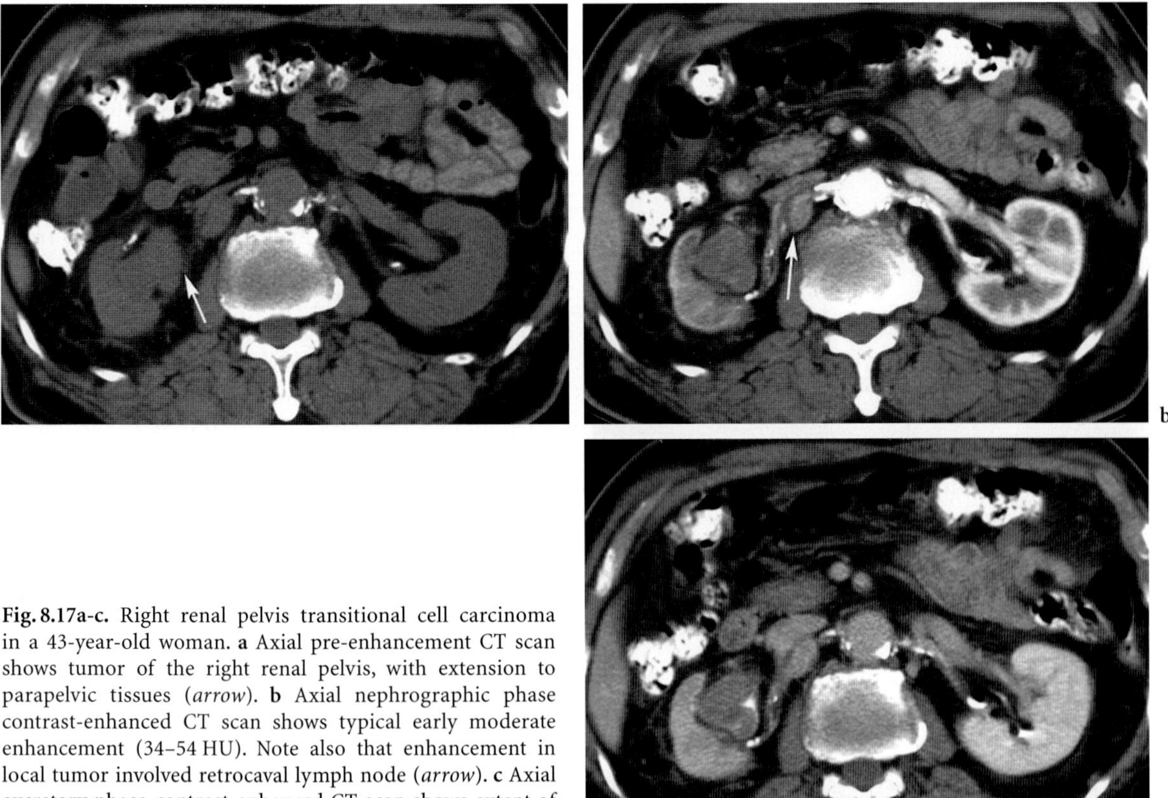

Fig. 8.17a-c. Right renal pelvis transitional cell carcinoma in a 43-year-old woman. **a** Axial pre-enhancement CT scan shows tumor of the right renal pelvis, with extension to parapelvic tissues (*arrow*). **b** Axial nephrographic phase contrast-enhanced CT scan shows typical early moderate enhancement (34–54 HU). Note also that enhancement in local tumor involved retrocaval lymph node (*arrow*). **c** Axial excretory phase-contrast-enhanced CT scan shows extent of tumor in the pelvis with a small amount of surrounding contrast visualized.

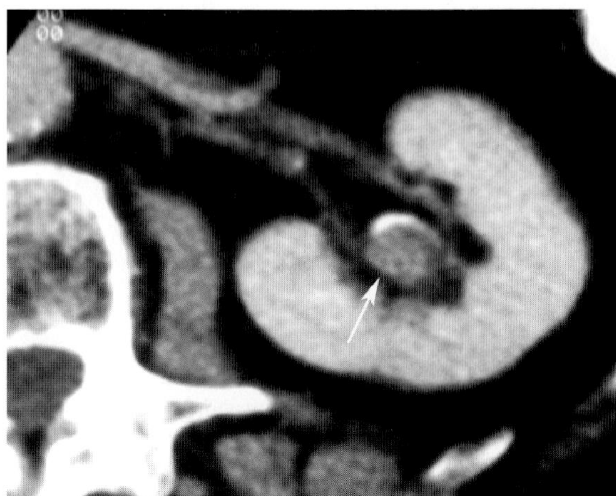

Fig. 8.18. Transitional cell carcinoma of the left upper pole in a 75-year-old woman. Axial excretory phase-contrast-enhanced CT scan shows focal mass (*arrow*) with surrounding contrast anteriorly within the collecting system.

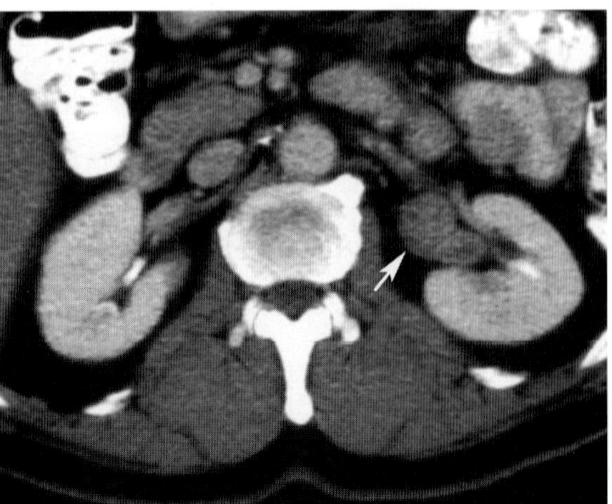

Fig. 8.19. Transitional cell carcinoma in a 72-year-old man with gross hematuria. Axial excretory phase-contrast-enhanced CT scan shows transitional cell carcinoma of the mid-pole calyx with extension into the renal pelvis (*arrow*).

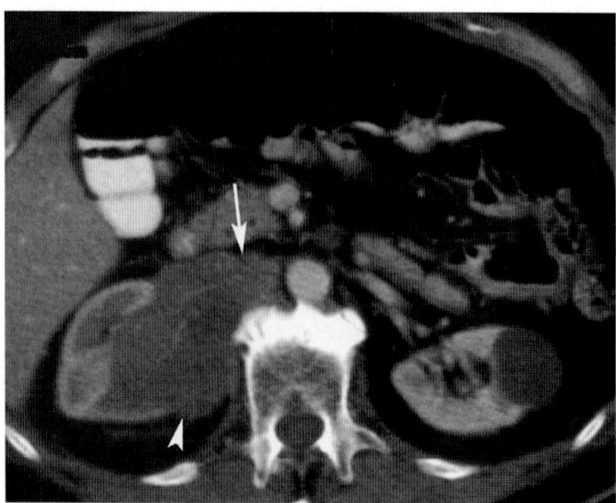

Fig. 8.20. Large transitional cell carcinoma in a 66-year-old man with frank hematuria and right flank mass. Axial contrast-enhanced CT scan shows a large transitional cell carcinoma of the right renal pelvis with perinephric/parapelvic extension (*arrowhead*) and invasion of the right renal vein and IVC (*arrow*).

cell carcinoma may appear nodular, especially on post-contrast imaging (Lang et al. 2003). Parenchymal invasion may be seen as a focal delay in all or part of the cortical nephrogram, although superimposed pyelonephritis or obstruction alone can also give these appearances (Fig. 8.22). Large infiltrating renal TCC may occasionally present with areas of necrosis and must be differentiated from lymphoma, metastases, and xanthogranulomatous pyelonephritis (XGP; Garant et al. 1998). Retention of contrast material in obstructed tubules may result in accentuated delayed enhancement of the renal parenchyma surrounding larger lesions.

Computed tomographic urography is capable of identifying lesions at an early stage, thereby allowing nephron-sparing surgery. It also allows demonstration of surrounding structures by reference to the source images. Adequate distension and opacification are fundamental factors in the thorough evaluation of the urothelium with CTU. The increased radiation exposure is estimated at only 50–80% over a complete IVU series (Lee et al. 1997). Although

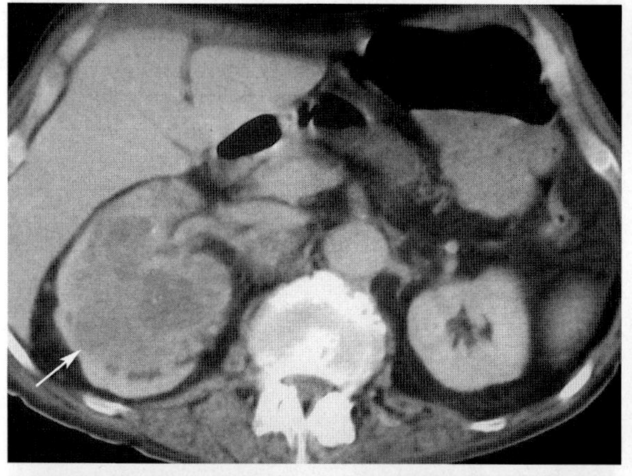

a

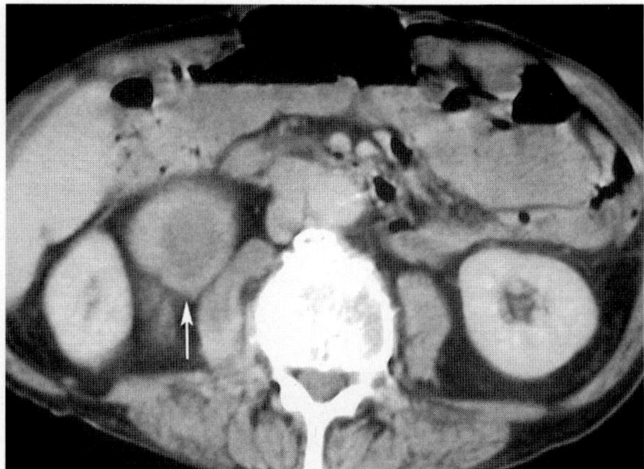

b

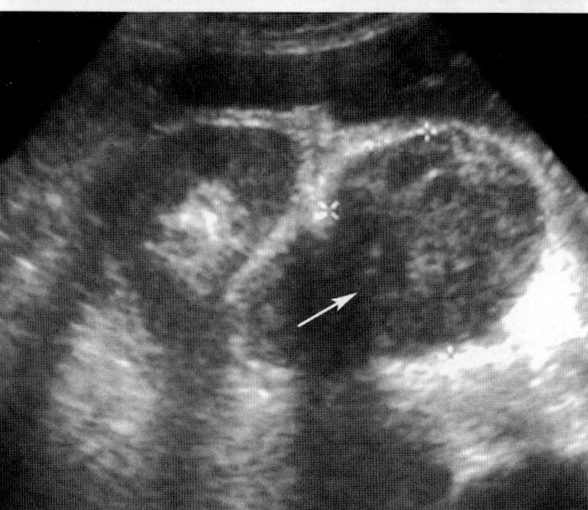

c

Fig. 8.21a-c. Transitional cell carcinoma of the right kidney in a 61-year-old man. **a** Axial contrast-enhanced CT scan shows large, enhancing soft tissue mass involving the pelvis of the right kidney with extension to involve the renal parenchyma (*arrow*) and perinephric tissues. The tumor expands centrifugally from the renal pelvis but there is preservation of the reniform contour. **b** Axial contrast-enhanced CT scan at a lower level demonstrates tumor extension into the proximal ureter with diffuse mural thickening and enhancement (*arrow*) and central clot. **c** Transverse US image at this level also shows diffuse tumor involvement of the ureter (*arrow*).

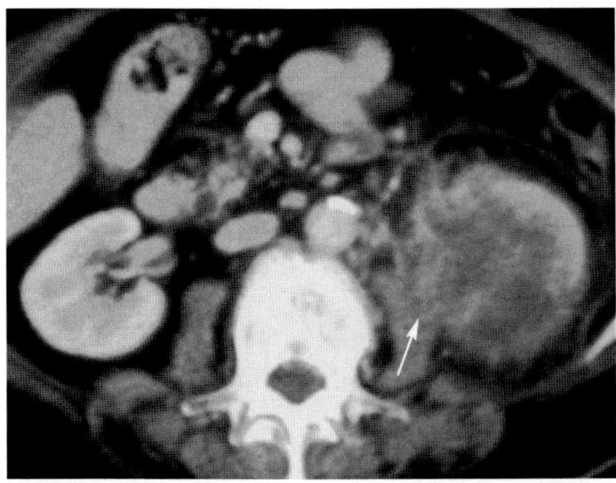

Fig. 8.22. Transitional cell carcinoma of the left kidney in a in a 67-year-old man. Axial contrast-enhanced CT scan shows tumor involving the upper pole of the left kidney with diffuse parenchymal infiltration and extension to involve the perinephric tissues and left psoas muscle (*arrow*).

reformatting and review of multiple images on different window settings is time consuming, CTU has the potential to stand alone as a comprehensive "one-stop" front-line study for hematuria and therefore detection of TCC.

8.6.5
Angiography

Angiography is not employed in the routine assessment of renal TCC but can distinguish TCC from RCC, which is often associated with neovascularization and tumoral arteriovenous shunting on angiography. Transitional cell carcinoma is typically hypovascular, occasionally demonstrating fine tortuous neovascularity or tumor blush. Encasement of vessels and a reduced intensity of the capillary nephrogram may be seen if TCC infiltrates the renal parenchyma. In rare cases where renal vein/IVC involvement is suspected, CT or duplex US are usually employed. Flow-sensitive MR imaging sequences have also been used in this role recently.

8.6.6
Magnetic Resonance Imaging

Magnetic resonance imaging is infrequently used in the primary diagnosis and assessment of renal TCC, and the MR imaging characteristics of this tumor are not well described. Magnetic resonance imaging, in general, has not played a leading role in renal tumor imaging, due to limitations in image quality, time-consuming sequences, and artifact susceptibility. Recently, however, the development of newer fast sequences has led to increased use. Magnetic resonance imaging has been shown to equal CT in the detection and diagnosis of renal masses (Cholankeril et al. 1986; Lang et al. 2003; Walter et al. 2003). Magnetic resonance imaging offers inherently high soft tissue contrast, is independent of excretory function, and multiplanar imaging permits direct image acquisition in the plane of tumor spread. The coronal plane is often advantageous because it allows evaluation of both kidneys, the renal vessels, the inferior vena cava, and the spine in a small number of slices.

Transitional cell carcinoma is of lower signal intensity than the normally hyperintense urine on T2-weighted sequences, permitting good demonstration of tumor in a dilated collecting system. Renal TCC, however, appears nearly isointense to renal parenchyma on T1-weighted and T2-weighted sequences, necessitating the use of contrast for accurate assessment of tumor extent (Kreft et al. 1997). Although TCC is a hypovascular tumor, moderate enhancement is seen post-gadolinium, although not to the same degree as the surrounding renal parenchyma (Figs. 8.23, 8.24). Differentiation between small renal calculi and tumor may occasionally be difficult unless definite gadolinium enhancement is seen in the tumor (Walter et al. 2003). Post-gadolinium imaging may be performed using 3D sequences to allow dynamic evaluation of the kidney. This allows assessment of renal vasculature in arterial and venous phases and the renal parenchyma in corticomedullary and nephrographic phases. Vascular invasion of renal vein/inferior vena cava (IVC), although rare, may also be demonstrated without gadolinium administration on T2-weighted or gradient-echo flow-sensitive sequences (Fig. 8.25). As with CT, however, limitations exist in detecting superficial invasion of the renal parenchyma, and small lesions may be missed because of motion artifacts (Kirkali and Tuzel 2003; Yousem et al. 1988). The MR imaging protocols to evaluate renal TCC should also include MRU, which may be static, or dynamic using gadolinium. Static MRU utilizing heavily T2-weighted sequences can permit accurate localization of obstruction (Fig. 8.26), although imaging of undilated systems may be suboptimal (Pretorius et al. 2000; Yousem et al. 1988). This technique is helpful in patients with impaired renal function, where iodinated contrast-enhanced urography is not possible. Contrast-enhanced T1-

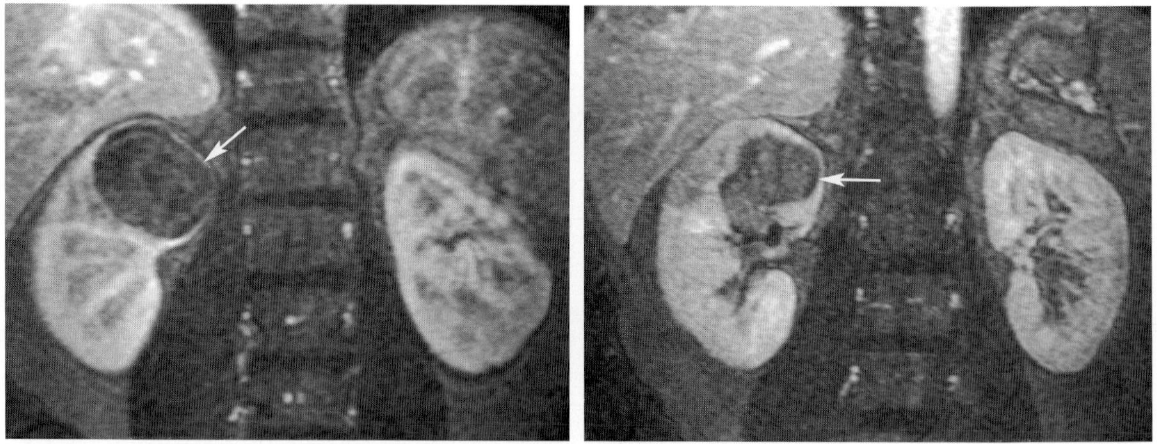

Fig. 8.23a,b. Renal transitional cell carcinoma in a 68-year-old woman. **a,b** Coronal contrast-enhanced 3D fast low-angle shot (FLASH) MRA source images in early phase of dynamic acquisition (TR=3.64 ms, TE=1.37 ms) demonstrate mildly enhancing tumor in the right renal pelvis and upper-pole calyx (*arrow*) with extension to involve upper-pole parenchyma but not the perirenal tissues.

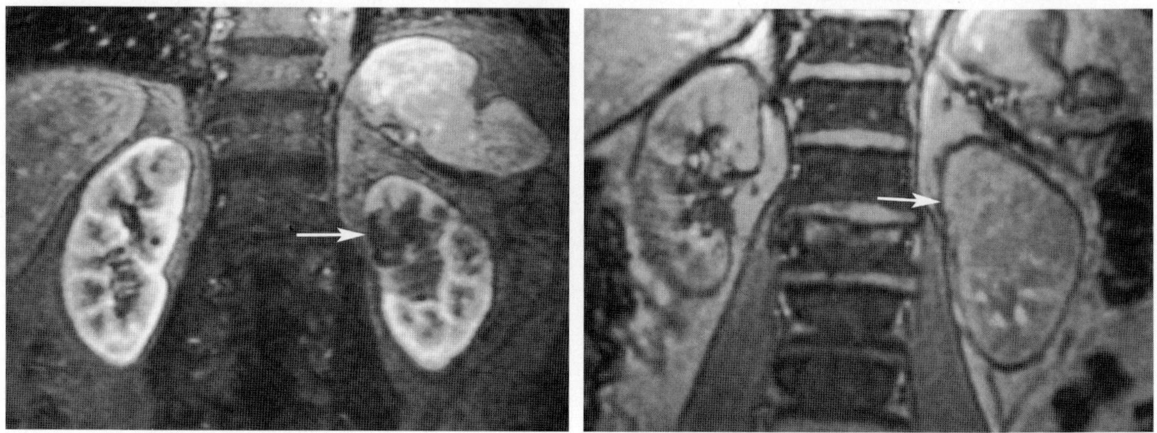

Fig. 8.24a,b. Renal transitional cell carcinoma in a 68-year-old woman. Coronal contrast-enhanced 3D fast low-angle shot (FLASH) MRA source images in **a** early and **b** late phases of dynamic acquisition (TR=3.64 ms, TE=1.37 ms) demonstrate moderately enhancing left upper-pole transitional cell carcinoma tumor (*arrow*).

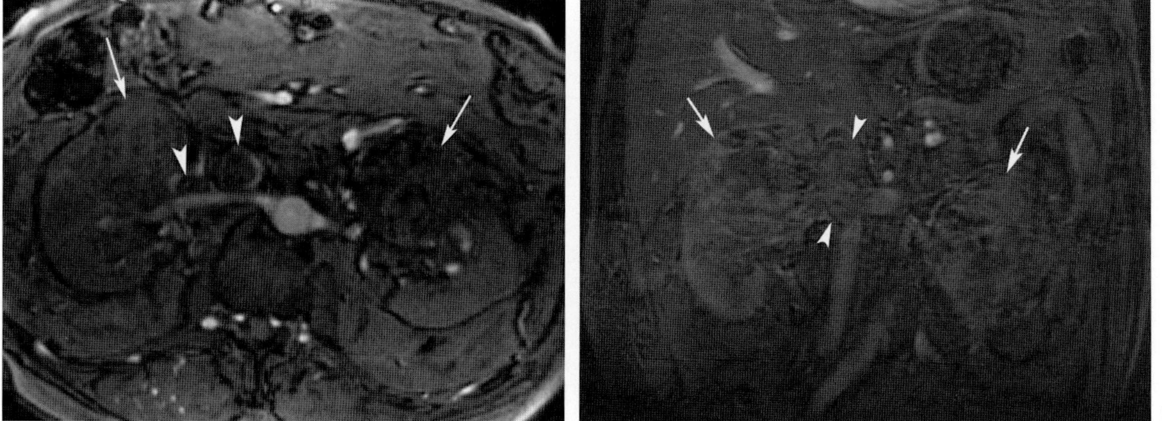

Fig. 8.25a,b. Transitional cell carcinoma in a 77-year-old man with hematuria. **a** Axial fat-suppressed fast-spin-echo T2-weighted (TR=8000 ms, TE=104 ms) and **b** coronal gradient-recalled acquisition in the steady state (GRASS; TR=30 ms, TE=8 ms) MR images demonstrate bilateral upper-pole transitional cell carcinoma (*arrows*) with right renal vein and inferior vena cava invasion (*arrowheads*).

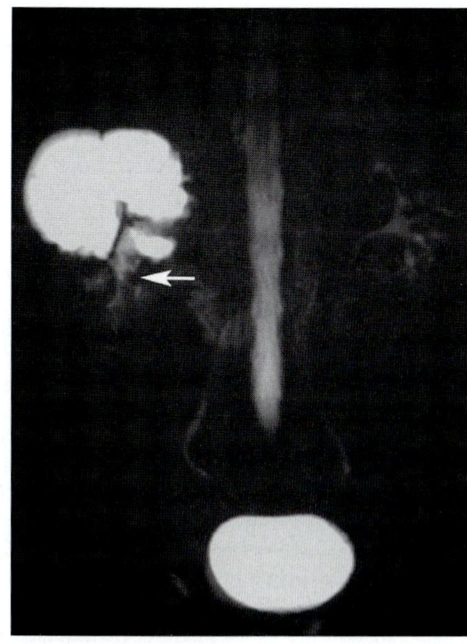

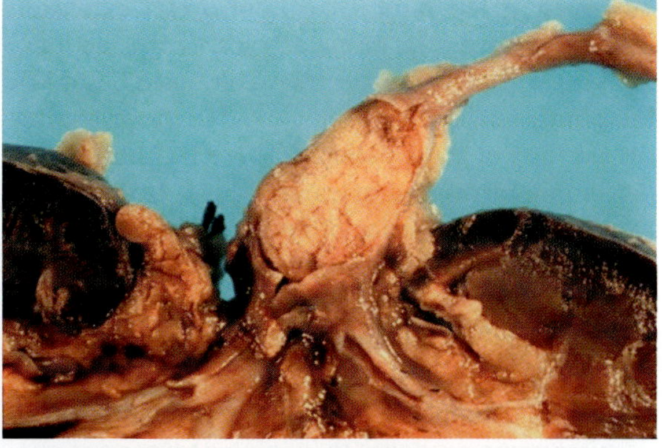

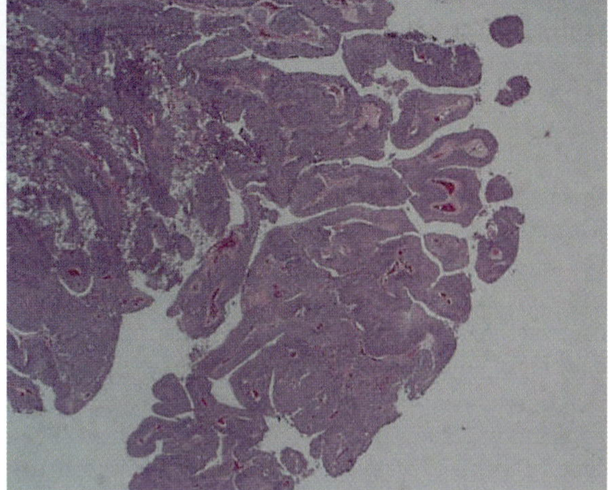

Fig. 8.26a-c. Renal pelvis transitional cell carcinoma in a 65-year-old man. **a** Coronal heavily half-Fourier acquisition single-shot turbo spin-echo (HASTE) T2-weighted MRU (TR=1500 ms, TE=116 ms) MIP image shows focal hydrone-phrosis of the right upper-pole calyx and irregularity of the pelvis and mid-calyx (*arrow*), consistent with transitional cell carcinoma. **b** Gross pathological section shows tumor in the right renal pelvis and proximal ureter. **c** Microscopic patho-logical section of tumor (hematoxylin and eosin stain; origi-nal magnification, ×40).

weighted MRU with/without diuretic provides dynamic imaging of the entire urinary tract and delayed acquisitions can be obtained at various time intervals depending on degree and level of obstruc-tion. Dynamic MRU also allows an estimate of renal function to be made. Post-processing of the data set to yield MIPs allows 3D rotation and viewing of sus-pected areas of disease without superimposition of other anatomic structures. This can be performed for both vascular structures and the collecting system; the latter, resembling conventional IVU studies, is readily acceptable to clinicians.

These comprehensive MR protocols can image all the anatomic components of the urinary tract in a single test and offer advantages over other tech-niques including lack of iodinated contrast medium and radiation exposure. Although MR imaging remains second to CT, it offers further non-invasive imaging of renal masses, which are not adequately characterized by other imaging modalities (WEEKS et al. 1995). The main disadvantage of MR imaging is the inability to reliably detect urinary tract cal-cifications, calculi, and air, which limits its use as a first-line test in the investigation of hematuria.

Although the sensitivity of renal parenchymal MR imaging with gadolinium for assessing renal masses and abnormalities of the nephrogram is consid-ered similar to that of CT, spatial resolution is poor compared with IVU or CTU, making it less likely to detect subtle urothelial malignancies (MILESTONE et al. 1990). Furthermore, the complete character-ization of renal masses may require multiple, time-consuming sequences pre- and post-gadolinium administration (KAWASHIMA et al. 2003).

8.7
Staging

Tumor stage at diagnosis influences the development of local recurrence and metastases, and hence over-all survival (MAHER et al. 2004; HALL et al. 1998). Furthermore, treatment and prognosis are largely determined by the depth of tumor infiltration, the degree of lymph node and distant metastases, and the histological tumor type, making exact staging imperative (Table 8.1). Conventional imaging methods, such as IVU and RP, cannot detect extension into the peripelvic fat or metastases. Cross-sectional imaging with dynamic contrast-enhanced CT or MR imaging is now routinely employed in the pre-surgical work-up of these patients. These techniques can determine intra- and extrarenal local extension of tumor and the presence of nodal or distant metastases with a high degree of accuracy. They are used in conjunction with ureterorenoscopy for staging prior to surgery. In most cases of renal TCC, CT has become routine in the further characterization of lesions demonstrated by other modalities and, despite varying reports on staging accuracy, is currently the preoperative imaging modality of choice (Tables 8.1, 8.2; Buckley et al. 1996; Chan et al. 2002; Scolieri et al. 2000; Urban et al. 1997a). As studies show higher detection rates for urothelial malignancies by CTU over IVU (Caoili et al. 2002), this technique is being advocated as a one-stop diagnostic and staging assessment of suspected urothelial malignancy. Although CT cannot distinguish between stages T0–TII tumor, it can differentiate early-stage TCC confined to the collecting system wall from advanced disease with local extension or distant metastases, which is important to define surgical management (McCarthy and Cowan 2002; Urban et al. 1997b). More advanced tumors infiltrating beyond the muscularis into the peripelvic fat typically show increased, inhomogeneous peripelvic density and stranding, although this finding may also be seen with superimposed infection, hemorrhage, or inflammation, and should be interpreted with caution to avoid overstaging (McCoy et al. 1991). Metastatic spread via urinary or hematogenous routes usually manifests as multifocal mucosal nodules or wall thickening, whereas direct invasion into the upper ureter generates a short or long stricture (Rothpearl et al. 1995). Extrarenal spread can occur at or through the renal hilum, and common sites of metastases include the lungs, retroperitoneum, lymph nodes, and bones. Renal vein or IVC invasion is occasionally seen and can be well demonstrated by comprehensive CTU protocols. The overall accuracy of CT in predicting the pathological stage ranges from 36 to 83% in the literature (Kim and Cho 2003), meaning ureterorenoscopy and biopsy remain essential additional tools for presurgical assessment.

As with CT, MR imaging can detect tumor involvement of the renal parenchyma, perinephric fat, and distant metastases. It therefore offers an alternative staging modality and has been shown to stage TCC lesions greater than 2 cm well (Kirkali and

Table 8.1. The TNM classification of renal transitional cell carcinoma

TNM	Histopathological findings
Tx	Primary tumor cannot be assessed
T0	No evidence of primary tumor
Ta	Papillary non-invasive carcinoma
Tis	Carcinoma in situ
T1	Tumor invades subepithelial connective tissue
T2	Tumor invades the muscularis
T3	Tumor invades beyond muscularis into periureteric fat or the renal parenchyma
T4	Tumor invades adjacent organs, pelvic/abdominal wall, or through the kidney into perinephric fat
Nx	Regional lymph nodes cannot be assessed
N0	No regional lymph node metastasis
N1	Metastasis in a single lymph node >2 cm or less in greatest dimension
N2	Metastasis in a single lymph node >2 cm but not >5 cm in greatest dimension, or multiple lymph nodes, none >5 cm in greatest dimension
N3	Metastasis in a lymph node >5 cm in greatest dimension
Mx	Distant metastases cannot be assessed
M0	No distant metastasis
M1	Distant metastasis

Table 8.2. Histopathological grading of renal transitional cell carcinoma

Grade	Histopathological grading
Gx	Grade of differentiation cannot be assessed
G1	Well differentiated
G2	Moderately differentiated
G3–G4	Poorly differentiated/undifferentiated

Tuzel 2003). T1-weighted images are used to determine tumor infiltration into the perirenal fat, and to show the endoluminal component. T1-weighted images are also good for detecting nodes, although an abnormal node can only be defined by size. T2-weighted images are used to determine the depth of tumor infiltration into the renal parenchyma and adjacent organs. Magnetic resonance imaging can help in differentiating perirenal changes, as fibrosis appears hypointense on T2-weighted sequences, particularly in long-standing cases (Pretorius et al. 2000). It is the preferred staging examination in patients who cannot tolerate iodinated contrast, and in whom multiplanar and vascular imaging is required for preoperative assessment.

8.8
Treatment

Because of the multifocal and metachronous nature of TCC, thorough assessment of the entire urothelium is required prior to treatment. Newly diagnosed renal lesions therefore require evaluation of the contralateral kidney and both ureters, usually with IVU and RP, and cystoscopic evaluation of the bladder (ROTHPEARL et al. 1995). The traditional treatment of renal TCC involves total nephroureterectomy with excision of the ipsilateral ureteral orifice and a contiguous cuff of bladder tissue (YOUSEM et al. 1988); however, the development of endoscopic and minimally invasive surgical techniques allows renal preservation in some patients, particularly those with a solitary kidney, bilateral tumor, poor renal function, low-grade tumor, or prohibitive operative risk, with results comparable to those of radical surgery (CHEN and BAGLEY 2000; KEELEY et al. 1997; KIRKALI and TUZEL 2003; TAWFIEK and BAGLEY 1997). Accurate radiological detection and tumor staging is therefore essential to determine appropriate surgical therapy, especially if conservative surgery is being considered, or the intensity of chemotherapy for advanced-stage tumors (ELLIOTT et al. 2001; TAWFIEK and BAGLEY 1997).

8.9
Follow-up

There is still no widely accepted protocol for the radiological follow-up of patients with primary TCC of the kidney (HESSION et al. 1999; URBAN et al. 1997a). Current data suggest that routine follow-up imaging strategies should be individually tailored based on primary tumor characteristics. In general, annual IVU and, if needed RP, is recommended, especially in the first 2 years after initial diagnosis (HERRANZ-AMO et al. 1999). As recurrent tumor may not be identified radiologically, RP and ureterorenoscopy should be sought if IVU fails to depict or adequately distend the entire upper tract, especially if cystoscopy is being performed or if there is a high index of suspicion. This vigilance is justified in order to detect early recurrence after conservative surgery or, in patients who have only one remaining kidney, to detect contralateral lesions at an early stage when local excision may be feasible. Due to the high rate of metachronous tumor in the bladder, frequent cystoscopy should also be performed. At our institution this is performed every 3 months for the first year, every 6 months for the second year, and yearly thereafter. If a metachronous bladder lesion is identified, a thorough assessment of the upper tracts is made and the cystoscopy cycle returns to that of every 3 months.

The advent of CTU as a diagnostic tool offers a potential alternative follow-up in these patients allowing assessment of the entire urothelium and also facilitating virtual cystoscopy to assess the bladder (ROTHPEARL et al. 1995). Computed tomographic tomography will likely become the primary radiological method of follow-up in these patients who require assessment of the entire urothelium, although cystoscopy is still necessary for direct bladder visualization and biopsy.

8.10
Conclusion

Transitional cell carcinoma is a common urological malignancy and in up to 5% of cases occurs in the kidney. The multicentric nature of TCC makes assessment of the entire urothelium essential prior to treatment. Vigilant urological and radiological follow-up is also warranted post-treatment to assess for metachronous lesions and recurrence. Conventional imaging modalities, such as IVU, RP, and US, still play a pivotal role in the assessment of hematuria in conjunction with endourological techniques. The recent advent of minimally invasive surgery that allows renal preservation makes accurate staging, usually with CT or MR imaging, mandatory to determine appropriate therapy. The technique of CTU has recently developed and offers superior detection of urinary tract tumors and calculi, as well as the ability to assess perirenal tissues and stage lesions, as a single comprehensive study. In the future, it is probable that CTU will become the standard investigation in the initial assessment and follow-up of patients with suspected TCC. Similar MR imaging protocols can also be used in patients not suitable for CTU, although detection of calculi may be suboptimal.

References

Barentsz JO, Jager GJ, Witjes JA, Ruijs JH (1996) Primary staging of urinary bladder carcinoma: the role of MRI and a comparison with CT. Eur Radiol 6:129–133

Buckley JA, Urban BA, Soyer P, Scherrer A, Fishman EK (1996) Transitional cell carcinoma of the renal pelvis: a retrospective look at CT staging with pathologic correlation. Radiology 201:194–198

Caoili EM, Cohan RH, Korobkin M, Platt JF, Francis IR, Faerber GJ, Montie JE, Ellis JH (2002) Urinary tract abnormalities: initial experience with multi-detector row CT urography. Radiology 222:353–360

Chan V, Pantanowitz L, Vrachliotis TG, Rabkin DJ (2002) CT demonstration of a rapidly growing transitional cell carcinoma of the ureter and renal pelvis. Abdom Imaging 27:222–223

Chen GL, Bagley DH (2000) Ureteroscopic management of upper tract transitional cell carcinoma in patients with normal contralateral kidneys. J Urol 164:1173–1176

Cholankeril JV, Freundlich R, Ketyer S, Spirito AL, Napolitano J (1986) Computed tomography in urothelial tumors of renal pelvis and related filling defects. J Comput Tomogr 10:263–272

Corrie D, Thompson IM (1987) The value of retrograde pyelography for fractionally visualized upper tracts on excretory urography in the evaluation of hematuria. J Urol 138:554–556

Elliott DS, Segura JW, Lightner D, Patterson DE, Blute ML (2001) Is nephroureterectomy necessary in all cases of upper tract transitional cell carcinoma? Long-term results of conservative endourologic management of upper tract transitional cell carcinoma in individuals with a normal contralateral kidney. Urology 58:174–178

Fielding JR, Silverman SG, Rubin GD (1999) Helical CT of the urinary tract. Am J Roentgenol 172:1199–1206

Garant M, Bonaldi VM, Taourel P, Pinsky MF, Bret PM (1998) Enhancement patterns of renal masses during multiphase helical CT acquisitions. Abdom Imaging 23:431–436

Gray Sears CL, Ward JF, Sears ST, Puckett MF, Kane CJ, Amling CL (2002) Prospective comparison of computerized tomography and excretory urography in the initial evaluation of asymptomatic microhematuria. J Urol 168:2457–2460

Grossfeld GD, Litwin MS, Wolf JS, Hricak H, Shuler CL, Agerter DC, Carroll PR (2001) Evaluation of asymptomatic microscopic hematuria in adults: the American Urological Association best practice policy, part I: definition, detection, prevalence, and etiology. Urology 57:599–603

Hadas-Halpern I, Farkas A, Patlas M, Zaghal I, Sabag-Gottschalk S, Fisher D (1999) Sonographic diagnosis of ureteral tumors. J Ultrasound Med 18:639–645

Hall MC, Womack S, Sagalowsky AI, Carmody T, Erickstad MD, Roehrborn CG (1998) Prognostic factors, recurrence, and survival in transitional cell carcinoma of the upper urinary tract: a 30-year experience in 252 patients. Urology 52:594–601

Herranz-Amo F, Diez-Cordero JM, Verdu-Tartajo F, Bueno-Chomon G, Leal-Hernandez F, Bielsa-Carrillo A (1999) Need for intravenous urography in patients with primary transitional carcinoma of the bladder? Eur Urol 36:221–224

Hession P, Flynn P, Paul N, Goodfellow J, Murthy LN (1999) Intravenous urography in urinary tract surveillance in carcinoma of the bladder. Clin Radiol 54:465–467

Joffe SA, Servaes S, Okon S, Horowitz M (2003) Multi-detector row CT urography in the evaluation of hematuria. Radiographics 23:1441–1446

Kawashima A, Glockner JF, King BF Jr (2003) CT urography and MR urography. Radiol Clin North Am 41:945–961

Keeley FX, Kulp DA, Bibbo M, McCue PA, Bagley DH (1997) Diagnostic accuracy of ureteroscopic biopsy in upper tract transitional cell carcinoma. J Urol 157:33–37

Keeley FX Jr, Bibbo M, Bagley DH (1997) Ureteroscopic treatment and surveillance of upper urinary tract transitional cell carcinoma. J Urol 157:1560–1565

Kim JK, Cho KS (2003) Pictorial review: CT urography and virtual endoscopy: promising imaging modalities for urinary tract evaluation. Br J Radiol 76:199–209

Kirkali Z, Tuzel E (2003) Transitional cell carcinoma of the ureter and renal pelvis. Crit Rev Oncol Hematol 47:155–169

Kreft BP, Muller-Miny H, Sommer T, Steudel A, Vahlensieck M, Novak D, Muller BG, Schild HH (1997) Diagnostic value of MR imaging in comparison to CT in the detection and differential diagnosis of renal masses: ROC analysis. Eur Radiol 7:542–547

Lang EK, Macchia RJ, Thomas R, Watson RA, Marberger M, Lechner G, Gayle B, Richter F (2003) Improved detection of renal pathologic features on multiphasic helical CT compared with IVU in patients presenting with microscopic hematuria. Urology 61:528–532

Lee TY, Ko SF, Wan YL, Cheng YF, Yang WC, Hsieh HH, Chen WJ, Eng HL (1997) Unusual imaging presentations in renal transitional cell carcinoma. Acta Radiol 38:1015–1019

Maher MM, Kalra MK, Rizzo S, Mueller PR, Saini S (2004) Multidetector CT urography in imaging of the urinary tract in patients with hematuria. Korean J Radiol 5:1–10

McCarthy CL, Cowan NC (2002) Multidetector CT urography (MD-CTU) for urothelial imaging (Abstract). Radiology 225 (Suppl):237

McCoy JG, Honda H, Reznicek M, Williams RD (1991) Computerized tomography for detection and staging of localized and pathologically defined upper tract urothelial tumors. J Urol 146:1500–1503

McNicholas MM, Raptopoulos VD, Schwartz RK, Sheiman RG, Zormpala A, Prassopoulos PK, Ernst RD, Pearlman JD (1998) Excretory phase CT urography for opacification of the urinary collecting system. Am J Roentgenol 170:1261–1267

Milestone B, Friedman AC, Seidmon EJ, Radecki PD, Lev-Toaff AS, Caroline DF (1990) Staging of ureteral transitional cell carcinoma by CT and MRI. Urology 36:346–349

Newhouse JH, Amis ES Jr, Bigongiari LR, Bluth EI, Bush WH Jr, Choyke PL, Fritzsche P, Holder L, Sandler CM, Segal AJ, Resnick MI, Rutsky EA (2000) Radiologic investigation of patients with hematuria. American College of Radiology. ACR Appropriateness Criteria. Radiology 215 (Suppl):687–691

O'Malley ME, Hahn PF, Yoder IC, Gazelle GS, McGovern FJ, Mueller PR (2003) Comparison of excretory phase, helical computed tomography with intravenous urography in patients with painless haematuria. Clin Radiol 58:294–300

Perlman ES, Rosenfield AT, Wexler JS, Glickman MG (1996) CT urography in the evaluation of urinary tract disease. J Comput Assist Tomogr 20:620–626

Pretorius ES, Wickstrom ML, Siegelman ES (2000) MR imaging of renal neoplasms. Magn Reson Imaging Clin N Am 8:813–836

Rothpearl A, Frager D, Subramanian A, Bashist B, Baer J, Kay C, Cooke K, Raia C (1995) MR urography: technique and application. Radiology 194:125–130

Scolieri MJ, Paik ML, Brown SL, Resnick MI (2000) Limitations of computed tomography in the preoperative staging of upper tract urothelial carcinoma. Urology 56:930–934

Silverman SG, Lee BY, Seltzer SE, Bloom DA, Corless CL, Adams DF (1994) Small (≤3 cm) renal masses: correlation of spiral CT features and pathologic findings. Am J Roentgenol 163:597–605

Szolar DH, Kammerhuber F, Altziebler S, Tillich M, Breinl E,

Fotter R, Schreyer HH (1997) Multiphasic helical CT of the kidney: increased conspicuity for detection and characterization of small (<3 cm) renal masses. Radiology 202:211–217

Tawfiek ER, Bagley DH (1997) Upper-tract transitional cell carcinoma. Urology 50:321–329

Urban BA, Buckley J, Soyer P, Scherrer A, Fishman EK (1997a) CT appearance of transitional cell carcinoma of the renal pelvis. Part 1. Early-stage disease. Am J Roentgenol 169:157–161

Urban BA, Buckley J, Soyer P, Scherrer A, Fishman EK (1997b) CT appearance of transitional cell carcinoma of the renal pelvis. Part 2. Advanced-stage disease. Am J Roentgenol 169:163–168

Walter C, Kruessell M, Gindele A, Brochhagen HG, Gossmann A, Landwehr P (2003) Imaging of renal lesions: evaluation of fast MRI and helical CT. Br J Radiol 76:696–703

Warshauer DM, McCarthy SM, Street L, Bookbinder MJ, Glickman MG, Richter J, Hammers L, Taylor C, Rosenfield AT (1988) Detection of renal masses: sensitivities and specificities of excretory urography/linear tomography, US, and CT. Radiology 169:363–365

Weeks SM, Brown ED, Brown JJ, Adamis MK, Eisenberg LB, Semelka RC (1995) Transitional cell carcinoma of the upper urinary tract: staging by MRI. Abdom Imaging 20:365–367

Wong-You-Cheong JJ, Wagner BJ, Davis CJ Jr (1998) Transitional cell carcinoma of the urinary tract: radiologic-pathologic correlation. Radiographics 18:123–142; quiz 148

Yousem DM, Gatewood OM, Goldman SM, Marshall FF (1988) Synchronous and metachronous transitional cell carcinoma of the urinary tract: prevalence, incidence, and radiographic detection. Radiology 167:613–618

9 Kidney Sarcomas

EMILY D. BILLINGSLEY and SANTIAGO RESTREPO

CONTENTS

9.1
Introduction

Primary sarcomas arising in the kidney, although quite rare, should be considered in the differential diagnosis of renal tumors. These tumors, of which there are various histological types, account for less than 1% of all renal malignancies (VOGELZANG et al. 1993). Primary renal sarcomas may arise from one or more of the progenitor cell lines of the connective tissues normally found within the kidney (Table 9.1).

E. D. BILLINGSLEY, MD
Chief Resident, Department of Radiology, Louisiana State University Health Sciences Center, 1542 Tulane Avenue, New Orleans, LA 70112, USA
S. RESTREPO, MD
Associate Professor of Radiology, Vice-Chairman of Research, Department of Radiology, Louisiana State University Health Sciences Center, 1542 Tulane Avenue, New Orleans, LA 70112, USA

Table 9.1. Cellular origin of primary renal sarcomas

Tissue type	Tumor
Smooth muscle	Leiomyosarcoma
Adipose tissue	Liposarcoma
Skeletal muscle	Rhabdomyosarcoma
Vascular	Angiosarcoma, hemangiopericytoma
Bone	Osteosarcoma
Cartilage	Chondrosarcoma
Myofibroblast	Malignant fibrous histiocytoma
Fibroblast	Fibrosarcoma
Neuroectoderm	Extraosseous Ewing sarcoma/primitive neuroectodermal tumor
Undifferentiated	Malignant mesenchymoma

Leiomyosarcoma is the most common histological subtype accounting for 50–60% of the primary renal sarcomas reported in the literature (GRIGNON et al. 1990). Less common entities, such as rhabdomyosarcoma, liposarcoma, malignant hemangiopericytoma, angiosarcoma, osteosarcoma, chondrosarcoma, malignant fibrous histiocytoma, fibrosarcoma, extraosseous Ewing sarcoma/primitive neuroectodermal tumor (PNET), and malignant mesenchymoma arising from the kidney, have also been reported but are exceedingly rare. Overall, the age at presentation with primary renal sarcoma ranges from 28 to 70, with the median age of 49 years. Forty percent of renal sarcomas contain central areas of necrosis at the time of diagnosis; average tumor size ranges from 5.5 to 23 cm. Prognosis is generally poor, and 90% of patients present with distant metastasis, pulmonary metastasis being the most common (LEVINE and KING 2000). Radiographically, most primary renal sarcomas are indistinguishable from renal cell carcinoma and histologically may be confused with renal cell carcinomas which contain tissues which have undergone sarcomatoid differentiation. For this reason, a case of sarcomatoid differentiation within a renal cell carcinoma is included in section 9.13, as this tumor is part of the differential diagnosis of primary sarcoma of the kidney. The diagnosis of primary renal sarcoma is made based on a combination of the imaging and histological characteristics of the tumor and often after extensive scrutiny to exclude more common tumors such as renal cell carcinoma.

9.2
Leiomyosarcoma

Renal leiomyosarcomas are the most common histological subtype of renal sarcomas, accounting for 58% of all primary renal sarcomas (Levine and King 2000). Arising from smooth muscle, these tumors originate from the renal capsule or from the smooth muscle of the renal pelvis or vasculature, including the renal vein or intraparenchymal

vasculature (Moazzam et al. 2002; Ng 1985). These tumors most commonly occur in the sixth decade of life (Chen and Lee 1997). Preponderance in women (7 of 10) has been reported, as well as preference for the right kidney (Deyrup et al. 2004).

Histopathologically, leiomyosarcoma appears as closely packed interlacing spindle-shaped cells with cellular atypia, and therefore can be confused with sarcomatoid differentiation within a renal cell carcinoma which also is composed primarily of spindle-shaped cells. Immunohistochemical stains of the cytoplasm of tumor cells of leiomyosarcoma are positive for vimentin and muscle-specific antigen, whereas those of the sarcomatoid variant of renal cell carcinoma are not (Moudouni et al. 2001). Renal leiomyosarcoma

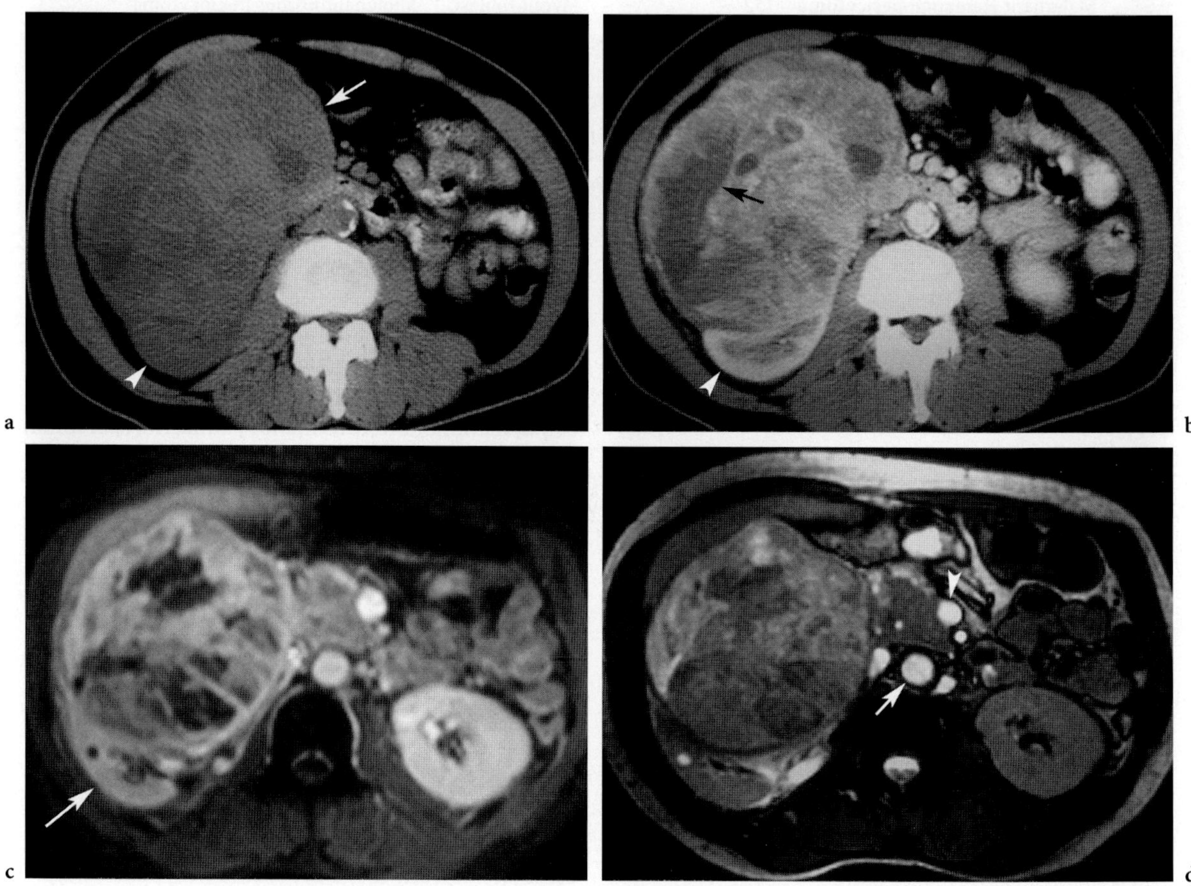

Fig. 9.1a-d. Leiomyosarcoma in a 60-year-old man. **a** Axial unenhanced CT scan demonstrates a large, heterogeneous soft tissue density mass arising from the anterior aspect of the right kidney at the midpolar region (*arrow*). The tumor is slightly hyperdense than the adjacent normal renal parenchyma, seen posteriorly (*arrowhead*). **b** Axial contrast-enhanced CT scan at the same level as **a** shows that the normally enhancing renal parenchyma posteriorly is clearly delineated (*arrowhead*) and the mostly solid mass is obviously arising from and splaying the kidney. Heterogeneous enhancement with hypodense areas is seen. These hypodense areas (*arrow*) are secondary to internal necrosis of the mass as it outgrows its vascular supply. **c** Axial fat-suppressed contrast-enhanced T1-weighted MR image demonstrates a heterogeneous, predominately hyperintense renal mass. The normal-appearing kidney is seen posteriorly (*arrow*). **d** Axial balanced fast-field-echo (FFE) T2-weighted MR image demonstrates a heterogeneous predominately hypointense mass. Extension of the tumor between the aorta (*arrow*) and the superior mesenteric artery (*arrowhead*) is demonstrated.

has been reported in a patient with tuberous sclerosis (FERNANDEZ DE SEVILLA et al. 1988) and malignant transformation of angiomyolipoma to leiomyosarcoma has also been reported (LOWE et al. 1992).

On unenhanced CT imaging, leiomyosarcomas are often higher in density than adjacent renal parenchyma and similar to paraspinal muscle density (Fig. 9.1). After administration of intravenous contrast, the solid components of these tumors demonstrate variable enhancement (Figs. 9.1, 9.2). Tumor calcification can occur in 10% of cases. Even though presentation with spontaneous rupture of a renal neoplasm is more commonly seen in large angiomyolipomas, leiomyosarcomas can present in this way (MOAZZAM et al. 2002). In such a case, the imaging findings correspond to those of a retroperitoneal hematoma. Computed tomography shows a large heterogeneous mass in the perinephric space with minimal postcontrast enhancement.

Magnetic resonance imaging characteristics of leiomyosarcoma, like the majority of primary renal sarcomas, include intermediate to hypointensity on T1-weighted MR imaging and intermediate to hyperintensity on T2-weighted MR imaging (Figs. 9.1, 9.2). Internal necrosis, especially when the tumor becomes large, is a common feature of this tumor (KAUSHIK and NEIFELD 2002). On T1-weighted MR images, the area of internal necrosis is hypointense, whereas on T2-weighted images, the area of necrosis is hyperintense (Fig. 9.2).

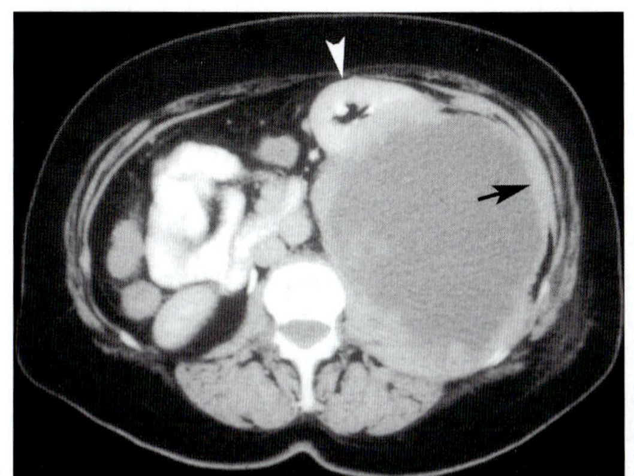

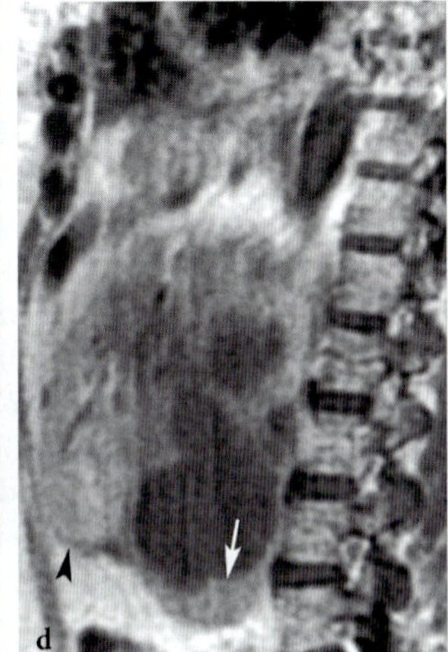

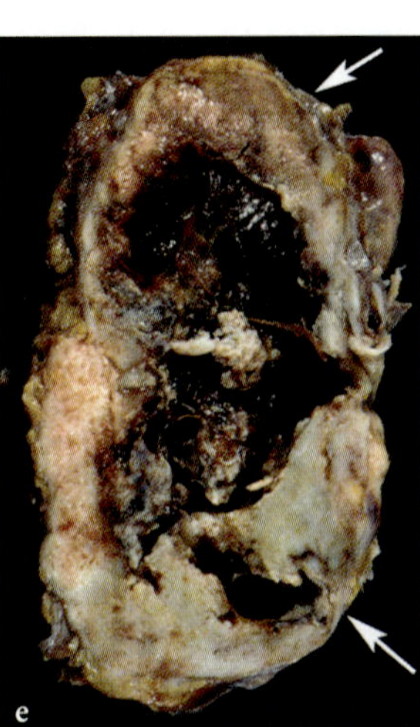

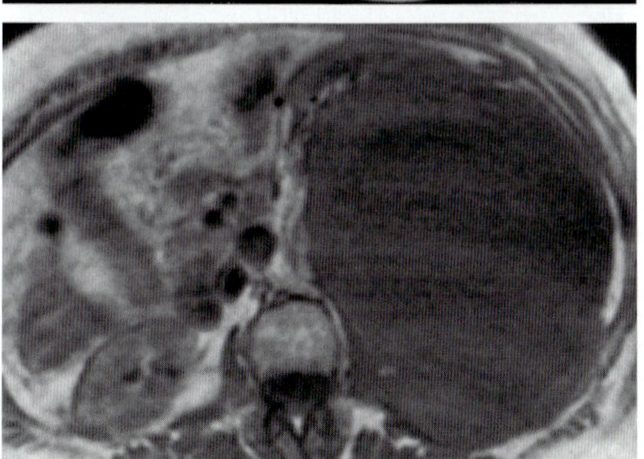

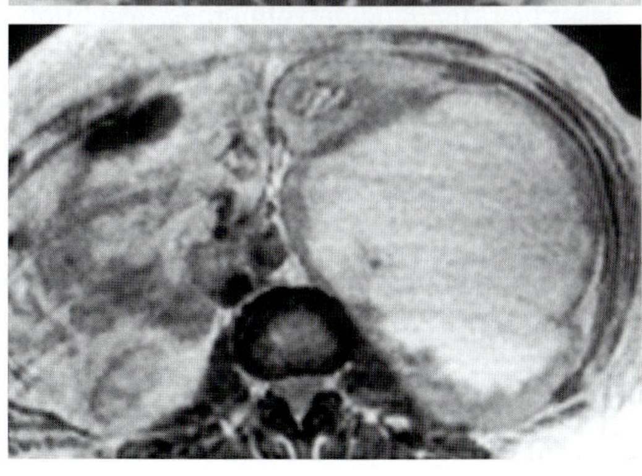

Fig. 9.2a-e. Leiomyosarcoma in a 40-year-old woman. **a** Axial contrast-enhanced CT scan with oral opacification demonstrates a large, mostly hypodense, mass occupying the left retroperitoneum. Note the internal nodularity of the peripheral rim of enhancing tissue (*arrow*) and splaying of the otherwise normal-appearing renal parenchyma seen anteriorly (*arrowhead*). Axial MR images show the left renal mass to contain central hypointensity on **b** T1-weighted spin echo and hyperintensity on **c** T2-weighted spin echo consistent with necrotic material and blood at its center. The left kidney is displaced anteriorly and the aorta displaced to the right by this large mass. **d** Sagittal contrast-enhanced T1-weighted MR image further illustrates the extensive necrotic center of this mass and nodularity at its periphery (*arrow*). The remaining normal portion of the kidney is seen anteriorly (*arrowhead*). **e** Cut surface of the surgical specimen after left nephrectomy confirms the highly necrotic central portion of the tumor and the nodular solid components at the periphery (*arrows*).

At nephrectomy, a tumor composed of nodular solid elements, and commonly areas of internal necrosis, is found (Fig. 9.2). Nephrectomy with adjuvant chemotherapy and postoperative radiation is currently the method of treatment; however, published clinical studies of the effectiveness of treatment and the prognosis are lacking (Moudouni et al. 2001). Intermediate- and high-grade tumors are aggressive neoplasms with poor prognosis.

9.3
Liposarcoma

Liposarcoma is one of the most common retroperitoneal tumors, often occurring in the perinephric space (Israel et al. 2002). Liposarcoma can arise from the retroperitoneal fat, including the perirenal fat within Gerota's fascia, or even the renal sinus fat, but are not usually primary neoplasms of the kidney. Because this tumor arises from the retroperitoneal space, a retroperitoneal liposarcoma will be seen displacing or encasing, but not invading, the renal parenchyma, as is illustrated in the selected CT images of two cases of retroperitoneal liposarcoma in Figs. 9.3 and 9.4. On the other hand, a primary renal liposarcoma will arise from and distort the architecture of the kidney. Rather than merely displacing the kidney, a primary renal liposarcoma will cause a defect in the renal parenchyma as it grows outward from the organ. In some cases, especially when the tumor is large, it can be difficult to determine whether a liposarcomatous mass is arising from or merely encasing the kidney. In a comprehensive review by Mayes et al. (1990), eight cases of liposarcoma with unequivocal involvement of the renal parenchyma were described. The histology of these tumors was reviewed, and the diagnosis of primary renal sarcoma was confirmed. In this case series, of the eight tumors occurring in patients from 33 to 68 years of age, there was no gender predominance.

On CT, both retroperitoneal and primary renal liposarcomas demonstrate a variety of appearances dependent on the differentiation of the fatty component of the tumor, ranging from well-differentiated tumors with fat-density Hounsfield units (HU) values to undifferentiated tumors that are difficult to distinguish radiographically from other sarcomas (Levine and King 2000). The differential diagnosis of these usually prominent fatty neoplasms should also include angiomyolipoma. In a review of 27 fat-containing tumors of the retroperitoneum, Israel et al. (2002) described the major imaging findings which are important to consider when differentiating angiomyolipoma from liposarcoma of the retroperitoneum. They noted that a defect in the renal parenchyma adjacent to the mass is commonly seen in exophytic angiomyolipomas, but not identified in the 12 cases of retroperitoneal liposarcoma reviewed. Liposarcoma arising in the retroperitoneum displaces and distorts the adjacent kidney, but the interface between the two is characteristically smooth. According to the same principle, primary renal sarcomas, because they arise from the kidney itself rather than the retroperitoneal space, disrupt the renal parenchyma, causing a defect similar to that described for angiomyolipomas. Additionally, Israel et al. (2002) noted that angiomyolipomas commonly contain enlarged vessels that can be seen on contrast-enhanced CT. By comparison, well-differentiated liposarcomas are less vascularized and those vessels that are present are not usually enlarged. Magnetic resonance imaging characteristics depend on the fat content of these tumors, which are hyperintense on both T1- and T2-weighted sequences (Fig. 9.5).

At nephrectomy, the lobulated fatty portion of this tumor is evident (Fig 9.5).

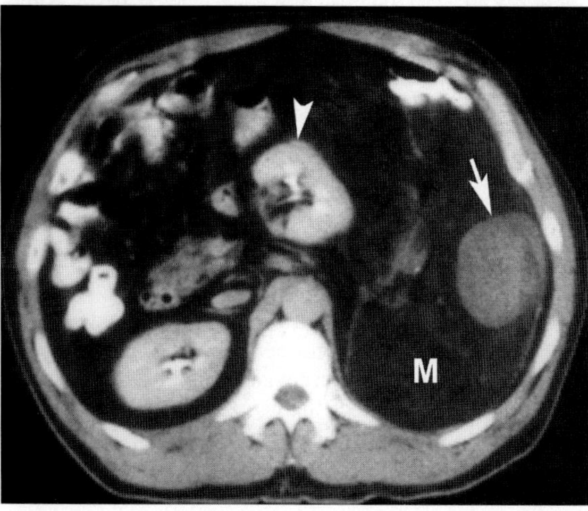

Fig. 9.3. Retroperitoneal liposarcoma in a 63-year-old man. Axial contrast-enhanced CT scan demonstrates a large retroperitoneal fat density mass (*M*) occupying the left renal fossa and retroperitoneal space. Within the mostly fatty tumor is a solid soft tissue component (*arrow*). The left kidney is significantly displaced anteriorly and medially (*arrowhead*), but there does not appear to be any disruption of the renal parenchyma. This tumor is a retroperitoneal liposarcoma, which is much more common than the primary renal liposarcoma.

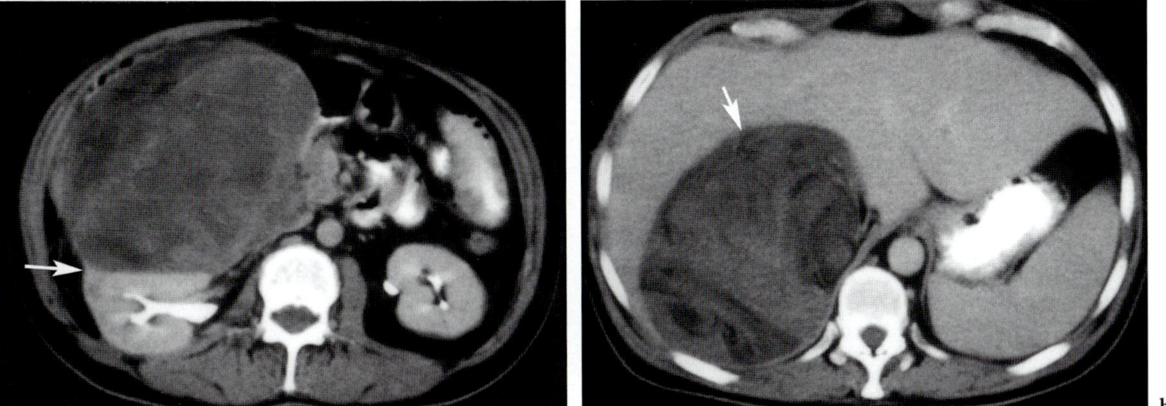

Fig. 9.4a,b. Retroperitoneal liposarcoma in a 53-year-old woman. **a** Axial contrast-enhanced CT scan shows a large, mostly fat density mass, displacing, compressing, and distorting the right kidney. Compared with the previous case of retroperitoneal liposarcoma seen in Fig. 9.3, this tumor is less well differentiated, containing soft tissue density whorls of tissue. Also note that the interface between the mass and the anterior margin of the right kidney is smooth (*arrow*). There is no defect in the renal parenchyma to suggest that the tumor is arising from the kidney, as would be seen in angiomyolipoma or primary renal liposarcoma. **b** This tumor is large, extending superiorly into the hepatorenal fossa (*arrow*) and displacing the right lobe of the liver anteriorly. Retroperitoneal liposarcoma demonstrates a propensity to spread throughout the retroperitoneal spaces.

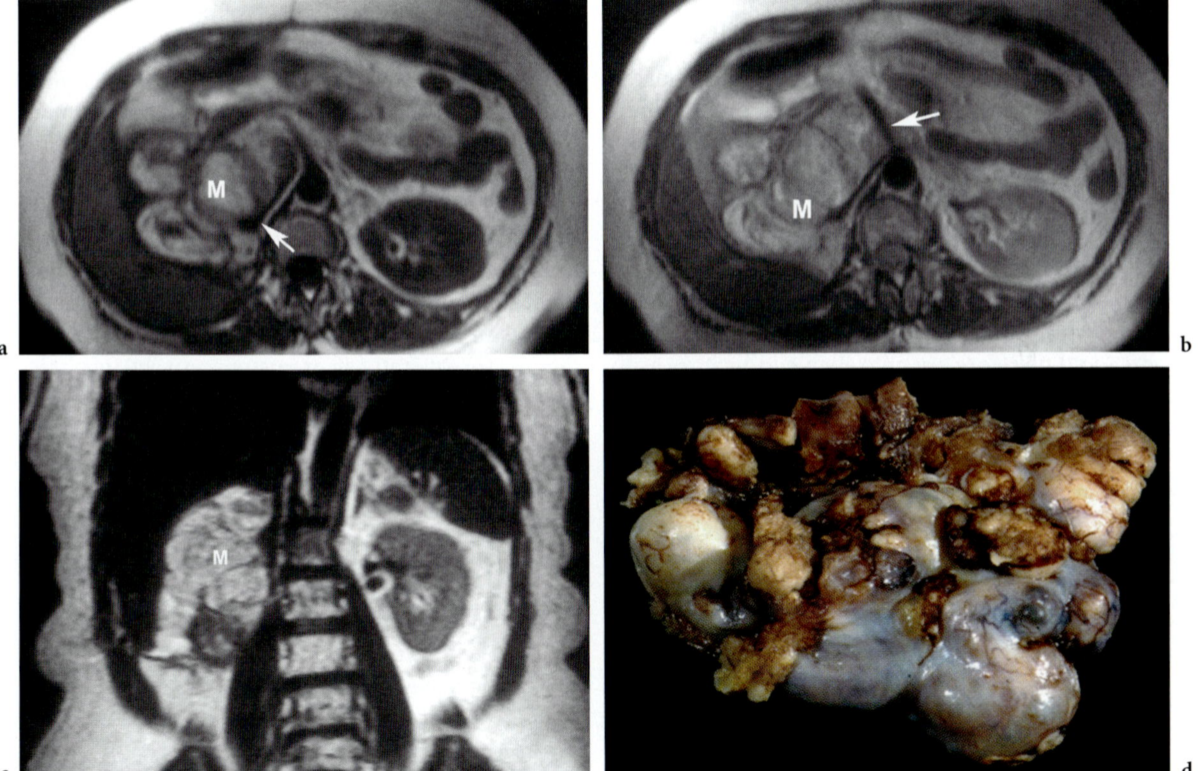

Fig. 9.5a-d. Capsular renal liposarcoma in a 48-year-old man. **a** Axial T1-weighted spin-echo MR image of a fat-containing, lobulated mass (*M*) arising from the right kidney causing significant compression of the inferior vena cava (*arrow*). No normal renal parenchyma remains. **b** Axial proton density-weighted MR image at the same level as **a** shows the inferior vena cava and left renal vein are significantly compressed by the mass (*M*), which extends medially to the level of the superior mesenteric artery (*arrow*). **c** Coronal T1-weighted spin-echo MR image demonstrates the lobulated fatty tumor of the right renal fossa (*M*) which has completely replaced the right kidney, growing superiorly into the hepatorenal fossa where it displaces the right lobe of the liver. **d** Gross surgical specimen shows the lobulated fatty tumor. The fatty components are yellowish, soft, and variegated. Histology is consistent with a liposarcoma arising from the renal capsule and invading the renal parenchyma.

9.4
Angiomyolipoma with Sarcomatoid Transformation

Angiomyolipomas are benign hamartomas of the renal parenchyma found in approximately 45–80% of patients with tuberous sclerosis, often multiple and bilaterally (Lowe et al. 1992). Angiomyolipomas may also present as unilateral, and often large, solitary tumors in a patient with no clinical signs of tuberous sclerosis. Given the prevalence of benign angiomyolipoma, especially in patients with tuberous sclerosis, a tumor arising from the kidney containing CT or MR imaging characteristics consistent with intratumoral fat is most likely a benign angiomyolipoma. The fat content with a negative density value (–10 to –100 HU) of these intraparenchymal renal lesions is readily apparent on thin-slice CT, and the diagnosis of angiomyolipoma is relatively certain except in rare cases of renal cell carcinoma containing intratumoral fat or, very rarely, primary renal liposarcoma.

Reported cases of renal angiomyolipoma containing a large soft tissue component made up of cells characteristic of sarcoma have been reported in the literature (Lowe et al. 1992). Upon histological examination of these tumors, cellular atypia is a common feature. These tumors most commonly contain spindle-shaped smooth muscle cells with variation in nuclear size and occasional mitosis, and may be confused with liposarcoma (Israel et al. 2002); however, aggressive features, such as cellular atypia, can also be seen in benign angiomyolipoma and therefore are not reliable indicators as to the potential malignant nature of these tumors. The propensity to invade adjacent structures, including the renal veins and local recurrence after incomplete surgical resection, is a well-documented feature of benign angiomyolipomas, and also is not helpful in distinguishing a benign angiomyolipoma from those with malignant sarcomatoid transformation. The true malignant nature of sarcomatoid transformation within a renal angiomyolipoma is noted in well-documented cases of distant metastasis to the lung and liver from malignant transformation of angiomyolipomas (Christiano et al. 1999; Cibas et al. 1998; Ferry et al. 1991; Kawaguchi et al. 2002; Martignoni et al. 2000). For this reason, it is important to include sarcomatoid transformation of an angiomyolipoma in the differential diagnosis of primary renal sarcoma. Figure 9.6 illustrates the CT and MR imaging characteristics of an angiomyolipoma with sarcomatoid transformation diagnosed in a 52-year-old woman who subsequently under-

went nephrectomy. At the time of surgery, liver metastases consistent with metastatic sarcomatous angiomyolipoma were discovered. The only consistent finding noted in the few cases of previously reported sarcomatoid transformation of angiomyolipoma is the presence of intratumoral fat. Both CT and MR imaging are capable of demonstrating the fat-density component of this tumor.

9.5
Rhabdomyosarcoma

Rhabdomyosarcoma is so named because of the malignant-appearing muscle cells within the tumor, which are identified by the presence of cross striations and immunohistochemical stains positive for desmin, myoglobin, and myogenin (Mainguene et al. 2003). Although rhabdomyosarcoma is primarily a tumor found in the soft tissues, primary rhabdomyosarcoma of the kidney in adults have also been reported but are exceedingly rare (Mainguene et al. 2003; Seabury et al. 1967; Srinivas et al. 1984). Weeks et al. (1991) reported eight cases of primary renal primitive neuroectodermal tumor similar clinicopathologically to malignant rhabdomyosarcoma, although the latter is noted to be more aggressive, with invasion of the renal veins, IVC, and adjacent soft tissues common. In one case series of three patients with primary renal rhabdomyosarcoma, despite aggressive treatment with combinations of radiation therapy (preoperatively or postoperatively), nephrectomy, and chemotherapy, all had distant metastasis at the time of diagnosis and died within 6 months of diagnosis (Srinivas et al. 1984).

Rhabdosarcomatous tumors of the kidney in children are better documented in the literature than those diagnosed in adults. Some authors have noted histologically malignant-appearing muscle cells in up to 50% of nephroblastomas (Wilms tumors) and consider embryonal renal rhabdomyosarcoma to represent an overgrowth of malignant muscle within a nephroblastoma (Beckwith and Palmer 1978; Seabury et al. 1967). In one case report, embryonal rhabdomyosarcoma, also referred to in the literature as cystic partially differentiated nephroblastoma, is described in infants with variegated mosaic aneuploidy and central nervous system malformations such as microcephalus, Dandy-Walker malformation, and cataracts (Furukawa et al. 2003).

Rhabdoid tumor of the kidney (RTK) is a rare, highly malignant renal tumor of childhood, recog-

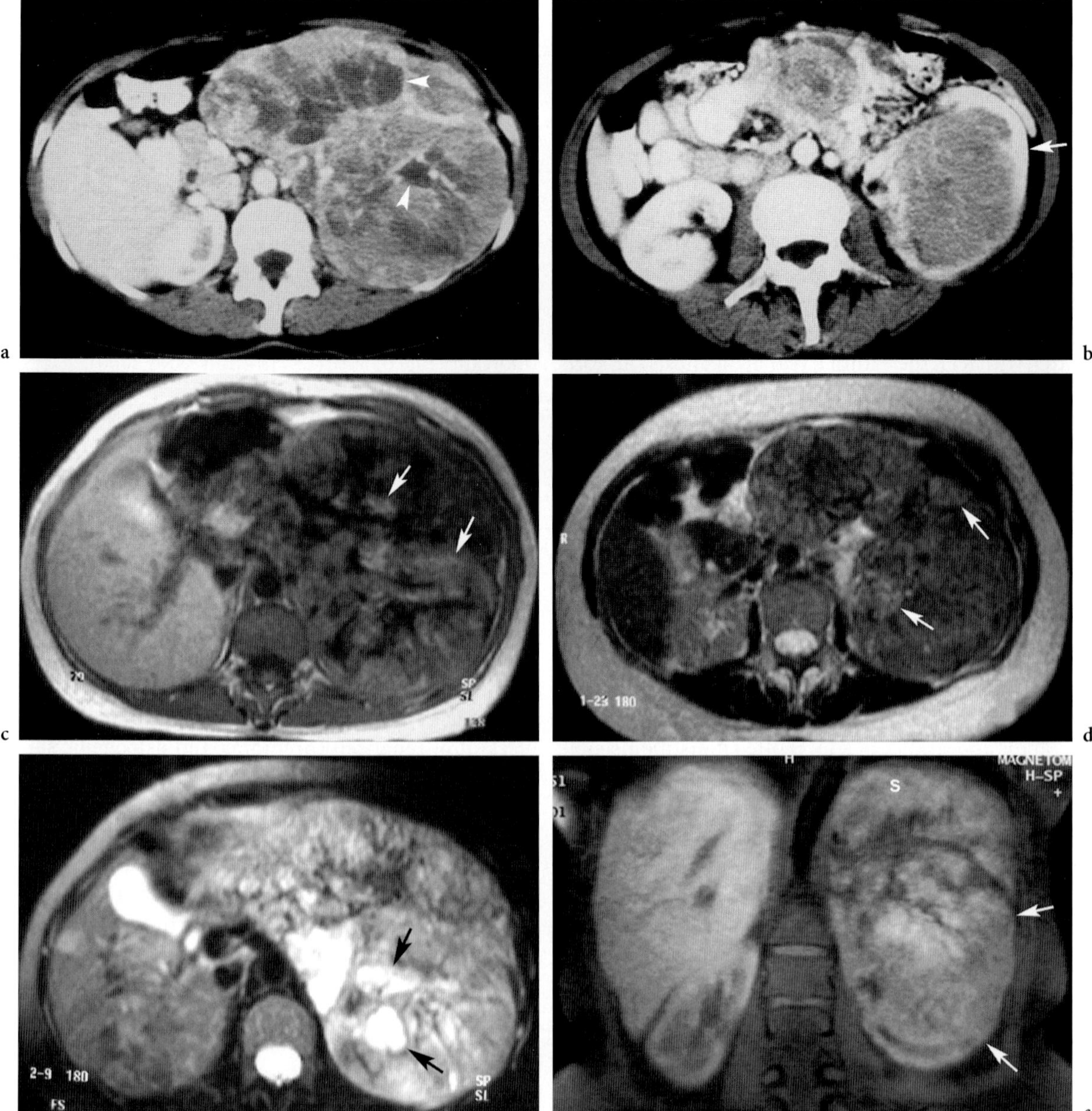

Fig. 9.6a-f. Angiomyolipoma with sarcomatoid transformation in a 52-year-old woman. **a,b** Axial contrast-enhanced CT scans show a large renal mass of the left kidney which extends across the midline of the abdomen. The mass contains tissues of differing degrees of enhancement, including areas of fat-density attenuation (*arrowheads*). There is a rim of normally enhancing renal parenchyma seen at the margins of the tumor in **b** (*arrow*). Axial **c** T1-weighted spin-echo and **d** T2-weighted spin-echo MR images demonstrate the complex nature of the solid left renal mass. Intratumoral fat appears hyperintense on the T1- and T2-weighted images (*arrows*). **e** Axial fat-suppressed FFE T2-weighted spin-echo MR image of the left renal mass demonstrates multiple hyperintense areas consistent with cystic fluid-filled spaces (*arrows*) similar in signal intensity to the fluid-filled gallbladder. Fat suppression is employed in this sequence to better characterize the fatty components of the tumor. **f** Coronal fat-suppressed contrast-enhanced T1-weighted MR image shows the large left renal mass (*arrows*) completely replacing the left kidney and displacing the spleen (*S*) superiorly; compare with the normal-appearing right kidney.

nized as a distinct entity (AGRONS et al. 1997). Rhabdoid tumor of the kidney accounts for 2% of childhood renal neoplasms (LOWE et al. 2000). It is unique among other renal tumors of childhood in its well-documented association with a second primary intracranial malignancy (WEEKS et al. 1989). As many as 10–15% of patients with RTK also have central nervous system lesions. Primitive neuroectodermal tumor, ependymoma, and cerebellar and brainstem astrocytoma have all been documented (LOWE et al. 2000). The implications of finding a brain lesion in a child with a renal tumor are significant, since most children with RTK die within 1 year of diagnosis (AGRONS et al. 1997). At presentation, nearly 80% have metastasis to the brain or lungs, and 18-month survival is less than 20% (LOWE et al. 2000). On the other hand, the diagnosis of Wilms tumor often incurs a favorable prognosis, with cure rates after nephrectomy and, in some cases, adjuvant chemotherapy, near 90% (LOWE et al. 2000). Compared with Wilms tumor, which is most commonly found in children at 36 months of age, and mesoblastic nephroma which is diagnosed at birth or in the neonatal period, the median age of diagnosis of RTK is 11 months (AGRONS et al. 1997). The male-to-female ratio is 1.5:1. Although the radiographic appearance of RTK is often indistinguishable from Wilms tumor, the pre-test predictive value for diagnosis of the former is low because of the rarity of RTK relative to Wilms tumor. Rhabdoid tumors can be identified on contrast-enhanced CT by their lobulated appearance. Often the tumor lobules are separated by intervening areas of low density necrosis and/or hemorrhage (CHUNG et al. 1995; LOWE et al. 2000). A unique feature of RTK is the presence of a subcapsular fluid collection, identified in 44% of the tumors reviewed by CHUNG et al. (1995).

9.6
Malignant Hemangiopericytoma

Hemangiopericytoma is a rare sarcoma arising from pericytes, the contractile cells that surround blood vessels and function in regulation of blood flow. These tumors occur in multiple areas in the body, the most common being the thigh. In a review of the literature, hemangiopericytoma of the kidney are reported in patients of 16–68 years and no gender predominance is noted (HEPPE et al. 1991).

Radiographically, hemangiopericytomas are highly vascular solid tumors which may resemble renal cell carcinoma or be homogeneous in density on CT.

Histopathologically, hemangiopericytomas show dilated branching capillaries referred to as the "staghorn" vascular pattern, lined by normal-appearing endothelial cells and surrounded by nests or whorls of spindle-shaped neoplastic pericyte cells (CHHIENG et al. 1999). These findings are not pathognomonic and similar architectural patterns are observed in other soft tissue neoplasms, such as malignant fibrous histiocytoma, chondrosarcoma, and leiomyosarcoma. Metastatic rates has been reported to be from 20 to 50% in hemangiopericytoma arising from all sites (HEPPE et al. 1991). Prognosis is generally poor, with an overall mortality rate of 50% (LEVINE and KING 2000).

9.7
Osteosarcoma

Primary renal osteosarcoma is an exceedingly rare tumor. It is believed to arise from undifferentiated mesenchymal cells of the kidney. Extensive ossification in a "sunburst" pattern, usually evident on routine radiographs, may suggest the diagnosis (O'MALLEY et al. 1991); however, the sarcomatoid variant of renal cell carcinoma and osteogenic sarcoma with metastasis to the kidney may also contain ossification (LEVINE and KING 2000; MICOLONGHI et al. 1984). Radiographic differentiation of these three malignancies is difficult. The sarcomatoid variant of renal cell carcinoma may be distinguished from primary renal osteosarcoma by the presence of a histologically detectable epithelial component and/or positive cytokeratin immunohistochemical staining in the former (O'MALLEY et al. 1991).

Renal tumor ossification is seen in osteogenic sarcoma of the bone metastasizing to the kidney, which is by far a more common malignancy than primary renal osteosarcoma. Elevated alkaline phosphatase levels may be helpful in distinguishing primary renal osteosarcoma from metastatic osteogenic sarcoma of the kidney when a calcified renal tumor is found in the absence of a clinical history of a primary tumor elsewhere or abnormal bone lesion on technetium nuclear bone scan (DANESHMAND et al. 2003).

9.8
Angiosarcoma

Angiosarcomas can be found anywhere in the body, although most commonly in the skin and subcutaneous tissues. There is a known association of vinyl chloride and Thorotrast exposure with an increased incidence of hepatic, cerebral, and pulmonary angiosarcoma (MAKK 1974). Few sufficiently well-documented cases of primary renal angiosarcoma exist in the English-language literature (ALLRED et al. 1981; PRINCE 1942). Microscopically, the tumor cells form closely packed sinusoidal vascular channels filled with blood and fibrin, lined by polygonal or spindle-shaped tumor cells (ALLRED et al. 1981). The presence of tumor cells lining the lumen of vascular channels distinguishes this tumor from the spindle cell variety of renal cell carcinoma and from the richly vascular hemangiopericytoma (ALLRED et al. 1981). Imaging characteristics are nonspecific.

9.9
Chondrosarcoma

First described as a skeletal tumor, reported cases of extraosseous mesenchymal chondrosarcoma arising from the kidney are found in the literature, the first case described by PITFIELD et al. in 1981. In all sites, these tumors present in patients, more commonly women, between 20 and 30 years of age (GOMEZ-BROUCHET et al. 2001). Although these tumors are relatively slow growing, they are also unpredictable. Development of metastasis to the liver and lungs 18 years after nephrectomy has been described in a case report of renal chondrosarcoma in a 39-year-old woman by MEHANNA et al. (2004). The CT imaging of primary renal chondrosarcoma most often demonstrate a large soft tissue tumor with central calcification. Often, the calcified renal mass can be seen radiographically (NATIV et al. 1985). Histologically, the tumor consists of islands of well-differentiated cartilage surrounded by undifferentiated and spindle-shaped cells (MALHOTRA et al. 1984).

9.10
Malignant Fibrous Histiocytoma and Fibrosarcoma

Malignant fibrous histiocytoma (MFH) is the most common soft tissue sarcoma occurring in adulthood, accounting for 20–40% of all soft tissue sarcomas (GIBBS et al. 2001). However, the incidence of MFH arising within the kidney is low; fewer than 50 cases have been reported in the literature (CHEN et al. 2003).

More commonly, MFH arises in the extremities or the retroperitoneum. Histologically, MFH is thought to arise from primitive mesenchymal cells with partial histiocytic differentiation that grow in a storiform or cartwheel-like growth pattern (SCRIVEN et al. 1984). Like other tumors with fibroblastic origin, including leiomyosarcoma, and fibrosarcoma, immunohistochemical stains for vimentin are positive (CHEN et al. 2003). The imaging characteristics are nonspecific and often similar to other primary renal sarcomas and renal cell carcinoma. In 50% of cases, necrosis or dystrophic calcification may also be seen. Intratumoral fat is rare. Magnetic resonance imaging is suited best for defining the anatomy of the tumor and its surrounding structures. Despite radical nephrectomy with wide excisional margins, MFH shows a greater than 50% tendency for local recurrence and distant metastases to the lungs and bone are common (CHEN et al. 2003).

Another uncommon malignant tumor of the kidney arising from fibrous tissue, usually of the renal capsule, is the renal fibrosarcoma (VALDES et al. 2003). This tumor occurs in adults, and the male-to-female ratio is equal (KANSARA and POWELL 1980). Sheets of spindle-shaped cells are seen microscopically, which can easily be misinterpreted as the much more common tumor, leiomyosarcoma; however, further evaluation with electron microscopy will reveal a prominent amount of collagen fibers interlaced with primitive-appearing mesenchymal cells suggestive of a fibrous rather than smooth muscle origin of the tumor. Staining with van Gieson and Mallory trichrome stains is helpful to confirm the presence of the collagenous fibers in the tissue and differentiate it from other renal tumors (KANSARA and POWELL 1980). Fibrosarcoma of the kidney is noted for its rapid rate of growth and aggressive behavior (ARES VALDES et al. 2003). Although it typically remains encapsulated, invasion of the renal veins is noted in 40% of published cases (KANSARA and POWELL 1980).

9.11
Malignant Mesenchymoma

Malignant mesenchymoma has been described as a tumor composed of two or more unrelated tissue types in addition to any fibrosarcomatous element. Specific tumor types, such as rhabdomyosarcoma with liposarcoma and rhabdomyosarcoma with osteosarcoma or chondrosarcoma, have been reported in the thigh and in the retroperitoneum.

Two previously reported cases of malignant mesenchymoma arising in the kidney demonstrate features of both leiomyosarcoma and osteosarcoma (QUINN et al. 1993).

9.12
Extraosseous Ewing Sarcoma/Primitive Neuroectodermal Tumor

Over 50 cases of renal primitive neuroectodermal tumor (PNET) have been reported in the literature (POMARA et al. 2004). It is often difficult to distinguish these tumors from extra-osseous Ewing sarcoma (EES), and also from malignant rhabdomyosarcoma, as these tumors are thought to arise from a common stem-cell precursor, although they demonstrate variable degrees of differentiation (RODRIGUEZ-GALINDO et al. 1997). These tumors are so similar, in fact, that EES and PNET have been shown to arise from a shared and unique chromosomal translocation in more than 90% of cases (POMARA et al. 2004). Primary renal PNET occurs most commonly in adolescents and young adults. The natural history of extra-skeletal PNET in all sites consists of a rapidly growing tumor with a propensity for early metastases to regional lymph nodes, bone, lung, and liver. Prognosis is poor, even for well-defined completely resectable tumors, because local recurrence after resection is common. Less than 55% of patients are disease free after 5 years (POMARA et al. 2004). Histological evaluation of both EES and PNET reveals small blue round cells arranged in perivascular lobules referred to as "Homer-Wright rosettes," interspersed with spindle-shaped cells and tumoral cells within the vascular lumens (POMARA et al. 2004). The appearance is similar to neuroblastoma, and immunohistochemical stains are often necessary for proper diagnosis (GONLUSEN et al. 2001). Immunohistochemical stains positive for the monoclonal antibody CD99 are noted in the cytoplasm of the malignant-appearing cells and highly suggestive of the diagnosis of EES/PNET (JIMENEZ et al. 2002; POMARA et al. 2004).

9.13
Sarcomatoid Differentiation of Renal Cell Carcinoma

Sarcomatoid change has been found to arise in all histological subtypes of renal cell carcinoma which include conventional/clear cell carcinoma, papillary renal carcinoma, chromophobe renal carcinoma, and collecting duct carcinoma, although it is not known whether there is predilection for sarcomatous change in any of these subtypes relative to the others (DE PERALTA-VENTURINA et al. 2001). Sarcomatoid change within a renal cell carcinoma is much more common than primary renal sarcoma; therefore, a thorough histological evaluation of multiple tumor sections should be employed to exclude sarcomatoid variant of renal cell carcinoma before a diagnosis of primary renal sarcoma is made.

Pathologically, the sarcomatoid variant of renal cell carcinoma contains the malignant spindle cell appearance similar to primary renal sarcomas. In a study of 101 sarcomatoid renal cell carcinomas by DE PERALTA-VENTURINA et al. (2001), the sarcomatoid component of the tumor resembled fibrosarcoma in 54%, malignant fibrous histiocytoma in 44%, rhabdomyosarcoma in 2% and undifferentiated sarcoma in the remaining tumors. The distinction between sarcomatoid variant of renal cell carcinoma and primary renal sarcoma depends on identifying an epithelial component of the tumor in the former. In sarcomatoid variant of renal cell carcinoma, the epithelial component is often easily identified histologically. The use of immunohistochemical stains for cytokeratin is also employed, although sometimes these are also positive in cases of leiomyosarcomas and, rarely, malignant fibrous histiocytoma (GRIGNON et al. 1990). In a review of more than 2000 cases of radical nephrectomies performed for renal cell carcinoma, CHEVILLE et al. (2004) reported the presence of a sarcomatoid component in 5% of the resected specimens.

Imaging characteristics are variable depending on the degree of differentiation of the tumor but are seldom helpful in distinguishing a renal cell carcinoma with sarcomatoid differentiation from a non-sarcomatous renal cell carcinoma. Diffusely calcified sarcomatoid renal cell carcinoma with osteosarcomatous differentiation has been reported as presenting with CT findings of a large calcified renal mass (DANESHMAND et al. 2003). Sarcomatoid change within a renal cell carcinoma indicates a highly aggressive neoplasm which frequently invades adjacent abdominal organs and regional lymph nodes (Fig. 9.7). The presence of a sarcomatous component was reported with a higher mortality and poorer prognosis, with a median survival of less than 1 year in most studies (CHEVILLE et al. 2004).

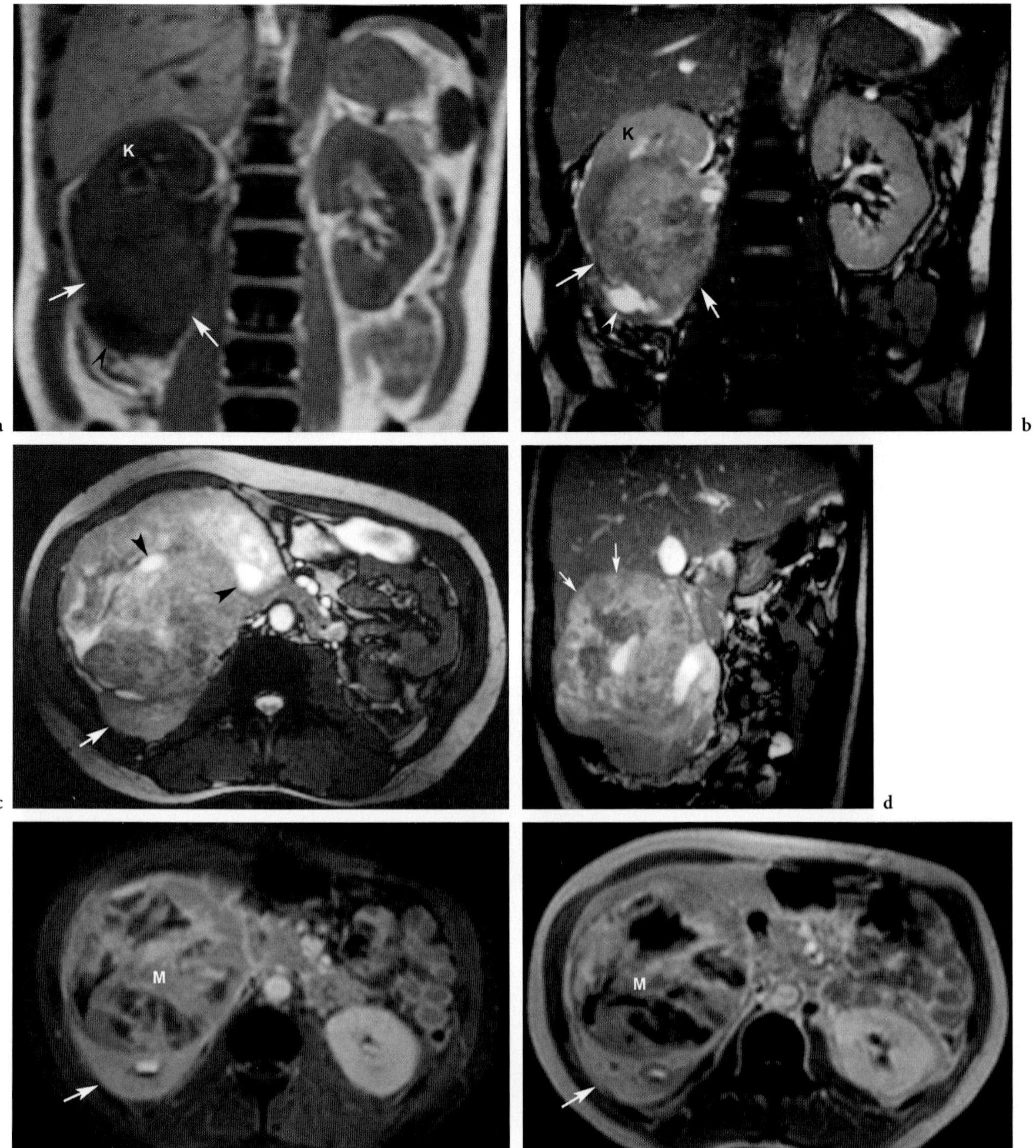

Fig. 9.7a-f. Sarcomatoid differentiation of renal cell carcinoma in a 65-year-old woman. Coronal **a** T1-weighted spin-echo and **b** balanced FFE T2-weighted MR images show the renal mass arising from the inferior pole of the right kidney (*arrows*). The normal renal parenchyma is seen at the superior pole (*K*). This predominately solid tumor contains a small area at its inferior aspect which is hyperintense on the T2-weighted images and hypointense on the T1-weighted images which may represent necrotic tissue or a cystic, fluid-filled space (*arrowhead*). **c** Axial balanced FFE T2-weighted MR image demonstrates the mass extending anteriorly from the right kidney and approaching the midline. A component of normal-appearing renal parenchyma (*arrow*) is seen posteriorly. Again demonstrated are the cystic spaces (*arrowheads*) within the mass. **d** Sagittal balanced FFE T2-weighted MR image shows that the right renal mass is replacing the renal parenchyma and extending into the subhepatic space (*arrows*). Axial **e** fat-suppressed contrast-enhanced T1-weighted and **f** contrast-enhanced T1-weighted MR images demonstrate the mostly solid mass arising from the right kidney. The complex nature of this mass (*M*) is demonstrated by the heterogeneous enhancement which appears as hyperintense areas after contrast administration, as compared with the homogeneous contrast enhancement of the normal contralateral kidney. A rim of normal renal parenchyma and contrast in the renal collecting system is seen posterior to the mass (*arrow*).

9.14
Conclusion

Primary renal sarcomas are rare entities which demonstrate aggressive local behavior and propensity for recurrence after surgical resection. The ominous nature of these lesions necessitates timely diagnosis and treatment. Before the diagnosis of primary renal sarcoma is made, the more common entities, such as sarcomatoid renal cell carcinoma or primary retroperitoneal sarcoma, should be considered. Diagnosis of renal cell sarcoma can be made with accuracy if three criteria, previously described by GRIGNON et al. (1990), are met:

1. The patient does not have a history of sarcoma elsewhere, to exclude metastatic disease.
2. The gross appearance of the tumor is compatible with origin in the kidney rather than involvement of the kidney by a retroperitoneal tumor.
3. Sarcomatoid variant of renal cell sarcoma is excluded.

Imaging characteristics of these neoplasms are highly variable, depending on the degree of differentiation of the tumor components. Both CT and MR imaging are useful in defining these characteristics, but the final diagnosis most often depends on histological and immunohistochemical evaluation.

References

Agrons GA, Kingsman KD, Wagner BJ, Sotelo-Avila C (1997) Rhabdoid tumor of the kidney in children: a comparative study of 21 cases. Am J Roentgenol 168:447–451

Allred CD, Cathey WJ, McDivitt RW (1981) Primary renal angiosarcoma. A case report. Hum Pathol 12:665–668

Ares Valdes Y, Ares Valdes N, Contreras Duvelgel DM (2003) Renal fibrosarcoma. Report of a case. Arch Esp Urol 56:1041–1043

Beckwith JB, Palmer NF (1978) Histopathology and prognosis of Wilms' tumor: results from the first national Wilms' tumor study. Cancer 41:1937–1948

Chen JH, Lee SK, Han WJ, Shen KH (2003) Primary giant cell malignant fibrous histiocytoma of the kidney with staghorn calculi. J Postgrad Med 49:246–248

Chen J, Lee S (1997) Renal leiomyosarcoma mimicking transitional cell carcinoma. Am J Roentgenol 169:312–313

Cheville JC, Lohse CM, Zincke H, Weaver AL, Leibovich BC, Frank I, Blute ML (2004) Sarcomatoid renal cell carcinoma: an examination of underlying histologic subtype and an analysis of associations with patient outcome. Am J Surg Pathol 28:435–441

Chhieng D, Cohen J, Waisman J, Fernandez G, Cangiarella J (1999) Fine-needle aspiration cytology of hemangiopericytoma: a report of five cases. Cancer 87:190–195

Christiano AP, Yang X, Gerber GS (1999) Malignant transformation of renal angiomyolipoma. J Urol 161:1900–1901

Chung CJ, Lorenzo R, Rayder S, Schemankewitz E, Guy CD, Cutting J, Munden M (1995) Rhabdoid tumors of the kidney in children: CT findings. Am J Roentgenol 164:697–700

Cibas ES, Goss GA, Kulke MH, Demetri GD, Fletcher CD (1998) Malignant epithelioid angiomyolipoma ("sarcoma ex angiomyolipoma") of the kidney: a case report and review of the literature. Am J Surg Pathol 83:1581–1592

Daneshmand S, Chandrasoma S, Lum C (2003) Sarcomatoid renal cell carcinoma with massive osteosarcomatous differentiation: an unusual image in clinical urology. Urology 61:1031–1032

De Peralta-Venturina M, Moch H, Amin M, Tamboli P, Hailemariam S, Mihatsch M, Javidan J, Stricker H, Ro JY, Amin MB (2001) Sarcomatoid differentiation in renal cell carcinoma: a study of 101 cases. Am J Surg Pathol 25:275–284

Deyrup AT, Montgomery E, Fisher C (2004) Leiomyosarcoma of the kidney. A clinicopathologic study. Am J Surg Pathol 28:178–182

Fernandez de Sevilla T, Muniz R, Palou J, Banus JM, Alegre J, Garcia A, Martinez-Vazquez JM (1988) Renal leiomyosarcoma in a patient with tuberous sclerosis. Urol Int 43:62–64

Ferry JA, Malt RA, Young RH (1991) Renal angiomyolipoma with sarcomatous transformation and pulmonary metastases. Am J Surg Pathol 15:21–40

Furukawa T, Azakami S, Kurosawa H, Ono Y, Ueda Y, Konno Y (2003) Cystic partially differentiated nephroblastoma, embryonal rhabdomyosarcoma, and multiple congenital anomalies associated with variegated mosaic aneuploidy and premature centromere division: a case report. J Pediatr Hematol Oncol 25:896–899

Gibbs JF, Huang PP, Lee RJ, McGrath B, Brooks J, McKinley B, Driscoll D, Kraybill WG (2001) Malignant fibrous histiocytoma: an institutional review. Cancer Invest 19:23–27

Gomez-Brouchet A, Soulie M, Delisle MB, Escourrou G (2001) Mesenchymal chondrosarcoma of the kidney. J Urol 166:2305

Gonlusen G, Ergin M, Paydas S, Bolat FA (2001) Primitive neuroectodermal tumor of the kidney: a rare entity. Int Urol Nephrol 33:449–451

Grignon DJ, Ayala AG, Ro JY, el-Naggar A, Papadopoulos NJ (1990) Primary sarcomas of the kidney. A clinicopathologic and DNA flow cytometric study of 17 cases. Cancer 65:1611–1618

Heppe RK, Donohue RE, Clark JE (1991) Bilateral renal hemangiopericytoma. Urology 38:249–253

Israel GM, Bosniak MA, Slywotzky CM, Rosen RJ (2002) CT differentiation of large exophytic renal angiomyolipomas and perirenal liposarcomas. Am J Roentgenol 179:769–773

Jimenez RE, Folpe AL, Lapham RL, Ro JY, O'Shea PA, Weiss SW, Amin MB (2002) Primary Ewing's sarcoma/primitive neuroectodermal tumor of the kidney: a clinicopathologic and immunohistochemical analysis of 11 cases. Am J Surg Pathol 26:320–327

Kansara V, Powell I (1980) Fibrosarcoma of the kidney. Urology 26:419–421

Kaushik S, Neifeld JP (2002) Leiomyosarcoma of the renal vein. Imaging and surgical reconstruction. Am J Roentgenol 179:276–277

Kawaguchi K, Oda Y, Nakanishi K, Saito T, Tamiya S, Nakahara K, Matsuoka H, Tsuneyoshi M (2002) Malignant transformation of renal angiomyolipoma: a case report. Am J Surg Pathol 26:523–529

Levine E, King BF Jr (2000) Adult malignant renal parenchymal neoplasms. Saunders, Philadelphia

Lowe BA, Brewer J, Houghton DC, Jacobson E, Pitre T (1992) Malignant transformation of angiomyolipoma. J Urol 147:1356–1358

Lowe LH, Isuani BH, Heller RM, Stein SM, Johnson JE, Navarro OM, Hernanz-Schulman M (2000) Pediatric renal masses: Wilm's tumor and beyond. Radiographics 20:1585–1603

Mainguene C, Choquenet C, Cucchi JM, Dupre F, Monticelli I, Michiels JF, de Pinieux G, Vieillefond A (2003) Primary pleomorphic rhabdomyosarcoma of the kidney in adults: an unusual tumor. Prog Urol 13:679–682

Makk L, Creech JL, Whelan JG Jr, Johnson MN (1974) Liver damage and angiosarcoma in vinyl chloride workers. J Am Med Assoc 64:230

Malhotra CM, Doolittle CH, Rodil JV, Vezeridis MP (1984) Mesenchymal chondrosarcoma of the kidney. Cancer 24:2495–2499

Martignoni G, Pea M, Rigaud G, Manfrin E, Colato C, Zamboni G, Scarpa A, Tardanico R, Roncalli M, Bonetti F (2000) Renal angiomyolipoma with epithelioid sarcomatous transformation and metastasis: demonstration of the same genetic defects in the primary and metastatic lesions. Am J Surg Pathol 24:889–894

Mayes DC, Fechner RE, Gillenwater JY (1990) Renal liposarcoma. Am J Surg Pathol 14:268–273

Mehanna D, Abu-Zidan FM, Rao S (2004) Liver metastasis in renal chondrosarcoma. Singapore Med J 45:183–185

Micolonghi TS, Liang D, Schwartz S (1984) Primary osteogenic sarcoma of the kidney. J Urol 131:1164–1166

Moazzam M, Ather MH, Hussainy AS (2002) Leiomyosarcoma presenting as a spontaneously ruptured renal tumor. A case report. BMC Urol 2:13

Moudouni SM, En-Nia I, Rioux-Leclerq N, Guille F, Lobel B (2001) Leiomyosarcoma of the renal pelvis. Scand J Urol Nephrol 35:425–427

Nativ O, Horowitz A, Lindner A, Many M (1985) Primary chondrosarcoma of the kidney. J Urol 134:120–121

Ng WD, Chan KW, Chan YT (1985) Primary leiomyosarcoma of the renal capsule. J Urol 133:834–835

O'Malley FP, Grignon DJ, Shepherd RR, Harker LA (1991) Primary osteosarcoma of the kidney. Report of case studies by immunohistochemistry, electron microscopy and DNA flow cytometry. Arch Pathol Lab Med 115:1262–1265

Pitfield J, Preston BJ, Smith PG (1981) A calcified renal mass: chondrosarcoma of the kidney. Br J Radiol 54:262

Pomara G, Cappello F, Cuttano MG, Rappa F, Morelli G, Mancini P, Selli C (2004) Primitive neuroectodermal tumor (PNET) of the kidney: a case report. BMC Cancer 4:3

Prince CL (1942) Primary angioendothelioma of the kidney: report of a case and brief review. J Urol 47:787

Quinn CM, Day DW, Waxman J, Krausz T (1993) Malignant mesenchymoma of the kidney. Histopathology 23:86–88

Rodriguez-Galindo C, Marina NM, Fletcher BD, Parham DM, Bodner SM, Meyer WH (1997) Is primitive neuroectodermal tumor (PNET) of the kidney a distinct entity? Cancer 79:2243–2250

Seabury JC (1967) Renal rhabdomyosarcoma. J Am Med Assoc 201:1043

Scriven RR, Thrasher TV, Smith DC, Stewart SC (1984) Primary renal malignant fibrous histiocytoma: a case report and literature review. J Urol 131:948–949

Srinivas V, Sogani PC, Hajdu SI, Whitmore WF Jr (1984) Sarcomas of the kidney. J Urol 132:13–16

Valdes YA, Valdes NA, Duvelgel C (2003) Renal fibrosarcoma. Report of a case. Arch Esp Urol 56:1041–1043

Vogelzang NJ, Fremgen AM, Guinan PD, Chmiel JS, Sylvester JL, Sener SF (1993) Primary renal sarcoma in adults. A natural history and management study by the American Cancer Society, Illinois Division. Cancer 71:804–810

Weeks DA, Beckwith JB, Mierau GW, Luckey DW (1989) Rhabdoid tumor of the kidney. A report of 111 cases from the national Wilms' tumor study pathology center. Am J Surg Pathol 13:439–458

Weeks DA, Beckwith JB, Mierau GW, Zuppan CW (1991) Renal neoplasms mimicking rhabdoid tumor of the kidney. A report from the National Wilms' Tumor Study Pathology Center. Am J Surg Pathol 15:1042–1054

10 Cystic Renal Masses

GARY M. ISRAEL

CONTENTS

10.1
Introduction

Cystic renal masses are common incidental findings when imaging the abdomen. Luckily, the overwhelming majority of them represent benign simple cysts and can be diagnosed confidently; however, more complicated cystic renal masses are sometimes identified, and differentiation of benign complex renal cysts from cystic renal neoplasms often presents a diagnostic challenge. In this chapter, the CT and MR imaging technique for assessing cystic renal masses, potential pitfalls in cystic renal mass evaluation, and the differentiation of benign and malignant cystic renal masses are reviewed.

10.2
Technique for CT and MR Imaging

The accurate diagnosis and characterization of a renal mass is dependent on many factors including

G. M. ISRAEL, MD
Associate Professor, Department of Diagnostic Radiology, Yale University School of Medicine, PO Box 208042, 333 Cedar Street, New Haven, CT 06520-8042, USA

the clinical history of the patient, the appearance of the renal mass, and the expertise of the radiologist. Unfortunately, the quality of the radiologic exam is frequently not emphasized; however this is a critical factor in making a correct diagnosis. The radiologist needs a firm understanding of what constitutes a high-quality exam and is responsible for ensuring that each exam be fully optimized.

Computed tomography (CT) is the modality of choice in evaluating a cystic renal mass and should be performed before and after intravenous contrast. At New York University Medical Center, a multidetector CT scan is used to evaluate all patients with a renal mass. Initially, unenhanced images are obtained and reconstructed to 4-mm-thick sections. Contrast-enhanced images are obtained using 150 ml of intravenous contrast injected at a minimum rate of 3 ml/s. Corticomedullary phase and nephrographic phase data sets are obtained using a scan delay of 40 and 100 s, respectively, and are reconstructed to 4-mm-thick slices. It is important to ensure that all of the imaging parameters (slice collimator, mAs, kVp, pitch) be kept constant between the unenhanced and contrast-enhanced (nephrographic phase) data sets to ensure that accurate Hounsfield unit (HU) readings of the mass are obtained. The corticomedullary data set can be further reconstructed into thinner overlapping slices for 3D imaging to depict the vascular anatomy.

Magnetic resonance imaging has been proven useful in characterizing cystic renal masses (ISRAEL et al. 2004). In patients who cannot receive iodinated intravenous contrast material because of allergy or renal insufficiency, MR imaging has the advantage of evaluating patients without exposure to potentially toxic contrast material. Gadolinium has been shown to be safe and well tolerated in patients with an iodinated contrast allergy and may be administered without concern for contrast-induced nephrotoxicity (NELSON et al. 1995; PRINCE et al. 1996; ROFSKY et al. 1991). For such patients MR imaging may be indicated, rather than CT. Patients with mildly reduced renal function (renal insufficiency but not on dialysis), a solitary kidney, or those who have undergone nephron-sparing surgery and, in need of serial follow-up exams, can receive a full dose of gadolinium without fear for the potential nephrotoxicity associated with iodinated contrast.

Renal MR imaging examinations are performed using a torso phased-array coil which increases the signal-to-noise ratio by a factor of two to three and allows for the use of smaller fields of view with concomitant increased spatial resolution. All sequences are performed during an end-expiratory breath-hold which has been shown to be more reproducible when compared with end-inspiration and assists in optimizing image co-registration for subtraction algorithms (HOLLAND et al. 1998). Unenhanced imaging includes a dual-echo axial breath-hold T1-weighted gradient-echo (GRE) sequence performed in phase and out of phase, a coronal breath-hold T2-weighted half-Fourier acquisition single-shot turbo spin-echo sequence, and an axial 3D frequency-selective fat-suppressed T1-weighted gradient-echo sequence (ROFSKY et al. 1999). After 20 ml of intravenous gadolinium followed by a 20-ml saline flush, the 3D sequence is repeated at multiple time points. For characterization of a renal mass, a scan delay of 3–5 min is suggested.

10.3
Renal Mass Enhancement

Using CT, HU measurements should be obtained and compared at the same location within the renal mass on the unenhanced and contrast-enhanced images. Formerly, a difference of 10 HU was suggested as evidence of enhancement (BOSNIAK 1986); however, this was based on HU readings using conventional (non-helical) CT scanners. With the development of helical CT, HU readings have become inconsistent (BOSNIAK and ROFSKY 1996). Presently, there is no unanimously accepted specific number which can be used as definitive and unequivocal evidence of enhancement within a renal mass. Some authors feel that the threshold of 10 HU should be increased to 15–20 HU (ABDULLA et al. 2002; BIRNBAUM et al. 2002; HENEGHAN et al. 2002; SIEGEL et al. 1999; ZAGORIA 2000), whereas others believe that a 10-HU threshold is still valid (BAE et al. 2000; CHUNG et al. 2004). In any event, it is important to be aware of the potential variability of HU readings, and it must be emphasized that whatever number is used

to determine enhancement, the determination must be unequivocal.

Some of the inconsistency of HU readings is likely secondary to pseudoenhancement, in which a simple renal cyst may show artificial apparent enhancement of 10 HU or more on contrast-enhanced CT (ABDULLA et al. 2002; BIRNBAUM et al. 2002; COULAM et al. 2000; HENEGHAN et al. 2002; MAKI et al. 1999). Pseudoenhancement is thought to be secondary to the image reconstruction algorithm used in helical scanners to adjust for beam-hardening effects. It is important to be aware of pseudoenhancement and to know when to suspect it. Pseudoenhancement most often occurs when the cyst is surrounded by renal tissue during the peak level of renal parenchymal enhancement. Many of these cysts are small (<2 cm) and completely intra-renal.

For MR imaging, a definitive method of determining enhancement in a renal mass has yet to be defined. In many cases, a qualitative comparison of the precontrast and postcontrast images is performed and straightforward enhancement is apparent; however, in some cases (such as a mass that is hyperintense on the precontrast images or in a hypovascular mass) enhancement is difficult, if not impossible, to appreciate if only subjective parameters are used. A promising method described by Ho et al. (2002) has shown that relative enhancement of renal masses can be measured on MR imaging using signal intensity readings obtained with region-of-interest measurements. Another method of demonstrating renal mass enhancement is image subtraction (HECHT et al. 2004; SUTO et al. 1989; LEE et al. 1996). Image subtraction is a postprocessing technique that has been used in MR imaging to facilitate the detection of enhancing masses on breast MR imaging and is used routinely for contrast-enhanced MR angiography. At New York University, image subtraction has been used successfully to assess enhancement characteristics of renal masses (HECHT et al. 2004) and has been proven very useful and reproducible in clinical practice.

Although the presence or absence of enhancement is the most important feature used to characterize cystic renal masses, this information must be combined with the morphological features of the wall and septa of the mass. Frequently, the hairline thin wall or septa of benign (nonsurgical) renal cysts appear to enhance when unenhanced and contrast-enhanced CT or MR images are compared side by side; however, it is not possible to quantify enhancement within these structures using region-of-interest (HU on CT or signal intensity units on MR imaging) measurements because they are so thin. This is referred to as "perceived" enhancement. On the other hand, the grossly thickened wall and septa or soft tissue within cystic renal neoplasms and indeterminate cystic renal masses show enhancement which can be quantified using region-of-interest (HU on CT or signal intensity units on MR imaging) measurements and is referred to as "measurable" enhancement.

10.4
Characterizing Cystic Renal Masses Using the Bosniak Classification

The incidental detection of cystic renal masses is common and therefore their accurate characterization is critical. In 1986 the Bosniak renal cyst classification (BOSNIAK 1986) was first introduced, providing a framework for evaluating cystic renal masses. With some modifications, the system has become well established and has proved helpful to radiologists and urologists in determining which lesions can safely be considered benign and which require surgical intervention or follow-up imaging (BOSNIAK 1997; ISRAEL and BOSNIAK 2003a; ISRAEL and BOSNIAK 2003b).

The Bosniak classification of renal cysts is based on an evaluation of the thickness and enhancement characteristics of the wall of the cyst, the presence, number, thickness, and enhancement characteristics of any septa which are present, the presence and amount of calcification within the wall or septa, the interface of the mass with the kidney, and the presence or absence of any enhancing soft tissue components. It can be simplified into three general categories: nonsurgical masses which do not need follow-up exams (categories I and II); nonsurgical masses in need of follow-up exams (category IIF); and surgical masses (categories III and IV).

Category I lesions are benign simple cysts which measure water density and do not enhance with intravenous contrast. They have a hairline thin wall and do not contain septa, calcifications, or solid components.

Category II masses are benign minimally complicated cystic lesions which may contain hairline thin septa but do not enhance with intravenous contrast, although minimal perceived (not measurable) enhancement of a hairline thin, smooth septum, or wall can sometimes be appreciated. Uniformly high-attenuation cysts (hyperdense cysts) which are less

than 3 cm and do not have measurable enhancement are included in this group. Fine calcification or a short segment of slightly thickened but smooth calcification may be present in the wall or septa (Fig. 10.1; ISRAEL and BOSNIAK 2003a).

Category IIF lesions are moderately complicated cysts which are thought to be benign but require follow-up examinations to prove benignity by demonstrating stability over time (ISRAEL and BOSNIAK 2003b). They may contain multiple hairline thin septa and/or minimal but smooth thickening of their wall or septa. As in category II cysts, these lesions may demonstrate perceived enhancement of their septa or walls, but they do not contain measurably enhancing structures. Completely intrarenal nonenhancing high-attenuation renal lesions (hyperdense cysts) ≥3 cm are also included in this category. Category IIF cysts may contain thick and nodular calcification (Figs. 10.2, 10.3; ISRAEL and BOSNIAK 2003a).

Category III lesions are complicated cystic lesions that have grossly thickened irregular or smooth walls or septa in which measurable enhancement can be clearly demonstrated (Fig. 10.4a). They may contain thick and irregular calcification similar to category IIF cysts; however, category III cysts demonstrate enhancement within the noncalcified portions of the mass, whereas category IIF cysts do not enhance (Fig. 10.5). Category III contains indeterminate lesions which could be benign or malignant and include chronic abscesses (Fig. 10.6) or chronically infected cysts, hemorrhagic cysts, benign

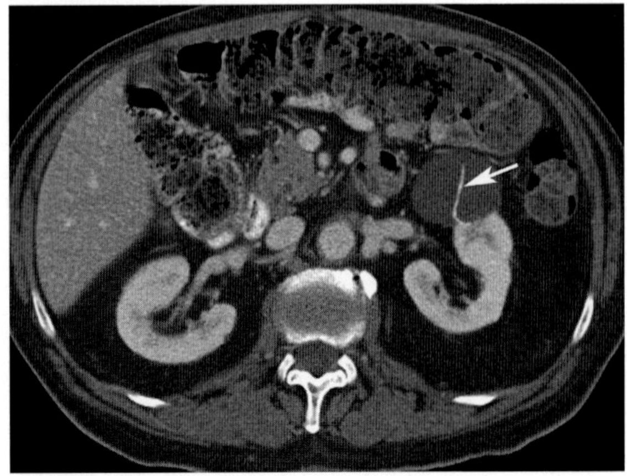

Fig. 10.1. Category II renal cyst in an 84-year-old man. Axial contrast-enhanced CT scan demonstrates a cystic renal mass in the left kidney. The cystic mass does not enhance, has a hairline thin wall, and contains a septation which has slightly thickened but smooth calcification (*arrow*) consistent with a Bosniak category II cyst.

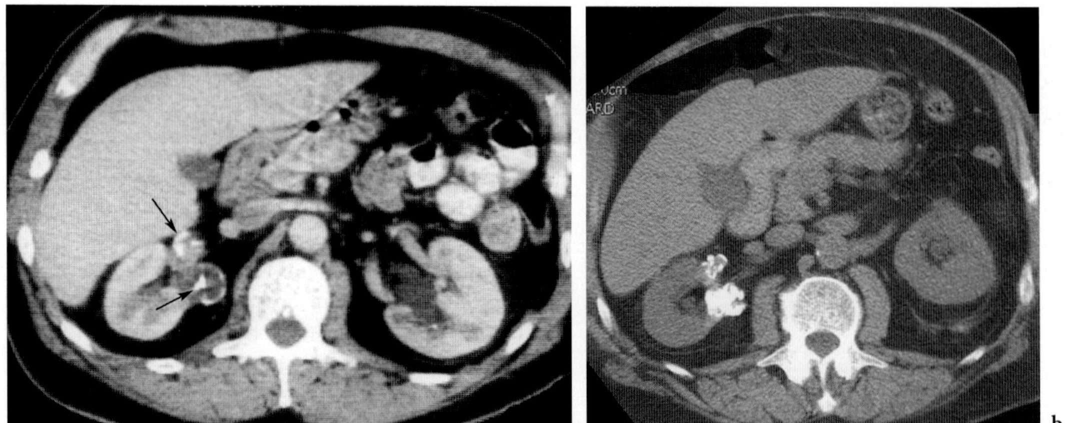

Fig. 10.2a,b. Category IIF renal cyst in a 61-year-old man with follow-up for over 17 years. **a** Axial contrast-enhanced CT scan obtained in 1981 demonstrates a bilobed cystic renal mass in the medial aspect of the right kidney. This mass contains thick and nodular calcification (*arrows*). Enhancement could not be demonstrated in any portion of the mass. **b** Axial unenhanced CT scan obtained in 1998 shows that the mass has not grown in size and has nearly completely filled in with calcification. On the contrast-enhanced images (not shown), enhancement could not be identified.

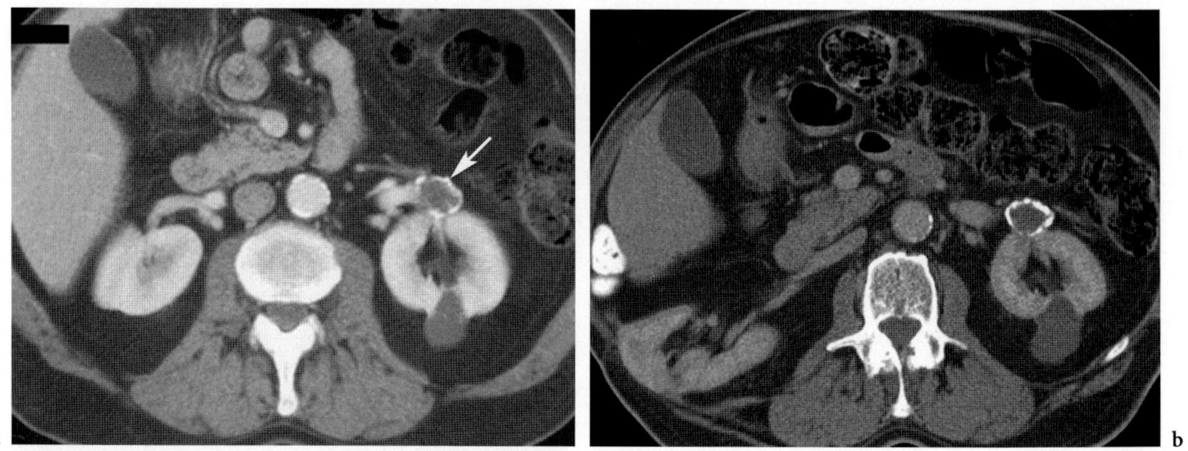

Fig. 10.3a,b. Category IIF renal cyst in a 72-year-old man with follow-up exams for 7 years. **a** Axial contrast-enhanced CT scan obtained in 1996 demonstrates a 2-cm mass with thick mural calcification (*arrow*) in the anterior aspect of the left kidney. There was no central enhancement within the mass. Note the simple cyst in the posterior aspect of the left kidney. **b** Axial contrast-enhanced CT scan obtained in 2003 shows that the mass is unchanged in size and the mural calcification is stable. Enhancement could not be demonstrated, consistent with a benign renal cyst. Note the post-operative appearance of the right kidney secondary to a partial nephrectomy for a renal cell carcinoma.

complex multiloculated cysts, benign multilocular cystic nephroma, or multiloculated cystic renal cell carcinoma. In most cases, they are considered surgical lesions; however, if an inflammatory mass is suspected (fever, flank pain, elevated white count), percutaneous aspiration and drainage may be performed to confirm the diagnosis of a renal abscess. Even though category III lesions are indeterminate, it is sometimes possible to suggest whether the lesion is more likely benign or malignant, based on the thickness of its wall and overall complexity. This,

combined with other aspects such as the size of the lesion and its location within the kidney, may affect the surgical approach by the urologist which can range from open or laparoscopic radical nephrectomy to open or laparoscopic partial nephrectomy. On gross inspection during surgery, these masses may also be "indeterminate" and their true nature can only be determined by histologic study.

Category IV lesions are malignant cystic masses in which enhancing soft tissue components are present (Figs. 10.7, 10.8).

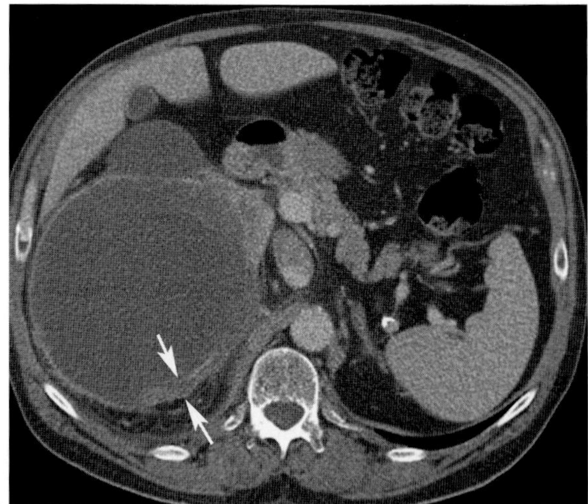

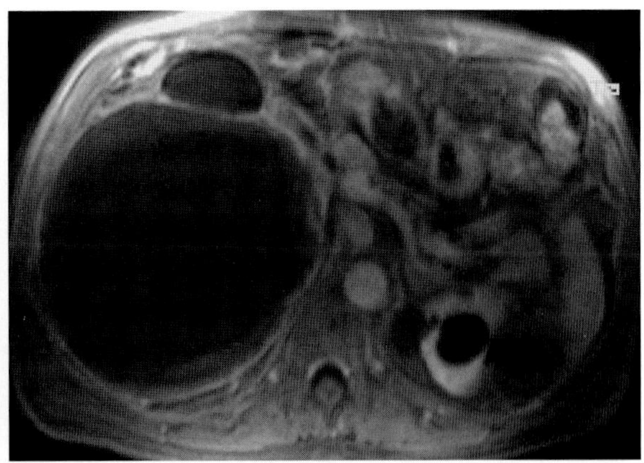

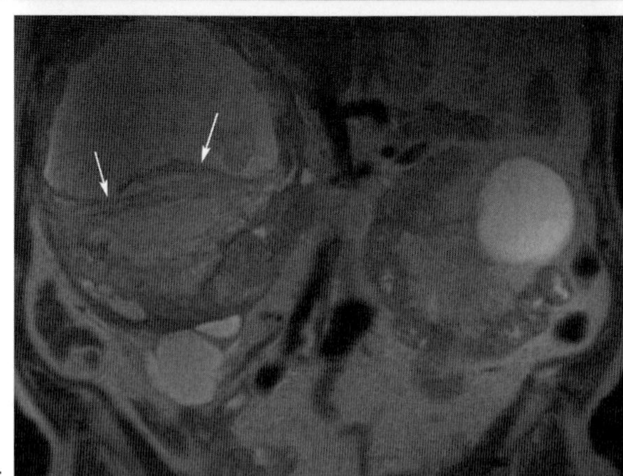

Fig. 10.4a–c. Category III cystic renal mass in a 76-year-old man. **a** Axial contrast-enhanced CT scan demonstrates a 15-cm complex cystic mass which has a thick irregular enhancing wall (*arrows*). There is no central enhancement within the mass. This mass is indeterminate and may represent a benign complex hemorrhagic cyst or a cystic neoplasm. At surgical pathology, a collecting duct carcinoma was diagnosed. **b** Axial fat-suppressed contrast-enhanced T1-weighted MR image demonstrates the complex cystic mass to have a thickened irregular enhancing wall without enhancement centrally, similar to the CT findings. **c** Coronal T2-weighted MR image demonstrates how the wall of the mass appears thicker and more irregular when compared with the contrast-enhanced CT image in **a** or the contrast-enhanced T1-weighted MR image in **b**. Also note the thick irregular structure (*arrows*) traversing the central portion of the mass, which is depicted on the T2-weighted MR image but cannot be seen on the CT or contrast-enhanced T1-weighted MR image.

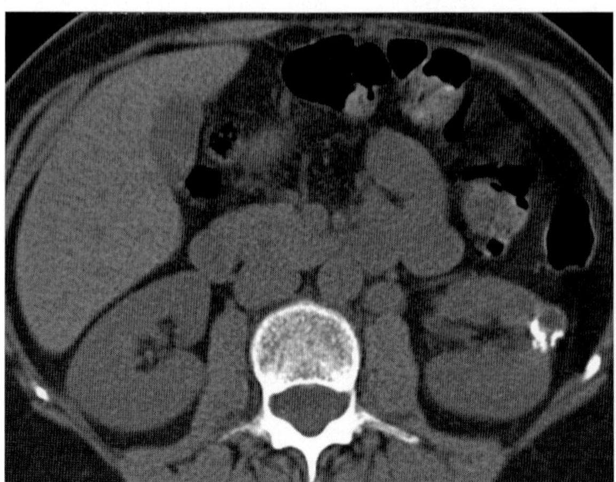

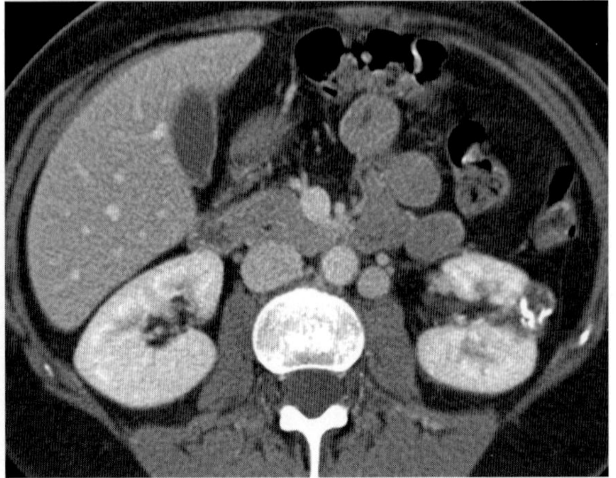

Fig. 10.5a,b. Complex calcified cystic renal mass in a 56-year-old woman. **a** Axial unenhanced CT scan demonstrates a 1.5-cm cystic mass in the left kidney which contains thick and irregular calcification along its posterior wall. The calcification in this cyst is typical of the type of calcification present in category IIF cysts. Centrally, this mass measured 22 HU. **b** Axial contrast-enhanced CT scan again demonstrates the complex calcified cystic mass. Hounsfield unit readings obtained in the same location as those on the unenhanced image show unequivocal enhancement to 53 HU, indicative of a surgical lesion. This enhancement is not present in category IIF cysts. The patient underwent a partial nephrectomy, and at surgical pathology, a renal cell carcinoma was diagnosed.

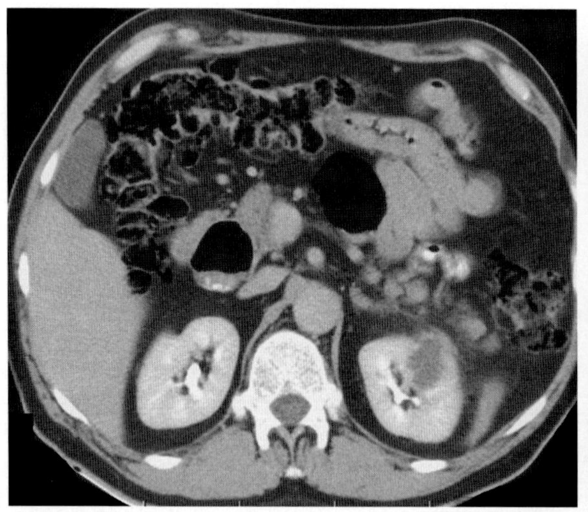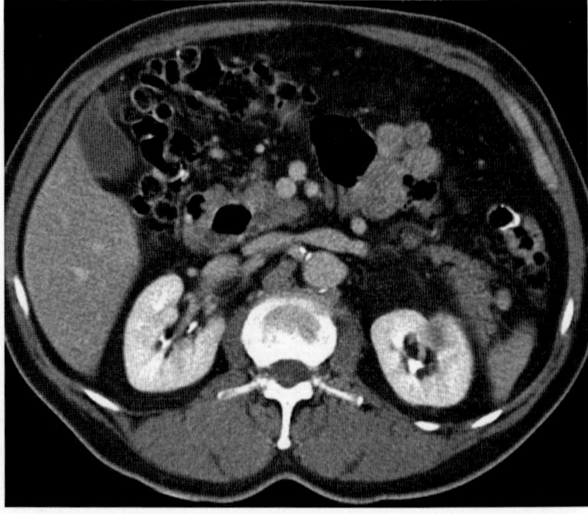

a   b

Fig. 10.6a,b. Complex cystic mass in a 52-year-old man with a low-grade fever. **a** Axial contrast-enhanced CT scan demonstrates a 2.5-cm cystic mass in the left kidney which has an enhancing thickened and irregular wall. Based only on the imaging findings, this is a category III cystic renal mass and may represent a benign or malignant lesion; however, when the imaging findings are combined with the patient's history of low-grade fever, a renal abscess becomes the most likely diagnosis. In this type of case, aspiration of the cystic renal mass may be performed. If purulent material is obtained from the lesion, a renal abscess is confirmed and the patient can be treated with antibiotics. **b** Axial contrast-enhanced CT image in the same patient after a 3-week course of antibiotics demonstrates nearly complete resolution of the renal abscess.

10.5
Comparing CT to MR Imaging

The Bosniak renal cyst classification is based only on CT findings; however, it is commonly applied to other imaging modalities, including MR imaging. Early experience suggests that MR imaging can be used reliably to evaluate most cystic renal masses using the Bosniak classification (ISRAEL et al. 2004); however, MR imaging may demonstrate some septa which are not depicted at CT, and may also show additional thickness of the septa and wall of some lesions, particularly on T2-weighted images (Fig. 10.4). The use of T2-weighted imaging in the evaluation of cystic renal masses is open to debate. While the exquisite contrast resolution of heavily T2-weighted images is helpful in characterizing simple renal cysts (even those <1 cm), its routine use in the evaluation of complex cystic renal masses has yet to be formally evaluated. T2-weighted images may demonstrate a more complex internal appearance of cystic renal masses when compared with T1-weighted images (with or without gadolinium) or CT images and it is uncertain how to incorporate this additional information into the overall evaluation of the mass. At this time, abnormalities depicted only on T2-weighted images should be interpreted with caution and compared carefully side by side

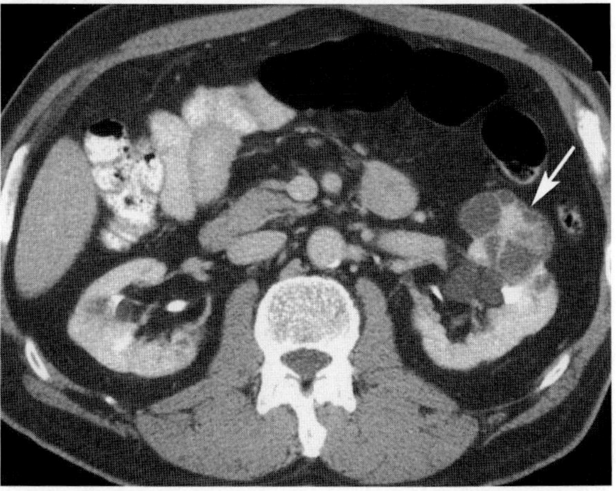

Fig. 10.7. Category IV left renal cyst in a 48-year-old man. Axial contrast-enhanced CT scan demonstrates a 4.5-cm complex cystic left renal mass which has a moderately thickened wall, grossly thickened septa, and enhancing soft tissue (*arrow*) centrally. At surgical pathology, a cystic renal cell carcinoma was diagnosed.

with the contrast-enhanced images to evaluate any enhancement within the structures depicted on the T2-weighted images.

Compared with contrast-enhanced CT, contrast-enhanced T1-weighted MR images have superior contrast resolution, and therefore MR imaging

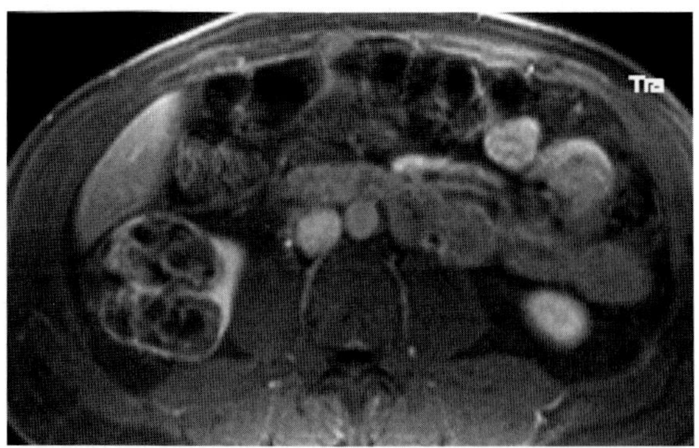

Fig. 10.8. Category IV right renal cyst in a 63-year-old man. Axial contrast-enhanced fat-suppressed T1-weighted MR image demonstrates a 6-cm complex cystic right renal mass with a grossly thickened and enhancing wall and septa and enhancing soft tissue components. A cystic renal cell carcinoma was diagnosed at surgical pathology.

may demonstrate definitive enhancement in renal lesions which show only equivocal enhancement on CT. In some cases it is possible that a cystic renal mass will be placed in a higher Bosniak category based on MR imaging than on CT. This is not a problem in cases in which patient management is not affected; however, it can create uncertainty in patient management in masses which appear as category IIF on CT but category III on MR imaging. Further experience is needed to determine the proper management of these types of cases, especially those that are borderline between categories IIF and III.

Although calcification of the wall or septa of cystic renal masses is common, it plays only a minor role in their overall evaluation (Israel and Bosniak 2003a). A potential shortcoming of MR imaging is its inability to depict calcification within the septa or wall of a cystic lesion. Theoretically, a unilocular cystic renal mass with a hairline thin wall containing a small amount of calcification (category II on CT) would be characterized as a simple cyst (category I) on MR imaging; however, this difference does not affect patient management and it is therefore unimportant. Furthermore, the diagnosis of malignancy or the decision to operate on a cystic mass should not be made on the basis of the presence or the amount of calcification (Israel and Bosniak 2003a), but depends on demonstrating enhancement in a grossly thickened wall or septa, or within soft tissue components of the mass; therefore, the inability of MR imaging to depict calcification in a cystic renal mass does not seem to be significant.

In some cases this can be advantageous. For instance, detecting enhancement in an irregularly thickened wall or septa of a heavily calcified cystic lesion on CT can be difficult because the calcification is closely associated with the noncalcified portion of the wall or septa, and prevents accurate HU measurements. On MR imaging, the calcification would not be depicted and the morphology of the noncalcified septa and wall could be better evaluated and any possible enhancement within these components can be better appreciated (Balci et al. 1999; Israel et al. 2004).

10.6
Role of Biopsy in Indeterminate Cystic Renal Mass

Some authors believe that renal mass biopsy is useful in evaluating the indeterminate cystic renal mass (Harisinghani et al. 2003; Lang et al. 2002), whereas others feel it is unreliable (Renshaw et al. 1997; Rybicki et al. 2003). When an indeterminate cystic renal mass (category III) is biopsied and a benign diagnosis is made, there will be uncertainty as to whether or not a sampling error is present. This is compounded by the fact that in some cystic renal cell carcinomas, the cystic architecture dominates the morphologic appearance of the tumor. In these cases, the overall population of malignant cells is small, and characterizing these masses as a renal malignancy may be difficult for the pathologist, even when the entire specimen is examined (Eble and Bonsib 1998). Furthermore, once a cystic renal mass is biopsied, the natural history of the mass has been changed. If it is decided to follow an indeterminate mass because of a benign biopsy result, it will be impossible to know if any change in the mass on the follow-up exam is secondary to a change in the nature of the mass or if it is a response to the previous instrumentation. Biopsy of an indeterminate cystic renal mass is an invasive procedure and most often seems unnecessary.

However, there are times in which percutaneous biopsy or aspiration of an indeterminate cystic renal mass may be warranted. If a renal abscess is suspected (because of a history of fever, leukocytosis, or urinary tract infection; Fig. 10.6), needle aspiration should be performed, and if pus is recovered, percutaneous drainage and treatment with antibiotics can be instituted; however, if blood or necrotic debris is recovered, surgical removal is indicated.

10.7
Other Cystic Renal Masses

10.7.1
Multilocular Cystic Nephroma

Multilocular cystic nephroma is a complex cystic renal mass which typically occurs in males during the first 2 years of life or in females younger than 5 years or between 40 and 60 years (WILLIAMSON and KING 2000). It contains multiple discrete cysts or locules and is surrounded by a fibrous capsule. The wall and septa of a multilocular cystic nephroma are typically grossly thickened (Fig. 10.9); therefore, it cannot be differentiated from a cystic renal cell carcinoma, and it is considered a surgical cystic renal mass (category III). Multilocular cystic nephroma may herniate into the renal pelvis, which is suggestive of this tumor.

10.7.2
Localized Cystic Disease of the Kidney

Localized cystic disease of the kidney is a benign condition in which multiple simple renal cysts are either clustered together or scattered diffusely throughout a kidney or portion of a kidney (SLYWOTZKY and BOSNIAK 2001). Superficially, this may resemble a multilocular cystic nephroma, a cystic renal neoplasm, or autosomal-dominant poly-

cystic kidney disease; therefore, familiarity with this entity is necessary to avoid mislabeling some patients with a hereditary condition and to avoid unnecessary surgery in others. The unilaterality of localized cystic disease of the kidney is an important initial observation which helps differentiate it from autosomal-dominant polycystic kidney disease, which typically affects both kidneys. In addition, liver and pancreatic cysts, and cerebral aneurysms, are associated with autosomal-dominant polycystic kidney disease, and not with localized cystic disease. Finally, a family history of renal disease (which should be present in autosomal-dominant polycystic kidney disease, but not in localized cystic disease) may also be helpful.

Since localized cystic disease represents clustered simple renal cysts, a capsule is not present; therefore, it is possible for normal renal parenchyma to insinuate itself between the adjacent cysts (Fig. 10.10). This is a distinguishing imaging feature which can be used to differentiate localized cystic disease from multilocular cystic nephroma and a cystic renal neoplasm, both of which have a capsule. After contrast administration, it is possible to identify the intervening renal parenchyma by scrolling through the lesion in real-time, at a workstation. It is imperative to be sure that this renal parenchyma enhance identically to the rest of the renal parenchyma, so that it is not confused with the thick enhancing septa within a multilocular cystic nephroma or multiloculated cystic renal cell carcinoma.

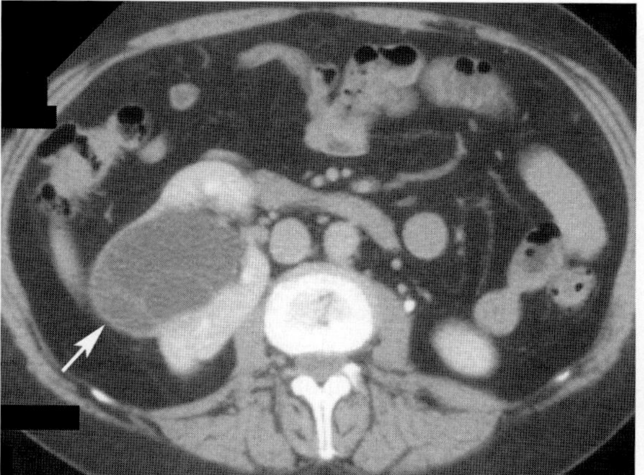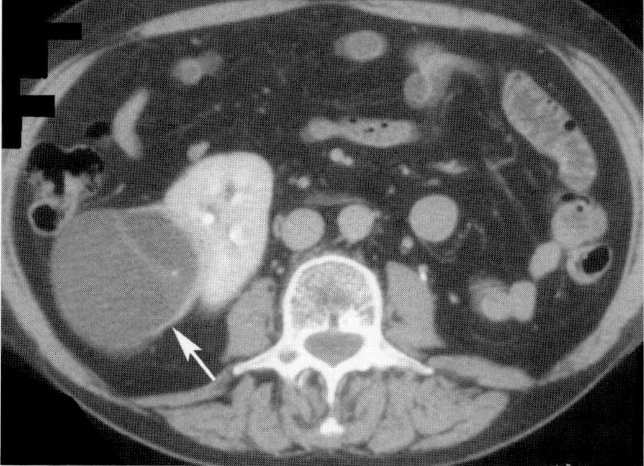

Fig. 10.9a,b. Indeterminate cystic renal mass in a 46-year-old woman. **a, b** Axial contrast-enhanced CT scans demonstrate a cystic renal mass in the right kidney which has a grossly thickened and enhancing wall (*arrow*) and a few moderately thickened septa. In **a**, the medial margin of the mass has extended into the renal sinus and herniated into the renal pelvis. While this is an indeterminate complex cystic mass (category III), the combination of its imaging findings along with the patient's gender and age suggest that this is a multilocular cystic nephroma; however, these findings are not specific for this diagnosis and a malignancy cannot be excluded. At surgical pathology, a multilocular cystic nephroma was diagnosed. (Image courtesy of S. McCarthy)

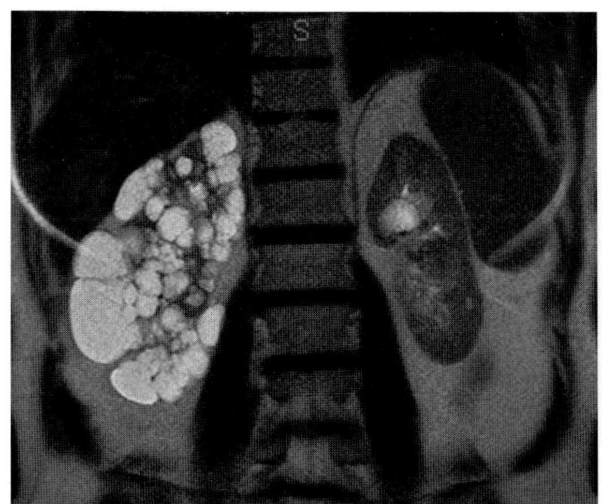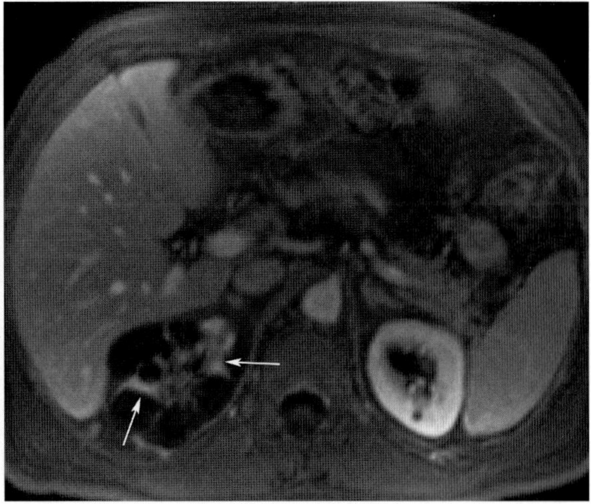

a

b

Fig. 10.10a,b. Localized cystic disease of the right kidney in a 68-year-old man. **a** Coronal T2-weighted MR image demonstrates innumerable cysts scattered throughout the right kidney without a surrounding capsule. Note that only a small parapelvic cyst and a tiny parenchymal cyst are present in the left kidney. **b** Axial contrast-enhanced fat-suppressed T1-weighted MR image demonstrates that normal renal parenchyma (which enhances identically to the parenchyma of the left kidney; *arrows*) has insinuated itself between the renal cysts. These findings are typical of localized cystic disease of the kidney. In this patient, there was no family history of renal disease or other manifestations to suggest autosomal-dominate polycystic kidney disease.

10.7.3
Calyceal Diverticulum

A calyceal diverticulum is a cystic structure, lined by transitional epithelium, which communicates with the collecting system of the kidney (Canales and Monga 2003). They are thought to be congenital, can be of variable size, and may occur anywhere in the kidney. They can be diagnosed by demonstrating a cystic renal mass which fills with contrast on intravenous pyelogram (IVP), CT, or MR imaging (Fig. 10.11). The neck of a diverticulum typically connects to the fornix of a calyx and is frequently narrow, which is why the calyceal diverticula usually fill with contrast during excretory-phase acquisitions. The narrow neck also contributes to chronic stasis of urine, which predisposes patients to develop calculi within the diverticulum and recurrent infection.

10.8
Conclusion

Even though the accurate diagnosis of a cystic renal mass is multifactorial, the quality of the examination (CT or MR imaging) is often not emphasized, and yet it is a significant factor in making a correct diagnosis. The techniques for high-quality CT and MR imaging have been reviewed and their role in the characterization of cystic renal masses has been summarized. The Bosniak renal cyst classification has proven helpful in classifying renal cysts into surgical and nonsurgical lesions and its application to MR imaging appears promising. In the future, with further experience using state-of-the-art CT and MR imaging, our ability to diagnose and manage complex cystic renal masses will further advance, leading to improved patient care.

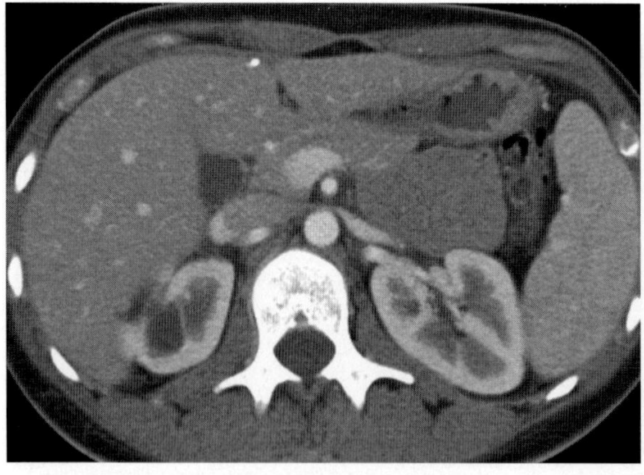

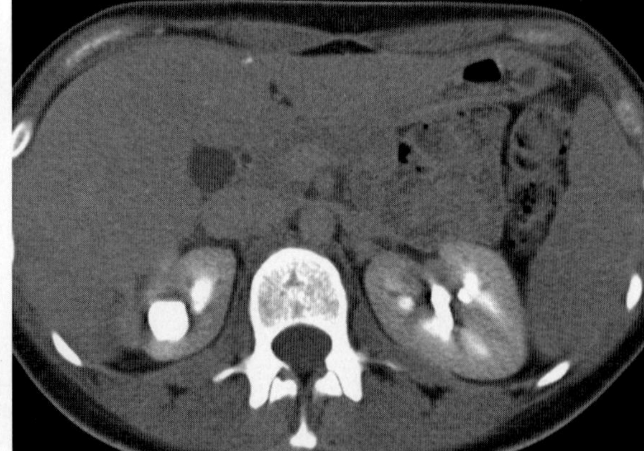

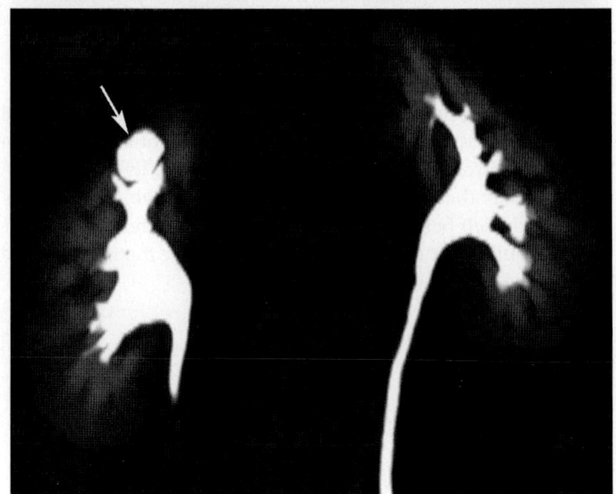

Fig. 10.11a-c. Calyceal diverticulum in a 23-year-old woman with a history of multiple urinary tract infections. **a** Axial contrast-enhanced CT scan obtained during the corticomedullary phase of enhancement demonstrates a small cystic structure at the upper pole of the right kidney. **b** Axial contrast-enhanced CT scan obtained during the excretory phase shows that the cystic structure fills with contrast material and is therefore connected to the collected system, diagnostic of a calyceal diverticulum. **c** Coronal maximum intensity projection (MIP) image produced from the excretory-phase CT data set shows the calyceal diverticulum (*arrow*) at the upper pole of the right kidney.

References

Abdulla C, Kalra MK, Saini S, Maher MM, Ahmad A, Halpern E, Silverman SG (2002) Pseudoenhancement of simulated renal cysts in a phantom using different multidetector CT scanners. Am J Roentgenol 179:1473–1476

Bae KT, Heiken JP, Siegel CL, Bennett HF (2000) Renal cysts: Is attenuation artifactually increased on contrast-enhanced CT images? Radiology 216:792–796

Balci NC, Semelka RC, Patt RH, Dubois D, Freeman JA, Gomez-Caminero A, Woosley JT (1999) Complex renal cysts: findings on MR imaging. Am J Roentgenol 172:1495–1500

Birnbaum BA, Maki DD, Chakraborty DP, Jacobs JE, Babb JS (2002) Renal cyst pseudoenhancement: evaluation with an anthropomorphic body CT phantom. Radiology 225:83–90

Bosniak MA (1986) The current radiological approach to renal cysts. Radiology 158:1–10

Bosniak MA (1997) Diagnosis and management of patients with complicated cystic lesions of the kidney. Am J Roentgenol 169:819–821

Bosniak MA, Rofsky NM (1996) Problems in the detection and characterization of small renal masses. Radiology 198:638–641

Canales B, Monga M (2003) Surgical management of the calyceal diverticulum. Curr Opin Urol 13:255–260

Chung EP, Herts BR, Linnell G, Novick AC, Obuchowski N, Coll DM, Baker ME (2004) Analysis of changes in attenuation of proven renal cysts on different scanning phases of triphasic MDCT. Am J Roentgenol 182:405–410

Coulam CH, Sheafor DH, Leder RA, Paulson EK, DeLong DM, Nelson RC (2000) Evaluation of pseudoenhancement of renal cysts during contrast-enahnced CT. Am J Roentgenol 174:493–498

Eble JN, Bonsib SM (1998) Extensively cystic renal neoplasms: cystic nephroma, cystic partially differentiated nephroblastoma, multilocular cystic renal cell carcinoma, and cystic hamartoma of renal pelvis. Semin Diagn Pathol 15:2–20

Harisinghani MG, Maher MM, Gervais DA, McGovern F, Hahn P, Jhaveri K, Varghese J, Mueller PR (2003) Incidence of malignancy in complex cystic renal masses (Bosniak category III): Should imaging-guided biopsy precede surgery? Am J Roentgenol 180:755–758

Hecht EM, Israel GM, Krinsky GA, Hahn WY, Kim DC, Belitskaya-Levy I, Lee VS (2004) Renal masses: quantitative analysis of enhancement with signal intensity measurements versus qualitative analysis of enhancement with image subtraction for diagnosing malignancy at MR imaging. Radiology 232:373–378

Heneghan JP, Spielmann AL, Sheafor DH, Kliewer MA, DeLong

DM, Nelson RC (2002) Pseudoenhancement of simple renal cysts: a comparison of single and multidetector helical CT. J Comput Assist Tomogr 26:90–94

Ho VB, Allen SF, Hood MN, Choyke PL (2002) Renal masses: quantitative assessment of enhancement with dynamic MR imaging. Radiology 224:695–700

Holland AE, Goldfarb JW, Edelman RR (1998) Diaphragmatic and cardiac motion during suspended breathing: preliminary experience and implications for breath-hold MR imaging. Radiology 209:483–489

Israel GM, Bosniak MA (2003a) Calcification in cystic renal masses: Is it important in diagnosis? Radiology 226:47–52

Israel GM, Bosniak MA (2003b) Follow-up CT of moderately complex cystic lesions of the kidney (Bosniak category IIF). Am J Roentgenol 181:627–633

Israel GM, Hindman N, Bosniak MA (2004) Evaluation of cystic renal masses: comparison of CT and MR imaging by using the Bosniak classification system. Radiology 231:365–371

Lang EK, Macchia RJ, Gayle B, Richter F, Watson RA, Thomas R, Myers L (2002) CT-guided biopsy of indeterminate renal cystic masses (Bosniak 3 and 2F): accuracy and impact on clinical management. Eur Radiol 12:2518–2524

Lee VS, Flyer MA, Weinreb JC, Krinsky GA, Rofsky NM (1996) Image subtraction in gadolinium-enhanced MR imaging. Am J Roentgenol 167:1427–1432

Maki DD, Birnbaum BA, Chakraborty DP, Jacobs JE, Carvalho BM, Herman GT (1999) Renal cyst pseudoenhancment: beam-hardening effects on CT numbers. Radiology 213:468–472

Nelson KL, Gifford LM, Lauber-Huber C, Gross CA, Lasser TA (1995) Clinical safety of gadopentetate dimeglumine. Radiology 196:439–443

Prince MR, Arnoldus C, Frisoli JK (1996) Nephrotoxicity of high-dose gadolinium compared with iodinated contrast. J Magn Reson Imaging 1:162–166

Renshaw AA, Granter SR, Cibas ES (1997) Fine-needle aspiration of the adult kidney. Cancer 81:71–88

Rybicki FJ, Shu KM, Cibas ES, Fielding JR, vanSonnenberg E, Silverman SG (2003) Percutaneous biopsy of renal masses: sensitivity and negative predictive value stratified by clinical setting and size of masses. Am J Roentgenol 180:1281–1287

Rofsky NM, Weinreb JC, Bosniak MA, Libes RB, Birnbaum BA (1991) Renal lesion characterization with gadolinium-enhanced MR imaging: efficacy and safety in patients with renal insufficiency. Radiology 180:85–89

Rofsky NM, Lee VS, Laub G, Pollack MA, Krinsky GA, Thomasson D, Ambrosino MM, Weinreb JC (1999) Abdominal MR imaging with a volumetric interpolated breath-hold examination. Radiology 212:876–884

Siegel CL, Fisher AJ, Bennett HF (1999) Interobserver variability in determining enhancement of renal masses on helical CT. Am J Roentgenol 172:1207–1212

Slywotzky CM, Bosniak MA (2001) Localized cystic disease of the kidney. Am J Roentgenol 176:843–849

Suto Y, Caner BE, Tamagawa Y, Matsuda T, Kimura I, Kimura H, Toyama T, Ishii Y (1989) Subtracted synthetic images in GD-DTPA enhanced MR. J Comput Assist Tomogr 13:925–928

Williamson B, King BF (2000) Benign neoplasms of the renal parenchyma. In Pollack HM, McClennan BL (eds) Clinical urography, 2nd edn. Saunders, Philadelphia, pp 1413–1439

Zagoria RJ (2000) Imaging of small renal masses: a medical success story. Am J Roentgenol 175:945–955

11 Collecting Duct Carcinoma

SEONG KUK YOON and SEO HEE RHA

CONTENTS

11.1
Introduction

Renal cell carcinoma (RCC) accounts for roughly 2–3% of adult malignancies and constitutes approximately 85% of all primary malignant renal tumors. The male-to-female annual incidence ratio for RCC is 1.5:1. The incidence is equivalent between whites and blacks. Although RCC may occur at any age, including childhood, there is a progressive increase in frequency with age. Patients usually present between the ages of 50 and 70 years, with a median age at diagnosis of 57 years (LEVINE and KING 2000). Rare types of RCC occurring in children have an appearance and behavior equivalent to those developing in adults.

S. K. YOON, MD, PhD
Assistant Professor, Department of Diagnostic Radiology, Dong-A University College of Medicine, 1, 3-Ga, Dongdaesin-Dong, Seo-Gu, Busan 602-715, South Korea
S. H. RHA, MD, PhD
Associate Professor, Department of Pathology, Dong-A University College of Medicine, 1, 3-Ga, Dongdaesin-Dong, Seo-Gu, Busan 602-715, South Korea

In 1976, MANCILLA-JIMENEZ et al. reported that atypical hyperplastic changes of adjacent collecting ducts were present in 3 of 34 papillary RCC and suggested that some papillary RCC may originate from collecting duct epithelium (SINGH and NABI 2002). The term Bellini duct carcinoma, reflecting the presumed site of origin, was first defined by CROMIE et al. (1979). It is also known by several synonyms: collecting duct carcinoma (CDC); medullary renal carcinoma; distal renal tubular carcinoma; and distal nephron carcinoma that arises from the cells of the distal nephron (KURODA et al. 2002). The detailed morphologic studies of THOENES et al. (1986) have delineated the major morphologic types of renal cell neoplasia and their histogenetic relationship to various segments of the renal tubular system, whereas chromophobe RCC and CDC have been categorized as distinct new entities in a new classification system of renal tumors (SRIGLEY and EBLE 1998). FLEMING and LEWI (1986) defined the diagnostic criteria and established collecting duct carcinoma of the kidney as a separate histologic entity arising in the renal medulla (NATSUME et al. 1997). The Heidelberg classification of renal tumors, introduced in 1997, identified five histologic types of renal cancer (conventional, papillary, chromophobe, collecting duct, and unclassifiable), according to their morphologic aspects and their chromosome alterations obtained by a cytogenetic analysis of the neoplastic karyotype (ANTONELLI et al. 2003). Since the First International Workshop on Renal Cell Carcinoma held by the World Health Organization, CDC has been also classified as an entity different from conventional (clear cell) renal carcinoma, papillary renal carcinoma, chromophobe renal carcinoma, and unclassified renal cell carcinoma. Each has distinct histomorphologic, ultrastructural, immunohistochemical, histochemical, and cytogenetic features. Conventional RCC is the most common cancer of the renal cortex, accounting for approximately 70% of cases. Most conventional RCCs contain clear cytoplasm, but some have eosinophilic or granular cytoplasm. Papillary RCC accounts for approximately

15% of RCC, including those previously referred to as chromophil RCC. Chromophobe RCC accounts for approximately 5% of cases of RCC. The cytoplasm contains numerous microvesicles that appear blue with Hale's colloidal iron stain. Unclassified RCC is reserved for cases that do not fulfill the criteria for the cancers described previously. These tumors are morphologically and genetically variable and are often high grade. Less than 2% of renal carcinomas are unclassified (Bostwick and Eble 1999).

The collecting duct is embryologically derived from the ureteric bud, whereas the remainder of the kidney develops from metanephric blastema. The ureteric bud also differentiates into ureter, renal pelvis, and calyces. The renal collecting ducts extend from the cortex to the tips of the renal papillae (Srigley and Eble 1998). Collecting duct carcinoma, or Bellini duct carcinoma, is a very rare, aggressive renal neoplasm that arises from the distal segment of the collecting ducts of Bellini in the renal medullary pyramids (Fig. 11.1), unlike the much more common variants of RCC which arise from the convoluted tubules (Sironi et al. 2003). Collecting duct carcinoma originates in the medullar collecting duct, which arises from the mesonephron. In contrast, the tubular structures of the kidney, which can be a point of origin for RCC, originate in the metanephric blastema (Auguet et al. 2000). Recognition of CDC remains somewhat controversial, and the tumor is typically described as containing irregular channels lined by highly atypical epithelium, often with a hob-nail cell appearance (Bostwick and Eble 1999). Collecting duct carcinoma is almost invariably centered in the renal medulla with or without extension into the renal cortex, renal pelvis, or hilar soft tissue. Its hypothesized origin from the collecting duct epithelium is supported by the presence of the collecting duct epithelium dysplasia far from the main tumor and reactivity of tumor cells with antibodies to high molecular weight cytokeratin and *Ulex europaeus* agglutinin-I (UEA-I; Gong et al. 2003).

The most common neoplasms arising from the collecting ducts are renal oncocytoma and chromophobe RCC, which appear to arise in the cortex from the intercalated cells of the proximal connecting segment of the collecting ducts. Collecting duct carcinoma is a much less common neoplasm that displays a tubulopapillary architecture, arises in the renal medulla (and later invades the renal cortex), and demonstrates infiltrating tubules with an associated desmoplastic reaction (Milowski et al. 2002). The microscopic appearance of the tumor is variable; thus, diagnosis based on histologic criteria

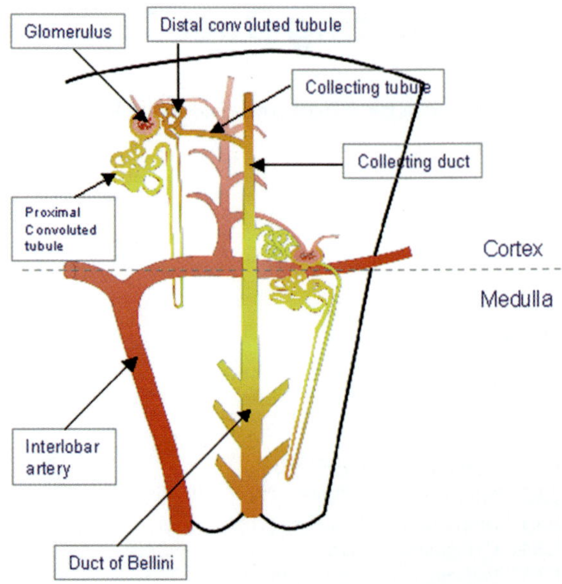

Fig. 11.1. Normal histologic anatomy of the kidney.

alone cannot be accurate, and immunohistochemical staining is needed to demonstrate the origin of the tumor (Kirkali et al. 1996). Because most CDC cases are published as case reports, it is difficult to characterize this entity.

In this chapter, we review the natural history, clinical course, pathologic and radiologic findings, treatment, and prognosis of typical CDCs.

11.2
Clinical Features

Collecting duct carcinoma is a rare variant of renal carcinoma associated with an aggressive course and an extremely poor prognosis. It is considered one of the most aggressive carcinomas of the renal tubular epithelium: 35–40% of patients with distant metastases and two-thirds of all patients are dead within 2 years of diagnosis (Gallob et al. 2001). Collecting duct carcinoma account for approximately 0.4–2.6% of all renal neoplasms. With regard to the incidence of CDC, Rumpelt et al. (1991) found six CDC (0.4%) among 1400 consecutive RCC. Most cases reported previously had a tendency to early dissemination and a fatal clinical course. Patients tend to be younger than those with classical RCC (median age at diagnosis of 43 years) and white (Milowski et al. 2002; Natsume et al. 1997). More men than women (ratio 2:1) are affected. There is no predominant laterality of the affected side. Patients with CDC usually have a family history of associated malignancies, including colon, pancreas, lung, ovary, and uterus malignancies (KURODA et al. 2002). Clinical manifestations of CDC, similar to those of RCC, are hematuria, flank pain, and palpable mass. Constitutional symptoms, such as fever, anorexia, and weight loss, are also common, but no particular paraneoplastic syndrome has been reported (AUGUET et al. 2000; PICKHARDT 1999).

The tumor typically follows an aggressive clinical course with most patients showing evidence of metastatic disease at presentation. The most common site of metastatic disease is the lymph nodes, including the cervical or supraclavicular lymph nodes and visceral metastases. Nodal involvement was reported in 77.8% and lung metastases in 44.4% of patients (PEYROMAURE et al. 2002). These findings are similar to those of DAVIS et al. (1995), who reported nodal involvement and lung metastasis rates of 78 and 27%, respectively. In their study tumors were also metastatic to the adrenal gland in 24% of cases and to the liver in 18%. In contrast to RCC, blastic bone metastases occur more frequently than lytic bone metastases in CDC. This rapid metastatic spread may be due to the tumor's central location, close to the renal hilus (MILOWSKI et al. 2002; PEYROMAURE et al. 2002). The growth pattern of CDC seems to be quite rapid, which would explain why it is almost always detected clinically (90% of our patients), especially when tumors are large (mean 94 mm). This is unlike other renal malignancies, which are increasingly more frequently discovered fortuitously (MEJEAN et al. 2003).

The association of CDC with sickle cell trait (SCT) has been noted by others. In one study 44.4% of patients were black and 55.6% had SCT. All black patients had SCT. In the series of DAVIS et al. (1995), which included 33 patients with CDC, all except 1 were black and had SCT (PEYROMAURE et al. 2002).

11.3
Pathology

There are five distinct subtypes of RCC: conventional (clear cell); papillary; chromophobe; collecting duct subtypes; and unclassified RCC. Each subtype has distinct histomorphologic, ultrastructural, immunohistochemical, histochemical, and cytogenetic features (GONG et al. 2003). A modern classification of renal epithelial neoplasms has been proposed that takes into account both the morphologic and genetic findings.

Collecting duct carcinoma is an adenocarcinoma consisting of two components. The first component is the main tumor mass, which is papillary with a fibrovascular core, whereas the second, invasive part is composed of glandular elements associated with marked desmoplastic reaction. The tumor cells are columnar, and show variable degrees of pleomorphism (NGUYEN and SCHUMANN 1997).

Several pathologic criteria define CDC. It has tubulopapillary architecture, arises in the renal medulla, and contains atypical hyperplastic changes in adjacent collecting tubules. Staining for high molecular weight cytokeratins and UEA-I lectin provides strong support for an origin in the collecting duct of the distal nephron. Some cytogenetic abnormalities have been identified, including loss of heterozygosity of 8p and 13q, which suggests that tumor suppressor genes on 8p and 13q may be involved in the pathogenesis of this variety of cancer (PEYROMAURE et al. 2002). The tumor can also have prominent papillary or sarcomatoid features, may contain mucin, and can resemble urothelial carcinoma with glandular differentiation or adenocarcinoma arising from the urothelium of the renal pelvis (GALLOB et al. 2001). The collecting duct is embryologically derived from the ureteric bud, which explains the urothelial features of some cases of CDC. The pathologic and immunohistochemical description as well as the cytogenetic abnormalities support the belief that CDC is more similar to urothelial carcinoma than to clear cell RCC (MILOWSKI et al. 2002).

Two other neoplasms considered to originate from the collecting ducts, renal medullary carcinoma (DAVIS et al. 1995) and low-grade CDC (MACLENNAN et al. 1997), have been described. Renal medullary carcinoma arises in young black patients with SCT, and has a reticular, yolk sac tumor-like, or adenoid cystic morphology. There is some overlap in histologic appearance between typical CDC and renal medullary carcinoma, with the latter seeming to form the aggressive end of the CDC spectrum (SRIGLEY and EBLE 1998). All patients with this tumor died of the disease; mean duration post-surgery was 15 months. Low-grade CDC presents a grossly solid or cystic, well-circumscribed, macroscopic appearance and is characterized by tubular formation of tumor cells with a hobnail cell appearance and low nuclear grade. This tumor seems to have a better prognosis than classic CDC (FUKUNAGA 1999). Collecting duct carcinoma appears to belong to a broad spectrum of distal CDC tumors with different morphologic traits and prognoses, which emphasizes the difficulty of diagnosing this condition.

11.3.1
Gross Morphology

Collecting duct carcinoma is usually located in the central region of the kidney and is poorly defined, with firm, gray-white, infiltrating tumors that develop from the medulla toward the cortex (Fig. 11.2). Of the tumors 87.5% are centered around the renal medulla and have irregular borders; however, not every renal tumor in the central location originates in the collecting ducts of the renal medulla (Fig. 11.3). The renal cortex was involved in 66.7% of the cases and the pelvocalyceal system in 44.4% of cases. Most common RCC is well delineated and centered on the cortex. Grossly, the tumor tends to be large at the time of diagnosis and may contain areas of necrosis. In large tumors, origin in the medulla is impossible to establish. In addition, although CDC demonstrates an infiltrative growth pattern initially, an expansile appearance may predominate as the tumor enlarges and extends beyond the renal capsule. The presence of a central, infiltrative component in such cases may be a useful finding. Collecting duct carcinoma ranges widely in size from 2.5 to 12 cm (mean 5 cm). Yellow areas of necrosis may be present. Some tumors have grown into the renal pelvis. Local extension may be grossly obvious with invasion of perirenal and renal sinus fat, and metastases to regional lymph nodes or the adrenal gland. Sometimes, gross renal

vein invasion may be seen (ANTONELLI et al. 2003; PICKHARDT 1999). The unaffected outer configuration of the kidney is explained by infiltrative interstitial, intratubular, and intravenous spreading (FUKUYA et al. 1996). A multicystic appearance secondary to dilated tubular structures is common.

11.3.2
Microscopic Findings

Typical CDC has a variety of growth patterns, including tubular (Fig. 11.4), papillary, tubulopapillary (Fig. 11.5), microcystic–papillary, pseudopapillary, cribriform, and solid patterns. Irregular angulated tubules infiltrate a desmoplastic stroma (Fig. 11.6). Microcystic change may be seen with the cysts irregular in contour and with small papillary infoldings (Fig. 11.7). RUMPELT et al. (1991) emphasized that the microcystic papillary pattern is diagnostically most important. The tubular architecture is markedly irregular, and anastomosing glands are often observed. Nuclear atypia are prominent, and significant atypical mitotic figures are also present. In addition to a desmoplastic stroma, there is commonly a brisk inflammatory infiltrate within and around the tumor. Extensive destruction of renal medullary and cortical tissue is often present. Marked vascular and lymphatic space invasion is common, and there is often permeation of hilar

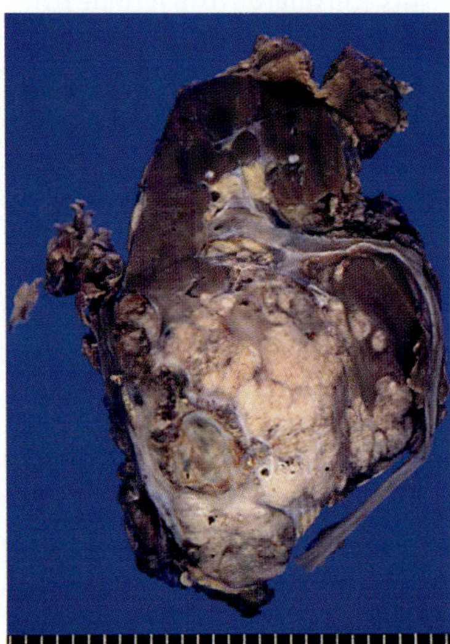

Fig. 11.2. Collecting duct carcinoma in a 45-year-old man. Gross specimen shows a poorly defined, grayish-white, multinodular protruding mass at the lower renal pole.

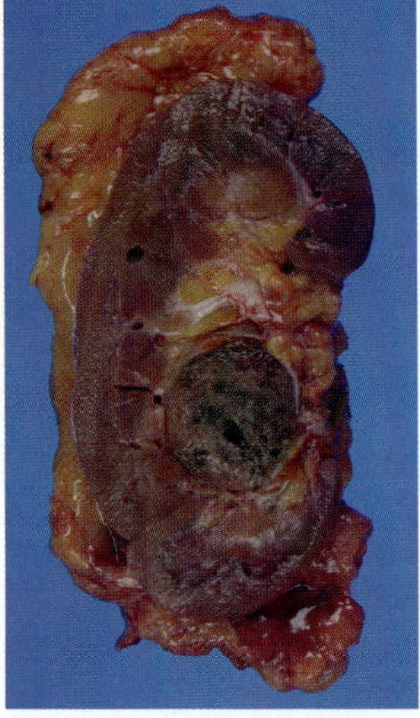

Fig. 11.3. Renal tumor in a central location in a 39-year-old woman. Gross specimen shows a well-marginated mass in the kidney. Chromophobe renal cell carcinoma was confirmed at histology. Central location does not always mean a collecting duct carcinoma.

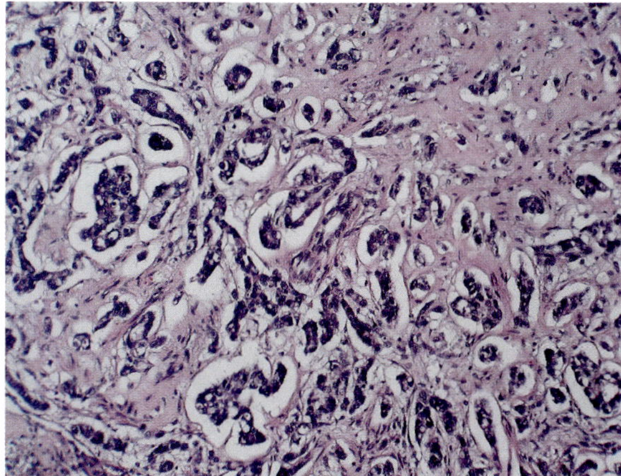

Fig. 11.4 Collecting duct carcinoma in a 45-year-old man. Photomicrograph shows a tubular growth pattern (hematoxylin and eosin stain; original magnification, ×200).

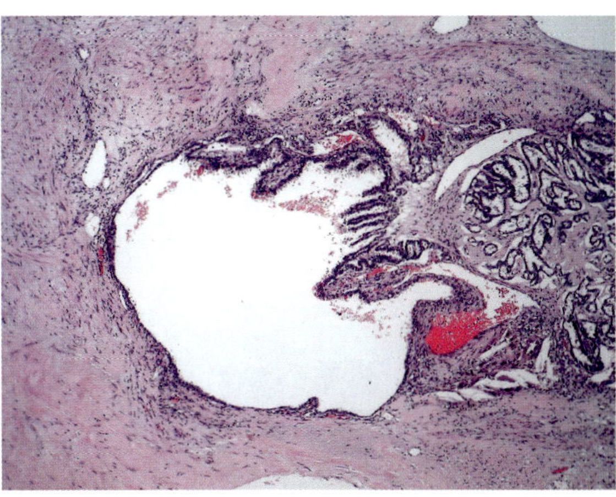

Fig. 11.5. Collecting duct carcinoma in a 45-year-old man. Photomicrograph shows tubulopapillary growth pattern (hematoxylin and eosin stain; original magnification, ×40).

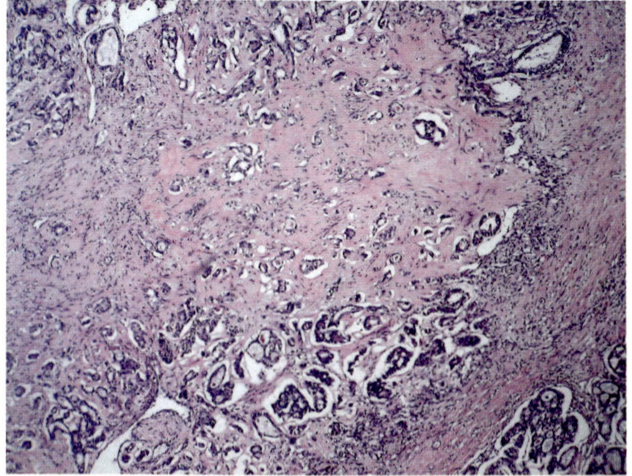

Fig. 11.6. Collecting duct carcinoma in a 45-year-old man. Photomicrograph shows an infiltrative growth with prominent desmoplastic reaction (hematoxylin and eosin stain; original magnification, ×100).

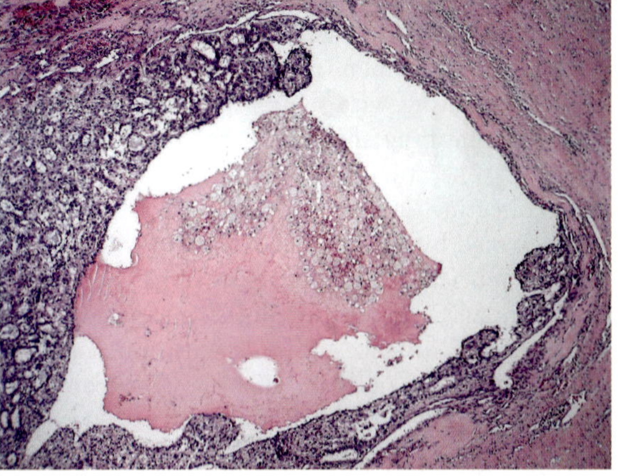

Fig. 11.7. Collecting duct carcinoma in a 45-year-old man. Photomicrograph of the collecting duct carcinoma depicts an intratumoral cystic area (hematoxylin and eosin stain; original magnification, ×40).

fat. The tumor biologic behavior is mostly aggressive with a high rate of local, lymphatic, and hematogenous spreading at diagnosis and a poor long-term prognosis. The tumor consists of an intermingling of clear, eosinophilic, or basophilic cells and polymorphic nuclei, often of hobnail appearance (Fig. 11.8); these are diagnostically helpful because hobnail cells are not seen in clear cell, papillary, or chromophobe RCC (SRIGLEY and EBLE 1998). Most CDCs have high-grade nuclear features. The plasma is lesser in amount and lacks the characteristic clear, granular and spindle cell types seen with RCC in which the nuclei are vesicular and firm and differentiation from metastatic lesions might be difficult, especially from ovarian and pancreatic origin tumors. The presence of dysplastic features

in the epithelium of collecting ducts near a tumor has been taken as evidence the tumor originated in the epithelium of the collecting ducts (Fig. 11.9; ANTONELLI et al. 2003; SINGH and NABI 2002). Collecting duct carcinoma with sarcomatoid transformation has been noted (AITA et al. 2003; KURODA et al. 2002).

11.3.3
Immunohistochemistry

Histopathologic differentiation of CDC from RCC is possible only by immunohistochemistry. In lectin histochemistry, *Ulex europaeus* agglutinin-I is commonly reactive. Peanut lectin is also often positive.

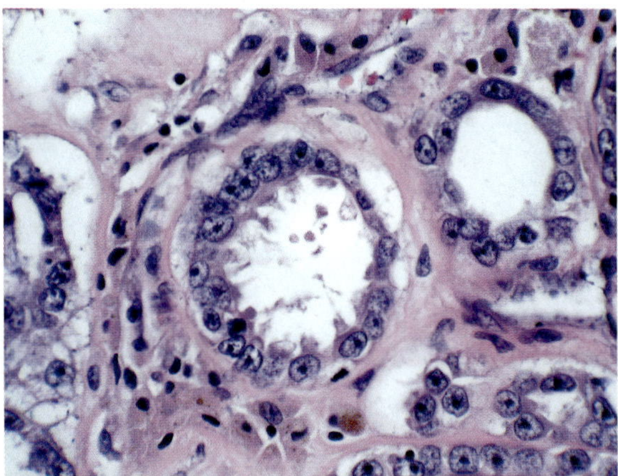

Fig. 11.8. Collecting duct carcinoma in a 62-year-old man. Photomicrograph reveals renal tubules lined by hobnail cells with high-grade nuclear atypism (hematoxylin and eosin stain; original magnification, ×400).

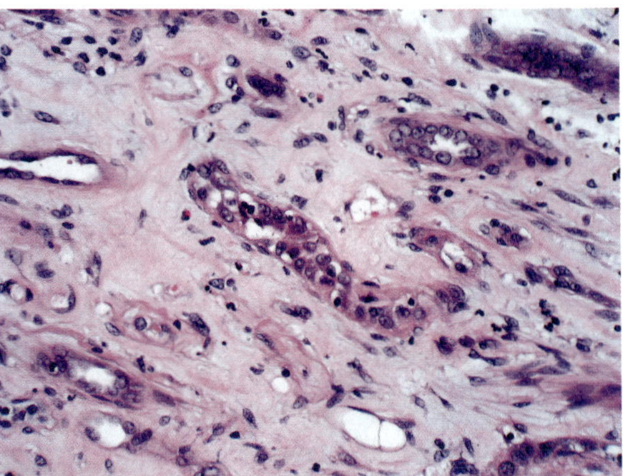

Fig. 11.9. Collecting duct carcinoma in a 62-year-old man. Photomicrograph shows a dysplastic epithelium of the collecting duct in the renal medulla (hematoxylin and eosin stain; original magnification, ×200).

High molecular weight keratin is commonly immunoreactive, and vimentin may also be reactive and negative staining with a proximal tubule marker (Leu-M1). Staining specifically for high molecular weight cytokeratins can provide further evidence for a collecting duct origin. The presence of mucin is confirmed by periodic acid–Schiff (PAS), Alcian blue, or mucicarmine staining in some cases. Such intracellular mucicarminophilic material is not seen with RCC; hence, staining with mucicarmine and PAS is useful in distinguishing CDC from RCC (Milowski et al. 2002; Singh and Nabi 2002).

11.3.4
Cytogenetics

Cytogenetically, CDC is characterized by a hypodiploid stem line, a high number of numerical and structural chromosome aberrations, and commonly, involvement of chromosome 1 and the autosomes (Antonelli et al. 2003).

11.3.5
Pathologic Criteria

Srigley and Eble (1998) described the typical CDC as a tubular or tubulopapillary tumor with desmoplastic stroma with inflammatory infiltrate and high nuclear grade. They proposed five major and four minor diagnostic criteria (Table 11.1).

Distinguishing CDC from papillary RCC is most important, because both tumors share some pathologic features, including a papillary architecture and positive reaction for distal nephron markers (Kuroda et al. 2002). Papillary RCC, medullary carcinoma, conventional RCC, transitional cell carcinoma, juxtaglomerular cell tumor, and metastatic carcinoma originating from other sites should be carefully considered and excluded when diagnosing CDC.

11.4
Radiologic Findings

Collecting duct carcinoma is usually centrally located and extensive with poorly defined borders. It frequently invades renal or hilar fat and vessels. These characteristics differ strongly from other types of RCC. For example, clear cell, chromophobe, and papillary carcinomas are usually located in the cortex and are well circumscribed with a distinctive cut surface appearance and color (Mejean et al. 2003). At diagnosis, CDC is frequently too large to allow a sharp definition of its location, but on image analysis, compared with RCC, it displays a very hypovascular and hypointense appearance.

Due to the rarity of CDC, radiographic findings have not been well established. Pickhardt et al. (2001) described the largest radiologic series in the literature. Imaging findings that support the diagnosis of CDC include a medullary location and an infiltrative appearance on CT, hyperechogenicity on ultrasound, hypointensity on T2-weighted MR images, distortion of the renal collecting system on urography, and hypovascularity on angiography. These tumors,

Table 11.1. Diagnostic criteria for collecting duct carcinoma

Major criteria	Minor criteria
Location in a medullary pyramid (small tumors)	Central location (large tumors)
Typical histology with irregular tubular architecture, desmoplasia, and high grade	Papillary architecture with wide, fibrous stalks, and desmoplastic stroma
Reactive with antibodies to high-molecular weight cytokeratin	Inflammatory stroma with numerous granulocytes
Reactive with *Ulex europaeus* lectin	Extensive renal, extrarenal, and vascular infiltration
Absence of urothelial carcinoma	

however, are often large at presentation and also have an expansile appearance and exophytic component that cannot be reliably distinguished from the more common cortical RCC. It cannot always be determined from radiologic images whether a renal tumor in a central location originated in the collecting ducts of the renal medulla.

Radionuclide studies seem to show uptake of Ga-67 in CDC, indicating that Ga-67 scintigraphy may be helpful for identifying this type of cancer preoperatively (PEYROMAURE et al. 2002).

11.4.1
Excretory Urography

Distortion of the intrarenal collecting system, with calyceal displacement and associated filling defects is observed. Medial displacement of the ureter can be seen. Focally prolonged cortical retention of contrast material may be seen on delayed film in the region that supports the medullary portion involved by tumor.

11.4.2
Ultrasound

Collecting duct carcinoma appears as a solid tumor with variable echogenicity compared with normal renal parenchyma, although most lesions are reported to be hyperechoic (Fig. 11.10). A hypoechoic rim is not identified at the tumor–parenchyma interface, indicating the absence of a pseudocapsule with this infiltrative neoplasm. Anechoic cystic areas are noted, representing either intratumoral cysts or cystic necrosis.

11.4.3
Computed Tomography

Collecting duct carcinoma generally shows a heterogeneous solid renal mass arising from the central kidney region with extension to the renal sinus. The

mean size of the tumors is 7.7 cm (range 1.5–19 cm). Most tumors exhibit involvement of the renal medulla (Fig. 11.11). Recognition of a medullary origin can be difficult in larger tumors. Replacement of the renal sinus fat or protrusion into the renal pelvis is present in many cases (Fig. 11.12). Occasionally, CDC reveals an exophytic appearance without involvement of the renal sinus (Fig. 11.13).

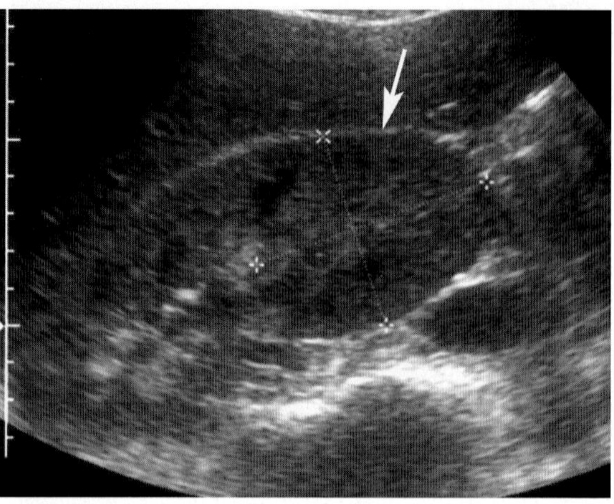

Fig. 11.10. Collecting duct carcinoma in a 45-year-old man. Longitudinal US image shows a poorly defined, hypoechoic mass (*arrow*) at the lower pole of the right kidney.

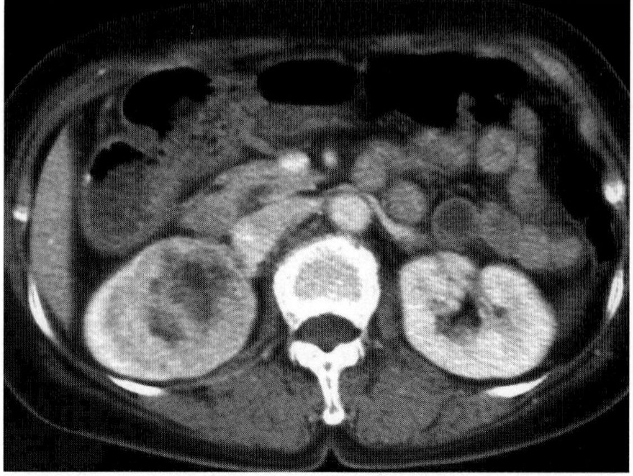

Fig. 11.11. Collecting duct carcinoma in a 55-year-old woman. Axial contrast-enhanced CT scan shows a poorly marginated enhancing mass in the renal medulla of the right kidney.

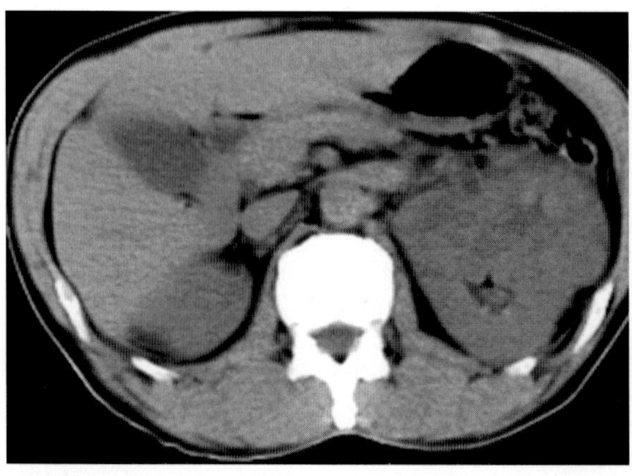 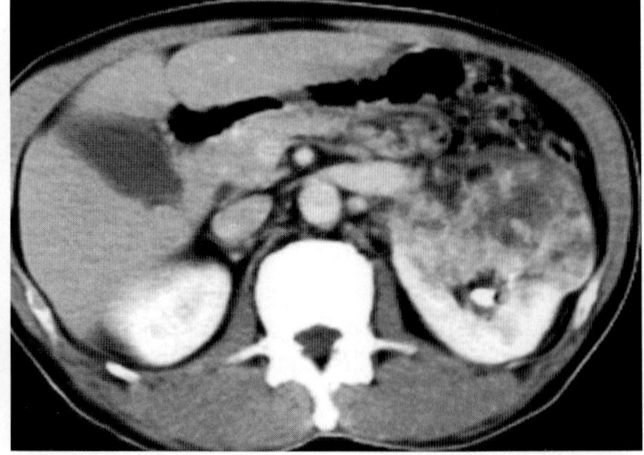

Fig. 11.12a,b. Collecting duct carcinoma in a 65-year-old man. **a** Axial unenhanced CT scan shows an ill-defined, inhomogeneous hypodense mass in the left kidney. **b** Axial contrast-enhanced CT scan shows a heterogeneous enhancing mass with protrusion into the left renal pelvis.

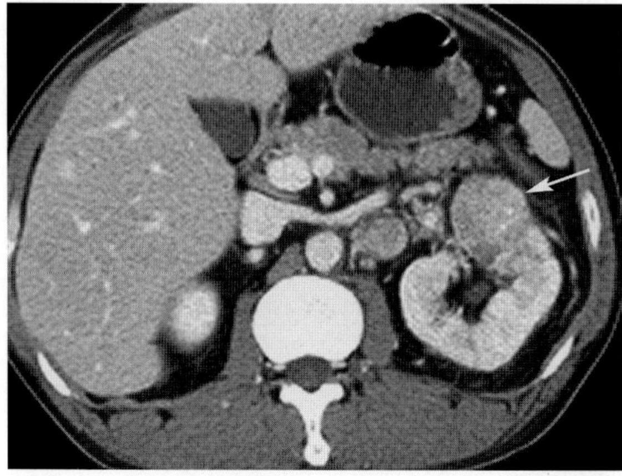 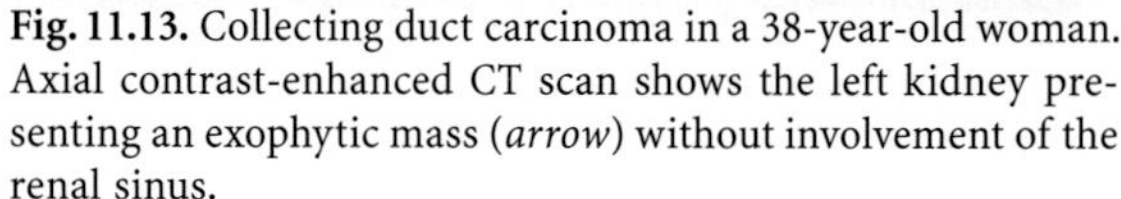 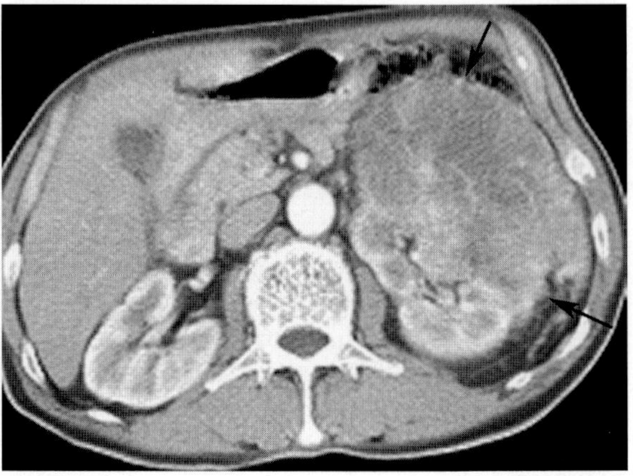

Fig. 11.13. Collecting duct carcinoma in a 38-year-old woman. Axial contrast-enhanced CT scan shows the left kidney presenting an exophytic mass (*arrow*) without involvement of the renal sinus.

Fig. 11.14. Collecting duct carcinoma in a 68-year-old man. Axial contrast-enhanced CT scan shows a cortical location and exophytic appearance of the left kidney mass (*arrows*).

In a few cases, however, the main location or center of the tumor is cortical or exophytic (Fig. 11.14).

Collecting duct carcinoma is classified into three types according to the predominate region of involvement and the pattern of the tumor growth: medullary location only; medullary location with cortical extension; and medullary location with renal sinus extension (Fig. 11.15). Smaller tumors are usually medullary only; however, in larger tumors, CDC is likely to extend into the renal cortex or renal sinus. The origin and growth patterns of CDC could explain CT findings that distinguish it from ordinary RCC, 94% of which show predominantly exophytic growth with distortion of the renal contour regardless of the size of the tumor (Fukuya et al. 1996).

Tumor margins are poorly circumscribed in most cases. An irregular, serrated tumor margin along the interface with the medullary portion of the kidney suggests infiltrative growth (Fig. 11.16). Sometimes, the tumor has several satellite cortical nodules (Mejean et al. 2003). Infiltrative growth is a much less common pattern in which tumor cells spread using the normal architecture as scaffolding for interstitial growth. In addition to infiltrative growth, expansile growth can be seen (Fig. 11.17). Most renal tumors other than CDC grow by radial expansion with displacement of the normal parenchyma, focal bulging of the renal contour, and pseudocapsule formation (Pickhardt et al. 2001). In many cases, the affected kidneys maintain a normal outer contour (Fig. 11.18). As the size of the tumor increases, an exophytic appearance may be seen (Fig. 11.19). Unlike the more common conventional RCC, contrast-enhanced CT scans of the CDC usually demonstrate a heterogeneous mass with min-

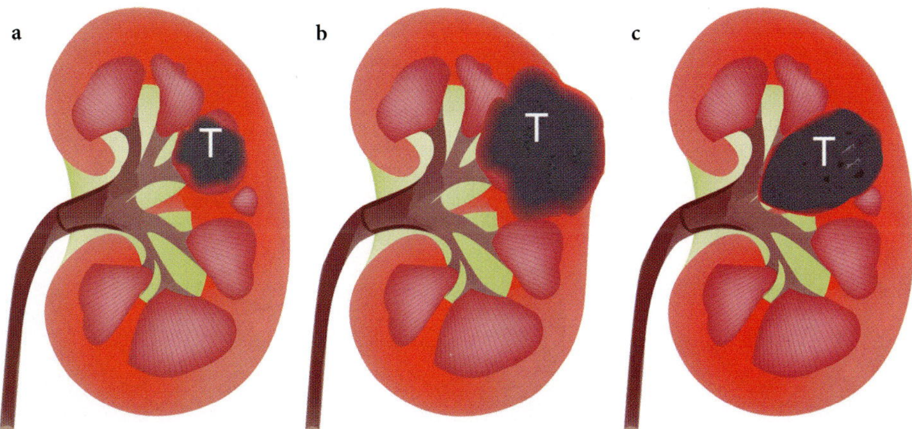

Fig. 11.15a-c. Collecting duct carcinomas are classified into three types according to the main location and the pattern of tumor growth (*T* tumor). **a** Medullary involvement only. **b** Medullary involvement with cortical extension. **c** Medullary involvement with renal sinus extension.

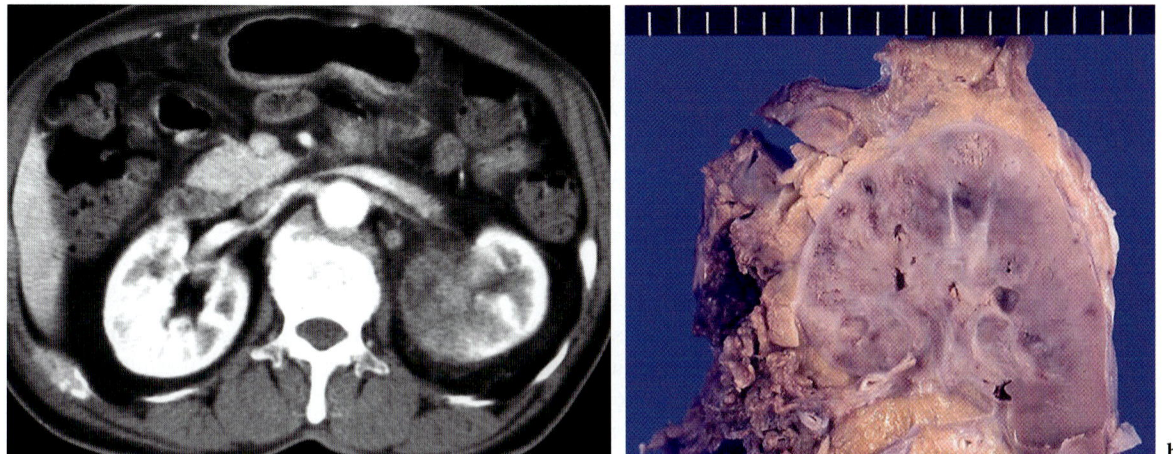

Fig. 11.16a,b. Collecting duct carcinoma in a 62-year-old man. **a** Axial contrast-enhanced CT scan shows left kidney ill-defined tumor with infiltrative growth pattern. **b** Gross specimen shows an infiltrative growth with poor demarcation in the renal medulla.

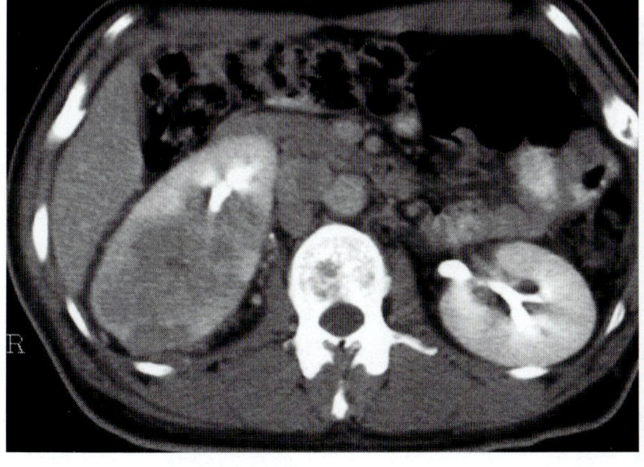

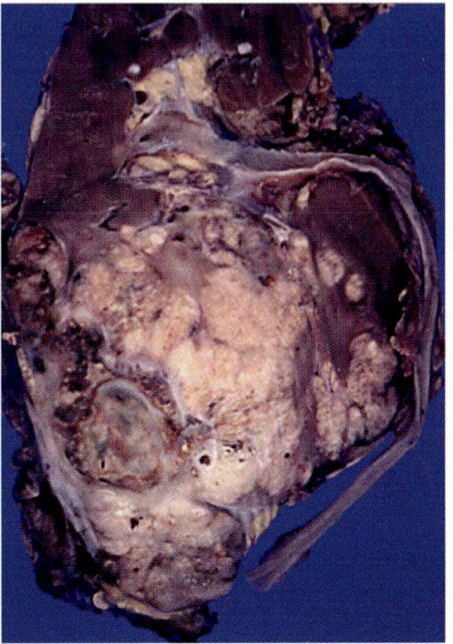

Fig. 11.17a,b. Collecting duct carcinoma in a 45-year-old man. **a** Axial contrast-enhanced CT scan shows an expansile growth in the right kidney with bulging tumor margins. **b** Gross specimen shows an ill-defined protruding mass at the lower pole.

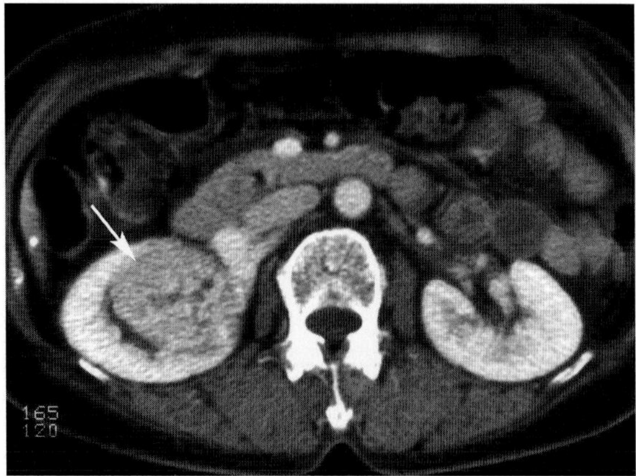

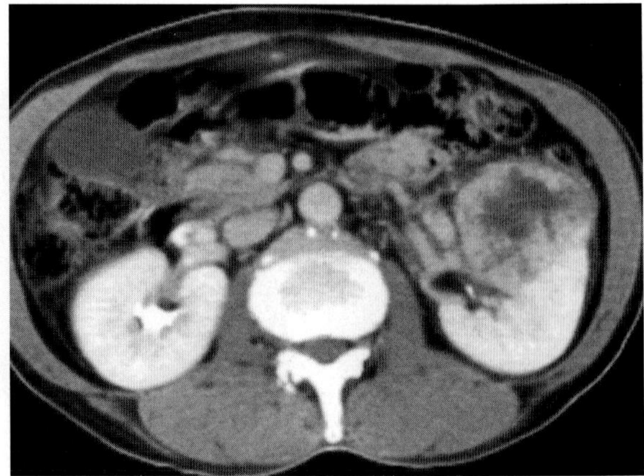

Fig. 11.18. Collecting duct carcinoma in a 62-year-old woman. Axial contrast-enhanced CT scan reveals a heterogeneous mass in the right kidney (*arrow*) with preservation of the renal outer contour.

Fig. 11.19. Collecting duct carcinoma in a 65-year-old man. Axial contrast-enhanced CT scan shows the left kidney tumor appears exophytic as collecting duct carcinoma enlarges.

imal or moderate enhancement (Figs. 11.20, 11.21). Gross extension to perinephric fat and vascular invasion are sometimes present (Fig. 11.22). Calcification is rare, unlike in conventional RCC (Fig. 11.23). A cystic component that resembles the more conventional cortical RCC, suggesting either intratumoral cyst or cystic necrosis, is frequently noted within the tumors (Fig. 11.24).

Many patients with CDC already have invasion into other sites, lymphadenopathy, or metastasis, when diagnosis is established. About 35-40% of patients have metastases at presentation. Regional lymph nodes (60–80%) (Fig. 11.25), lung (Fig. 11.26) or adrenal glands (25%), bone, and liver are common metastatic sites. Lymph node metastasis and inferior vena caval thrombosis are also present. Metastases to bone appear osteolytic or osteoblastic appearance (Fig. 11.27; KURODA et al. 2002).

In summary, medullary location, involvement of the renal sinus, infiltrative growth, preservation of renal contour, and weak enhancement are CT findings most commonly seen in patients with CDC of the kidney.

11.4.4
Magnetic Resonance Imaging

Collecting duct carcinoma appears isointense to normal renal parenchyma on T1-weighted spin-echo images and hypointense to normal renal parenchyma on T2-weighted spin-echo images. As with CT, weak enhancement is noted on contrast-enhanced T1-weighted image (Fig. 11.28). The lack of a visible marginal hypointense rim indicates that there is no pseudocapsule. In general, RCC appears

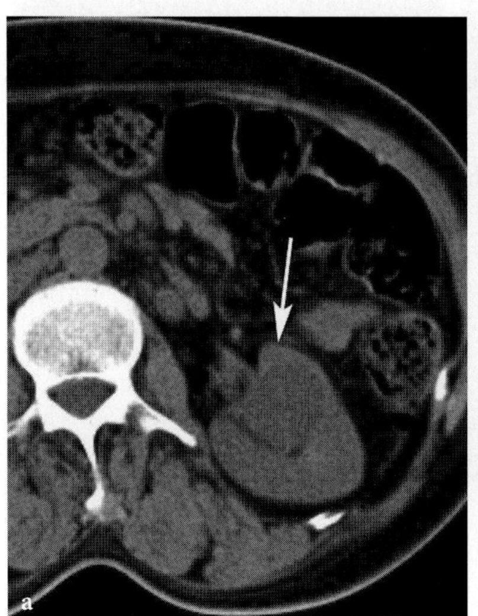

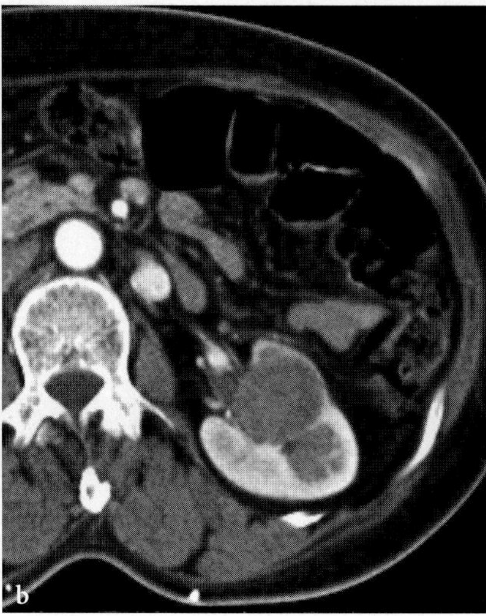

Fig. 11.20a,b. Collecting duct carcinoma in a 49-year-old man. **a** Axial unenhanced CT scan shows a hypodense mass (*arrow*) at the left renal medulla. **b** Axial contrast-enhanced CT scan shows minimal enhancement of the tumor.

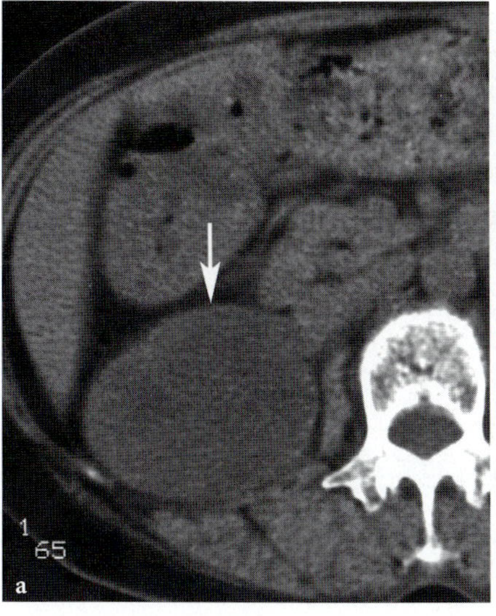
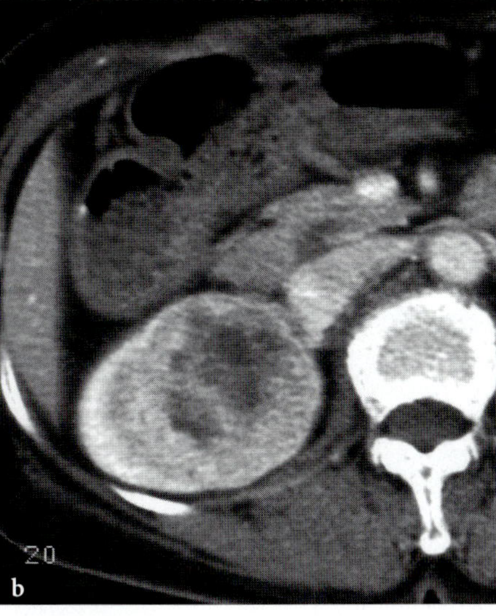

Fig. 11.21a,b. Collecting duct carcinoma in a 64-year-old woman. **a** Axial unenhanced CT scan shows a hypodense mass (*arrow*) with preservation of the right renal contour. **b** Axial contrast-enhanced CT scan shows moderate, heterogeneous enhancement of the tumor.

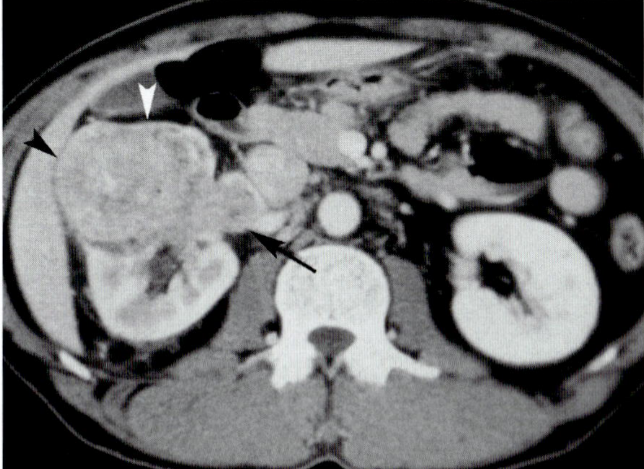
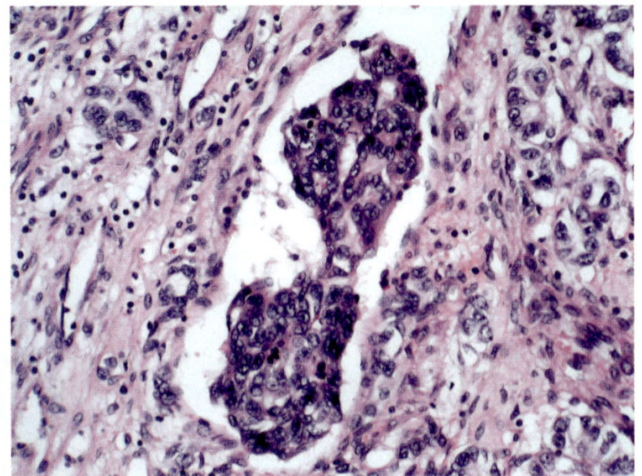

Fig. 11.22a,b. Collecting duct carcinoma in a 55-year-old man. **a** Axial contrast-enhanced CT scan shows an anterior exophytic mass in the right kidney (*arrowheads*) and hypodense thrombus (*arrow*) in the right renal vein. **b** Photomicrograph demonstrates tumor emboli and vascular invasion (hematoxylin and eosin stain; original magnification, ×200).

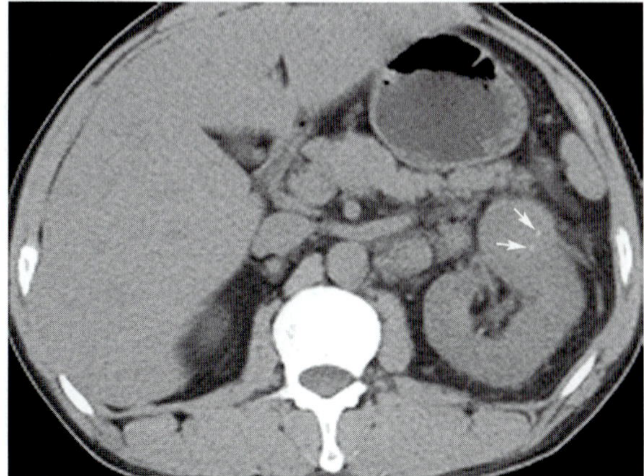

Fig. 11.23. Collecting duct carcinoma in a 38-year-old woman. Axial unenhanced CT scan reveals multiple tiny calcifications (*arrows*) within the exophytic tumor in the left kidney.

slightly hypointense to normal renal parenchyma on T1-weighted images and slightly hyperintense on T2-weighted images. Hypointensity on T2-weighted images appears to favor CDC, especially with a centrally located tumor (PICKHARDT et al. 2001).

11.4.5
Angiography

Selective renal angiography shows the tumors to be hypovascular compared with normal renal parenchyma; however, with CT it remains difficult to differentiate CDC from other infiltrating tumors of the kidney such as lymphoma, metastasis, sarcomatoid carcinoma, and calyceal urothelial tumors with renal spread, and from xanthogranulomatous pyelo-

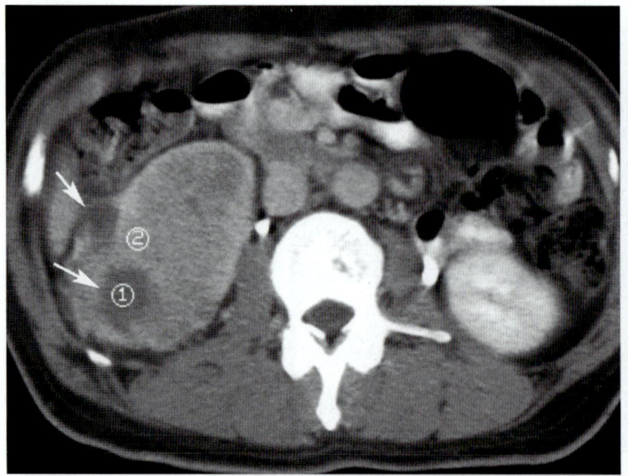
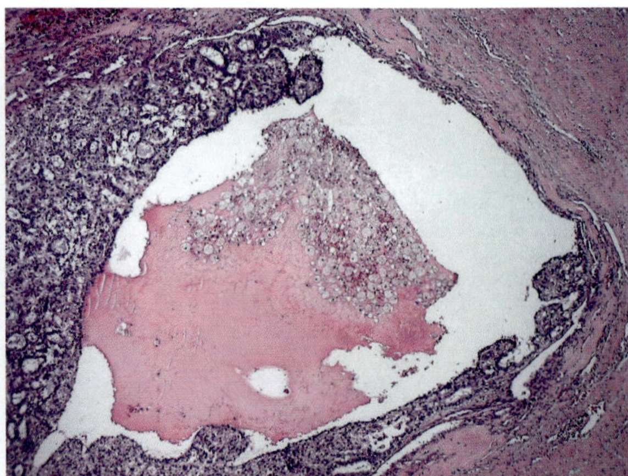

a   b

Fig. 11.24a,b. Collecting duct carcinoma in a 45-year-old man. **a** Axial contrast-enhanced CT scan shows multiple cystic lesions (*arrows*) within the poorly defined tumor in the right kidney. **b** Photomicrograph depicts an intratumoral cystic area (hematoxylin and eosin stain; original magnification, ×40).

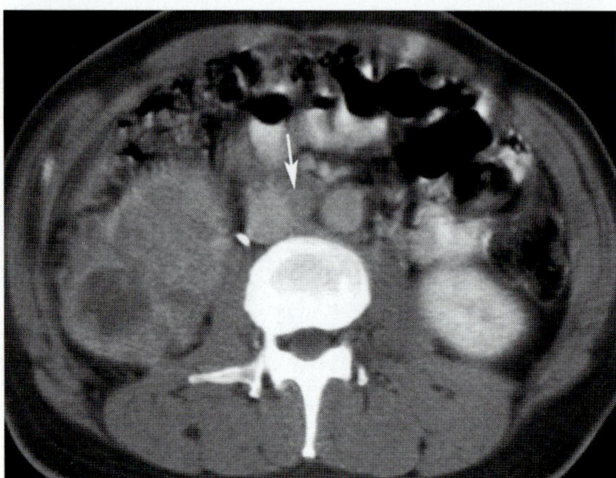

Fig. 11.25. Collecting duct carcinoma in a 45-year-old man. Axial contrast-enhanced CT scan shows a heterogeneous mass in the right kidney and mildly enhancing interaorticocaval lymphadenopathy (*arrow*).

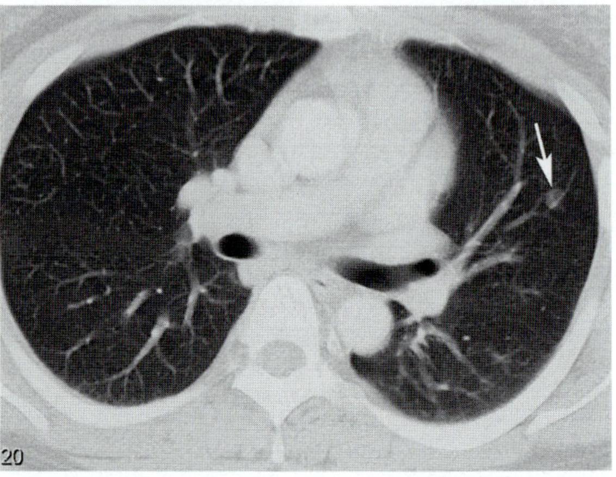

Fig. 11.26. Collecting duct carcinoma in a 55-year-old woman. Axial chest CT scan at lung window shows a small hematogenous metastatic left pulmonary nodule (*arrow*).

nephritis. A single infiltrating renal tumor should suggest the diagnosis of CDC (Mejean et al. 2003).

11.4.6
Differential Diagnosis

Differential diagnoses for centrally located renal lesions with infiltrative features include invasive transitional cell or squamous cell carcinoma of the renal collecting system, renal lymphoma, renal metastases, invasive RCC involving the columns of Bertin, mesoblastic nephroma, renal medullary carcinoma, and bacterial pyelonephritis (Pickhardt 1999). Although only about 6% of cortical RCC is truly infiltrative, RCC nonetheless represents a sig-

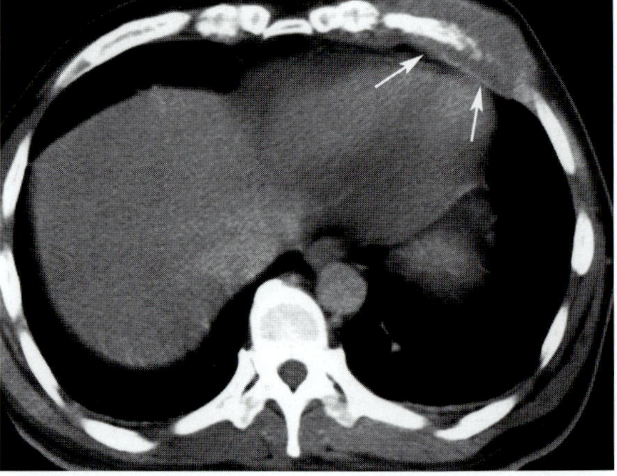

Fig. 11.27. Collecting duct carcinoma in a 45-year-old man. Axial CT scan shows rib destruction with metastatic soft tissue mass (*arrows*).

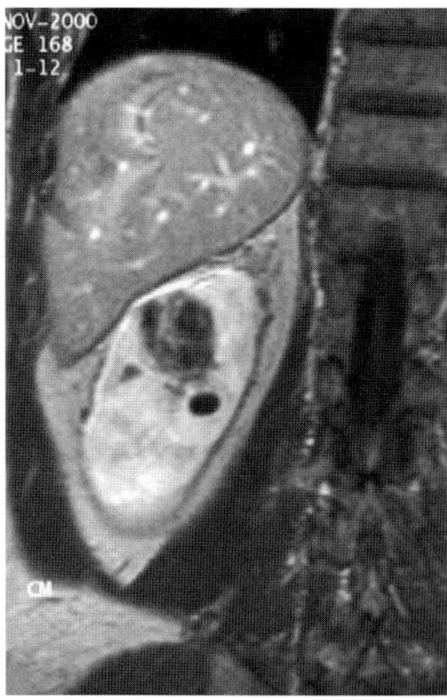

Fig. 11.28. Collecting duct carcinoma in a 69-year-old man. Coronal contrast-enhanced T1-weighted MR image reveals a poorly enhancing tumor with internal enhancing areas in the right kidney.

nificant proportion of infiltrative tumors given its overall abundance. Distinguishing between cortical RCC and collecting duct carcinoma on preoperative imaging studies has prognostic significance.

It is important to keep in mind that a central location in the kidney does not mean that a tumor originates in the collecting ducts of the renal medulla.

11.5
Treatment

The standard treatment for CDC of the kidney is radical nephrectomy; however, it is not clear if such a radical operation is needed for small CDC (Matsumoto et al. 2001). Collecting duct carcinoma shows aggressive behavior and advanced stage at the time of presentation, causing death in two-thirds of the patients within 2 years of surgery, so that a systemic multidrug therapy is necessary in the majority of patients (Sironi et al. 2003).

11.6
Prognosis

The overall prognosis of CDC is generally poor. About two-thirds of patients with CDC die of carcinoma

within 2 years of diagnosis. Many patients with CDC already have invasion into other sites or metastases when the diagnosis is established. Approximately 35–40% of patients have metastases at presentation. Common metastatic sites include regional lymph nodes, adrenal glands, bone, lung, and liver. Lymph node metastasis and inferior vena caval thrombosis are also known to occur, as in RCC. Metastases to bone often appear osteoblastic radiographically. The rapid metastatic spread and aggressiveness of CDC may be due to its central or perihilar location (Kuroda et al. 2002; Singh and Nabi 2002).

Patients usually present at an advanced clinical stage and have a poor prognosis. There is no standard treatment regimen for patients who present with metastatic disease (Kirkali et al. 1996). Treatment for CDC based on surgical excision alone does not appear to improve the prognosis and can be a source of perioperative and early postoperative complications, which are rare in the context of RCC (Mejean et al. 2003). Patients treated with radical nephrectomy, radiation, chemotherapy, or immunotherapy have shown mixed results, but the number of patients is too small to draw any useful conclusion and the prognosis is generally worse than with other types of RCC (Kuroda et al. 2002). Close follow-up is recommended regardless of the stage; however, McLennan et al. (1997) have described a series of unusual low-grade tubulocystic renal cancers with a good prognosis (Fig. 11.29).

11.7
Conclusion

Collecting duct carcinoma is an aggressive subtype of RCC derived from the renal medulla. The tumor occurs in a wide age range, predominately in men. The usual histologic pattern is that of a tubular or tubulopapillary carcinoma with a desmoplastic stroma. Imaging features suggestive of this diagnosis include a medullary origin and an infiltrative growth pattern. This type of cancer is associated with an extremely poor prognosis. At presentation CDC is metastatic to regional lymph nodes. The characteristic location, typical histologic and radiologic appearance, and reportedly poor prognosis differentiate CDC from the more common RCC. Death usually occurs within 2 years. Various treatments have been proposed but with disappointing results, including radiation therapy, immunotherapy and some combinations of chemotherapy.

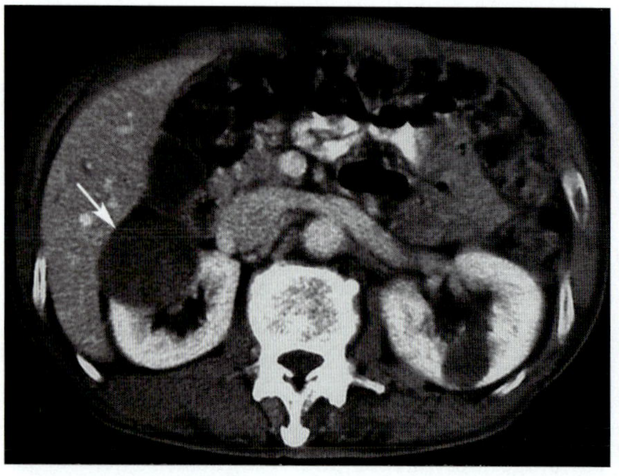
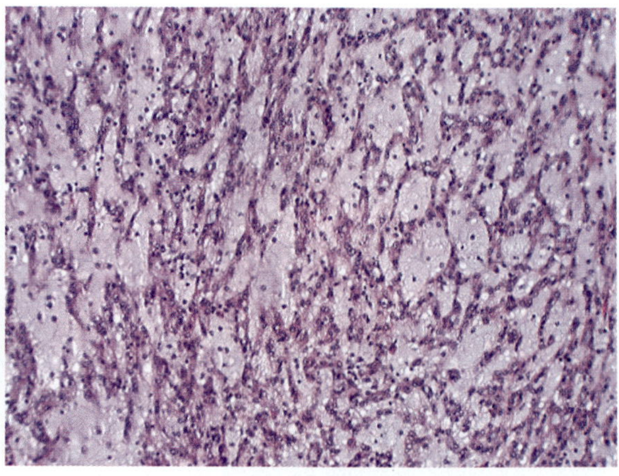

Fig. 11.29a,b. Collecting duct carcinoma in a 60-year-old man. **a** Axial contrast-enhanced CT scan shows a hypodense tumor with poor enhancement in the right kidney. **b** Photomicrograph shows mucin-containing tumor cells with tubulopapillary growth (hematoxylin and eosin stain; original magnification, ×100). Low-grade, tubular, mucinous renal carcinoma of possible collecting duct origin was confirmed by radical nephrectomy.

References

Aita K, Tanimoto A, Fujimoto Y et al. (2003) Sarcomatoid collecting duct carcinoma arising in the hemodialysis-associated acquired cystic kidney: an autopsy report. Pathol Int 53:463–467

Antonelli A, Portesi E, Cozzoli A et al. (2003) The collecting duct carcinoma of the kidney: a cytogenetical study. Eur Urol 43:680–685

Auguet T, Molina JC, Lorenzo A et al. (2000) Synchronus renal cell carcinoma and Bellini duct carcinoma: a case report on a rare coincidence. World J Urol 18:449–451

Bostwick DG, Eble JN (1999) Diagnosis and classification of renal cell carcinoma. Urol Clin North Am 26:627–635

Cromie WJ, Davis CJ, DeTure FA (1979) Atypical carcinoma of kidney: possibly originating from collecting duct epithelium. Urology 13:315–317

Davis CJ, Mostofi FK, Sesterhenn IA (1995) Renal medullary carcinoma: the seventh sickle cell nephropathy. Am J Surg Pathol 19:1–11

Fleming S, Lewi HJ (1986) Collecting duct carcinoma of the kidney. Histopathology 10:1131–1141

Fukunaga M (1999) Sarcomatoid collecting duct carcinoma. Arch Pathol Lab Med 123:338–341

Fukuya T, Honda H, Goto K et al. (1996) Computed tomographic findings of Bellini duct carcinoma of the kidney. J Comput Assist Tomogr 20:399–403

Gallob JA, Upton MP, DeWolf WC et al. (2001) Long-term remission in a patient with metastatic collecting duct carcinoma treated with taxol/carboplatin and surgery. Urology 58:1058i–1058iii

Gong Y, Sun X, Haines GK et al. (2003) Renal cell carcinoma, chromophobe type, with collecting duct carcinoma and sarcomatoid components. Arch Pathol Lab Med 27:e38–e40

Kirkali Z, Celebi I, Akan G et al. (1996) Bellini duct (collecting duct) carcinoma of the kidney. Urology 47:921–923

Kuroda N, Toi M, Hirol M et al. (2002) Review of collecting duct carcinoma with focus on clinical and pathobiological aspects. Histol Histopathol 17:1329–1334

Levine E, King BF (2000) Adult malignant renal parenchymal neoplasms. In: Pollack HM, McClennan BL (eds) Clinical urology. Saunders, Philadelphia, pp 1440–1559

MacLennan GT, Farrow GM, Bostowick DG (1997) Low-grade collecting duct carcinoma of the kidney: report of 13 cases of low-grade mucinous tubulocystic renal carcinoma of possible collecting duct origin. Urology 50:679–684

Mancilla-Jimenez R, Stanley RJ, Blath RA (1976) Papillary renal cell carcinoma: a clinical, radiologic, and pathologic study of 34 cases. Cancer 38:2469–2480

Matsumoto H, Wada T, Aoki A et al. (2001) Collecting duct carcinoma with long survival treated by partial nephrectomy. Int J Urol 8:401–403

Mejean A, Roupret M, Larousserie F et al. (2003) Is there a place for radical nephrectomy in the presence of metastatic collecting duct (Bellini) carcinoma? J Urol 169:1287–1290

Milowski MI, Rosmarin A, Tickoo SK et al. (2002) Active chemotherapy for collecting duct carcinoma of the kidney. A case report and review of the literature. Cancer 94:111–116

Natsume O, Seiichiro O, Futami T et al. (1997) Bellini duct carcinoma: a case report. Jpn J Clin Oncol 27:107–110

Nguyen GK, Schumann GB (1997) Cytopathology of renal collecting duct in urine sediment. Diagn Cytopathol 16:446–449

Peyromaure M, Thiounn N, Scotte F et al. (2002) Collecting duct carcinomas of the kidney: a clinicopathological study of 9 cases. J Urol 170:1138–1140

Pickhardt PJ (1999) Collecting duct carcinoma arising in a solitary kidney: imaging findings. Clin Imaging 23:115–118

Pickhardt PJ, Siegel CL, McLarney JK (2001) Collecting duct carcinoma of the kidney: Are imaging findings suggestive of the diagnosis? Am J Roentgenol 176:627–633

Rumpelt HJ, Störkel S, Moll R et al. (1991) Bellini duct carcinoma: further evidence for this rare variant of renal cell carcinoma. Histopathology 18:115–122

Singh I, Nabi G (2002) Bellini duct carcinoma: review of diagnosis and management. Int Urol Nephrol 34:91–95

Sironi M, Delpiano C, Claren R et al. (2003) New cytological findings on fine-needle aspiration on renal collecting duct carcinoma. Diagn Cytopathol 29:239–240

Srigley JR, Eble JN (1998) Collecting duct carcinoma of kidney. Semin Diagn Pathol 15:54–67

Thoenes W, Störkel S, Rumpelt HJ (1986) Histopathology and classification of renal cell tumors (adenomas, oncocytomas and carcinomas). The basic cytological and histopathological elements and their use for diagnostics. Pathol Res Pract 181:125–143

12 Renal Sinus Neoplasms

Sung Eun Rha and Jae Young Byun

CONTENTS

12.1
Introduction

The renal sinus is the medial compartment of the kidney that surrounds the kidney's pelvocalyceal system and communicates with the perinephric space (Figs. 12.1, 12.2). The major branches of the renal artery and vein along with the major and minor calyces of the collecting system are located within the renal sinus. The remainder of the sinus is filled with adipose tissue, lymphatic channels, nerve fibers of the autonomic nervous system, and varying quantities of fibrous tissue (Amis 2000; Amis and Cronan 1988; Davidson et al. 1999; Zagoria and Tung 1997b). Of these constituents, fat is the largest single component of the renal sinus and is readily seen with ultrasound (US), computed tomography (CT), and magnetic resonance (MR) imaging. The quantity of fat in the renal sinus normally and gradually increases with age and obesity (Fig. 12.3; Zagoria and Tung 1997b). Observation of renal sinus fat is important for detecting small tumors in that area, as well as for determining the exact tumor staging.

Renal sinus involvement of tumors is significant because the renal sinus contains numerous lymphatics and veins that may permit dissemination of a tumor otherwise regarded as renal limited. Because there is no fibrous capsule separating the renal cortex of the columns of Bertin from the renal sinus fat, a renal tumor may continue unrestricted into the sinus fat, which is rich in veins and lymphatics (Bonsib et al. 2000). Although renal sinus involvement is not currently used in either the Robson or TNM staging systems, the centrally located renal

S. E. Rha, MD
Assistant Professor, Department of Radiology, Kangnam St. Mary's Hospital, College of Medicine, The Catholic University of Korea, 505 Banpo-Dong, Seocho-Ku, Seoul 137-040, South Korea
J. Y. Byun, MD
Professor and Chairman, Department of Radiology, Kangnam St. Mary's Hospital, College of Medicine, The Catholic University of Korea, 505 Banpo-Dong, Seocho-Ku, Seoul 137-040, South Korea

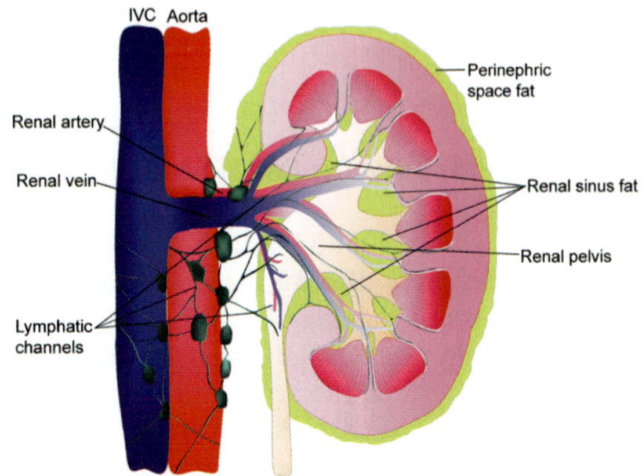

Fig. 12.1. Diagrammatic illustration shows the normal anatomy and major constituents of the renal sinus. Note that fat is the largest component of the renal sinus. (With permission from Rha et al. 2004)

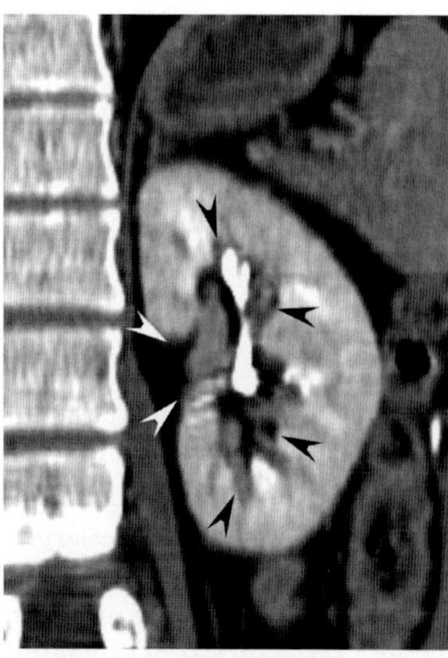

Fig. 12.2. Normal CT anatomy of the renal sinus in a 57-year-old man. Coronal contrast-enhanced CT scan obtained during the excretory phase clearly shows the extent of the renal sinus (*arrowheads*). (With permission from RHA et al. 2004)

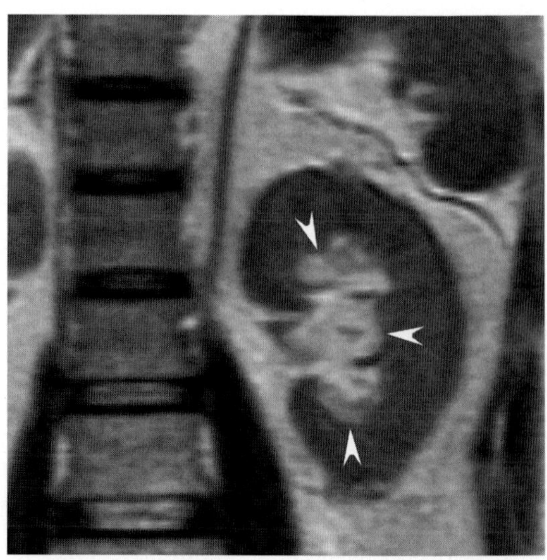

Fig. 12.3. Magnetic resonance imaging anatomy of renal sinus in a 73-year-old man with renal sinus lipomatosis. Coronal turbo spin-echo T2-weighted MR image (TR=6500 ms, TE=120 ms) shows prominent fat in the left renal sinus (*arrowheads*).

tumors in the renal sinus may affect surgical planning and prognosis of the renal tumors.

A broad spectrum of benign and malignant neoplasms exist involving the renal sinus, either arising primarily from sinus structures or secondarily extending into the sinus from the adjacent cortex or retroperitoneum. Tumors involving the renal sinus can be classified depending on their origins into four subgroups: (a) epithelial tumors of the renal pelvis; (b) mesenchymal tumors of the renal sinus; (c) renal parenchymal tumors projecting into the renal sinus; and (d) retroperitoneal tumors extending to the renal sinus.

12.2
Imaging Modalities for Renal Sinus Tumors

Various imaging modalities can be used for the evaluation of tumors affecting the renal sinus; these include excretory urography, US, CT, MR imaging, and angiography. Each modality can provide useful information regarding the detection, characterization, and extent of tumors.

Excretory urography is useful for evaluating the involvement of the renal collecting system. Most neoplastic conditions of the renal sinus are focal and are termed parapelvic (the prefix "para" means "alongside" or "beside"). These abnormalities cause focal displacement and compression of the pelvocalyceal system on excretory urography and a circumscribed mass on cross-sectional images. Irregular pelvocalyceal deformity suggests direct invasion by malignant tumors or unusual inflammatory conditions. A very large tumor displaces the kidney laterally and may cause anterior rotation. Conversely, disorders that diffusely surround the pelvocalyceal system are termed peripelvic (the prefix "peri" means "around"). The representative peripelvic neoplastic condition is renal lymphoma infiltrating the renal sinus, which causes generalized effacement and stretching of the pelvocalyceal system on excretory urography, mimicking renal sinus lipomatosis or renal sinus cyst (DAVIDSON et al. 1999).

Ultrasound functions as the initial screening modality for noninvasive imaging of the kidney and is useful in distinguishing cystic from solid space-occupying tumors when excretory urography detects the lesions. Normal renal sinus is imaged as an area of increased echo with variable contours due to the fat–parenchyma interface (Fig. 12.4). A collapsed renal pelvis may be indistinguishable from echogenic renal sinus fat. Despite good results with US, there are limitations, especially with small lesions when the renal sinus lesion is poorly defined or the echo pattern is similar to or the same as the adjacent renal sinus fat or adjacent renal parenchyma (ROSENFIELD et al. 1979).

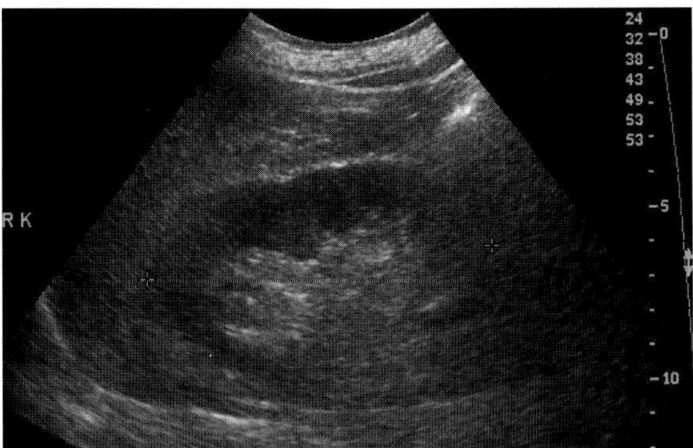

Fig. 12.4. Normal US anatomy of the renal sinus in a 73-year-old man with renal sinus lipomatosis. Longitudinal US image of right kidney shows prominent renal sinus as a central hyperechoic area with variable contours due to the fat–parenchyma interface.

Computed tomography is the most sensitive, efficient, and comprehensive imaging modality for evaluating the kidneys and is the problem-solving technique for a wide variety of renal sinus tumors. The recent development of multidetector CT provides dramatically increased speed of scan acquisition and improved spatial resolution through the use of thinner collimation. Multiplanar reconstruction images can allow exact determination of the extent of complex renal sinus tumors (Jeffrey 2004). In general, the coronal plane is the most useful for the evaluation of renal sinus lesions because it provides a comprehensive view of the kidney including the renal sinus (Pozzi-Mucelli et al. 2004).

Magnetic resonance imaging is an alternative to CT for the evaluation of renal sinus tumors as it allows detailed tissue characterization of complicated renal sinus tumors and direct multiplanar images with the same image resolution in the coronal, sagittal, and axial planes, and it can also be used in patients with renal failure or contrast material allergies (Pozzi-Mucelli et al. 2004).

12.3
Epithelial Tumors of the Renal Pelvis

Malignant tumors arising from the urothelium of the renal pelvis constitute only 5% of urinary tract neoplasms. Approximately 90% of pelvocalyceal cancers are transitional cell carcinomas and the remaining 10% are squamous cell carcinomas. These tumors are centered in the renal pelvis and

secondarily invade the renal sinus fat and renal parenchyma (Pickhardt et al. 2000).

12.3.1
Transitional Cell Carcinoma

Transitional cell carcinoma of the renal pelvis is epidemiologically similar to that of the bladder: there is male predominance; typical patient age at diagnosis is the sixth or seventh decade of life; and tobacco and industrial carcinogens are risk factors (McLaughlin et al. 1983). Hematuria is the principal symptom and multifocality is a significant problem for patients with transitional cell carcinomas in the upper urinary tract. Nearly 50% of patients have a history of urothelial carcinoma of the bladder or ureters or later develop urothelial carcinoma.

Depending on the gross morphologic features, transitional cell carcinomas are classified into papillary, infiltrating, and mixed papillary and infiltrating. Eighty-five percent of renal pelvis transitional cell carcinomas are papillary. Papillary transitional cell carcinomas are characterized by their frondlike morphologic structure, with the fronds lined by a thick layer of transitional epithelium. Infiltrating tumors are characterized by thickening and induration of the renal pelvic wall. If the renal pelvis is involved, there is often invasion into the renal parenchyma (Wong-You-Cheong et al. 1998). Pathologically, stage I transitional cell carcinomas of the renal pelvis are limited to the uroepithelium and lamina propria mucosae. Stage II tumors invade to, but not beyond, the muscularis. Stage III tumors infiltrate into the renal parenchyma or the peripelvic fat. Stage IV tumor is defined by local extrarenal extension, lymph node involvement, or distant metastasis (Wong-You-Cheong et al. 1998).

On excretory urography, transitional cell carcinomas of the renal pelvis may show imaging findings such as intraluminal filling defects due to tumor or blood, amputated calyces resulting from malignant stricture, hydronephrosis caused by tumor obstruction of the ureteropelvic junction, or nonfunctioning kidney. Ultrasound shows a poorly defined soft tissue mass replacing the renal sinus fat (Fig. 12.5; Wong-You-Cheong et al. 1998).

Typical CT findings include a sessile or flat solid mass in the renal calyces and/or pelvis, or focal renal pelvic wall thickening or infiltrating mass (Baron et al. 1982). Obstruction occurs earlier or later in the natural history of a given tumor

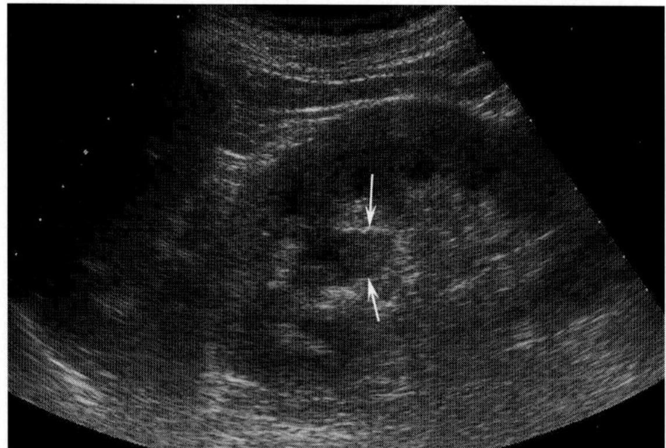

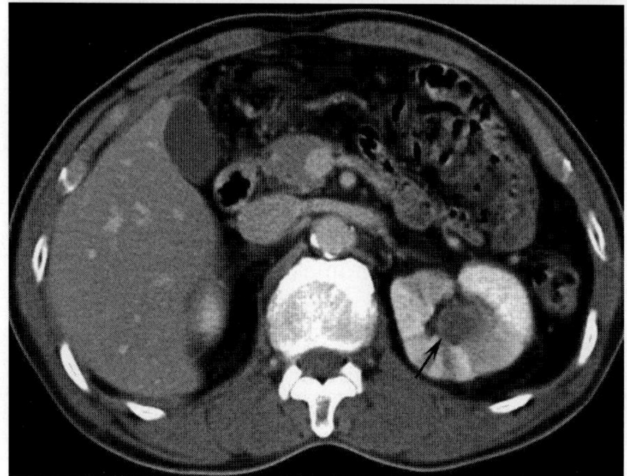

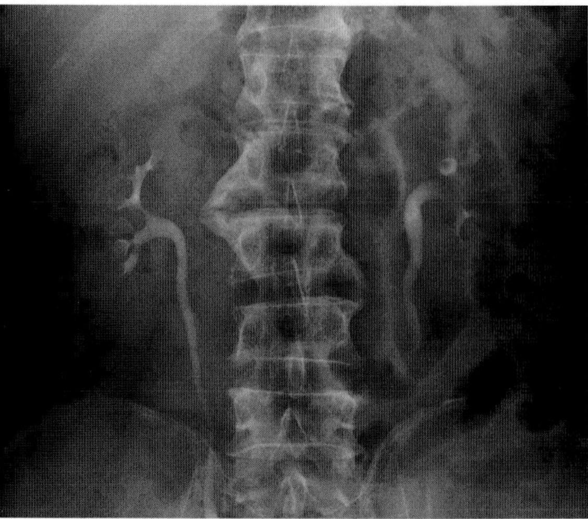

Fig. 12.5a-c. Transitional cell carcinoma in a 65-year-old man with intermittent gross hematuria. **a** Longitudinal US image shows an ill-defined hypoechoic lesion (*arrows*) in the central echo complex of the superior aspect of the left kidney. **b** Excretory urography shows no opacification of the upper-pole calyx of the left kidney. **c** Axial contrast-enhanced CT scan shows a soft tissue mass (*arrow*) in the left renal sinus and coarse striations of a diminished nephrogram of the left kidney. On pathologic examination, papillary transitional cell carcinoma was found in the renal pelvis and upper-pole calyx with focal infiltration into the renal parenchyma.

depending on its anatomic location and pattern of growth. On CT and MR imaging, early-stage transitional cell carcinoma of the kidney, stage I or II, is a central solid mass in the renal pelvis that expands centrifugally with compression of the renal sinus fat and appears separated from the renal parenchyma either by renal sinus fat or excreted contrast material (Fig. 12.6); however, CT has limited ability to differentiate between stage I and stage II carcinomas (URBAN et al. 1997a). On the contrary, invasive transitional cell carcinoma, stage III or IV, obliterates the renal sinus fat and infiltrates into the surrounding parenchyma, typically not disturbing its reniform contour (Fig. 12.7, 12.8; URBAN et al. 1997b). This growth pattern is helpful for differentiating transitional cell carcinoma from renal cell carcinoma, which tends to grow by expansion. Differentiation from renal cell carcinoma is usually suggested when CT reveals the relatively central location of the tumor, its centrifugal expansion or invasion of the kidney, its hypovascular nature, or a combination of these findings (KAWASHIMA and GOLDMAN 2000).

12.3.2
Squamous Cell Carcinoma

Approximately 10% of renal pelvic tumors are squamous cell carcinomas. Squamous cell carcinomas are strongly associated with renal calculi, and chronic irritation of the urothelium appears to be an important etiologic factor in the development of squamous cell carcinoma (BLACHER et al. 1985). Imaging findings of squamous cell carcinomas are indistinguishable from those of transitional cell carcinomas (Fig. 12.9); however, when compared with the transitional cell carcinomas, squamous cell carcinoma of the kidney tends to appear with predominantly extraluminal tumor extension rather than purely intraluminal tumor growth on CT (NARUMI et al. 1989). The presence of a renal stone in association with a geographic infiltrating renal lesion with a large renal sinus component implies the diagnosis of squamous cell carcinoma (Fig. 12.10; WIMBISH et al. 1983). Most squamous cell carcinomas of the renal pelvis are high stage. Extensive infiltration of the renal parenchyma is common and survival for 5 years is rare (BLACHER et al. 1985).

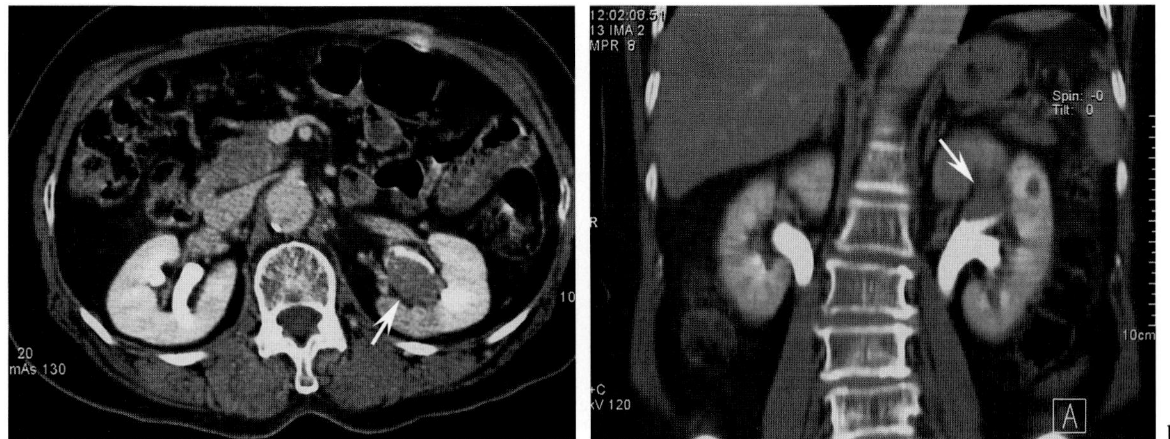

Fig. 12.6a,b. Transitional cell carcinoma of the renal pelvis in a 73-year-old woman with a 1-month history of left flank pain and intermittent gross hematuria. **a** Axial contrast-enhanced CT scan shows an ill-defined low-density mass lesion (*arrow*) in the renal pelvis of the left kidney. **b** Coronal reformatted contrast-enhanced CT scan obtained during the excretory phase shows the tumor involvement of the renal pelvis and upper calyces (*arrow*) and clearly demonstrates the extent of this renal pelvis tumor. Note that the renal sinus fat is not obliterated and the renal contour is preserved. On pathologic examination, papillary transitional cell carcinoma was found in the renal pelvis and upper-pole calyx without invasion into the renal parenchyma.

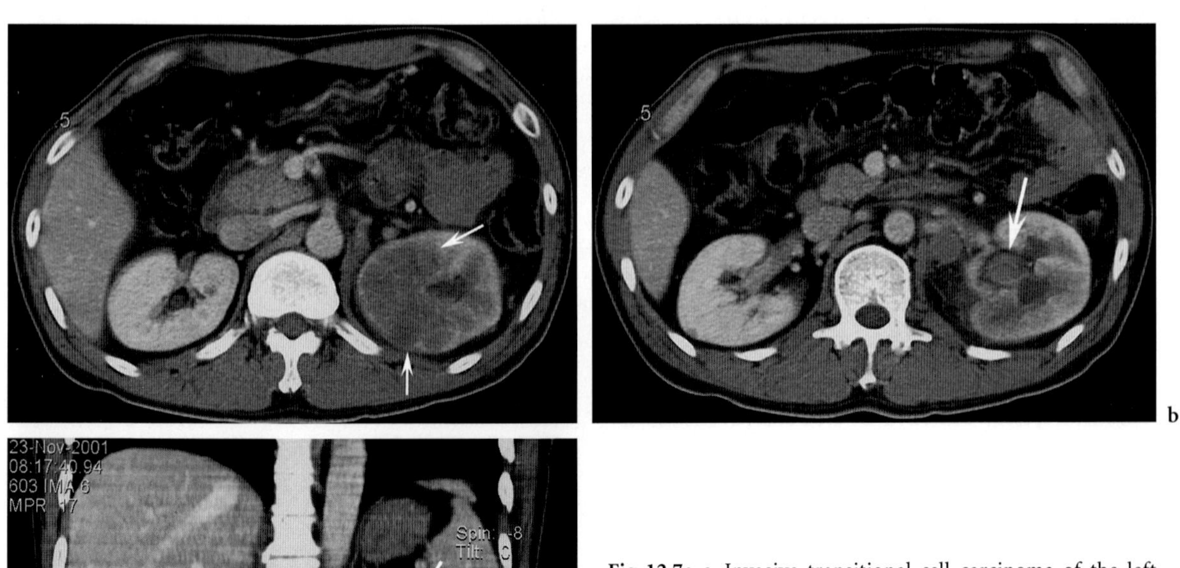

Fig. 12.7a-c. Invasive transitional cell carcinoma of the left kidney in a 46-year-old man. **a** Axial contrast-enhanced CT scan obtained during the nephrographic phase shows an ill-defined low-density mass (*arrows*) involving the renal parenchyma. Note that the renal contour is preserved. **b** Axial contrast-enhanced CT scan caudad to (**a**) shows a soft tissue density mass (*arrow*) occupying the renal pelvis. An enlarged retroperitoneal lymph node is also seen in the left para-aortic space. **c** Coronal reformatted contrast-enhanced CT scan obtained during the nephrographic phase shows the tumor involvement of the renal pelvis (*black arrow*) and upper parenchyma (*white arrow*).

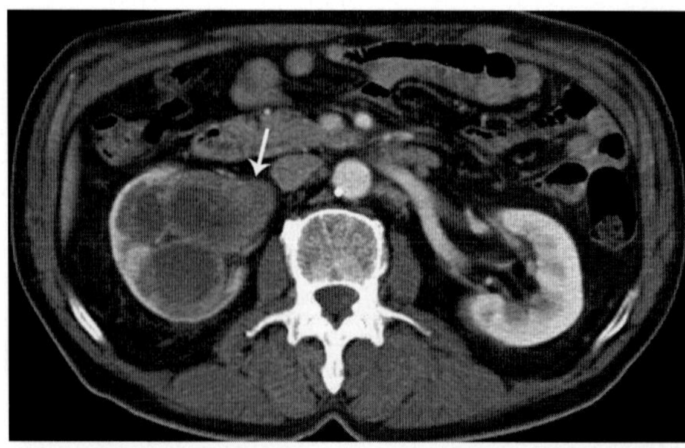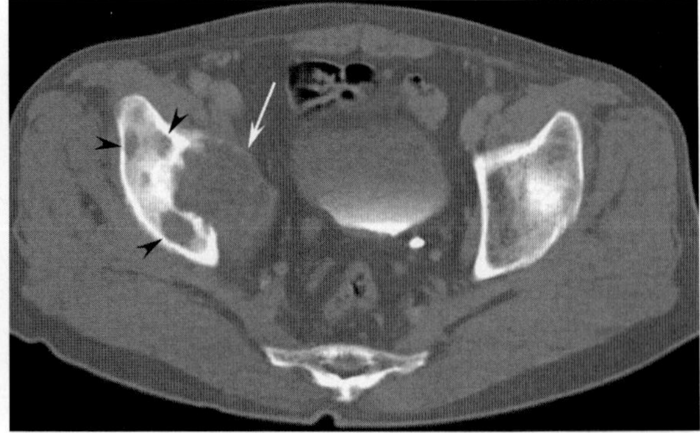

Fig. 12.8a,b. Invasive transitional cell carcinoma with bone metastasis in a 64-year-old man. **a** Axial contrast-enhanced CT scan obtained during the nephrographic phase shows an ill-defined hypodense tumor (*arrow*) in the dilated renal pelvis growing into the renal parenchyma while preserving the reniform outline of the right kidney. **b** Axial CT scan at the level of the sacrum shows a large expansile mass (*arrow*) with multifocal bone destruction in the right iliac bone (*arrowheads*).

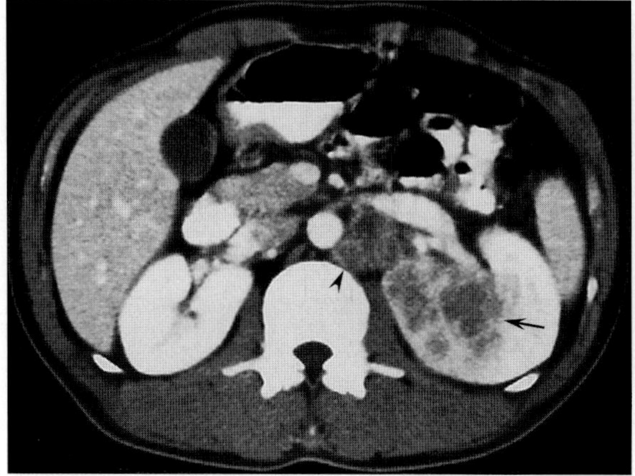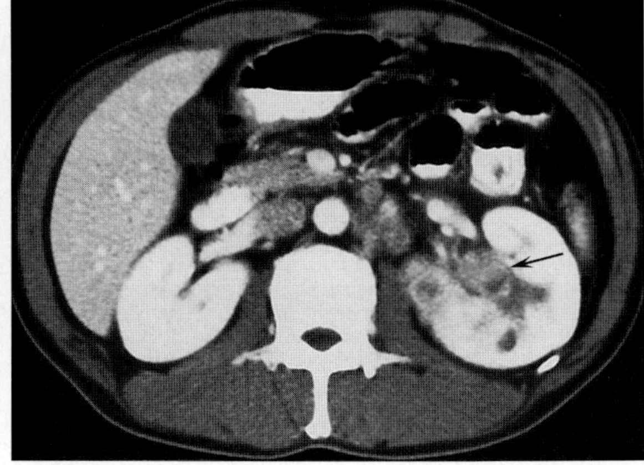

Fig. 12.9a,b. Squamous cell carcinoma in a 57-year-old man. **a** Axial contrast-enhanced CT scan obtained during the nephrographic phase shows centrally located ill-defined tumor (*arrow*) in the left kidney and left para-aortic lymphadenopathy (*arrowhead*). **b** Axial contrast-enhanced CT scan 1 cm caudad to (**a**) shows tumor infiltrating into the renal sinus (*arrow*). This tumor cannot be differentiated from transitional cell carcinoma by this CT finding.

12.4
Mesenchymal Tumors of the Renal Sinus

Primary mesenchymal origin tumors of the kidney are rare but may develop in the renal sinus space as well as in the renal capsule and renal parenchyma. The malignant renal neoplasms of pure mesenchymal origin are leiomyosarcoma, fibrosarcoma, liposarcoma, hemangiopericytoma, malignant fibrous histiocytoma, etc. (Choi et al. 1996; Shirkhoda and Lewis 1987). Leiomyosarcoma is the most common malignant tumor of primary mesenchymal origin neoplasms (Shirkhoda and Lewis 1987). The previously reported benign tumors should be known for their differential diagnosis purpose and include hemangioma, fibroma, leiomyoma, angiomyolipoma, neurogenic tumor, teratoma, etc. (Borrego et al. 1995; Cormier et al. 1989; Dasgupta et al. 1998; Ewald et al. 1982; Lee et al. 2000; Metro et al. 2000; Yoon et al. 1997; Yusim et al. 2001; Walther 1997).

Imaging findings of these rare tumors are usually nonspecific; however, the common imaging findings of primary mesenchymal origin tumors of the renal sinus are that the mass is relatively well circumscribed, the epicenter of the mass is located at the renal sinus, the mass is surrounded by attenuated renal parenchyma, and the renal pelvis is stretched over the tumor with or without hydronephrosis. It is important to make an accurate preoperative diagnosis of benign mesenchymal tumor because the treatment of choice is surgical or endoscopic excision,

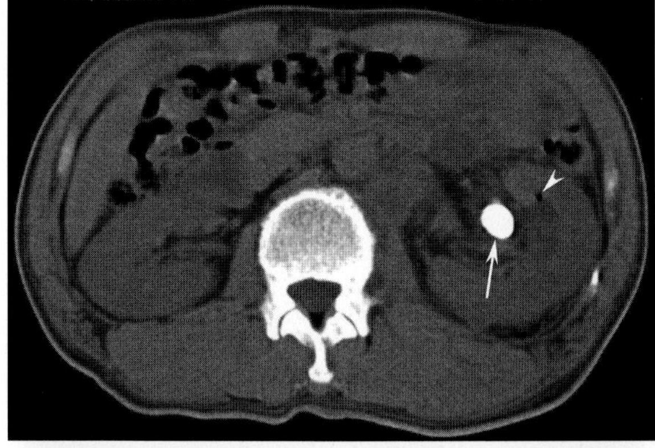

a

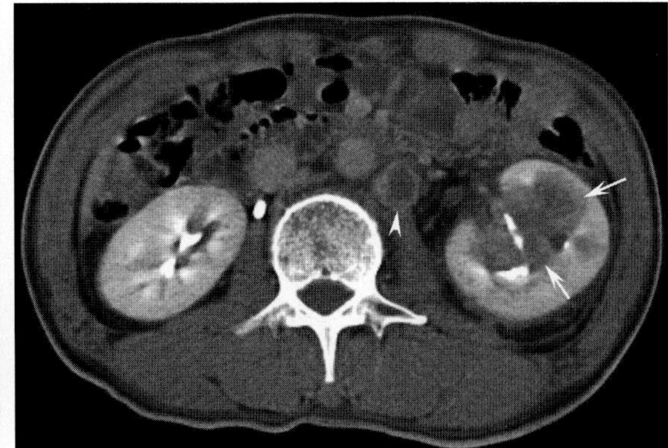

b

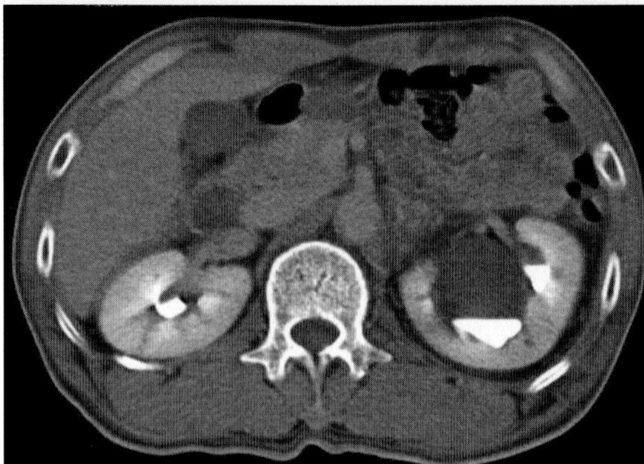

c

Fig. 12.10a-c. Squamous cell carcinoma in a 50-year-old man with chronic calculus disease and left flank pain. **a** Axial unenhanced CT scan shows a hyperdense stone (*arrow*) in the left renal pelvis. A tiny air bubble (*arrowhead*) is seen in the renal sinus due to the previously performed percutaneous nephrostomy. **b** Axial contrast-enhanced CT scan obtained during the excretory phase shows an infiltrative mass (*arrows*) in the renal pelvis extending to the renal parenchyma. Note the metastatic lymph nodes (*arrowhead*) in the para-aortic space. **c** Axial contrast-enhanced CT scans obtained during the excretory phase cephalad to (**b**) shows the dilated upper-pole calyceal system and delayed excretion of contrast material. (With permission from Rha et al. 2004)

but a preoperative differential diagnosis is difficult to make and these kinds of tumors are usually misdiagnosed preoperatively as the more common renal cell carcinomas or transitional cell carcinomas and are consequently treated with nephroureterectomy or radical nephrectomy, even in the benign cases (Yusim et al. 2001).

12.4.1
Leiomyosarcoma

Leiomyosarcoma of kidney, although a rare neoplasm, represents 2–3% of all malignant renal tumors. The origin of the renal leiomyosarcoma is generally from the interlacing bundles of smooth muscle in the inner layer of the renal capsule, in the wall of the renal pelvis, and within vessels of the renal parenchyma. About 33–58% of renal sarcomas are leiomyosarcoma (Shirkhoda and Lewis 1987). When the leiomyosarcoma is located within the renal parenchyma, it is difficult to differentiate from renal cell carcinoma. Conversely, in the case of the renal sarcoma originating within the renal sinus, the renal parenchyma appears draped over

the tumor. If a huge, well-encapsulated neoplasm originates from the renal sinus, the diagnosis of renal sarcoma should be considered (Fig. 12.11). Renal sarcoma generally has a poor prognosis and requires aggressive therapy, usually with radical nephrectomy and chemotherapy (Davis et al. 1992). The lungs are the most frequent site of metastases.

12.4.2
Hemangiopericytoma

Hemangiopericytoma is an uncommon neoplasm that can occur in the kidney as well as in several other organs. Only 22 cases of renal hemangiopericytoma have ever been reported. Affected patients range in age from 18 to 68 years (mean age 42 years). Pathologically, hemangiopericytoma arises from the renal capsule as well as from renal parenchyma. Only one case of hemangiopericytoma occurring in the renal sinus has been reported (Fig. 12.12; Choi et al. 1996). The prognosis of renal hemangiopericytoma is generally poor, with an overall mortality rate of 50% (Heppe et al. 1991).

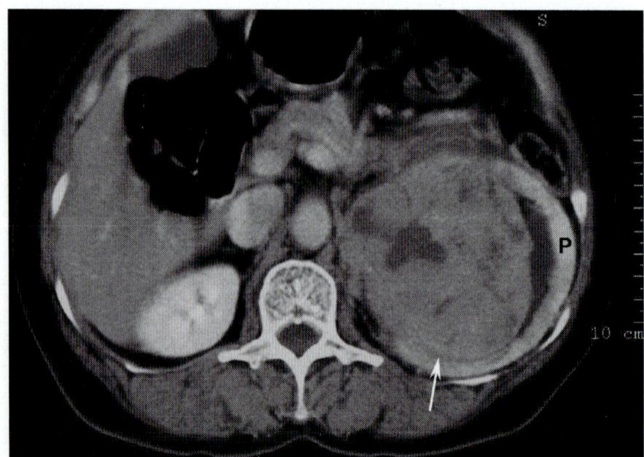

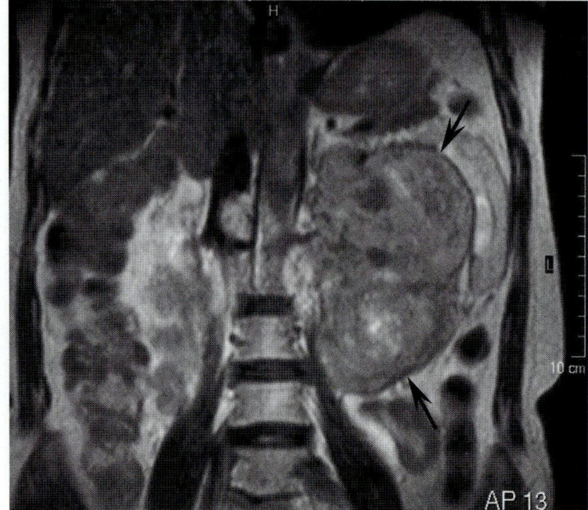

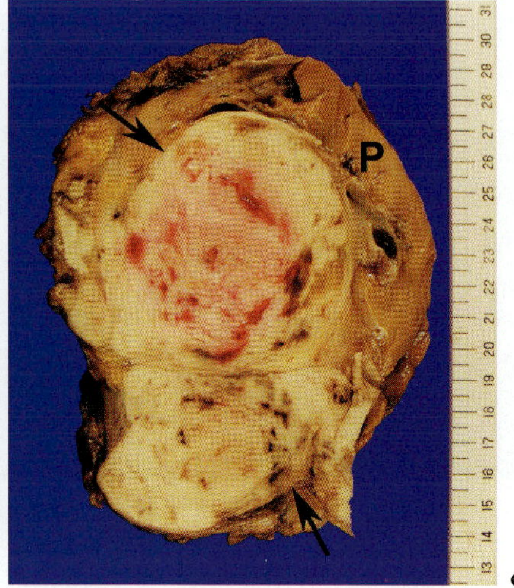

Fig. 12.11a-c. Leiomyosarcoma in the left renal sinus in a 65-year-old woman with left flank pain and a palpable left abdominal mass. **a** Axial contrast-enhanced CT scan shows a large heterogeneous-density mass (*arrow*) expanding the left renal sinus. The renal parenchyma (*P*) is markedly compressed and displaced laterally. **b** Coronal turbo spin-echo T2-weighted MR image (TR=6500 ms, TE=120 ms) clearly demonstrates the location and extent of the tumor (*arrows*). **c** Photograph of the surgical specimen shows a relatively well-defined tumor mass (*arrows*), 13×9×8 cm in size, located at the renal sinus. The mass shows a solid and compact cut surface with central hemorrhage and necrosis. The mass is confined to the sinus and does not invade the renal parenchyma or the pelvis. The adjacent renal parenchyma (*P*) is compressed by the tumor mass. (With permission from Rha et al. 2004)

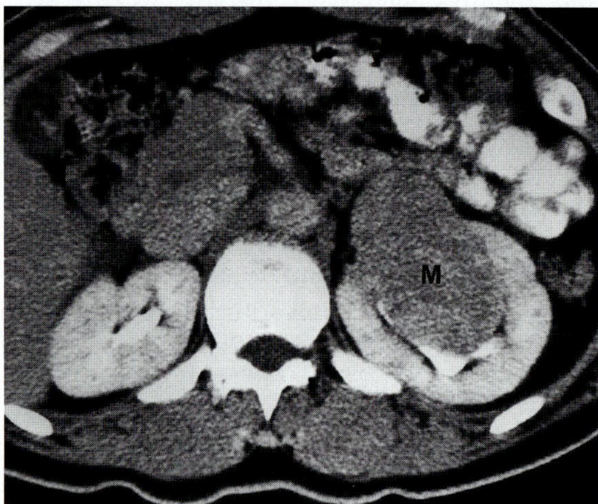

Fig. 12.12. Hemangiopericytoma in the left renal sinus in a 30-year-old woman with generalized weakness. Axial contrast-enhanced CT scan shows a large, well-defined, soft-tissue-density mass (*M*) occupying the central portion of the left renal sinus and compressing the opacified pelvocalyceal systems. (With permission from Rha et al. 2004)

12.4.3
Differential Diagnosis

It is essential to determine preoperatively the differential diagnosis of a variety of mesenchymal tumors, especially the benign tumors. Although this can be difficult, every effort should be made to arrive at the correct diagnosis.

Although renal hemangioma can be found in any part of the kidney, it usually occurs in the mucosa or subepithelial tissue of the pelvis (48.7%), in the pyramid (42.1%), and in the cortex of the kidney (9.2%; Virgili 2003). It is one of the benign causes of hematuria in young adults. Renal pelvis hemangiomas vary in size from microscopic to 10 cm or more but usually measure 1–2 cm. There are no specific clinical or radiologic findings for hemangiomas. Interestingly, even though this mass is a vascular tumor, the hemangioma may not enhance on contrast-enhanced CT scans depending on intratumoral hemorrhage or thrombosis of the vessels perfusing the mass. Renal hemangioma should be included in the differential diagnosis, especially when CT shows little enhancement of the renal mass located at the pelvocalyceal junction or in the inner medulla (Fig. 12.13; LEE et al. 2000).

Renal leiomyoma is an uncommon benign tumor but is the most common among benign mesothelial tumors encountered in the genitourinary tract with an incidence of about 5% at autopsy (YUSIM et al. 2001). It originates from the smooth muscle found in the renal capsule, renal pelvis, and vasculature. Computed tomography findings are variable from purely cystic to entirely solid lesions depending on their variable consistency (Fig. 12.14; DASGUPTA 1998).

12.5
Renal Parenchymal Tumors Projecting into the Renal Sinus

Most renal parenchymal tumors grow by expansion, manifesting as ball-like masses (ZAGORIA and TUNG 1997a). The medially growing renal parenchymal mass may project into the renal sinus and compress or infiltrate the renal sinus fat. The representative tumors are renal cell carcinoma and benign multilocular cystic nephroma.

12.5.1
Renal Cell Carcinoma

Renal cell carcinomas are the most common malignant renal parenchymal neoplasms. Most renal cell carcinomas grow by expansion and commonly extend into the renal sinus, leading to focal hydronephrosis or calyceal displacement (Figs. 12.15, 12.16; ZAGORIA and TUNG 1997a). The clinical significance of renal cell carcinoma extending into the renal sinus is that the imaging appearance may be similar to that of transitional cell carcinoma, and tumor staging influences surgical management. Unlike transitional cell carcinoma, renal cell carcinoma has a tendency to extend into the venous system (Fig. 12.17). Although indications for partial nephrectomy are constantly changing, the most suitable indication for partial nephrectomy is a renal tumor smaller than 3 cm without invasion of the renal sinus fat, perinephric fat, or renal collecting system, particularly in patients with diminished renal function, and a solitary kidney or bilateral renal malignancy (PRETORIUS et al. 1999). Invasion of renal sinus fat indicates that partial nephrectomy cannot successfully and completely remove the renal mass. Three-dimensional CT or MR imaging helps to delineate the precise location of the renal mass and its relationship to the collecting system and renal vessels.

12.5.2
Multilocular Cystic Nephroma

Multilocular cystic nephromas are benign multiseptated cystic tumors originating from the renal parenchyma. These tumors have a biphasic age distribution, occurring predominantly in boys and middle-aged women. The gross finding of multilocular cystic nephroma is a solitary, well-

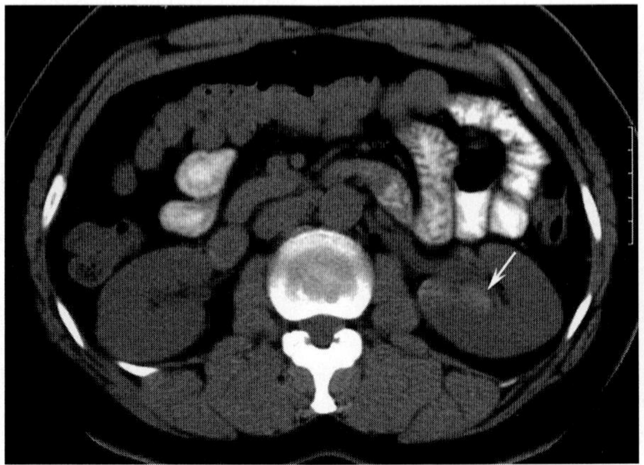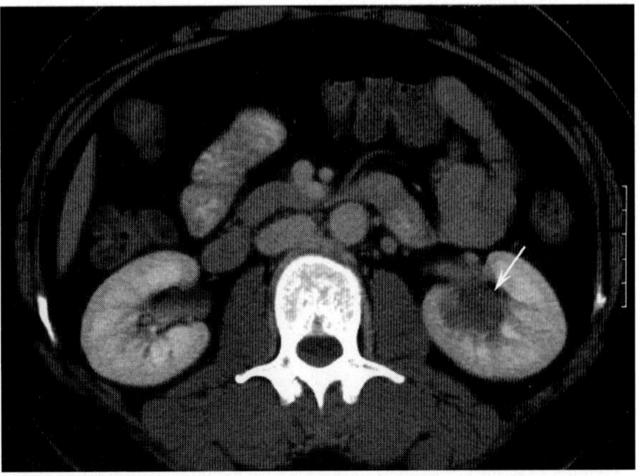

a   b

Fig. 12.13a,b. Venous hemangioma in the left renal sinus in a 33-year-old man with gross hematuria and left flank pain. **a** Axial unenhanced CT scan shows a well-defined hyperdense lesion (*arrow*) adjacent to the left renal pelvis. **b** Axial contrast-enhanced CT scan shows a poorly enhancing, hypodense mass (*arrow*). Because of the possibility of malignancy, a left nephrectomy was performed. At pathologic examination, the lesion was composed of multiple vascular channels of variable sizes beneath the pelvic mucosa. (With permission from RHA et al. 2004)

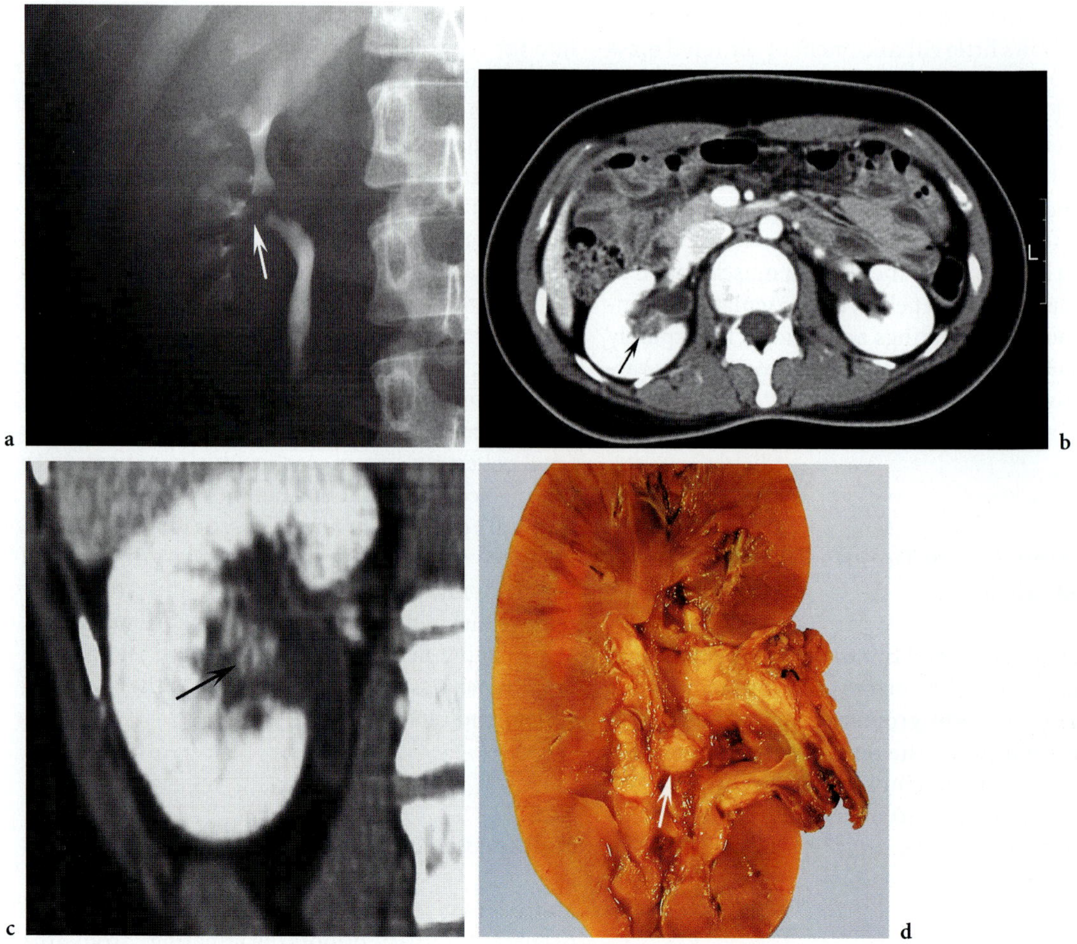

Fig. 12.14a-d. Leiomyoma involving the renal sinus in a 28-year-old woman with gross hematuria. **a** Excretory urography shows a focal smooth mass effect on the pelvocalyces of the right kidney (*arrow*). **b** Axial contrast-enhanced CT scan obtained during the nephrographic phase shows a small soft-tissue-density mass (*arrow*) obliterating the sinus fat in the right kidney along the posterior margin of the right renal pelvis. **c** Coronal reformatted CT scan demonstrates a round soft-tissue-density mass lesion (*arrow*) in the right renal sinus and mild dilation of the pelvocalyceal system. **d** Photograph of the surgical specimen shows a well-defined round mass (*arrow*) in the renal sinus. Microscopic examination reveals a renal leiomyoma in the right renal sinus. (With permission from RHA et al. 2004)

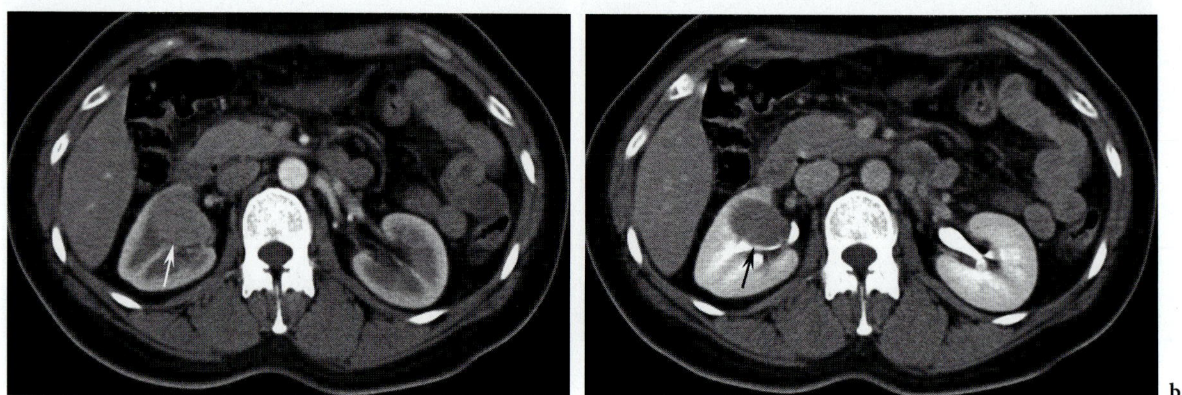

Fig. 12.15a,b. Renal cell carcinoma located near the renal sinus in a 43-year-old woman. **a** Axial contrast-enhanced CT scan obtained during the corticomedullary phase shows a large, well-defined, soft-tissue-density mass (*arrow*) in the central portion of the right kidney. **b** Axial contrast-enhanced CT scan obtained during the excretory phase shows the mass indenting the opacified pelvocalyceal systems (*arrow*). Pathology confirmed chromophobe-type renal cell carcinoma near the renal sinus without invasion of the renal vein or renal pelvis.

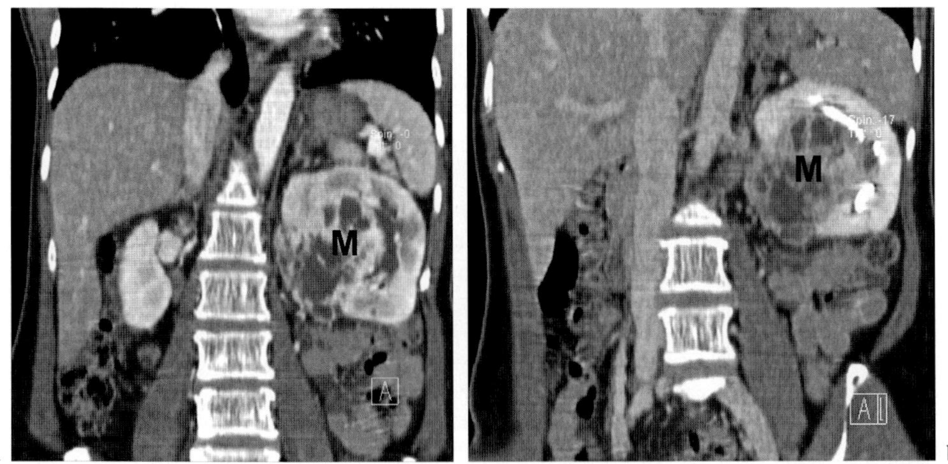

Fig. 12.16a,b. Centrally located renal cell carcinoma in a 56-year-old woman. Coronal reformatted contrast-enhanced CT scans obtained during **a** the corticomedullary phase and **b** the excretory phase show a large lobulated heterogeneous density mass *(M)* involving the left renal sinus.

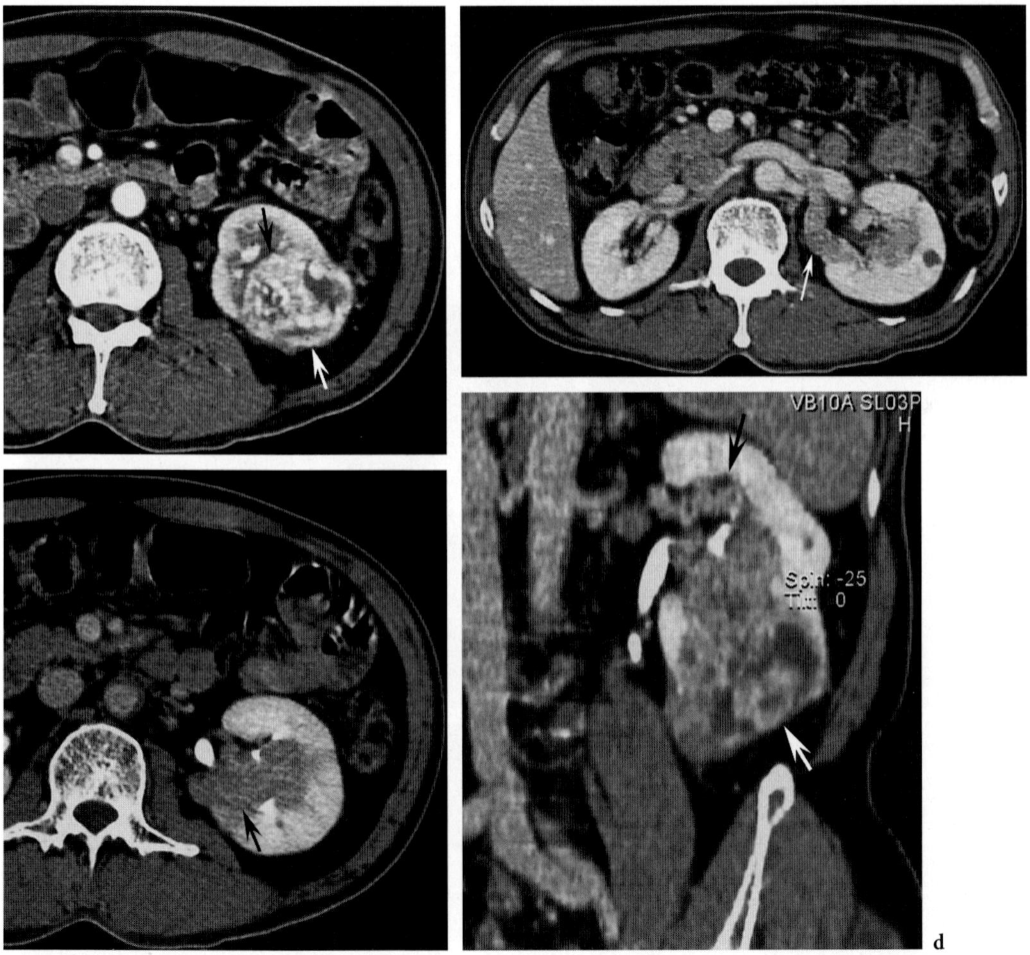

Fig. 12.17a-d. Renal cell carcinoma extension into the renal sinus in a 51-year-old man with gross hematuria. **a** Axial contrast-enhanced CT scan shows a lobulated heterogeneously enhancing tumor *(arrows)* involving the lower pole of the left kidney. **b** Axial contrast-enhanced CT scan obtained 1 cm cephalad to **a** shows the posterior segmental branch of the left renal vein occupied by the tumor thrombus *(arrow)*. **c** Axial contrast-enhanced CT scan obtained 2 cm cephalad to **a** shows the tumor extending to the left renal sinus *(arrow)*. **d** Coronal reformatted contrast-enhanced CT obtained during the excretory phase clearly shows the tumor involvement of the renal sinus and the extent of the renal cell carcinoma *(arrows)*. These findings were confirmed at radical nephrectomy. The pathologic stage was T3b N0. (With permission from RHA et al. 2004)

circumscribed, multiseptated mass of noncommunicating fluid-filled loculi, surrounded by a thick fibrous capsule and compressed renal parenchyma (MADEWELL et al. 1983). Interestingly, this lesion frequently herniates into the renal sinus, causing a filling defect in the renal pelvis and sometimes obstructive caliectasia (MADEWELL et al. 1983), but this sign is nonspecific and may be present in case of Wilms tumor or renal cell carcinoma. On imaging studies, multilocular cystic nephroma presents as a well-defined encapsulated cystic mass containing numerous thick septa (Fig. 12.18; ZAGORIA and TUNG 1997b). Although the typical findings are present, the possibility of cystic renal cell carcinoma or Wilms' tumor cannot be entirely excluded; therefore, surgery is indicated, even when the diagnosis of multilocular cystic nephroma is strongly suspected (CASTILLO et al. 1991).

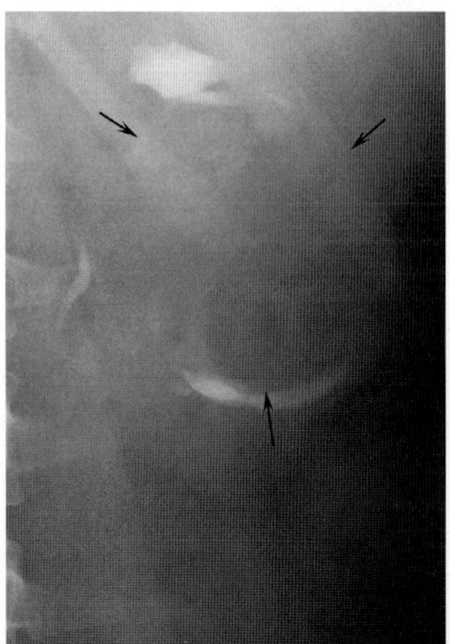

Fig. 12.18a-e. Multilocular cystic nephroma in a 32-year-old man. **a** Excretory urography shows marked splaying of the upper and lower calyceal systems (*arrows*) with mild dilation of the upper pole calyx. **b** Longitudinal US image of the left kidney shows a multiloculated cystic mass in the lower pole of the left kidney. **c** Axial contrast-enhanced CT scan obtained during the excretory phase shows a well-defined multi-chambered cystic mass in the left kidney. **d** Axial true fast imaging with steady-state precession MR image (TR=6.3 ms, TE=3.0 ms, flip angle 70°) again shows a hyperintense cystic mass in the left kidney. Note the numerous fine septations without solid components. **e** Coronal contrast-enhanced T1-weighted MR image (TE=130 ms, TE=4.1 ms) clearly shows herniation of the cystic mass (*arrow*) into the renal sinus. (With permission from RHA et al. 2004)

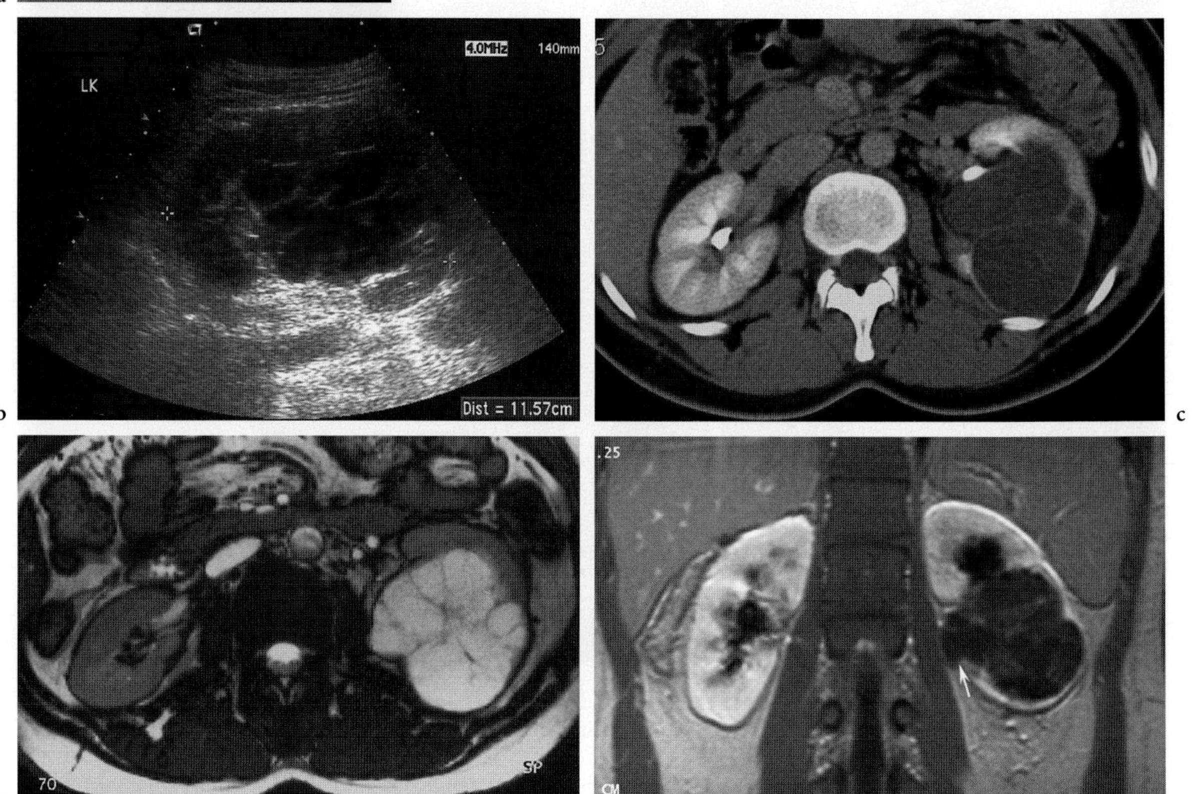

12.6
Retroperitoneal Tumors Extending to the Renal Sinus

12.6.1
Lymphoma

As the renal sinus is a medial extension of the perinephric space, any retroperitoneal tumor can extend to the renal sinus (Fig. 12.19). The representative example is a lymphoma. Retroperitoneal lymphoma with contiguous extension into the renal sinus is a common manifestations of lymphoma (URBAN and FISHMAN 2000). These patients present with a large, bulky retroperitoneal mass that envelops and surrounds the normal constituents of the renal sinus, often with contiguous spread into the perinephric space (Fig. 12.20). This situation is most common in patients with advanced non-Hodgkin lymphoma. The renal vessels remain patent despite tumor encasement, a finding that is characteristic for lymphoma. Conversely, obstructive hydronephrosis is often caused by direct involvement of the renal collecting system (JAFRI et al. 1982; URBAN and FISHMAN 2000). Renal lymphoma can also infiltrate the renal sinus or the renal parenchyma, maintaining its reniform shape (Fig. 12.21). On CT and US, lymphomatous masses are characteristically homogeneous. On CT, the mass enhances less. Renal lymphoma is usually hypoechoic on US, a finding that reflects tissue homogeneity. On MR imaging, renal lymphoma tends to be hypointense relative to the renal cortex on T1-weighted images and hetero-

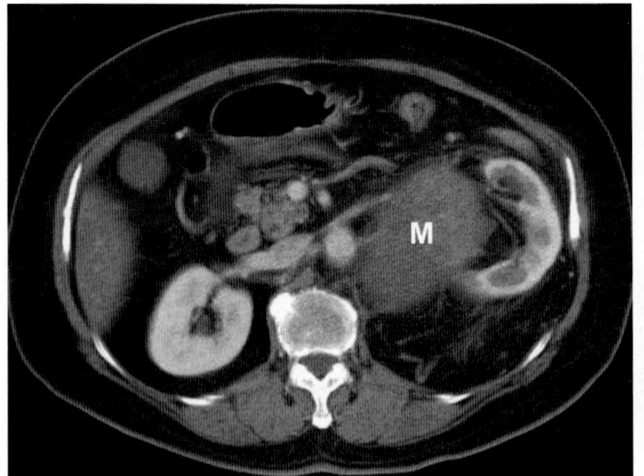
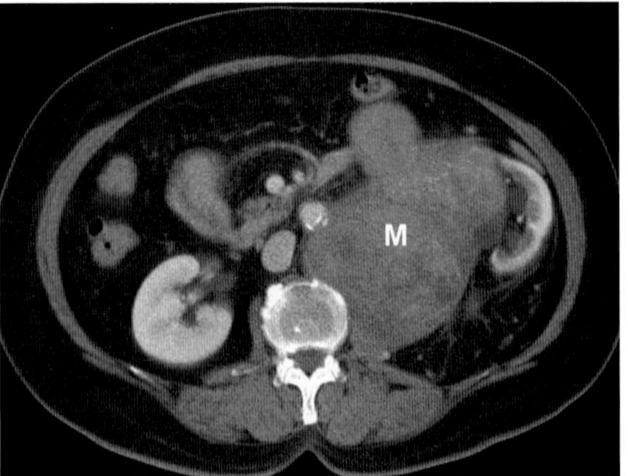

a

b

Fig. 12.19a,b. Retroperitoneal spindle cell tumor extending to the renal sinus in a 63-year-old woman. a, b Axial contrast-enhanced CT scans show a bulky lobulated soft-tissue-density mass (M) in the left para-aortic space and extending to the left renal sinus. It causes dilation of the left renal pelvis and calyces.

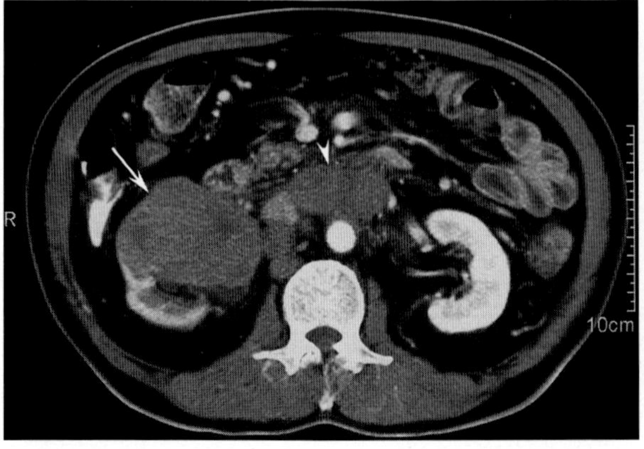
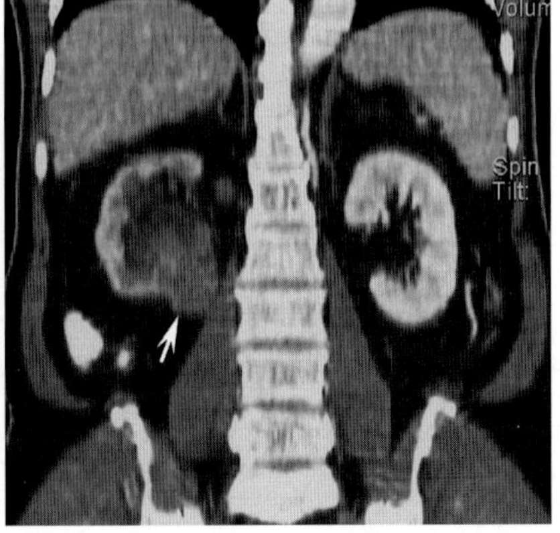

a

b

Fig. 12.20a,b. Lymphoma involving the renal parenchyma and renal sinus in a 56-year-old man with generalized weakness. a Axial contrast-enhanced CT scan shows a large relatively homogeneous mass (arrow) involving the right renal parenchyma and renal sinus. Note the multiple enlarged retroperitoneal lymph nodes (arrowhead). b Coronal reformatted CT scan obtained during the nephrographic phase shows the extent of the lymphoma mass (arrow) and mild hydronephrosis of the right kidney. (With permission from RHA et al. 2004)

geneously hypointense or isointense on T2-weighted images. Minimal enhancement is generally detected, although renal lymphoma enhances considerably less than normal renal parenchyma.

12.6.2
Metastasis

Metastasis to the sinus lymph nodes occurs either as part of a generalized retroperitoneal process or as an isolated involvement, as with primary gonadal tumors, because of rich supply of perforating capsular vessels and lymphatics into the renal sinus (Fig. 12.22; DAVIDSON et al. 1999).

12.7
Conclusion

A broad pathologic spectrum of tumors can occur in the renal sinus. The diagnosis and exact preoperative staging of renal sinus tumors relies on a multimodality imaging approach that includes excretory urography, US, CT, MR imaging, and angiography. Ultrasound is an excellent noninvasive technique to confirm whether such a mass is cystic or solid. If US findings suggest a solid mass, CT or MR imaging is used as a problem-solving technique and for evaluation of the staging or to determine the extent of the lesion. In general, the coronal plane of cross-sectional imaging is the most useful for the evaluation of renal sinus lesions, because it provides a comprehensive view of complicated renal sinus pathology. Familiarity with the imaging features and differential diagnoses of various renal sinus tumors will facilitate prompt, accurate diagnosis and treatment.

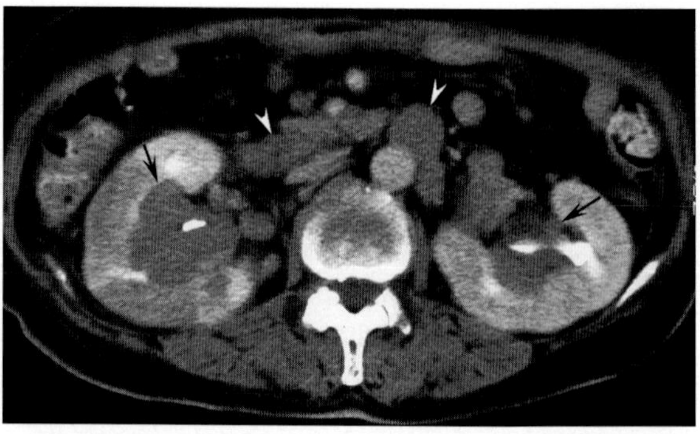

Fig. 12.21. Peripelvic lymphoma in a 63-year-old woman. Axial contrast-enhanced CT scan shows soft tissue density masses involving the renal sinus of both kidneys (*arrows*). Multiple retroperitoneal lymph nodes (*arrowheads*) are also seen.

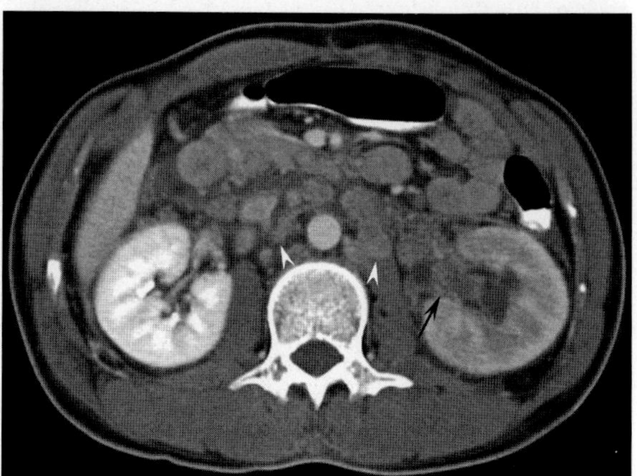

Fig. 12.22. Metastatic lymphadenopathy from ascending colon cancer involving the left renal sinus in a 36-year-old man. Axial contrast-enhanced CT scan shows multiple soft-tissue-density lymph nodes (*arrowheads*) in the retroperitoneum extending to the left renal sinus (*arrow*) with mild obstructive hydronephrosis of the left kidney.

References

Amis ES Jr (2000) Cysts of the renal sinus. In: Pollack HM, McClennan BL (eds) Clinical urography, 2nd edn. Saunders, Philadelphia, pp 1404–1412

Amis ES Jr, Cronan JJ (1988) The renal sinus: an imaging review and proposed nomenclature for sinus cysts. J Urol 139:1151–1159

Baron RL, McClennan BL, Lee JK et al. (1982) Computed tomography of transitional cell carcinoma of the renal pelvis and ureter. Radiology 144:125–130

Blacher EJ, Johnson DE, Abdul-Karim FW et al. (1985) Squamous cell carcinoma of renal pelvis. Urology 25:124–126

Bonsib SM, Gibson D, Mhoon M, Greene GF (2000) Renal sinus involvement in renal cell carcinomas. Am J Surg Pathol 24:451–458

Borrego J, Cuesta C, Allona A et al. (1995) Myxoid neurofibroma of the renal sinus. Actas Urol Esp 19:415–418

Castillo OA, Boyle ET Jr, Kramer SA (1991) Multilocular cysts of kidney: a study of 29 patients and review of literature. Urology 37:156–162

Choi YJ, Hwang TK, Kang SJ et al. (1996) Hemangiopericytoma of renal sinus expanding to the renal hilum: an unusual presentation causes misinterpretation as transitional cell carcinoma. J Korean Med Sci 11:351–355

Cormier P, Patel SK, Turner DA et al. (1989) MR imaging

findings in renal medullary fibroma. Am J Roentgenol 153:83–84

Dasgupta P, Sandison A, Parks C et al. (1998) Case report: Renal leiomyoma with unusual calcification. Clin Radiol 53:857–858

Davidson AJ, Hartman DS, Choyke PL et al. (1999) Renal sinus and periureteral abnormalities. In: Davidson AJ, Hartman DS, Choyke PL et al. (eds) Davidson's radiology of the kidney and genitourinary tract, 3rd edn. Saunders, Philadelphia, pp 431–455

Davis R, Vaccaro JA, Hodges GF (1992) Renal leiomyosarcoma: plea for aggressive therapy. Urology 40:168–171

Ewald N, Cukier J, Roth A et al. (1982) Teratoma of the renal sinus. Apropos of a case. J Urol (Paris) 88:553–554

Heppe RK, Donohue RE, Clark JE (1991) Bilateral renal hemangiopericytoma. Urology 38:249–253

Jafri SZ, Bree RL, Amendola MA et al. (1982) CT of renal and perirenal non-Hodgkin lymphoma. Am J Roentgenol 138:1101–1105

Jeffrey RB Jr (2004) Clinical impact of multidetector CT. In: Fishman EK, Jeffrey RB Jr (eds) Multidetector CT. Principles, techniques, and clinical applications. Lippincott Williams and Wilkins, Philadelphia, pp 53–58

Kawashima A, Goldman SM (2000) Neoplasms of the renal collecting system, pelvis, and ureters. In: Pollack HM, McClennan BL (eds) Clinical urography, 2nd edn. Saunders, Philadelphia, pp 1560–1641

McLaughlin JK, Blot WJ, Mandel JS et al. (1983) Etiology of cancer of the renal pelvis. J Natl Cancer Inst 71:287–291

Lee HS, Koh BH, Kim JW et al. (2000) Radiologic findings of renal hemangioma: report of three cases. Korean J Radiol 1:60–63

Madewell JE, Goldman SM, Davis CJ Jr et al. (1983) Multilocular cystic nephroma: a radiographic–pathologic correlation of 58 patients. Radiology 146:309–321

Metro MJ, Ramchandani P, Banner MP et al. (2000) Angiomyolipoma of the renal sinus: diagnosis by percutaneous biopsy. Urology 55:286

Narumi Y, Sato T, Hori S et al. (1989) Squmous cell carcinoma of the uroepithelium: CT evaluation. Radiology 173:853–856

Pickhardt PJ, Lonergan GJ, Davis CJ Jr et al. (2000) Infiltrative renal lesions: radiologic–pathologic correlation. Radiographics 20:215–243

Pozzi-Mucelli R, Rimondini A, Morra A (2004) Radiologic evaluation in planning surgery of renal tumors. Abdom Imaging 29:312–319

Pretorius ES, Siegelman ES, Ramchandani P et al. (1999) Renal neoplasms amenable to partial nephrectomy: MR imaging. Radiology 212:28–34

Rha SE, Byun JY, Jung SE et al. (2004) The renal sinus: pathologic spectrum and multi-modality imaging approach. Radiographics 24 (Suppl 1):S117–S131

Rosenfield AT, Taylor KJ, Dembner AG et al. (1979) Ultrasound of renal sinus: new observations. Am J Roentgenol 133: 441–448

Shirkhoda A, Lewis E (1987) Renal sarcoma and sarcomatoid renal cell carcinoma: CT and angiographic features. Radiology 162:353–357

Urban BA, Fishman EK (2000) Renal lymphoma: CT patterns with emphasis on helical CT. Radiographics 20:197–212

Urban BA, Buckley J, Soyer P et al. (1997) CT appearance of transitional cell carcinoma of the renal pelvis. Part 1. Early-stage disease. Am J Roentgenol 169:157–161

Urban BA, Buckley J, Soyer P et al. (1997) CT appearance of transitional cell carcinoma of the renal pelvis. Part 2. Advanced-stage disease. Am J Roentgenol 169:163–168

Virgili G, Stasi SM di, Bove P et al. (2003) Cavernous hemangioma of the renal hilum presenting as an avascularized solid mass. Urol Int 71:325–328

Walther PJ (1997) Uncommon neoplasms of the kidney. In: Raghavan D, Scher HI, Leibel SA, Lange PH (eds) Principles and practice of genitourinary oncology. Lippincott-Raven, Philadelphia, pp 897–909

Wimbish KJ, Sanders MM, Samuels BI et al. (1983) Squamous cell carcinoma of the renal pelvis: case report emphasizing sonographic and CT appearance. Urol Radiol 5:267–269

Wong-You-Cheong JJ, Wagner BJ, Davis CJ Jr (1998) Transitional cell carcinoma of the urinary tract: radiologic–pathologic correlation. Radiographics 18:123–142

Yoon YD, Byun JY, Jee WH et al. (1997) Imaging diagnosis in various renal sinus lesions. J Korean Radiol Soc 37:509–514

Yusim IE, Neulander EZ, Eidelberg I et al. (2001) Leiomyoma of the genitourinary tract. Scand J Urol Nephrol 35:295–299

Zagoria RJ, Tung GA (1997) Renal masses. In: Zagoria RJ, Tung GA (eds) Genitourinary radiology: the requisites. Mosby, St. Loius, pp 81–121

Zagoria RJ, Tung GA (1997) The renal sinus, pelvocalyceal system, and ureter. In: Zagoria RJ, Tung GA (eds) Genitourinary radiology: the requisites. Mosby, St. Louis, pp 152–191

13 Small Renal Neoplasms

Nancy S. Curry

CONTENTS

13.1
Introduction

A subset of renal parenchymal neoplasms, lesions under 3 cm in greatest diameter, presents special challenges to the radiologist, pathologist, and urologist. These lesions became significant as CT came into use because masses of this size frequently escaped the capability of standard excretory urography (EXU), even with tomography, to detect them (Amendola et al. 1988; Curry et al. 1986; Jamis-Dow et al. 1996). The relative sensitivities of EXU, ultrasound (US), and incremental (non-helical) CT for detecting renal lesions under 3 cm in diameter are 67, 79, and 94%, respectively (Warshauer et al. 1988). Before CT and US were in routine use, only 5% of renal cell carcinomas (RCC) were discovered at this small size (Smith et al. 1989). In the decade from the mid-1980s to the mid-1990s, however, the number of imaging studies performed nearly doubled, with the result that one-half to two-

thirds of small RCCs are now detected incidentally on cross-sectional imaging (Hsu et al. 2004; Volpe et al. 2004).

13.2
Pathology

Autopsy series have shown a 7–23% incidence of renal tumors 3 cm in diameter or less (Petersen et al. 1992). The most common cause of a solid renal mass under 3 cm in diameter is RCC, accounting for about 68–90% of resected tumors of this size (Jinzaki et al. 2000; Levine et al. 1989; Silverman et al. 1994). The remainder of the lesions in these series proved to be oncocytoma, metanephric adenoma, leiomyoma, angiomyolipoma (AML), transitional cell carcinoma, and lymphoma. Oncocytomas are derived from proximal tubular cells and have finely granular, eosinophilic cytoplasm. They are difficult to distinguish from malignant tumors since oncocytes may be found in RCC. Metanephric adenoma, an uncommon but distinct type of benign renal epithelial tumor composed of small tubular structures with papillary infoldings, has been recognized and reported with increased frequency (Fielding et al. 1999; Jinzaki et al. 2000). Other non-cystic, non-neoplastic abnormalities, such as focal renal infection, infarction, malakoplakia and rare heterotopic tissue (extramedullary hematopoiesis, adrenal rests, and endometriosis), may mimic renal neoplasms.

Tumors less than 2 cm in diameter, removed during partial nephrectomy, have about one chance in three of benign pathology (Steinberg et al. 2003). Sectioning of the kidneys in a series of 500 unselected necropsies in a Portuguese population revealed that 39% contained cysts, 18% medullary fibrous nodules, 4% cortical adenomas, 1% leiomyomas, and < 1% contained lipomas, fibromyolipomas, and capsular fibromas (Reis et al. 1988). Most of these lesions were less than 1 cm in diameter.

N. S. Curry, MD
Professor of Radiology and Urology, Department of Radiology, Medical University of South Carolina, 169 Ashley Avenue, Charleston, SC 29425, USA

The choice of 3 cm to define a "small" renal neoplasm is an arbitrary one, based on controversy in the pathologic literature regarding whether benign renal adenoma is a distinct entity from a small renal carcinoma. Large renal cancers have to be small at some point in their evolution, but unlike the well-known colon polyp to carcinoma progression, there is no predictable adenoma–carcinoma sequence for renal parenchymal neoplasms. Both tumors arise from the proximal convoluted tubule and pathologic features lack clear-cut criteria to differentiate them (BENNINGTON 1973). BELL's analysis of 65 renal tumors established that the likelihood of metastases increases as the size of a renal tumor increases (BELL 1950). That series revealed only three tumors with diameters less than 3 cm (4.6%) that showed evidence of metastasis at autopsy. While some pathologists interpreted these statistics as a rationale for considering such small lesions benign, most currently classify small renal tumors as potentially malignant or pre-malignant lesions (BENNINGTON 1973; BENNINGTON 1987; SOMEREN et al. 1989). Some researchers who argue that since the term "adenoma" implies a benign neoplasm, its use to describe small renal tumors should be abandoned. DNA content analysis of small renal tumors supports the hypothesis that at least some of these tumors have the potential for aggressive behavior because they demonstrate DNA aneuploidy, a feature shared by larger RCCs (ELLIS et al. 1992).

13.3
Growth Characteristics

The histologic distribution of small renal carcinomas is similar to that of larger tumors, with the clear cell subtype accounting for about 70% of cases (Fig. 13.1), papillary 20% (Fig. 13.2), chromophobe 5% (Fig. 13.3), and sarcomatoid lesions occurring less frequently (HSU et al. 2004). Most are low-grade, low-stage tumors with variable growth rates (Fig. 13.4). In BOSNIAK's series, 40 patients with renal neoplasms 3.5 cm in diameter or smaller were followed from 1.75 months to 8.5 years (mean 3.25 years; BOSNIAK et al. 1995). A mean linear growth rate of 0–1.1 cm/year (mean 0.36 cm/year) was established for these lesions and no metastases occurred in the observation period. Most of the tumors (75%) grew no more than 0.5 cm/year. Twenty-six of these tumors were resected. Most were Fuhrman grade I lesions, whereas four were

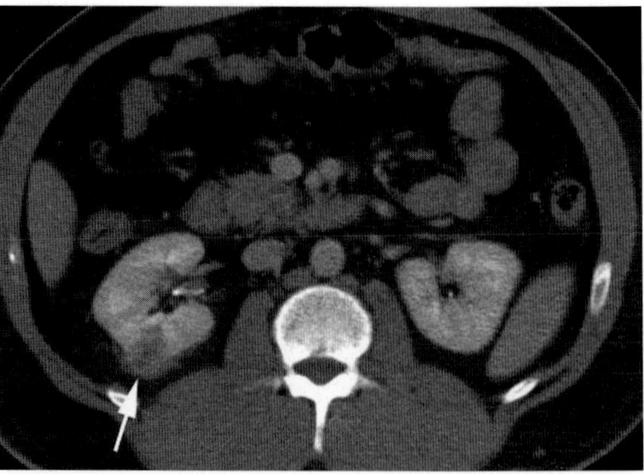

Fig. 13.1. Clear cell carcinoma in a 33-year-old man with right flank pain and history of renal calculi. Axial contrast-enhanced CT scan reveals a 2.5 cm right renal enhancing solid mass (89 HU; *arrow*). A Fuhrman nuclear grade II/IV clear cell carcinoma was resected.

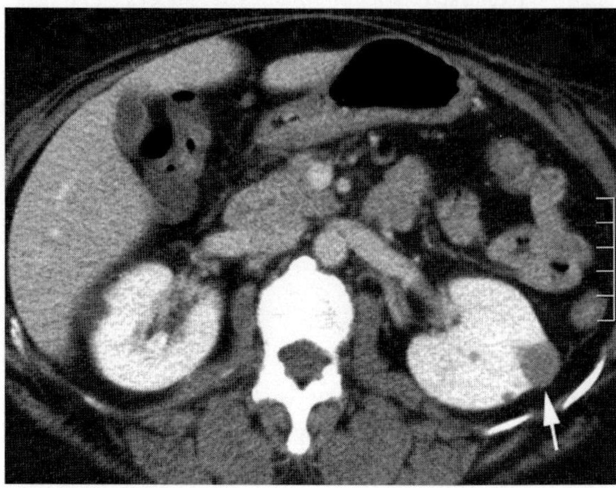

Fig. 13.2. Papillary RCC in a 63-year-old woman with left flank pain and hematuria. Axial contrast-enhanced CT scan reveals a homogeneous 2 cm left renal mass (83 HU; *arrow*). A partial nephrectomy was performed.

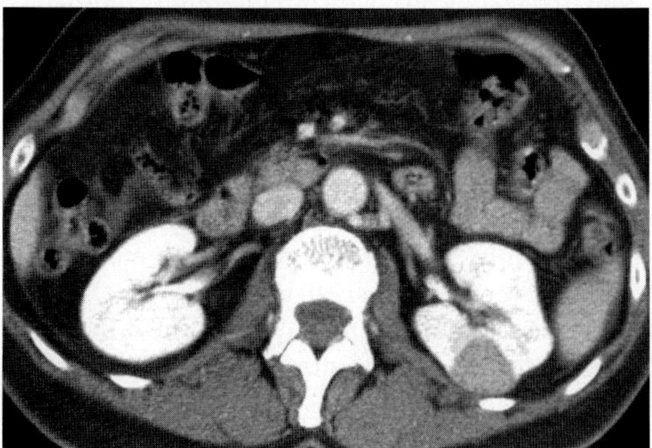

Fig. 13.3. Chromophobe RCC in a 70-year-old woman. Axial contrast-enhanced CT scan shows incidental 2.7 cm left renal mass which enhanced 71 HU over baseline scan. (With permission from CURRY 2002)

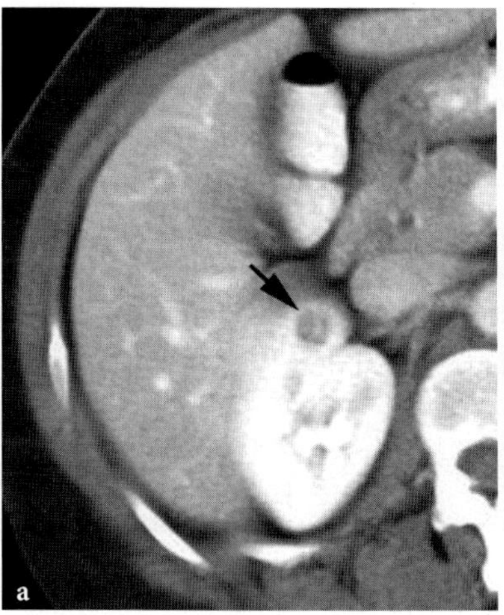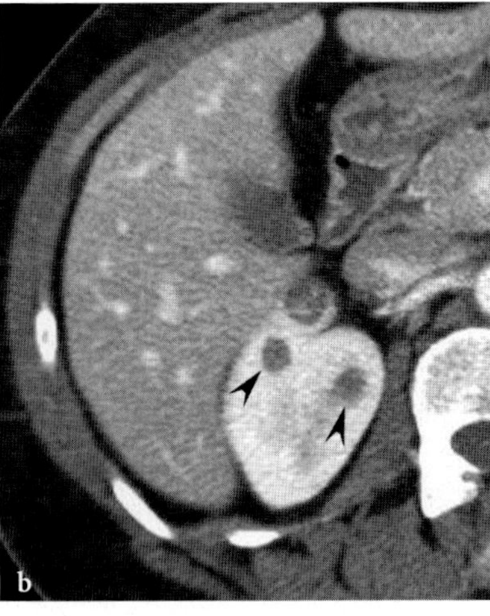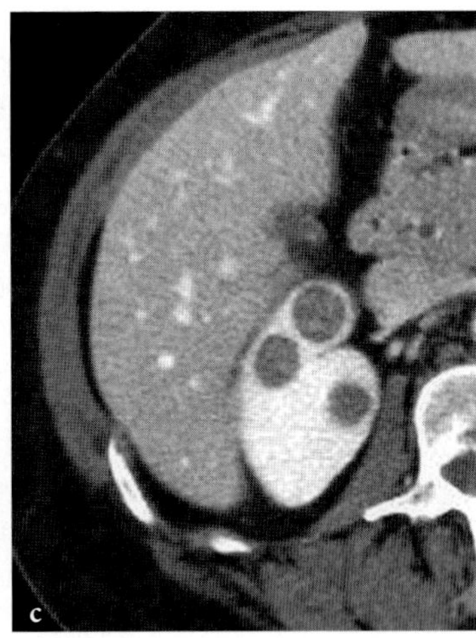

Fig. 13.4a-c. Growth of RCC in a 55-year-old woman post-left nephrectomy for clear cell carcinoma. No history of hereditary or familial renal cancer syndromes. **a** Axial contrast-enhanced CT scan shows 7 mm tumor in the anterior right kidney (*arrow*). **b** Axial contrast-enhanced CT scan 2 years later shows that the lesion grew to 12 mm in diameter and two smaller lesions appeared (*arrowheads*). **c** Axial contrast-enhanced CT scan 4 years after the first scan (**a**) shows that the anterior mass increased to 18 mm diameter. The resected lesions were all clear cell carcinoma. Additional masses were treated with radiofrequency ablation.

grade II. Even the three tumors which grew more rapidly, at 1.0–1.1 cm/year never metastasized, and two of these were grade II.

A prospective study presented the follow-up of 32 tumors in 29 patients with renal masses less than 4 cm in diameter who either refused or were unfit for surgery (Rendon et al. 2000). These patients were examined with serial abdominal imaging with US, CT, or MR imaging exams. Median follow-up was 27.9 months (range 5.3–143 months) with three or more observations per patient. Average overall growth rate was 0.1 cm/year. Five of these tumors were ultimately resected due to increases in size, and four were removed due to patient anxiety despite no change in size. Eight tumors were RCCs and one was an oncocytoma. Four of the RCCs were Fuhrman grade II, and two each were grades III and IV. Despite the fact that 11 of 32 masses (34%) doubled in volume within 1 year or achieved a diameter of 4 cm, none of the patients developed metastases or died of RCC. The authors concluded that one-third of small renal neoplasms grow under observation, but that growth is slow or undetectable in the majority. Rather than immediate surgery for small renal neoplasms, the authors proposed a period of cautious initial observation in selected patients, especially the elderly or infirm, with surgery reserved for those patients with rapid doubling times.

While the vast majority of renal tumors this size behave in a benign fashion, there have been multiple reports of metastases associated with them

(Amendola et al. 1988; Bell 1950; Curry et al. 1986; Hajdu and Thomas 1967; Talamo and Shonnard 1980). Aizawa et al. (1987) reported a retrospective study of 40 RCCs under 3 cm of which 7 (17.5%) had remote metastases at surgery or autopsy. Those which metastasized were associated with a more infiltrative growth pattern, solid or alveolar microscopic structure, granular or spindle cell type, atypical nuclei, lower nephron origin, and advanced patient age. Prognosis is poor once metastases have occurred with 5-year survival in the range of 5–10%.

A study of patients with renal cancer associated with uremic acquired cystic disease showed that some high-grade tumors doubled in volume in less than 6 months, with growth most pronounced in a solid pattern, grade III sarcomatous lesion (Takebayashi et al. 2000). Due to the variable growth rate of these neoplasms, the authors recommend an initial follow-up CT at 3 months to detect the most aggressive lesions, and again at 1-year intervals. Surgical resection was recommended for lesions with volume doubling times of less than 1 year, and immediate removal of tumors with volume doubling times of less than 6 months.

In another series illustrating the potential for aggressive clinical behavior of small renal carcinomas, 5 of 74 patients (7%) with tumors under 3 cm treated by radical nephrectomy had positive nodes or distant metastases at diagnosis (Eschwege et al. 1996). A report by Hsu et al. (2004) showed that of 50 renal lesions 3 cm or smaller, 19 tumors (38%)

had extension outside the renal capsule at the time of surgery (T3 or T4) and 14 (28%) possessed a high nuclear grade (Fuhrman grade III or IV). The majority (70%) of them were clear cell carcinoma with the rest (28%) composed of papillary or chromophobe tumors. This tendency toward higher grade and stage at presentation is distinctly greater than reported in previous series.

13.4
CT Imaging

13.4.1
Technical Considerations

Multiphasic helical CT is the standard methodology of renal mass detection and characterization, with US and MR imaging playing secondary roles. Even before the development of multidetector helical scanners, 95% of renal masses 8–15 mm in diameter and 74% of lesions smaller than 8 mm were detectable (Szolar et al. 1997). The current generation of 16-slice scanners allows much faster scanning, providing very thin-section images with reconstruction capabilities that allow even earlier detection and better characterization of renal masses.

Given an adequate intravenous bolus of contrast material, even very tiny renal lesions <5 mm are clearly visible. Characterization is much more difficult than detection, however, as it is necessary to accurately distinguish small simple cysts from solid renal neoplasms. This was a particular problem before helical CT scanners became widely available in the 1990s. Renal cysts are very common in older individuals. They are usually round, homogeneous, well-defined from the adjacent parenchyma, and have no calcification or significant wall thickening. Unfortunately, some renal tumors, particularly the smaller ones, share these features. It is never safe, therefore, to assume that lesions with these characteristics are simple cysts by their appearance alone (Fig. 13.5).

An objective way of assuring that a lesion is a cyst is to place an electronic cursor within it, which is easily accomplished at the CT console or with a picture-archiving system. Simple cyst fluid registers 0–20 Hounsfield units (HU; Bosniak and Rofsky 1996). When a mass shows higher values, comparison between pre-contrast and post-contrast images is crucial to determine if there is significant enhancement of the lesion. A cyst may exhibit density greater than water on the initial scan if it has

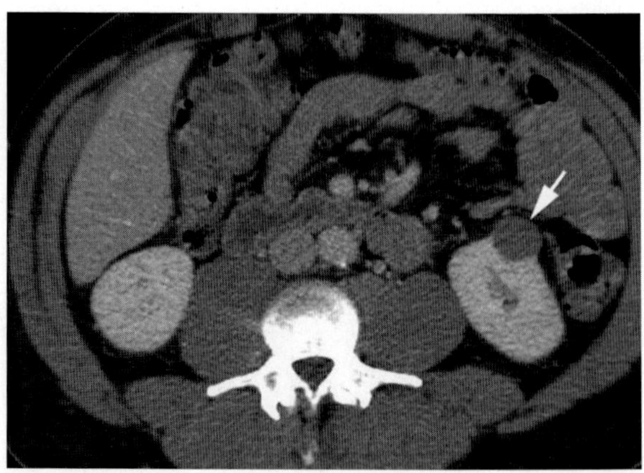

Fig. 13.5. Papillary type clear cell carcinoma in a 41-year-old man with flank pain. Axial contrast-enhanced CT scan shows a left 2.6 cm renal mass (*arrow*) which is homogeneous and superficially resembles a simple renal cortical cyst. It measured 45 HU, however, and showed enhancement of 20 HU from baseline unenhanced CT scan (not shown). Resected tumor was a papillary-type clear cell carcinoma, Fuhrman grade II/IV.

undergone internal hemorrhage. It would not be expected to change after intravenous contrast material is administered, however. An increase in density of more than 10–15 HU is considered evidence that tumoral microcirculation is distributing contrast within it (Fig. 13.6). In some cases, when a renal mass is incidentally detected on a single-phase CT performed for reasons unrelated to the kidneys, delayed images at 10 min can be obtained to see if the lesion de-enhances. Any hyperdense internal content within a hemorrhagic cyst would be expected to stay at the same density on delayed scans, whereas a neoplasm would be expected to show a decrease in density as the contrast washes out of it (Macari and Bosniak 1999).

One of the few clearly recognizable solid renal tumors on CT is AML, because the macroscopic fat content of this tumor has a characteristic negative density value (Figs. 13.7, 13.8). Even very small amounts of fat are detectable by pixel mapping. Unfortunately, in a small minority of these tumors, the muscle or angiomatous components predominate and these AMLs therefore cannot be distinguished from RCC (Fig. 13.9).

13.4.2
Lesion Pseudoenhancement

Unfortunately, the renal parenchyma surrounding a simple cyst has its own microcirculation distrib-

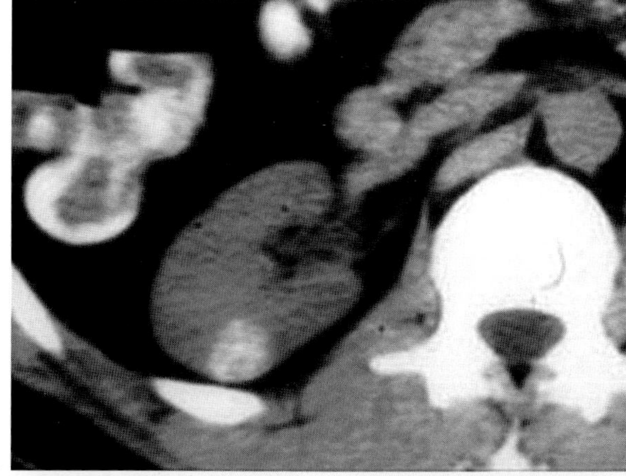

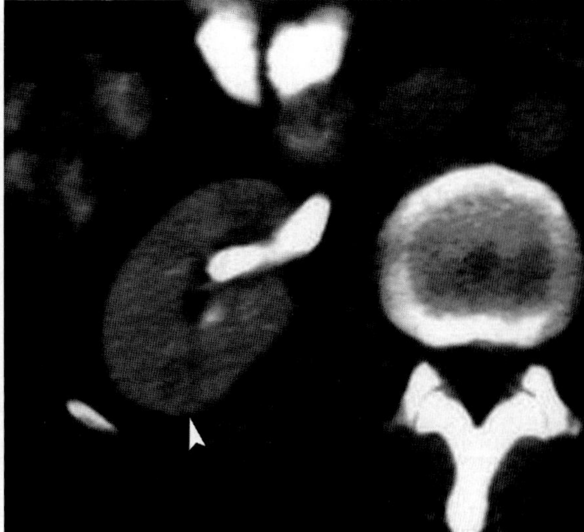

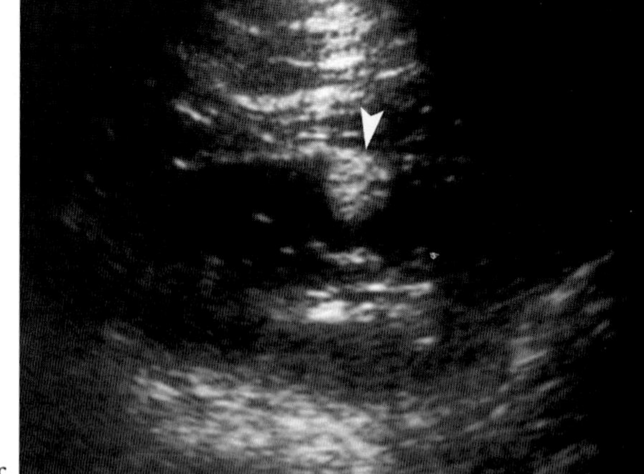

Fig. 13.6a-c. Hyperdense nodule in a 44-year-old man with surgically proven renal papillary adenocarcinoma. a Axial unenhanced CT scan shows incidentally found 1.8 cm hyperdense nodule (79 HU) in the right kidney. b Axial contrast-enhanced CT scan shows near isodensity with the enhancing renal parenchyma on excretory phase image (*arrowhead*). The lesion increased by 20 HU. c Sagittal US of the right kidney shows a highly echogenic lesion (*arrowhead*). (With permission from CURRY 1995; image courtesy of D. Cammoun)

uting contrast material. If the lesion does not fully occupy the slice in the craniocaudal plane, the inclusion of normal parenchyma in the measured density will create a partial volume effect, i.e., pseudoenhancement.

Pseudoenhancement is usually not a problem with large renal masses whose visibility on multiple sequential images allow cursor readings precisely at the z-axis center. It is still a problem, however, when small masses appear on only a few contiguous axial images. An optimized CT technique is crucial in the evaluation of small renal masses. With current helical scanners, a maximum slice thickness of 5 mm should be used. Four-, 8-, and 16-slice multidetector scanners allow 2.5- to 1.25-mm sections. These sections are usually fused to 5-mm thickness for primary viewing, but indeterminate small lesions can often be resolved by creating overlapping 1.25-mm reconstructions (Fig. 13.10). In a recent report, multidetector CT images of kidneys scanned at 4×2.5-mm collimation were used to compare two types of reconstruction: 3 mm at 1.5-mm increments (with overlap) and the standard protocol of 5-mm thick-

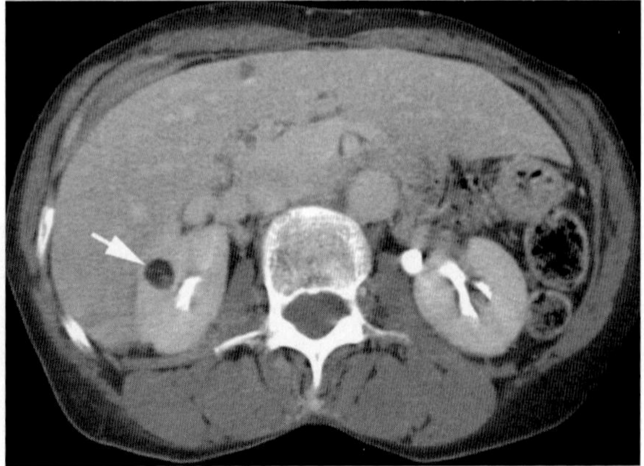

Fig. 13.7. Incidental small sporadic angiomyolipoma of the right kidney in a 69-year-old woman. Axial contrast-enhanced CT scan shows a lesion with very low density (–61 HU; *arrow*) consistent with macroscopic fat.

ness at 5-mm increments (without overlap). Twenty-eight additional lesions were detected using the thin-section overlapping protocol (JINZAKI et al. 2004).

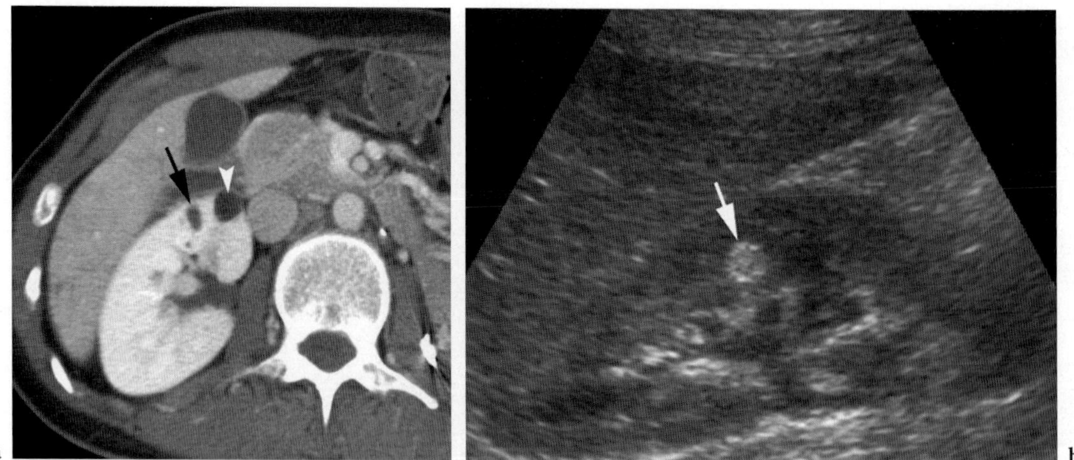

Fig. 13.8a,b. Tuberous sclerosis in a 37-year-old woman. **a** Axial contrast-enhanced CT scan shows two small (5 and 10 mm) angiomyolipomas of the right kidney that measured –70 HU (*arrow*) and –80 HU (*arrowhead*). **b** Sagittal ultrasound shows a hyperechoic 1-cm angiomyolipoma in another part of the same right kidney (*arrow*).

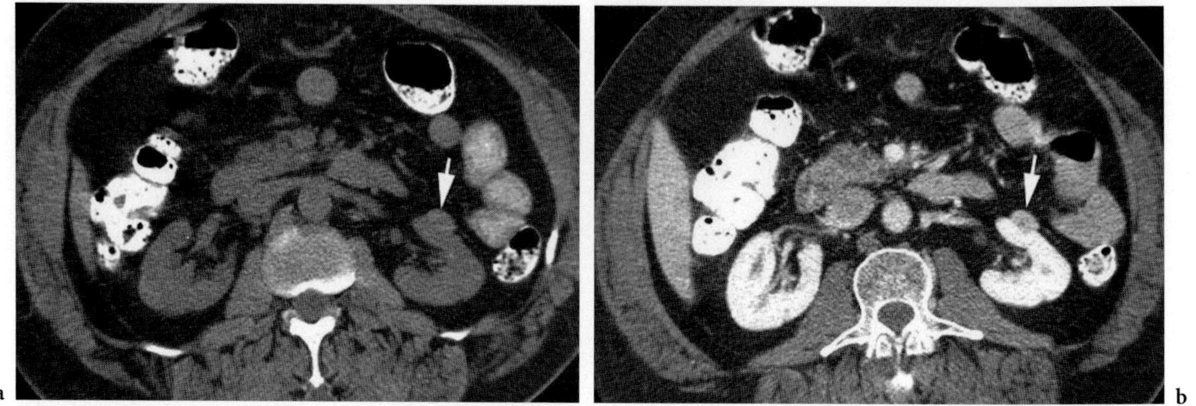

Fig. 13.9a,b. Angiomyolipoma without macroscopic fat in a 61-year-old woman. **a** Axial unenhanced CT scan shows a 1.7×1.4 cm exophytic lesion of the anterior left kidney (*arrow*). The lesion measures 66 HU. **b** Axial contrast-enhanced CT scan at the same level as **a** shows tumor enhancement to 103 HU (*arrow*). Laparoscopically resected tumor showed microscopic fat only.

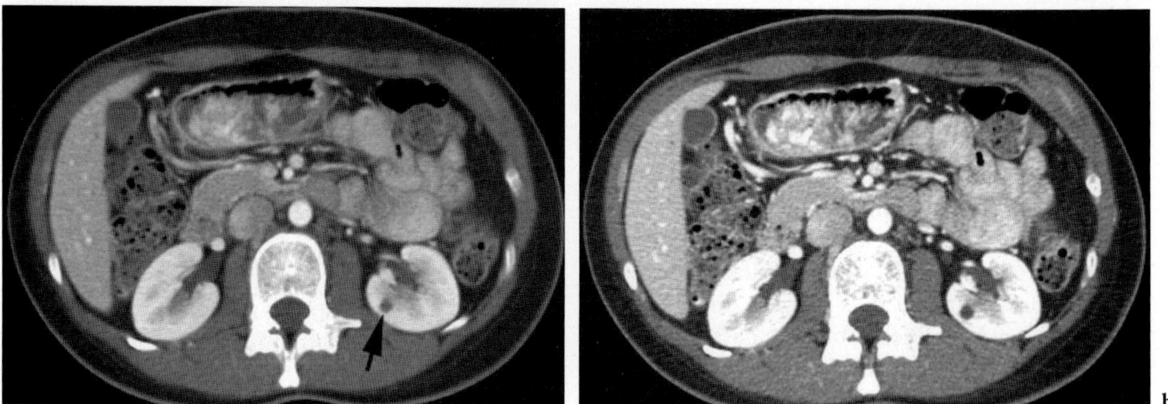

Fig. 13.10a,b. Simple cyst in a 42-year-old woman with breast cancer in whom an overlapping thin-section reconstruction on 16-slice MDCT was performed to evaluate an indeterminate small renal mass. **a** Axial contrast-enhanced CT scan shows 6 mm hypodensity in the left kidney (*arrow*) which measures 48 HU, not consistent with a simple cyst. **b** Axial 1.25-mm reconstructed CT image with repeat measurement of 6 HU confirms that the lesion is a cyst.

Despite the ability to create very thin sections, however, there is still a problem with pseudoenhancement in very small lesions in the range of 5–15 mm in diameter for both single-detector helical CT and multidetector scanners, both in vitro and in vivo (BAE et al. 2000; BIRNBAUM et al. 2002). A recent in vitro study suggests that the problem is greater with multidetector CT (MDCT), particularly those with matrix array detector design, and that the effect is more pronounced the smaller the lesion and the greater the surrounding enhancement (ABDULLA et al. 2002). For cysts smaller than 1 cm in diameter, density differences of 12–33 HU can be seen at high background density. Scanning fluid-filled tubular phantoms, ABDULLA et al. (2002) showed that the partial-volume effect was probably not responsible. They speculated that beam-hardening effects and differing reconstruction algorithms are responsible and suggested allowing a higher limit to the level of pseudoenhancement. BIRNBAUM et al. (2002) also suggest raising the threshold level of enhancement to 20 HU when characterizing lesions <1.5 cm. This approach would, however, reduce the sensitivity of the examination to detect hypovascular renal tumors. It is known that well-differentiated papillary RCCs show relatively low contrast enhancement because of their intrinsic hypovascularity (HERTS et al. 2002; JINZAKI et al. 2000).

This element of uncertainty is reflected in a clinical study of interobserver variability in assessing lesions for enhancement, an effect most frequently observed for lesions in the range of 1.0–1.5 cm in size (SIEGEL et al. 1999). JINZAKI's study showed that with the use of MDCT and thin overlapping reconstructions, 84% (38 of 45) of masses between 5 and 10 mm could be characterized as cysts using the established contrast-enhanced threshold value of 20 HU (JINZAKI et al. 2000). Even this methodology has its limits, however. Although 5 mm and smaller lesions were detectable, most below that size could not be characterized.

13.4.3
Multiphasic CT Imaging

Another advantage of the development of multislice CT is the ability to image the kidneys in different physiologic stages of contrast excretion. There are several time-dependent post-contrast phases of enhancement which provide information germane to renal mass evaluation. The early arterial phase is reserved for cases in which surgical planning requires information on the number and location of vessels supplying the mass. The subsequent early cortical nephrogram phase exhibits well-defined corticomedullary differentiation with intense cortical opacification contrasting with the unopacified medulla. This is the phase commonly seen in CT studies of the abdomen in which the kidneys are not the primary focus. Thereafter, a uniform nephrogram phase develops as the medulla opacifies, and finally, an excretory phase occurs as the pyelocalyceal structures begin to fill with contrast.

The conspicuity of different types of renal tumor varies with the degree of vascularity and location in the parenchyma. Small hypovascular masses are difficult to discern in the early cortical phase unless they extend into the adjacent cortex (Fig. 13.11). Some small hypervascular tumors may enhance to

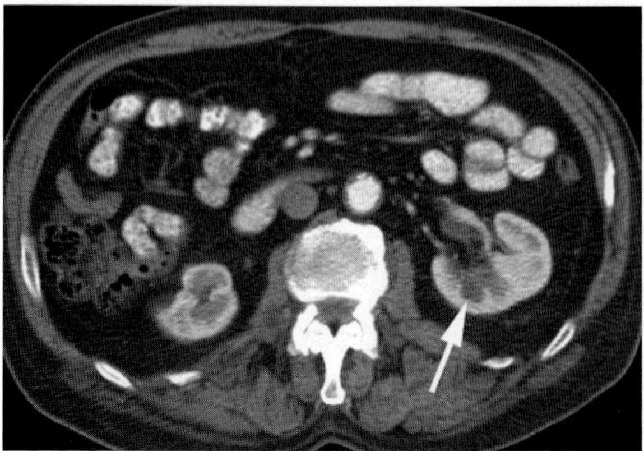
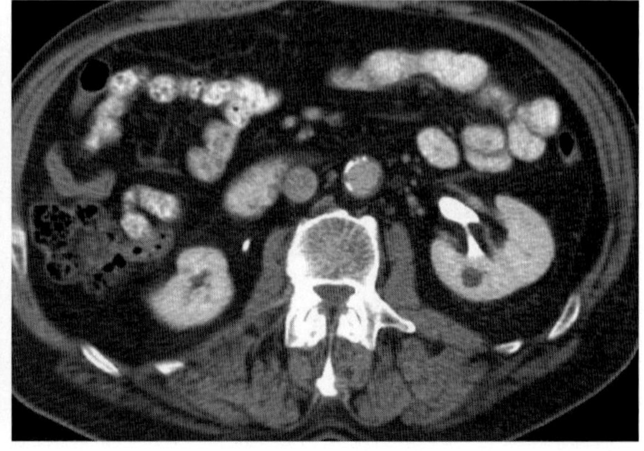

a   b

Fig. 13.11a,b. Conspicuity of small medullary masses on early vs later phase of excretion in a 47-year-old man undergoing CT for evaluation of hematuria. **a** Axial contrast-enhanced CT scan at early corticomedullary differentiation phase of contrast excretion shows 1 cm hypodensity in the posterior left kidney (*arrow*) which blends into the unopacified medulla. **b** The lesion is easily identified on excretory phase imaging and reconstructed thin sections determined it is a cyst.

the same degree as the opacified adjacent cortex, effectively camouflaging themselves from detection (Fig. 13.12). In end-stage kidneys with poor perfusion, however, small tumors may be more conspicuous since there is a higher achievable density difference between the tumor and diminished background parenchymal enhancement (Fig. 13.13; Takebayashi et al. 1999). Tumors with similar histology may exhibit differing enhancement characteristics depending on the degree of associated vascularity and necrosis (Fig. 13.14).

The excretory phase is most useful in the identification and staging of upper tract transitional cell carcinoma (Fig. 13.15). This tumor appears as a central area of high density in the renal pelvis or infundibulum on scans without contrast. After intravenous contrast, it exhibits only mildly increased density, corresponding to the hypovascular nature of these tumors. In the excretory phase transitional cell carcinoma creates solid or irregular filling defects in the expanded collecting system. Larger or infiltrative lesions may involve the adjacent parenchyma (Urban et al. 1997).

The phases of enhancement described above overlap and are variable in onset and duration depending on injection rate, volume of contrast used, and

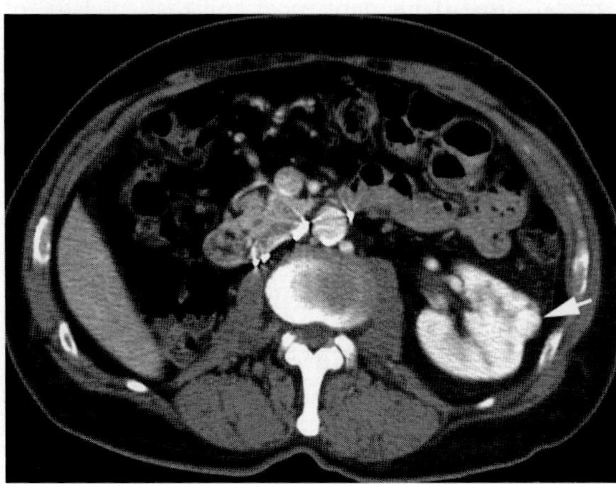

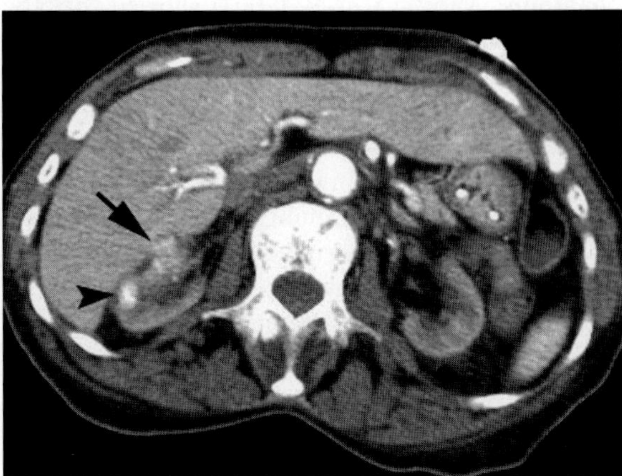

Fig. 13.12. Hypervascular mass difficult to discern on early phase of enhancement in a 79-year-old man. Axial contrast-enhanced CT scan shows intensely enhancing 1.8 cm mass (*arrow*), protruding from the lateral cortex of the left kidney, which nearly matches the adjacent normal renal cortex. Clear cell carcinoma treated by laparoscopic cryoablation.

Fig. 13.13. Conspicuous hypervascular masses in a 66-year-old woman with end-stage renal disease. Axial contrast-enhanced CT scan at early arterial phase shows renal atrophy bilaterally with poor cortical perfusion. An intensely enhancing 9 mm nodule is present in the right kidney (*arrowhead*) with a larger, but less enhancing, lesion anterior to it (*arrow*).

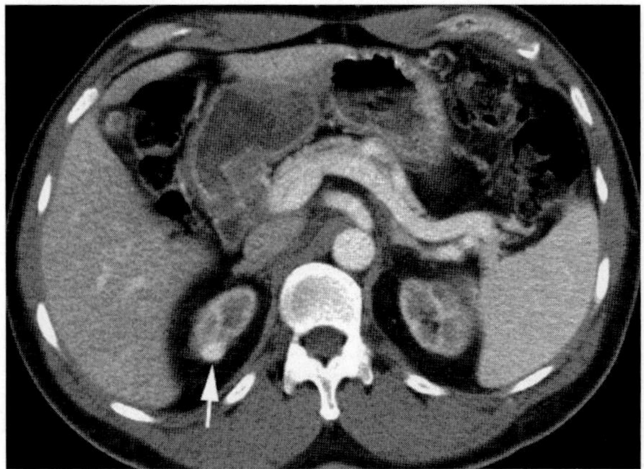

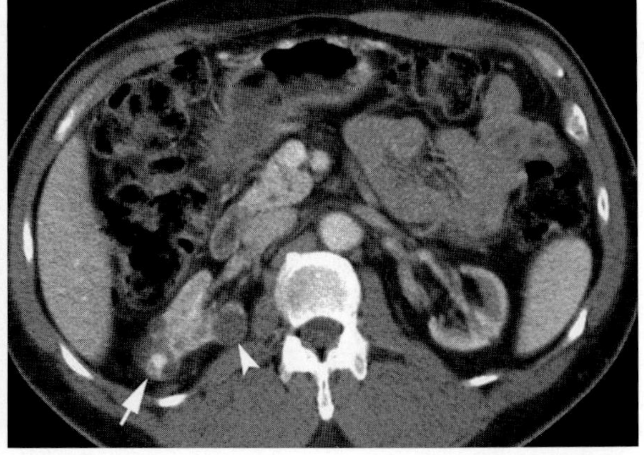

a

b

Fig. 13.14a,b. End-stage renal disease in a 57-year-old woman on dialysis with hematuria. **a** Axial contrast-enhanced CT scan shows a homogeneously enhancing 7 mm nodule in the right upper pole (*arrow*). **b** Axial contrast-enhanced CT scan at mid-kidney level shows a heterogeneously enhancing nodule within a partially cystic mass posteriorly (*arrow*) and a poorly enhancing mass medially (*arrowhead*); all three were clear cell carcinomas. (With permission from Curry 2002)

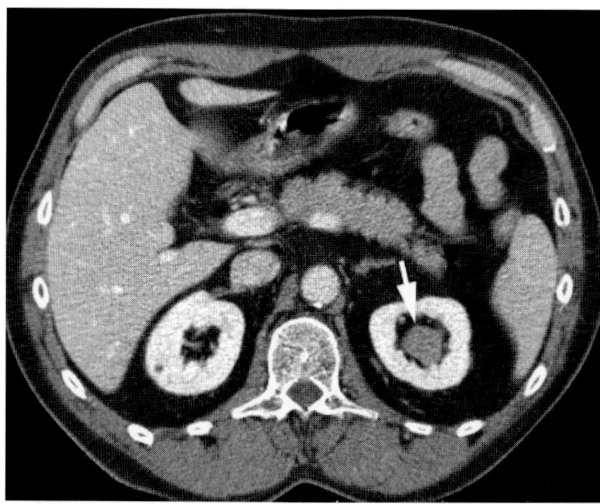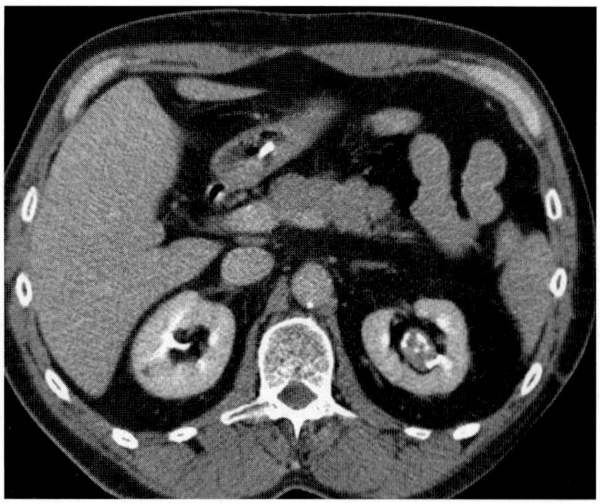

Fig. 13.15a,b. Transitional cell carcinoma in a 65-year-old man with gross painless hematuria. **a** Axial contrast-enhanced CT scan shows a central lesion in the left kidney (*arrow*) surrounded by renal sinus fat with density higher than urine (30 HU). **b** Excretory phase CT scan shows contrast filling interstices of tumor of the upper renal pelvis.

patient factors such as cardiac output. Probably the highest tumor detection yield is obtained when CT imaging is used in the homogeneous nephrographic phase (SILVERMAN et al.1994; SZOLAR et al. 1997; YUH and COHAN 1999).

13.4.4
CT Characteristics of Small Renal Masses

There is scant information on the CT features of small RCCs. In a review of CT features of 78 pathologically proven RCC tumors, eight were 3 cm in diameter or less (ZAGORIA et al. 1990); of these, one showed evidence of necrosis and one had distant metastases. The majority of small tumors in this series had a distinct tumor–parenchymal interface and none exhibited calcification. The authors therefore cautioned that small malignant renal tumors often have a benign appearance on incremental (non-helical) CT.

A Japanese study of 36 small RCC tumors compared cellular architecture with CT findings (YAMASHITA et al. 1992). The solid lesions (mostly clear cell carcinomas) were iso- or hypodense on unenhanced CT, whereas the papillary or tubular types (all granular cell) were iso- to slightly hyperdense (Fig. 13.6). Most of the tumors were homogeneous in appearance both before and after contrast, but 10 (28%) showed intratumoral necrosis, differing from ZAGORIA et al. (1990) study. Solid architecture tumors showed significantly higher contrast enhancement

than the papillary or tubular tumors. Calcification was rare, occurring in only one tumor.

A later study retrospectively evaluated imaging characteristics of 35 renal masses under 3 cm in size obtained with more advanced helical CT techniques (SILVERMAN et al. 1994). Twenty-seven of these masses proved to be RCC and the others were transitional cell carcinoma (2), leiomyoma (1), angiomyolipoma (1), and benign cysts (4). The findings were similar to incremental CT in that most of the small RCCs were non-calcified homogeneous masses which showed an initial density of 20 HU or greater and enhanced with contrast by at least 10 HU. Septations were underestimated in three cases and septate lesions were interpreted as solid in two cases. The authors concluded that many of the difficulties in the analysis of renal masses are not solved by helical CT imaging.

In 2000, a study of 40 surgically resected renal neoplasms evaluated enhancement patterns using a double-phase helical CT protocol (JINZAKI et al. 2000). The study found that the degree of enhancement in the corticomedullary differentiation phase correlated with microvessel density and that not all tumors with homogeneous enhancement showed necrosis or hemorrhage on histologic evaluation. Although enhancement patterns differed among the subtypes of RCC, with clear cell carcinomas showing greater peak enhancement in this phase than chromophobe or papillary RCC, it was not possible to differentiate benign oncocytomas from metanephric adenomas in the series. This result is not

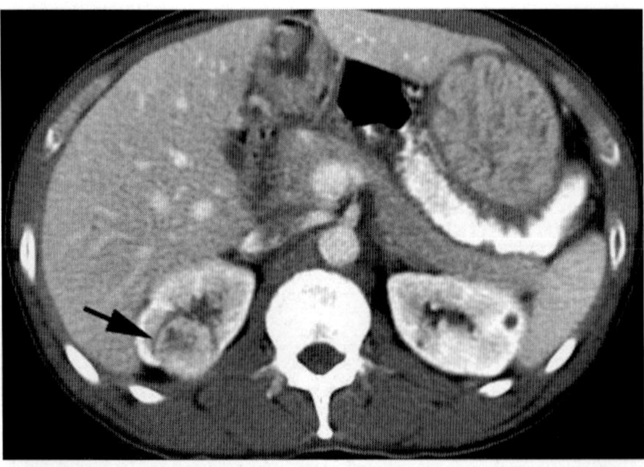

Fig. 13.16. Hypervascular tumor in a 54-year-old man. Axial contrast-enhanced CT scan shows 2.5 cm mass in the upper pole of the right kidney (*arrow*). Pathologist could not distinguish between oncocytoma or chromophobe RCC because the resected tumor had features supportive of both types of tumor.

surprising, given that it is difficult for pathologists to determine whether a neoplasm with oncocytic features is benign or malignant (Figs. 13.16, 13.17).

In a study on differentiation of subtypes of RCC using biphasic and monophasic helical CT, KIM et al. (2004) found that heterogeneous or predominantly peripheral enhancement was typical of small clear cell carcinomas, whereas most papillary and chromophobe tumor subtypes showed homogeneous enhancement.

Another 2004 study of renal masses evaluated with MDCT showed that the newer scanner technology and thin overlapping reconstructions make it easier to distinguish cysts, reducing the number of indeterminate small renal masses. It has not been proven, however, that solid lesions or cystic lesions with septa or nodularity <1 cm in size can be characterized (JINZAKI et al. 2004).

13.5
MR Imaging of Small Renal Masses

Magnetic resonance imaging was not used initially as the primary method of investigation of renal masses, in part because of limitations in detection with conventional spin-echo sequences. Since the signal intensity of solid tumors can resemble that of normal renal parenchyma on both T1- and T2-weighted images, there is only a 63% renal tumor detection rate at a size less than 3 cm in diameter (SEMELKA et al. 1991). This limitation, coupled with other factors such as slow scan times, limited availability and cost, initially restricted MR imaging to patients with renal failure and iodine or contrast sensitivity (Figs. 13.18, 13.19); however, recent advances in MR imaging with dynamic gadolinium enhancement, fat suppression, and surface coils, have made detection and characterization of small lesions possible (Fig. 13.20; PRETORIUS et al. 1999). In a retrospective review of MR imaging signal characteristics of 35 lesions of this size (20 RCCs and 15 benign lesions), enhancement made it simple to differentiate hypervascular RCCs from hypovascular tumors and benign lesions (SCIALPI et al. 2000). Hypovascular tumors and benign lesions could not be distinguished, however, on simple observation and required quantitative evaluation of signal intensity profiles and contrast-to-noise ratios.

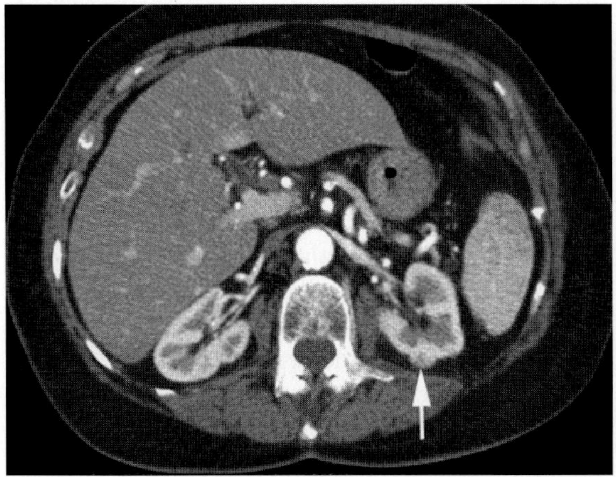

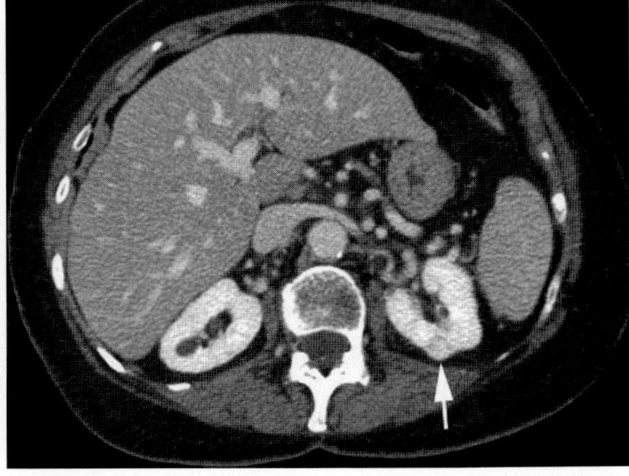

a b

Fig. 13.17a,b. Oncocytoma in a 75-year-old woman with history of breast carcinoma. **a** Axial contrast-enhanced CT scan at corticomedullary differentiation phase incidentally detects a 1.5 cm left renal mass (*arrow*). **b** This mass is better seen at nephrogram phase (*arrow*). Core biopsy pathology prior to radiofrequency ablation was consistent with oncocytoma rather than granular cell or chromophobe carcinoma.

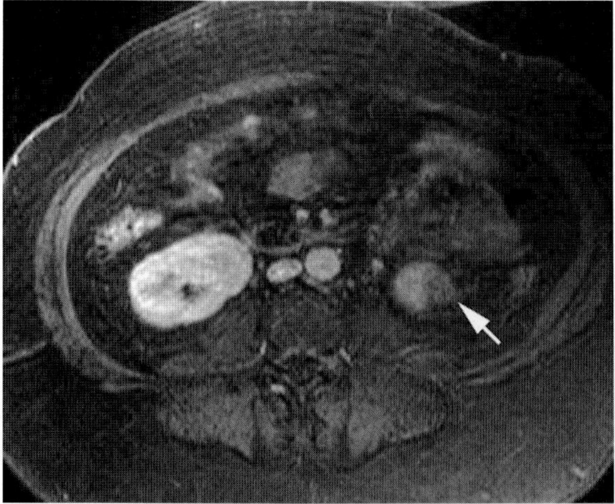

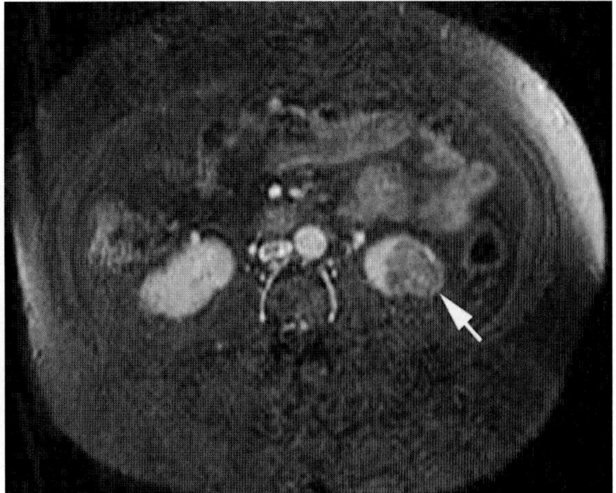

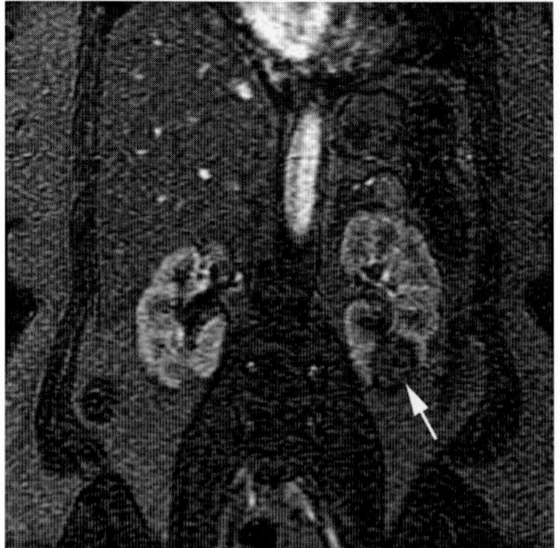

Fig. 13.18a-c. Hyperdense lesion in the lower pole of the left kidney on unenhanced CT (not shown) in a 57-year-old woman with renal insufficiency. a Axial delayed post-gadolinium fat-suppressed T1-weighted MR image shows a 2.1×1.8 cm heterogeneously enhancing mass of the left lower pole (*arrow*). b A similar image obtained 3 years later shows an increase in size of the mass to 3.1×2.4 cm (*arrow*). c Coronal immediate post-gadolinium fat-suppressed T1-weighted MR image shows tumor extent (*arrow*). (With permission from CURRY 2002)

13.6
Ultrasound of Small Renal Masses

Ultrasound is less accurate in detecting and characterizing small renal neoplasms than CT or MR imaging. A study of 20 patients with von Hippel-Lindau disease, genetically predisposed to developing cysts and solid tumors of the kidney, showed that US was able to detect only 70% of lesions 2 cm in diameter, whereas CT detected 95% (JAMIS-DOW et al. 1996). Size was a more important factor than cystic vs solid nature. Most RCCs are hypoechoic to normal renal parenchyma, but some are isoechoic and therefore undetectable unless they protrude significantly from the kidney surface. Nearly one-third of small RCC tumors are hyperechoic and may be mistaken for a benign AML (Fig. 13.6; FORMAN et al. 1993). In these cases the presence of an anechoic rim or central cystic areas are US features which suggest RCC over AML (SIEGEL et al. 1996).

13.7
Fine-Needle Aspiration and Biopsy of Small Renal Masses

Fine-needle aspiration and core biopsy are useful techniques in the evaluation of extrarenal tumors but are not routinely used in the kidney. Most studies show that imaging diagnosis is more accurate, and complications, although rare, such as hemorrhage, pneumothorax, or needle-tract seeding, may occur (ZAGORIA 2000). Fine-needle aspirates of small renal lesions may not yield enough tissue for definitive diagnosis and cellular heterogeneity and the potential for sampling error contribute to uncertainty (CAMPBELL et al. 1997). Core biopsies do not yield any improved benefit in the kidney. A prospective series determining the accuracy of core biopsies of renal lesions obtained intraoperatively reported a false-negative rate of 20% and a false-positive rate of 34% (DECHET et al. 1999). A retrospective study of percu-

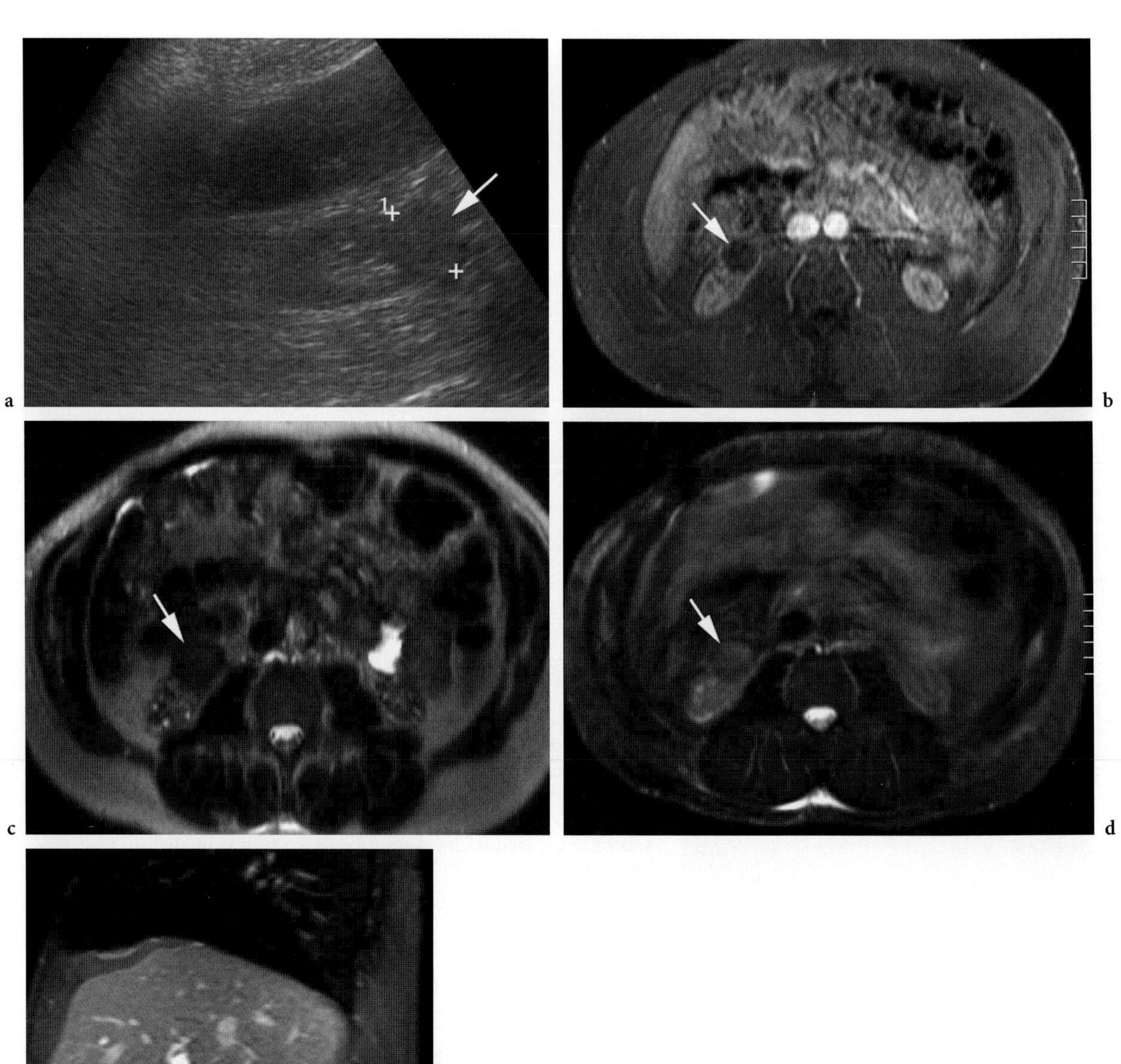

Fig. 13.19a-e. End-stage renal disease and renal transplant in a 46-year-old man with chronic hematuria. **a** Transverse US image shows a 2.4 cm echogenic lesion in the small, native right kidney (*arrow*). **b** Axial contrast-enhanced fat-suppressed T1-weighted, **c** axial non fat-suppressed T2-weighted, **d** axial fat-suppressed T2-weighted, and **e** sagittal contrast-enhanced fat-suppressed T1-weighted MR images show a non hyperenhancing, non-fatty mass of the right lower pole (*arrow*), which proved at nephrectomy to be a chromophobe type RCC with papillary growth pattern (Fuhrman grade II/IV).

taneous biopsies of renal masses showed that four of ten false-negative results for RCC occurred in lesions of 3 cm diameter or less (RYBICKI et al. 2003).

There may, however, be a role for biopsy in the case of small lesions whose imaging evaluation is equivocal and in which the patient has been referred for percutaneous ablation of a presumed cancer. Since as many as 37% of patients referred for such treatment may have benign masses, biopsy may be appropriate to avoid an invasive procedure (TUNCALI et al. 2004). Biopsy of renal masses is also appropriate in problem cases, such as the presence of a non-renal primary tumor or lymphoma where treatment decisions would be altered by the outcome (Figs. 13.21–13.24).

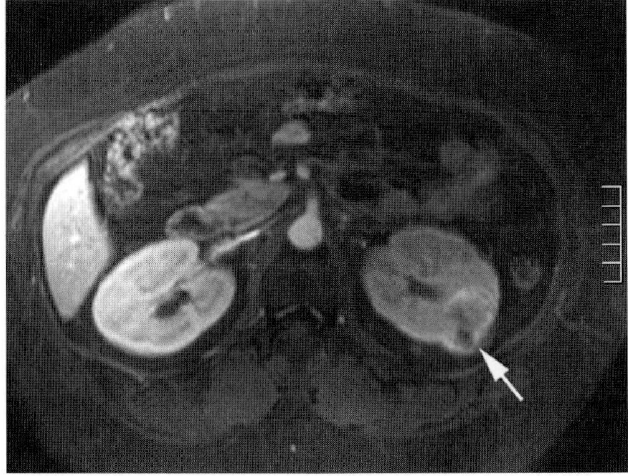

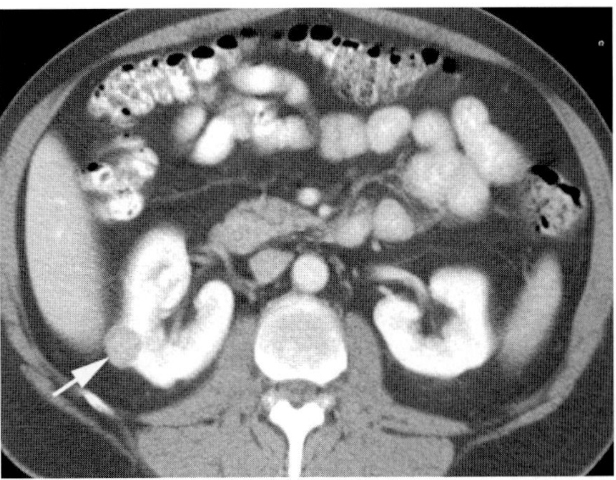

Fig. 13.20. Complex left upper pole renal lesion on ultrasound exam (not shown) in a 53-year-old woman with pancreatitis. Axial contrast-enhanced fat-suppressed T1-weighted MR image shows a 2.5 cm left heterogeneously enhancing mass which proved to be a Fuhrman grade III clear cell carcinoma at surgery (*arrow*).

Fig. 13.21. Renal cell carcinoma in a 51-year-old man with melanoma of the ear. Axial contrast-enhanced CT scan shows 1.9 cm tumor of the right kidney (*arrow*). Pathology yielded a clear cell carcinoma (Fuhrman grade I/IV).

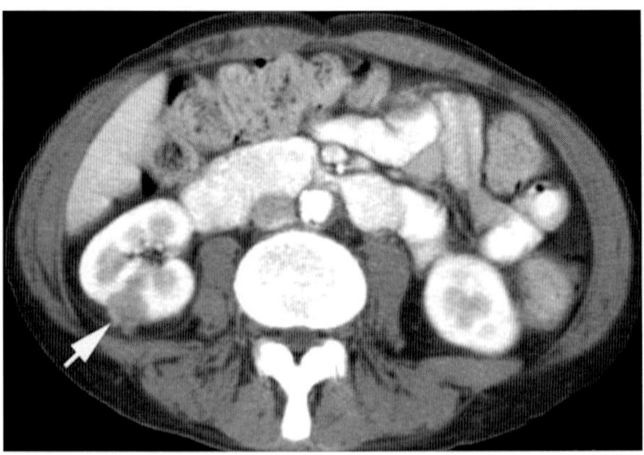

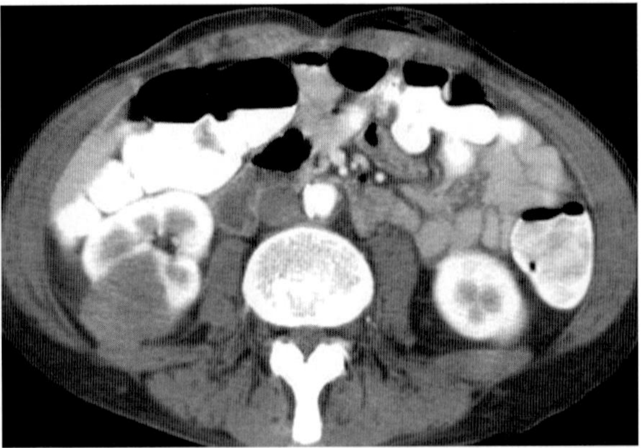

Fig. 13.22a,b. Renal metastasis from small cell lung cancer in a 51-year-old man. **a** Initial axial contrast-enhanced CT scan shows solitary small right posterior renal mass (*arrow*). **b** Axial contrast-enhanced CT scan one month later shows the mass increased strikingly in size.

13.8
Treatment Options

Small renal neoplasms may be treated by wedge resection, partial nephrectomy, laparoscopic surgery, or percutaneous tumor ablation techniques such as cryotherapy and radiofrequency ablation. The percutaneous approaches reduce morbidity and convalescence time. They are still invasive procedures, however, and not all small renal neoplasms are destined to behave aggressively. If the object of surgery is to remove a tumor which is life threatening, there ought to be guidelines for selecting which lesions should be treated and which should undergo careful observation.

Is the detection of very small solid renal lesions of 1–1.5 cm size important? Does resection/ablation of neoplasms of this size lead to a cancer-free, longer life? These questions about the effect of discovery on mortality point to biases built into such speculation (BLACK and LING 1990; BOSNIAK 1995). If the lesion is destined to grow slowly and the patient dies of unrelated causes, length of time bias is introduced. If the lesion is of questionable malignant potential, overdiagnosis bias exists. If very small lesions are by nature highly aggressive, and destined to end the patient's life, finding them earlier probably does not influence the ultimate outcome (lead-time bias).

BOSNIAK (1995) advocates observation for lesions less than 2 cm in diameter in patients who are

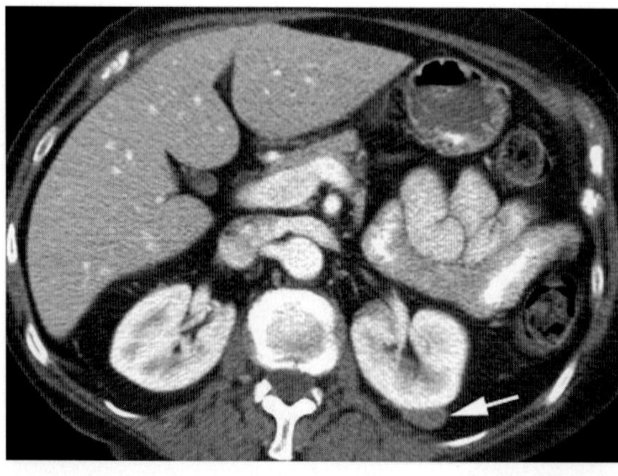

Fig. 13.23 Isolated renal lymphoma in a 71-year-old woman with abdominal pain. Axial contrast-enhanced CT scan shows a small left renal mass (*arrow*). The mass was percutaneously biopsied and was found to be B-cell non-Hodgkin lymphoma.

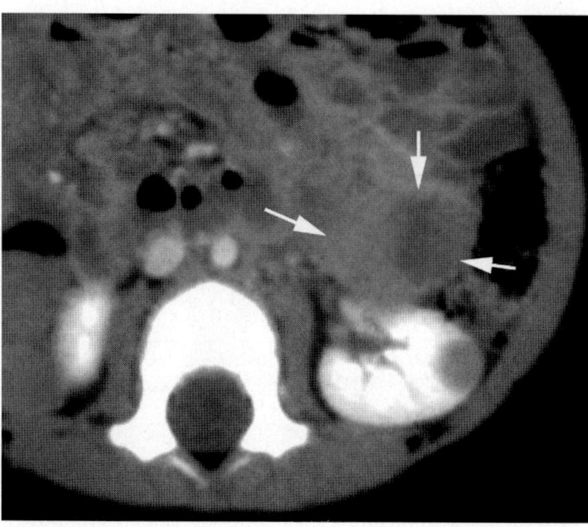

Fig. 13.24 Metastatic neuroblastoma in an 18-month-old boy presenting with leg pain. Axial contrast-enhanced CT scan shows an enhancing (83 HU) 1 cm solid lesion in the left kidney. A metastasis was present in the femur. The lower margin of an adrenal mass extends anterior to the kidney (*arrows*). Lesions were biopsy proven. (With permission from Curry 1995)

elderly or poor surgical risks. He would extend this to 2.5–3.0 cm during the observation period so that growth rate can be assessed periodically. He suggests follow-up studies at 6- to 12-month intervals, with the interval determined by growth rate. If the lesion is growing significantly and resection can be performed, surgery would then be justified. He warns, however, that observation should be reserved for homogeneous, well-defined, non-necrotic tumors, since necrotic tumors tend to be more aggressive. Observation is not justified in a young, healthy

patient who is found to have a tumor of >1.5–2.0 cm. Although these masses may show indolent growth, they should be resected at discovery to avoid the risk that the lesion will grow rapidly and metastasize.

13.9
Conclusion

Radiologists frequently encounter small renal masses in daily practice. Most are small benign cysts which are difficult to characterize because of their size. With modern cross-sectional imaging techniques, however, it is possible to distinguish most of these from true renal neoplasms. The small renal neoplasms that contain fat or reside within the collecting system of the kidney are easily identified and managed appropriately. The remainder of enhancing, small solid renal masses continue to be a challenge. Since their histologic make-up and biologic behavior cannot be accurately predicted by imaging, a choice of nephron-sparing surgical or percutaneous ablation techniques vs "watchful waiting" are rational options for management. The appropriate course of action depends heavily on individual patient factors.

References

Abdulla C, Kalra MK, Saini S et al. (2002) Pseudoenhancement of simulated renal cysts in a phantom using different multidetector CT scanners. Am J Roentgenol 179:1473–1476

Aizawa S, Suzuki M, Kikuchi Y et al. (1987) Clinicopathological study on small renal cell carcinomas with metastases. Acta Pathol Jpn 37:947–954

Amendola MA, Bree RL, Pollack HM et al. (1988) Small renal cell carcinomas: resolving a diagnostic dilemma. Radiology 166:637–641

Bae KT, Heiken JP, Siegel CL et al. (2000) Renal cysts: Is attenuation artifactually increased on contrast-enhanced CT images? Radiology 216:792–796

Bell ET (ed) (1950) Tumors of the kidney. In: Renal diseases. Lea and Febiger, Philadelphia

Bennington JL (1973) Cancer of the kidney: etiology, epidemiology, and pathology. Cancer 32:1017–1029

Bennington JL (1987) Renal adenoma. World J Urol 5:66–70

Birnbaum BA, Maki DD, Chakraborty DP et al. (2002) Renal cyst pseudoenhancement evaluation with an anthropomorphic body CT phantom. Radiology 225:83–90

Black WC, Ling A (1990) Is earlier diagnosis really better? The misleading effects of lead time and length time biases. Am J Roentgenol 155:625–630

Bosniak MA (1995) Observation of small incidentally detected renal masses. Semin Urol Oncol 13:267–272

Bosniak MA, Rofsky NM (1996) Problems in the detection and characterization of small renal masses. Radiology 198:638–641

Bosniak MA, Birnbaum BA, Krinsky GA et al. (1995) Small renal parenchymal neoplasms: further observations on growth. Radiology 197:589–597

Campbell SC, Novick AC, Herts B et al. (1997) Prospective evaluation of fine needle aspiration of small, solid renal masses: accuracy and morbidity. Urology 50:25–29

Curry NS (1995) Small renal masses (lesions smaller than 3 cm): imaging evaluation and management. Am J Roentgenol 164:355–362

Curry NS (2002) Imaging the small solid renal mass. Abdom Imaging 27:629–636

Curry NS, Schabel, SI, Betsill WL (1986) Small renal neoplasms: diagnostic imaging, pathologic features, and clinical course. Radiology 158:113–117

Dechet CB, Sebo T, Farrow G et al. (1999) Prospective analysis of intraoperative frozen needle biopsy of solid renal masses in adults. J Urol 162:1282–1285

Ellis WJ, Bauer KD, Oyasu R et al. (1992) Flow cytometric analysis of small renal tumors. J Urol 148:1774–1777

Eschwege P, Saussine C, Steichen B et al. (1996) Radical nephrectomy for renal cell carcinoma 30 mm or less: long-term follow-up results. J Urol 155:1196–1199

Fielding JR, Visweswaran A, Silverman S et al. (1999) CT and ultrasound features of metanephric adenoma in adults with pathologic correlation. J Comput Assist Tomogr 23:441–444

Forman HP, Middleton WD, Melson GL et al. (1993) Hyperechoic renal cell carcinomas: increase in detection at US. Radiology 188:431–434

Hajdu SI, Thomas AG (1967) Renal cell carcinoma at autopsy. J Urol 97:978–982

Herts BR, Coll DM, Novick AC et al. (2002) Enhancement characteristics of papillary renal neoplasms revealed on triphasic helical CT of the kidneys. Am J Roentgenol 178:367–372

Hsu RM, Chan DY, Siegelman SS (2004) Small renal cell carcinomas: correlation of size with tumor stage, nuclear grade, and histologic subtype. Am J Roentgenol 182:551–557

Jamis-Dow CA, Choyke PL, Jennings SB et al. (1996) Small (≤3 cm) renal masses: detection with CT versus US and pathologic correlation. Radiology 198:785–788

Jinzaki M, Tanimoto A, Mukai M et al. (2000) Double-phase helical CT of small renal parenchymal neoplasms: correlation with pathologic findings and tumor angiogenesis. J Comput Assist Tomogr 24:835–842

Jinzaki M, McTavish JD, Zou KH et al. (2004) Evaluation of small (≤3 cm) renal masses with MDCT: benefits of thin overlapping reconstructions. Am J Roentgenol 183:223–228

Kim JJ, Kim TK, Han JA et al. (2004) Differentiation of subtypes of renal cell carcinoma on helical CT scans. Am J Roentgenol 178:1499–1506

Levine E, Huntrakoon M, Wetzel CH (1989) Small renal neoplasms: clinical pathologic and imaging features. Am J Roentgenol 153:69–73

Macari M, Bosniak MA (1999) Delayed CT to evaluate renal masses incidentally discovered at contrast-enhanced CT: demonstration of vascularity with deenhancement. Radiology 213:674–680

Petersen RO (1992) Kidney: neoplastic disorders. In: Petersen RO (ed) Urologic pathology. Lippincott, Philadelphia, p 77

Pretorius ES, Siegelman ES, Ramchandani P et al. (1999) Renal neoplasms amenable to partial nephrectomy: MR imaging. Radiology 212:28–34

Reis M, Faria V, Lindoro J et al. (1988) The small cystic and noncystic noninflammatory renal nodules: a postmortem study. J Urol 140:721–723

Rendon RA, Stanietzky N, Panzarella T et al. (2000) The natural history of small renal masses. J Urol 164:1143–1147

Rybicki FJ, Shu KM, Cibas ES et al. (2003) Percutaneous biopsy of renal masses: sensitivity and negative predictive value stratified by clinical setting and size of masses. Am J Roentgenol 180:1281–1287

Scialpi M, DiMaggio A, Midiri M et al. (2000) Small renal masses: assessment of lesion characterization and vascularity on dynamic contrast-enhanced MR imaging with fat suppression. Am J Roentgenol 175:751–757

Semelka RC, Hricak H, Stevens SK et al. (1991) Combined gadolinium-enhanced and fat saturation MR imaging of renal masses. Radiology 178:803–809

Siegel CL, Middleton WD, Teefey SA et al. (1996) Angiomyolipoma and renal cell carcinoma: US differentiation. Radiology 198:785–788

Siegel CL, Fisher AJ, Bennett HF (1999) Interobserver variability in determining enhancement of renal masses on helical CT. Am J Roentgenol 172:1207–1212

Silverman SG, Lee BY, Seltzer SE et al. (1994) Small (≤to 3 cm) renal masses: correlation of spiral CT features and pathologic findings. Am J Roentgenol 163:597–605

Smith SJ, Bosniak MA, Megibow AJ et al. (1989) Renal cell carcinoma: earlier discovery and increased detection. Radiology 170:699–703

Someren A, Zaatari GS, Campbell WG et al. (1989) Tumors of differentiated tubular epithelium: renal "adenoma" and adenocarcinoma. In: Someren A (ed) Urologic pathology with clinical and radiologic correlations. Macmillan, New York, pp 162–163

Steinberg AP, Lin CH, Matin S et al. (2003) Impact of tumor size on laparoscopic partial nephrectomy: analysis of 163 patients (Abstract). J Urol 169 (Suppl):174a

Szolar DH, Kammerhuber F, Altzieber S et al. (1997) Multiphasic helical CT of the kidney: increased conspicuity for detection and characterization of small (<3 cm) renal masses. Radiology 201:211–217

Takebayashi S, Hidai H, Chiba T et al. (1999) Using helical CT to evaluate renal cell carcinoma in patients undergoing hemodialysis: value of early enhanced images. Am J Roentgenol 172:429–433

Takebayashi S, Hidai H, Chiba T et al. (2000) Renal cell carcinoma in acquired cystic kidney disease: volume growth rate determined by helical computed tomography. Am J Kidney Dis 36:759–766

Talamo TS, Shonnard JW (1980) Small renal adenocarcinoma with metastases. J Urol 124:132–134

Tuncali K, van Sonnenberg E, Shankar S et al. (2004) Evaluation of patients referred for percutaneous ablation of renal tumors: importance of a preprocedural diagnosis. Am J Roentgenol 183:575–582

Urban BA, Buckley J, Soyer P et al. (1997) CT appearance of transitional cell carcinoma of the renal pelvis. Am J Roentgenol 169:157–168

Volpe A, Panzarella T, Rendon RA et al. (2004) The natural history of incidentally detected small renal masses. Cancer 100:738–745

Warshauer DM, McCarthy SM, Street L et al. (1988) Detection of renal masses: sensitivities and specificities of excretory urography/linear tomography, US and CT. Radiology 169:363–365

Yamashita Y, Takahashi M, Watanabe O et al. (1992) Small renal cell carcinoma: pathologic and radiologic correlation. Radiology 184:493–498

Yuh BI, Cohan RH (1999) Detecting and characterizing renal masses during helical CT. Am J Roentgenol 173:747–755

Zagoria RJ (2000) Imaging of small renal masses: a medical success story. Am J Roentgenol 175:945–955

Zagoria RJ, Wolfman NT, Karstaedt N et al. (1990) CT features of renal cell carcinoma with emphasis on relation to tumor size. Invest Radiol 25:261–266

14 Unusual Kidney Cancers

Kyeong Ah Kim and Cheol Min Park

CONTENTS

14.1
Introduction

Renal cell carcinoma (RCC) is the most common solid renal neoplasm. It accounts for 3% of adult malignancies. Clear cell (conventional) carcinoma is the most common pathologic subtype of RCC. Usually, RCC is a hypervascular, solid, solitary mass

K. A. Kim, MD
Assistant Professor, Department of Radiology, Korea University Guro Hospital, 97 Gurodong-Gil, Guro-Ku, Seoul 152-703, South Korea
C. M. Park, MD
Professor, Department of Radiology, Korea University Guro Hospital, 97 Gurodong-Gil, Guro-Ku, Seoul 152-703, South Korea

with contour bulging. In this chapter, we illustrate and discuss the imaging features of unusual RCCs. Renal cell carcinoma can show different features according to the pathologic tumor subtype (papillary, chromophobe, collecting duct, sarcomatoid). Preoperative diagnosis of cyst-associated RCC (cyst-adenocarcinoma, multilocular cystic RCC, acquired cystic disease of the kidney, adult polycystic kidney disease) is very difficult, especially in cases of RCC originating in a cyst. Multiple or bilateral presentation of RCC occurs in less than 5% of cases. In addition, RCCs may demonstrate unusual findings such as infiltrative growth mimicking transitional cell carcinoma, fatty component mimicking angiomyolipoma (AML), severe perinephric infiltration, and extensive calcifications mimicking inflammation or other tumor. Renal cell carcinomas can be associated with hereditary disease such as von Hippel-Lindau disease. We also correlate radiologic findings with pathologic findings.

14.2
RCC According to Pathologic Subtypes

14.2.1
Classification

Significant advances in the appropriate classification of RCCs have resulted from the application of immunohistochemistry, electron microscopy, cytogenetics, and molecular genetics. Table 14.1 presents a classification of RCCs modified from that proposed at a consensus meeting in 1997 and followed in its essentials in the 2004 World Health Organization system (WHO; Eble et al. 2004; Storkel et al. 1997). Each subtype is associated with a different prognosis and tumor behavior. Patients with papillary RCC or with chromophobe RCC have a higher 5-year survival rate than those with conventional RCC of the same stage (Reuter and Presti 2000; Bosnib 1999).

Table 14.1. Classification of renal cell carcinoma

Clear cell
Papillary
Chromophobe cell
Collecting duct
Medullary
Mucinous tubular and spindle cell
Unclassified

14.2.2
Clear Cell Type

The clear cell type is the most common histologic variant of RCC, accounting for approximately 70% of cases. Grossly, most clear cell RCCs are solitary and randomly distributed in the renal cortex. On section, areas of necrosis, cystic degeneration, hemorrhage, and calcification are commonly present. Histologically, cells interspersed with abundant, thin-walled blood vessels that result in a sinusoidal vascular pattern characterize the clear cell type of RCC (Murphy et al. 2004).

At imaging, the expansile growth of RCC is manifested as a relatively well-marginated, solitary mass. A focal contour bulge in the renal surface is typical. Usually, RCC is a hypervascular solid mass (Fig. 14.1). On helical CT scans, clear cell RCCs show stronger enhancement than the other subtypes in the corticomedullary and the excretory phase (Kim et al. 2002). After injection of contrast material, they usually show heterogeneous enhancement. Most larger tumors and some small tumors show areas of necrosis or hemorrhage. Unenhanced CT demonstrates well calcification in the tumor.

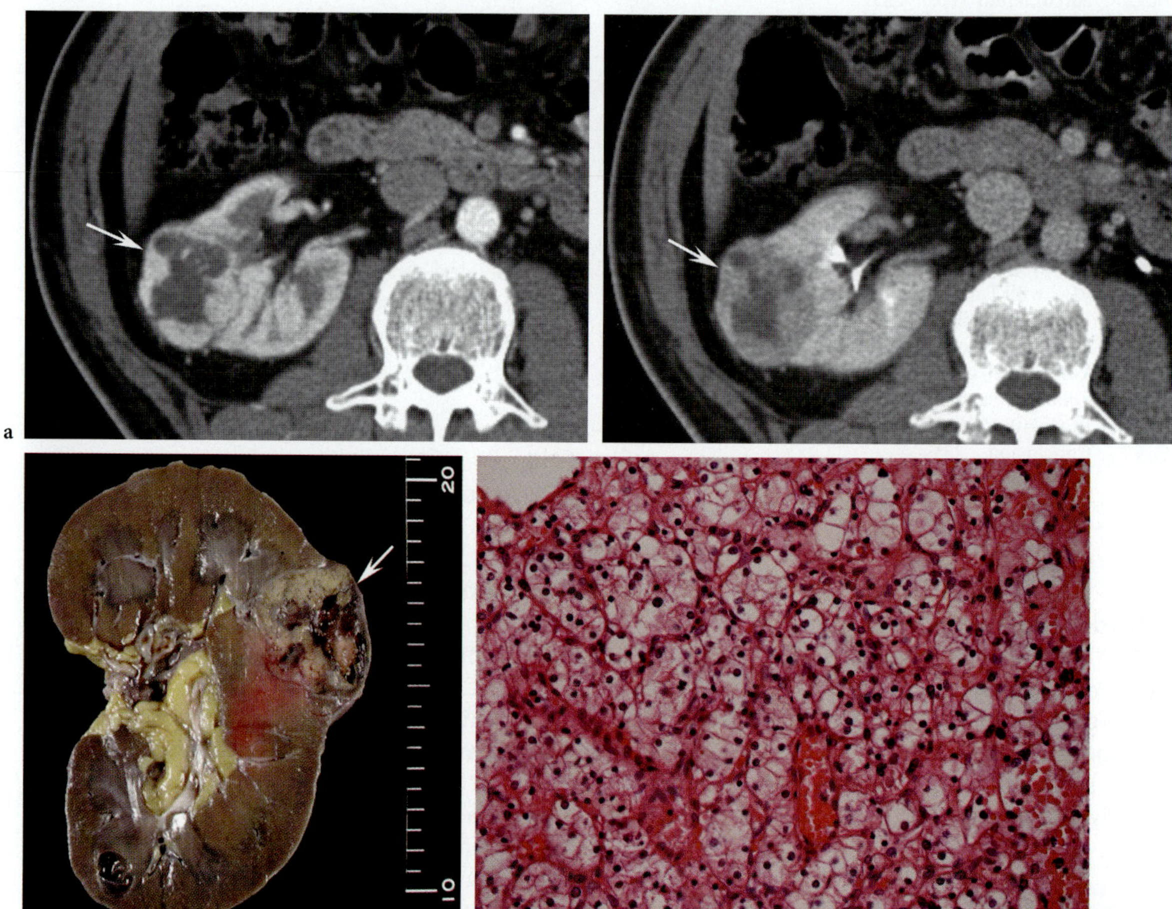

Fig. 14.1a-d. Clear cell (conventional) renal cell carcinoma in a 48-year-old man. Axial contrast-enhanced CT scans in **a** corticomedullary and **b** excretory phases show expansile hypervascular mass (*arrow*) in right kidney. This lesion shows heterogeneous enhancement. **c** Gross specimen shows exophytic mass (*arrow*) with hemorrhage and necrosis. **d** Microscopic examination shows solid nests of cells that are separated by a prominent sinusoidal vascular network (Hematoxylin and eosin stain; original magnification, ×200).

14.2.3
Papillary Type

Papillary RCC, a histologically distinct type, comprises 10–15% of RCCs. Papillary RCCs are variable in size, and small tumors must be distinguished from true renal cortical adenomas. The classification of RCCs defines any papillary tumor larger than 0.5 cm as a carcinoma (STORKEL et al. 1997). Grossly, the papillary type of RCC is well circumscribed and eccentrically situated in the renal cortex. More than 80% of tumors are confined to the cortex within the renal capsule at the time of nephrectomy. Intratumoral hemorrhage and necrosis are seen in two-thirds of cases, a finding that correlates with the radiographic finding of reduced or absent tumor vascularity (PRESS et al. 1984). Compared with other types of RCC, they are more often associated with cortical adenomas and are more often multiple. Histologically, papillary RCC is almost always surrounded by a fibrous capsule. The tumor is characterized by a single layer or pseudostratified layers of cells arranged on fibrovascular stalks (MURPHY et al. 2004).

Computed tomography features closely correlate with the previously established clinicopathologic and angiographic appearances. Papillary RCC demonstrates low stage at presentation in most cases (stages I or II), and has a high frequency of calcification and less enhancement (diminished vascularity) than typical RCC on CT scans (Fig. 14.2). There is no consistent ultrasound (US) pattern. On the basis of these observations, a prospective CT diagnosis of papillary RCC is reasonable. This is particularly important when nephron-sparing surgery is a clinical consideration (PRESS et al. 1984). Homogeneity and low tumor-to-parenchyma enhancement ratios on the parenchymal-phase scans correlate significantly with papillary RCC. Heterogeneity and tumor enhancement ratios do not correlate with the nuclear grade of the carcinoma (HERTS et al. 2002).

14.2.4
Chromophobe Cell Type

This is a variant with distinctive histologic and cytogenetic features. The primary purpose of separating this lesion from other renal neoplasms is to distinguish it from benign oncocytoma (THOENES et al. 1988). As currently defined, chromophobe cell RCCs constitute approximately 5% of renal neoplasms. All reported lesions have been well-circumscribed and solitary. The cut surfaces are typically pale yellow, tan, or brown, and may closely mimic an oncocytoma. Histologically, there are two major patterns of growth, referred to as the classic and the eosinophilic types. Microvesicles may concentrate around the nucleus, producing a distinctive perinuclear halo. This is an important distinguishing feature from oncocytoma (MURPHY et al. 2004).

The clinicopathologic characteristics of chromophobe RCC include hypovascularity/avascularity on angiography, low rate of laboratory abnormalities, low stage/low grade, and a favorable prognosis compared with the common types of RCC (ONISHI et al. 1996).

Unenhanced CT scans show attenuation equal to or slightly lower than that of renal parenchyma, and on early and delayed phase contrast-enhanced scans, attenuation is low in all cases (Fig. 14.3). There is neither venous nor lymph node involvement, and no distant metastasis. Even where the nuclear grade is higher, a well-demarcated solid mass is observed, the tumor stage is lower and the prognosis is better (CHO et al. 2002).

On helical CT scans, conventional (84%), papillary (74%), and collecting duct (100%) RCCs tend to show heterogeneous or predominantly peripheral enhancement, whereas chromophobe RCCs (69%) usually show homogeneous enhancement. Perinephric change and venous invasion are not noted in chromophobe RCC, although both are common in collecting duct RCC (KIM et al. 2002).

14.2.5
Collecting Duct Type

Collecting duct tumors constitute less than 1% of malignant epithelial renal neoplasms in adults (SRIGLEY and EBLE 1998). In the WHO classification, the tumor is grouped with RCC but is designated carcinoma of the collecting ducts of Bellini, reflecting its presumed site of origin (EBLE et al. 2004). Grossly, collecting duct carcinomas are predominantly localized to the medulla but may invade the cortex. They tend to distort adjacent calyces and the renal pelvis. Hemorrhage, with or without necrosis, is typically present. Histologically, the classic collecting duct type of RCC is composed of a mixture of dilated tubules and papillae. Usually, collecting duct carcinomas infiltrate the adjacent renal parenchyma, producing a striking desmoplastic response.

Collecting duct carcinoma (CDC) is an aggressive malignancy, associated with an extremely poor prog-

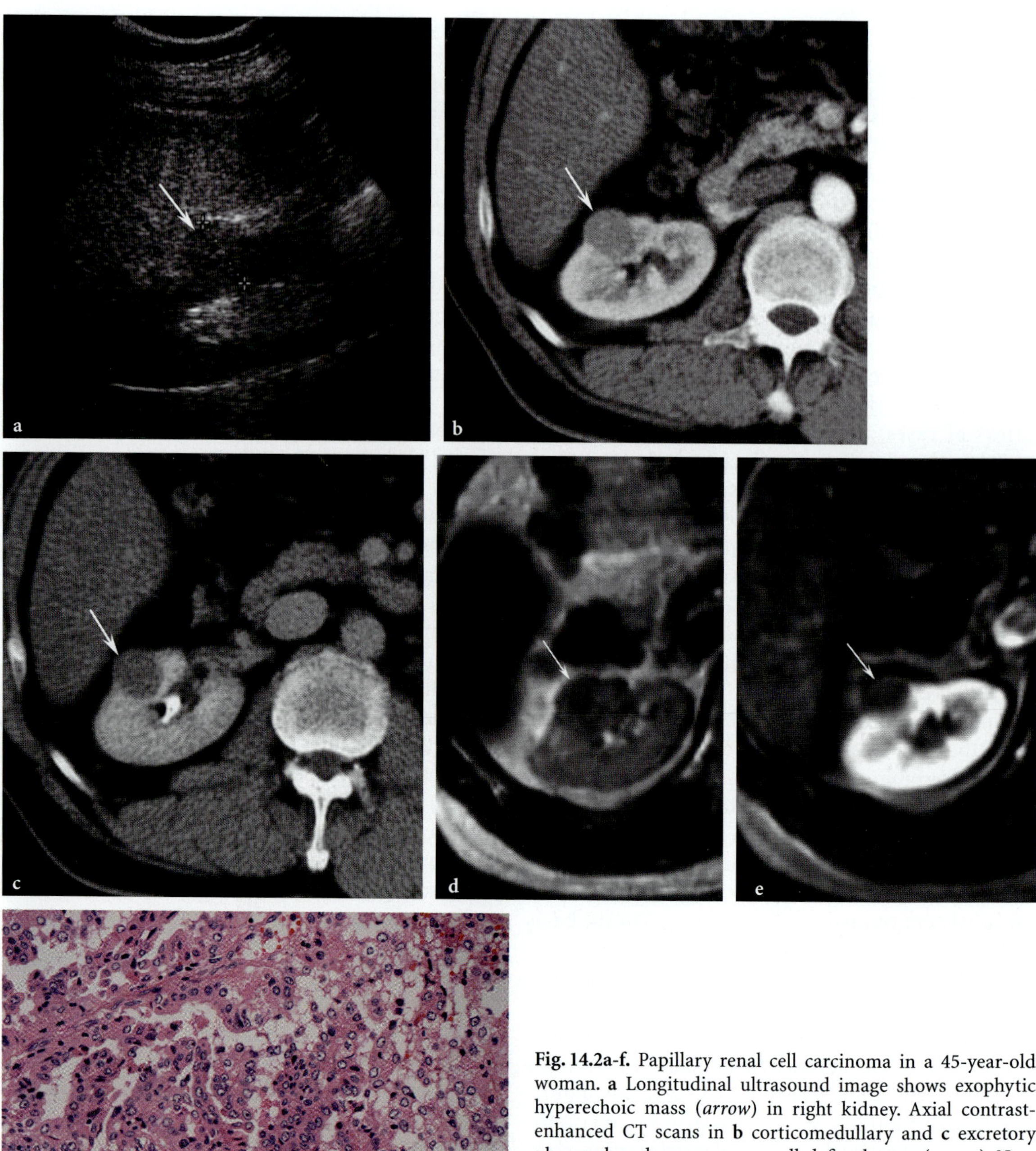

Fig. 14.2a-f. Papillary renal cell carcinoma in a 45-year-old woman. **a** Longitudinal ultrasound image shows exophytic hyperechoic mass (*arrow*) in right kidney. Axial contrast-enhanced CT scans in **b** corticomedullary and **c** excretory phases show homogeneous well-defined mass (*arrow*). Note that the mass does not enhance well. **d** Axial T2-weighted and **e** contrast-enhanced T1-weighted MR images show homogeneous mass (*arrow*) with poor contrast enhancement. **f** Microscopic examination shows rows of cuboidal or low columnar cells that are arranged around fibrovascular fronds (Hematoxylin and eosin stain; original magnification, ×200).

nosis. At presentation CDC is metastatic to regional lymph nodes in approximately 80% of cases, to the lung or adrenal gland in 25% and to the liver in 20%. Median survival after nephrectomy has been reported to be 22 months (DIMOPOULOS et al. 1993).

FUKUYA et al. (1996) reported the CT findings of five cases of CDC. In all cases the affected kidneys maintained the normal outer contours. In four cases the renal masses protruded into the central sinuses. Contrast enhancement was minimal in four cases.

The tumors varied in size from 1.5 to 19 cm (mean 7.7 cm). Medullary involvement was present on CT in 94%, but cortical involvement or an exophytic component was also present in 88 and 59%, respectively.

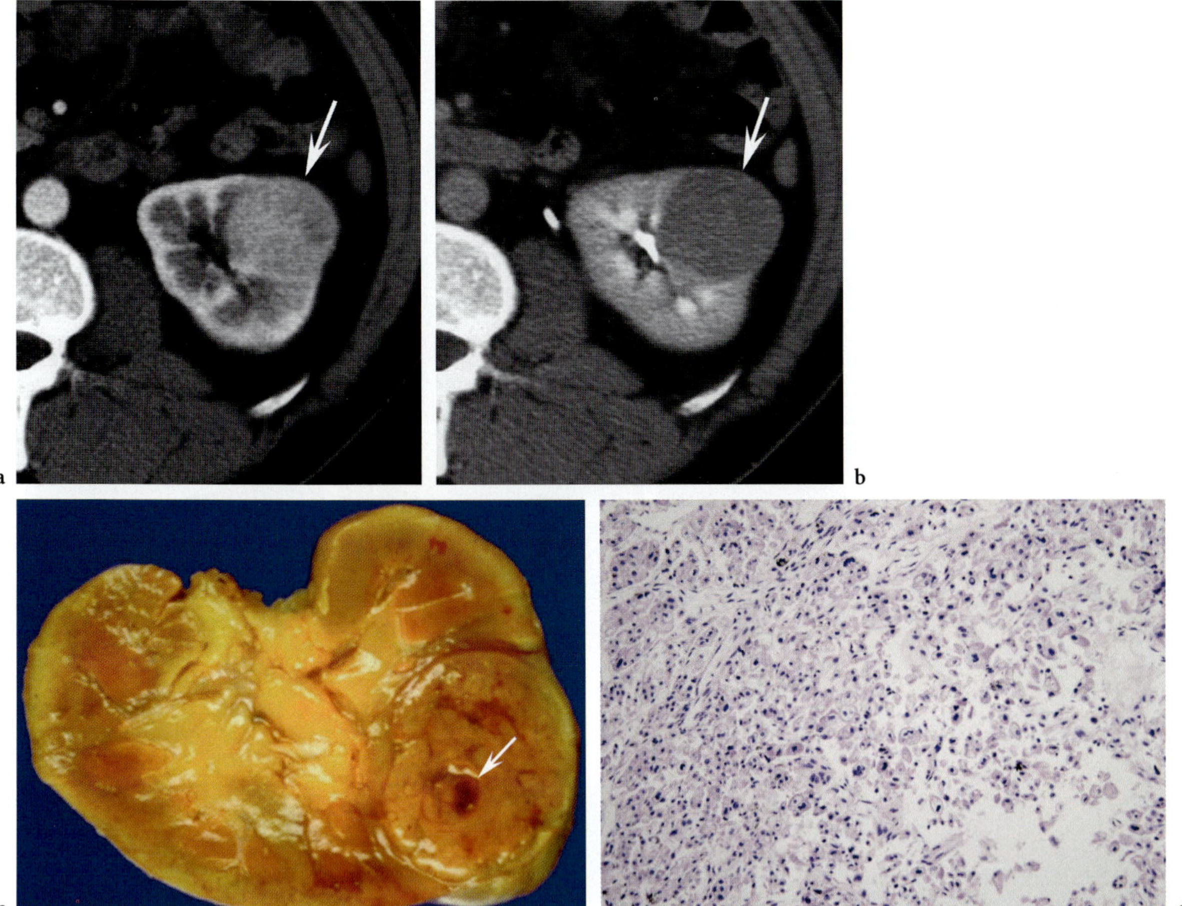

Fig. 14.3a-d. Chromophobe renal cell carcinoma in a 47-year-old man. Axial contrast-enhanced CT scans in **a** corticomedullary and **b** excretory phases show well-demarcated smooth margined mass (*arrow*) in left kidney. There is no evidence of extension to adjacent structures or regional lymphadenopathy. **c** Gross specimen shows well-circumscribed tumor with pale tan color and small punctuate area of hemorrhage (*arrow*). **d** Microscopic examination shows poorly staining cells with a reticular cytoplasm characterized by a perinuclear halo and peripheral cytoplasm rich in mitochondria (Hematoxylin and eosin stain; original magnification, ×200).

The reniform contour of the kidney was preserved in 41% and correlated with a smaller tumor size. Tumors showed an infiltrative appearance on CT in 65%, but an expansile component was also present. A cystic component was present on CT in 35%. On sonography, the solid tumor component was hyperechoic to normal renal parenchyma in most cases. On MR imaging, all tumors were hypointense on T2-weighted imaging. On urography, all lesions distorted the intrarenal collecting system. On angiography, all tumors were hypovascular. Medullary involvement and an infiltrative appearance are common findings on cross-sectional imaging and may suggest the diagnosis of CDC (Fig. 14.4). In large tumors, however, these features are frequently overshadowed by an exophytic or expansile component that cannot be distinguished from the more common cortical RCC (PICKHARDT et al. 2001).

14.2.6
Medullary Type

Medullary RCC is a distinctive clinicopathologic entity that apparently occurs exclusively in patients with sickle cell hemoglobinopathies, almost always the sickle cell trait (SWARTZ et al. 2002). The tumor is believed to originate in the collecting ducts but is not considered a subtype of CDC in classification schemes. Renal medullary carcinoma confers a dismal prognosis, with advanced metastatic disease common at presentation and an overall mean survival after surgery of slightly less than 4 months. Metastatic involvement of regional lymph nodes, liver, and lung are common associated findings (DAVIS et al. 1995).

The radiologic appearance of renal medullary carcinoma is that of a prototypical infiltrative lesion. An

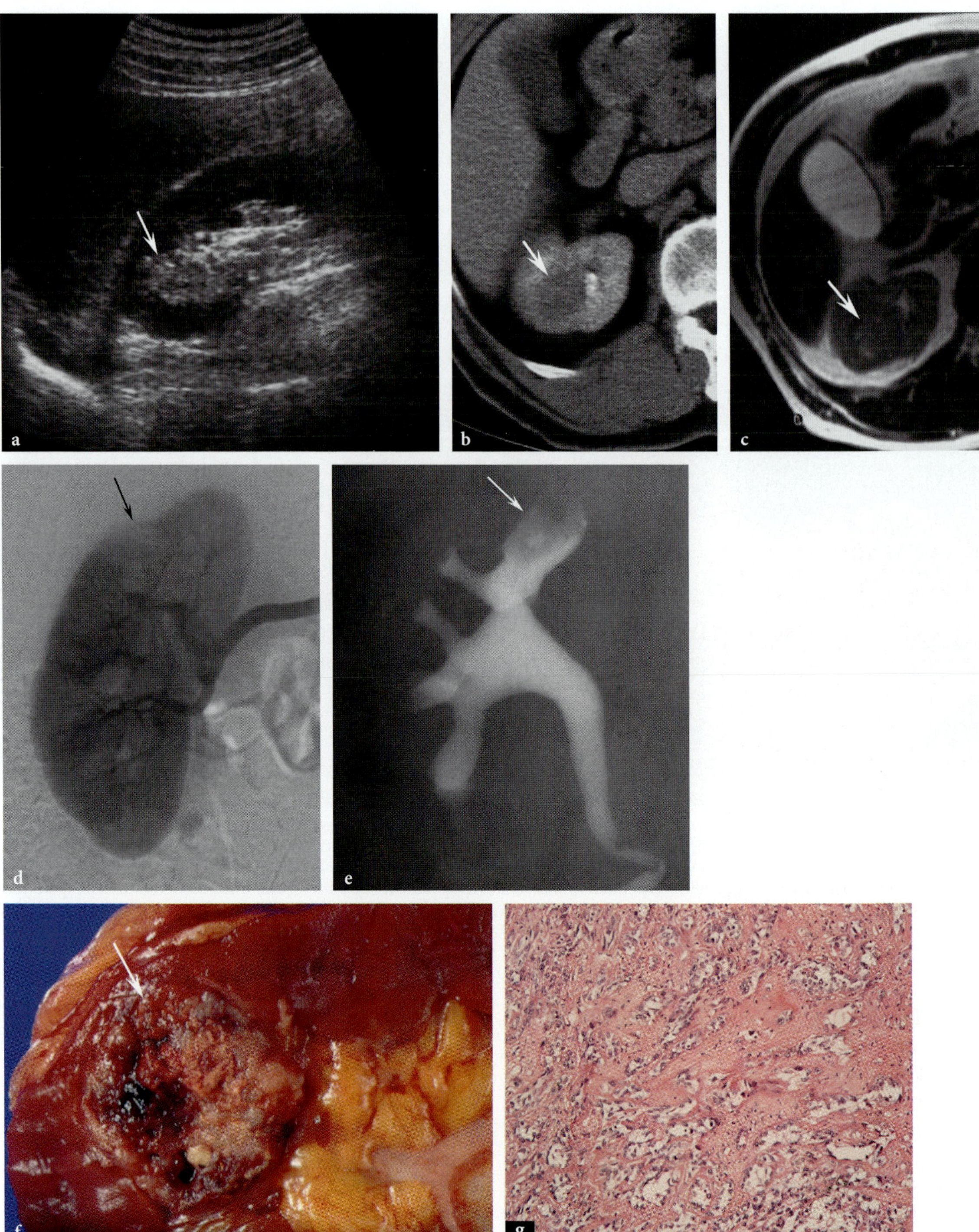

Fig. 14.4a-g. Collecting duct renal cell carcinoma in a 70-year-old man. **a** Longitudinal ultrasound image shows a hyperechoic mass (*arrow*) in upper pole of right kidney. No hypoechoic rim is identified. **b** Axial contrast-enhanced CT scan in excretory phase shows lesion (*arrow*) enhances to lesser degree than surrounding parenchyma. **c** Axial T2-weighted MR image shows lesion (*arrow*) to be low in signal intensity without hypointense rim. **d** Selective renal angiography shows the tumor to be hypovascular (*arrow*) compared with normal renal parenchyma. **e** Anteroposterior excretory urogram shows distortion of the intrarenal collecting system (*arrow*). **f** Gross specimen shows relatively well-defined lobulating mass (*arrow*) with central hemorrhage in the renal medulla. Although mass appears grossly expansile, no pseudocapsule was present at pathologic review. **g** Microscopic examination shows irregular tubules with branching lumens embedded in desmoplastic stroma and lined by atypical epithelial cells (Hematoxylin and eosin stain; original magnification, ×200).

ill-defined mass centered in the renal medulla with extension into the renal sinus and cortex is characteristic. Caliectasis may be seen, presumably as a result of the sinus invasion. Larger tumors expand the kidney but tend to maintain its reniform shape. The tumors are heterogeneous on US and contrast-enhanced CT, reflecting characteristic tumor necrosis (DAVIDSON et al. 1995).

14.2.7
Sarcomatoid Type

Sarcomatoid RCC is not a distinct histologic entity but rather represents high-grade transformation in different subtypes of RCC. Foci of high-grade spindle cells, often reminiscent of a malignant fibrous histiocytoma, can occur in all histologic subtypes of RCC, and current classifications do not recognize tumors with these features as a distinct subtype (EBLE et al. 2004). Nevertheless, the presence of a sarcomatoid component in an RCC is widely considered to be a poor prognostic sign. Sarcomatoid areas are present in 1.0–6.5% of RCCs (PERALTA-VENTURINA et al. 2001). Grossly, the sarcomatoid type of RCC is large and invasive. The inconspicuous lesions that present with large metastases are distinctly unusual. The presence of a bulging, lobulated, soft, gray-white, fleshy component should alert the surgeon to the possibility of a sarcomatous element. Histologically, the sarcomatoid component is characterized by interlacing or whorled bundles of spindle cells, sometimes in a storiform pattern.

The imaging features of sarcomatoid type RCC are not well characterized in the literature (Fig. 14.5). The more common subtypes – clear cell, papillary, and chromophobe cell – typically appear as well-defined masses and may form a capsule of connective tissue and compressed atrophic renal parenchyma as the tumor grows. Occasionally, the tumor appears ill-defined and infiltrative. This appearance is more typical of the uncommon sarcomatoid subtype (Fig. 14.6) but may be seen with the other subtypes as well.

14.2.8
Hypovascular or Avascular RCC

Over 80% of RCCs are iso- and/or hypervascular and have a typical tumor blush after the arterial injection of a contrast agent (WEYMAN et al. 1980). This angiographic feature is an important radiologic finding when discriminating RCCs from the other types of renal tumor. In contrast, the remaining RCCs show hypovascular or even avascular imaging on renal angiography. Although some cases of these negative angiographic findings are difficult to diagnose as RCC, the introduction of new imaging modalities, such as CT, MR imaging, and US, has led to substantial improvement in the accuracy of diagnosis (LONDON et al. 1989).

ONISHI et al. (2002) studied hypovascular or avascular RCCs, with special reference to their histopathological characteristics. Papillary RCC was the most frequently observed hypovascular or avascular renal tumor (34.9%; Fig. 14.2). The vascularity differed among the variants, i.e., some cases had a basophilic and solid variant with avascular features, whereas the remaining cases had wide stromal organization showing hypovascular features. The second most frequently observed hypovascular or avascular RCC was chromophobe cell carcinoma (27.8%; Fig. 14.3). No difference in vascularity was detected between variants, except for two cases with sarcomatoid changes (avascular features). The third most frequently observed hypovascular or avascular RCC was cyst-associated RCC (23%). All RCCs originating in a cyst showed avascular features, and the remaining cystic RCCs showed hypovascular features. The remaining hypovascular or avascular RCCs were cases of clear cell carcinoma accompanied by sarcomatoid changes (6.3%), spindle cell carcinoma (4.0%), and collecting duct carcinoma (4.0%). Tumor-related neovascularity is thought to be closely related to the density of the surrounding structural organization of the tumor cells, such as the fibrovascular channels and the fibrous stalks containing vascular septa. Hypovascular or avascular RCCs can be categorized as non-clear cell carcinoma and some clear cell carcinoma accompanied by sarcomatoid changes.

14.2.9
Infiltrative Growth Pattern of RCC

Neoplasms account for a considerable number of infiltrative renal lesions seen on imaging studies (AMBOS et al. 1977; HARTMAN et al. 1988). Specific entities that appear infiltrative include a variety of uncommon tumors (e.g., renal medullary carcinoma); however, infiltrative growth may also be an atypical manifestation of RCC (Figs. 14.6, 14.7). Other neoplasms that may exhibit infiltrative growth include epithelial neoplasms of the renal parenchyma, collecting duct carcinoma, renal medullary

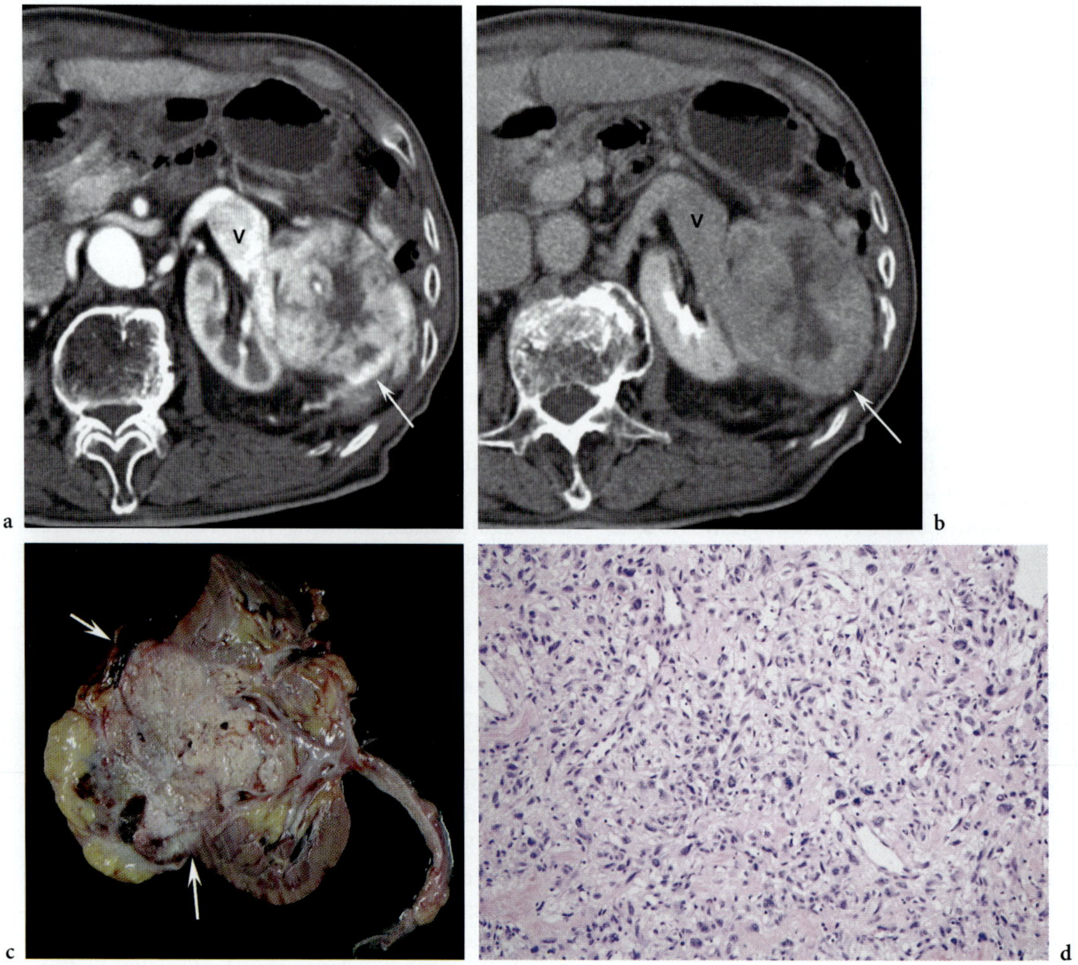

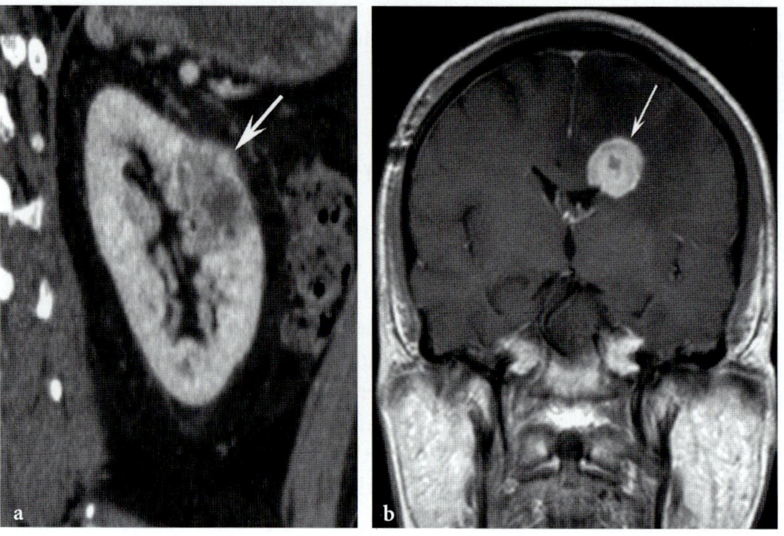

Fig. 14.5a-d. Sarcomatoid-type clear cell renal cell carcinoma in an 81-year-old man. Axial contrast-enhanced CT scans in **a** corticomedullary and **b** excretory phases show a exophytic growing hypervascular mass in left kidney. There is thrombosis and invasion of left renal vein (*V*) and perinephric fat invasion (*arrow*). **c** Gross specimen shows a large tumor (*arrows*) with bulging, lobulated, pale gray-white cut surface. **d** Microscopic examination shows nests of clear cell carcinoma mixed with sarcomatoid elements (Hematoxylin and eosin stain; original magnification, ×200).

Fig. 14.6a,b. Infiltrative growth pattern of sarcomatoid type renal cell carcinoma in a 41-year-old man. **a** Sagittal reconstruction contrast-enhanced CT image shows a poorly defined heterogeneous mass (*arrow*) in the left kidney involving the medulla and cortex, effacing or abutting the renal sinus. **b** Coronal brain MR scan shows a well-enhancing mass (*arrow*) with peritumoral edema in left frontal lobe. This patient presented with brain metastasis.

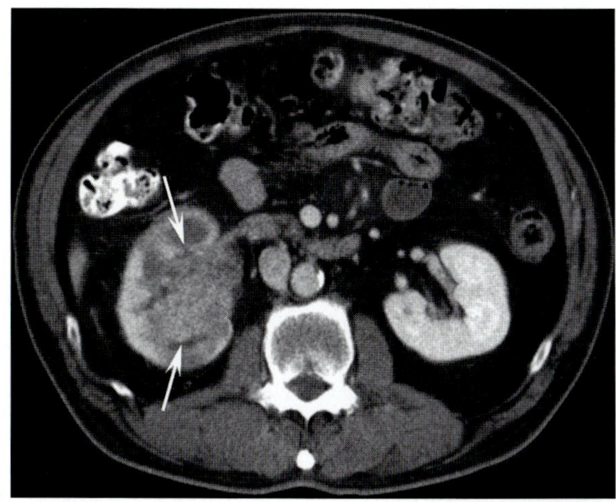
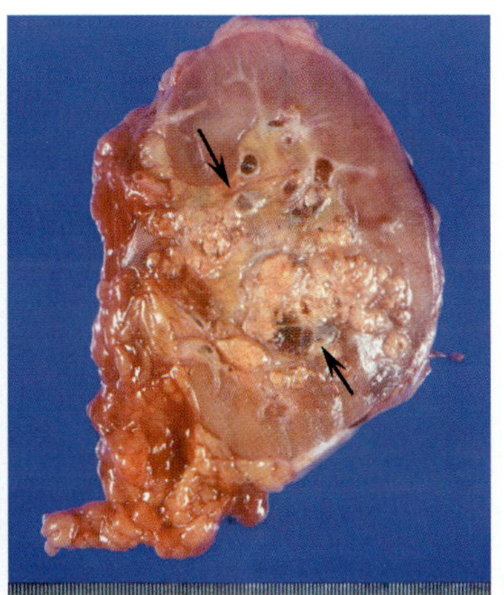

Fig. 14.7a,b. Infiltrative growth pattern of clear cell renal cell carcinoma in a 55-year-old man. a Axial contrast-enhanced CT scan in excretory phase shows a heterogeneous, poorly defined mass (*arrows*) in the right kidney with preserved reniform. b Gross specimen shows a poorly demarcated whitish solid mass (*arrows*). The tumor invades the renal vein and peripelvic soft tissue.

carcinoma, renal pelvic carcinomas, renal sarcomas, lymphoproliferative diseases, metastatic disease, and several pediatric tumors. Some renal tumors may demonstrate both infiltrative and expansile features at radiologic and pathologic examination. In these cases, an infiltrative component may indicate more aggressive behavior (PICKHARDT et al. 2000).

One study found that, regardless of tumor size, 94% of cortical RCCs exhibit an expansile appearance with exophytic growth that disrupts the reniform contour (ZAGORIA et al. 1990). Infiltrative growth is a much less common pattern, whereby tumor cells spread using the normal renal architecture as scaffolding for interstitial growth. The margin between an infiltrative tumor and kidney is often poorly defined because of a broad zone of transition. Infiltrative lesions may enlarge the kidney but usually maintain the reniform contour. These growth patterns can often be distinguished on cross-sectional imaging through analysis of tumor morphology, particularly the interface between the tumor and the normal kidney. Although only about 6% of cortical RCCs are truly infiltrative, they nonetheless represent a significant proportion of infiltrative tumors given their overall abundance (PICKHARDT et al. 2000; ZAGORIA et al. 1990).

Urothelial tumors of the renal pelvis, namely invasive transitional cell carcinoma and squamous cell carcinoma, also tend to involve the kidney by infiltration. A centrally located collecting duct carcinoma with invasion into the renal pelvis may be indistinguishable from an invasive transitional cell carcinoma of the renal pelvis. The distinction, however, has significant implications for treatment

because nephroureterectomy is indicated for urothelial carcinomas, but nephrectomy is performed for renal parenchymal malignancies (PICKHARDT et al. 2001).

14.3
Cyst-Associated RCC

Renal cell carcinomas are often associated with cysts. In most cases, the cyst is of the common variety generally considered a cortical retention cyst, but associations with both acquired and hereditary polycystic diseases have been well documented (GARDNER 1984; KUMAR et al. 1980).

14.3.1
Cystic Changes in RCC

Extensively cystic renal tumors are not classified as separate pathologic entities but must be discussed because they may present diagnostic challenges. Overall, cystic change occurs in up to 15% of RCCs. Radiologically, these tumors are classified into four categories: (a) cysts resulting from an intrinsic multilocular pattern of growth; (b) cysts resulting from an intrinsic unilocular pattern of growth (Fig. 14.8); (c) cysts resulting from cystic degeneration of a previously solid tumor (Fig. 14.9); and (d) cystic RCC originating in a preexisting, benign cyst (HARTMAN et al. 1986). It is important to differentiate multilocular cystic RCC from this group, due to distinctive

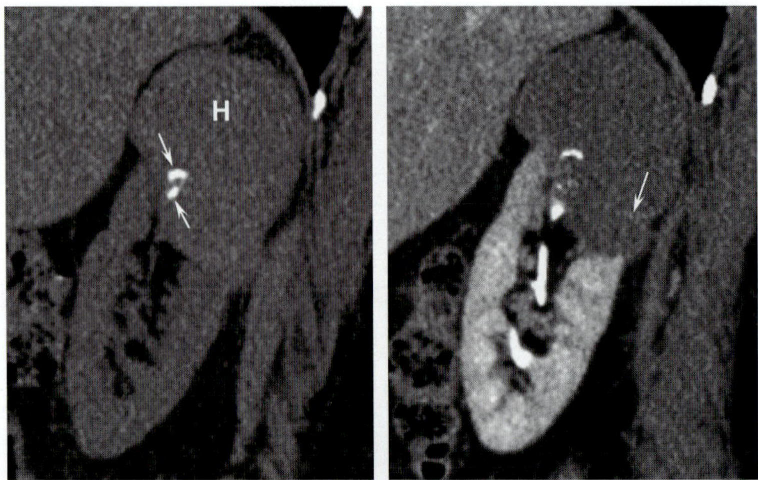

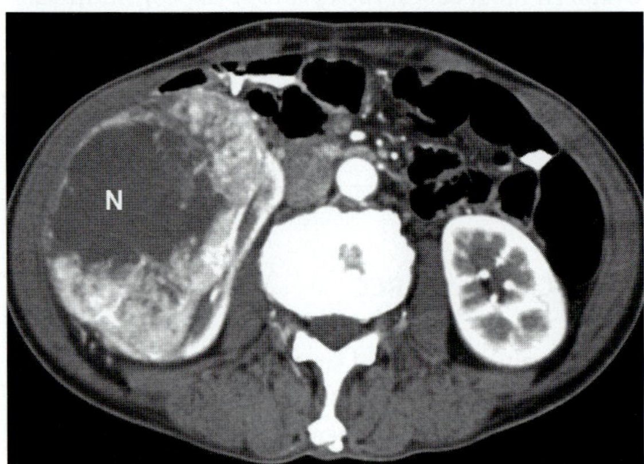

Fig. 14.8a-c. Cystic renal cell carcinoma in a 58-year-old woman. a Sagittal reconstruction unenhanced CT image shows a cystic lesion with internal high-density hemorrhage (*H*) and focal calcifications (*arrows*). b Sagittal reconstruction contrast-enhanced CT scan on excretory phase shows no definite solid enhancing portion within the cystic lesion. There is suspicious subtle septal enhancement (*arrow*). c Gross specimen consists of a previously ruptured cyst. The inner surface shows diffuse irregular and trabecular appearance.

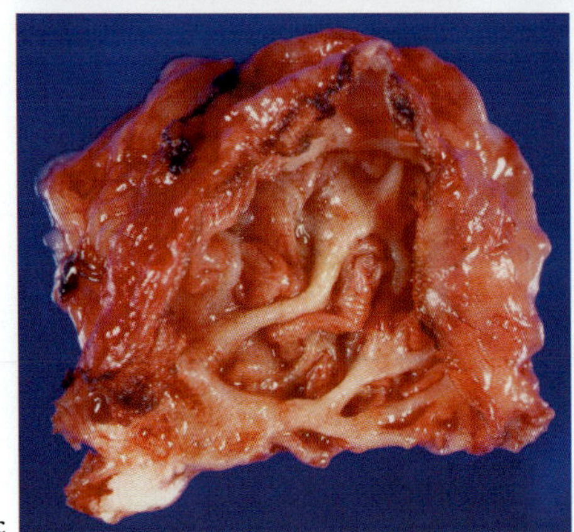

Fig. 14.9. Cystic necrosis of renal cell carcinoma in a 68-year-old woman. Axial contrast-enhanced CT scan shows a large hypervascular mass with central low-attenuation necrosis (*N*) in right kidney.

clinicopathologic characteristics of these tumors (Murphy et al. 2004).

In cases resulting from cystic necrosis of a previously solid tumor, the cysts may contain old and recent hemorrhage as well as necrotic tissue. Generally, malignancy should be suspected when any cystic mass in the kidney contains hemorrhagic or necrotic material, and extensive sampling is warranted. In such cases, identifiable tumor may be scant and the identification of any clear cell or papillary areas indicates the presence of malignancy. The presence of extensive cystic necrosis has been reported to be associated with a poor prognosis (Brinker et al. 2000).

Macrocystic multilocular RCC shows a multiloculated configuration on US and contrast-enhanced CT. Angiography reveals neovascularity peripherally or within the tumor. Microcystic multilocular RCC does not fulfill the criterion for a cystic mass on US: they are irregularly hyperechoic. There is little enhancement on postcontrast CT and only slight neovascularity on angiography. Unilocular RCC shows a cystic mass with an irregular wall or mural nodules on US and contrast-enhanced CT. Necrotic RCC shows various sonographic findings from anechoic to irregular echoic. The appearance on CT varies from cystic with mural nodules to a multi-loculated or irregular architecture. Neovascularity is seen in the periphery in most tumors (YAMASHITA et al. 1994).

Bosniak classification is useful for differentiating cystic renal masses in categories I–IV (BOSNIAK 1997b). There were too few samples to allow meaningful conclusions to be drawn for category II renal masses. It is critical to differentiate between complicated cysts of categories II and III because of the major implications for prognosis and clinical management (KOGA et al. 2000).

14.3.2
Multilocular Cystic RCC

In approximately 5% of clear cell RCCs, multiple cysts are the predominant pathologic finding (MURAD et al. 1991). These so-called cystic or multilocular cystic RCCs (MCRCCs) are considered a subtype of the clear cell variety. The tumors are well circumscribed, with noncommunicating cysts separated by irregular, thick, fibrous septa, reminiscent of a multilocular cyst. The correct interpretation is achieved by the recognition of the presence of small aggregates of low-grade clear cells in the walls of the cysts. The septa are fibrotic or hyalinized and may be calcified, with or without ossification. The criteria for diagnosis of multilocular cystic RCC include: (a) growth as an expansile mass surrounded by a fibrous pseudocapsule; (b) a tumor composed of cysts and septa without expansile solid nodules; and (c) septa containing aggregates of clear cells (EBLE and BOSNIB 1998). The MCRCCs must be distinguished from RCCs with cystic change; the latter may have expansile clear cell masses in their cyst walls or papillary excrescences covered by clear cells.

On US and CT, MCRCC appears as a well-defined multilocular cystic mass with serous, proteinaceous, or hemorrhagic fluid, with no expansile solid nodules in the thin septa, and sometimes with small slightly enhanced solid areas constituting less than 10% of the entire lesion (Fig. 14.10). When radiologic examinations demonstrate a cystic renal mass of this kind in adult men, MCRCC should be included in the differential diagnosis (KIM et al. 2000).

YAMASHITA et al. (1995) found that the radiologic appearance of MCRCCs of smaller size do not fulfill the previously documented criteria of MCRCCs. Although multiple cysts were seen within the tumors pathologically, MCRCCs of smaller sizes appeared solid on radiologic examinations; however, contrast enhancement or neovascularity was very slight.

14.3.3
RCC in Acquired Cystic Disease of the Kidney

There is an estimated tenfold increase in the risk of RCC for patients with chronic renal failure and a 50-fold increased risk with acquired cystic kidney disease (ISHIKAWA et al. 1990; MATAS et al. 1975). The frequency of RCC varies directly with both the duration of dialysis and the number of cysts (MATSON and COHEN 1990). Patients are younger than the usual patients with RCC (HUGHSON et al. 1986). The number of cysts is important for establishing a diagnosis of RCC associated with acquired cystic disease: at least five cysts are necessary for diagnosis of acquired cystic disease. In most cases of RCC associated with acquired cystic disease, there is focal hyperplasia of the epithelium, with or without atypia. These atypical epithelial proliferations harbor cytogenetic abnormalities and are hypothesized to represent early neoplastic lesions (CHEUK et al. 2002).

A significant difference in mean attenuation values between carcinomas and renal parenchymas is seen on images with early enhancement but not on those with delayed enhancement. Early contrast-enhanced helical CT is superior to delayed enhanced helical CT for revealing RCC in end-stage kidney disease (Fig. 14.11; TAKEBAYASHI et al. 1999).

Sonographic angiography is useful for the detection of small nodules in patients with chronic renal failure but does not allow differentiation of malignant from benign lesions (TAKASE et al. 1994).

14.3.4
RCC in Polycystic Kidney Disease

Intracystic epithelial hyperplasia occurs in up to 90% of polycystic kidneys and various tumors are identified in up to 25% of cases, but almost all are small and well differentiated, with the histologic features of cortical adenomas (GREGOIRE et al. 1987). Renal cell carcinoma is rare in adult polycystic kidneys and probably occurs with no greater frequency than might be expected based on the prevalence of the two conditions.

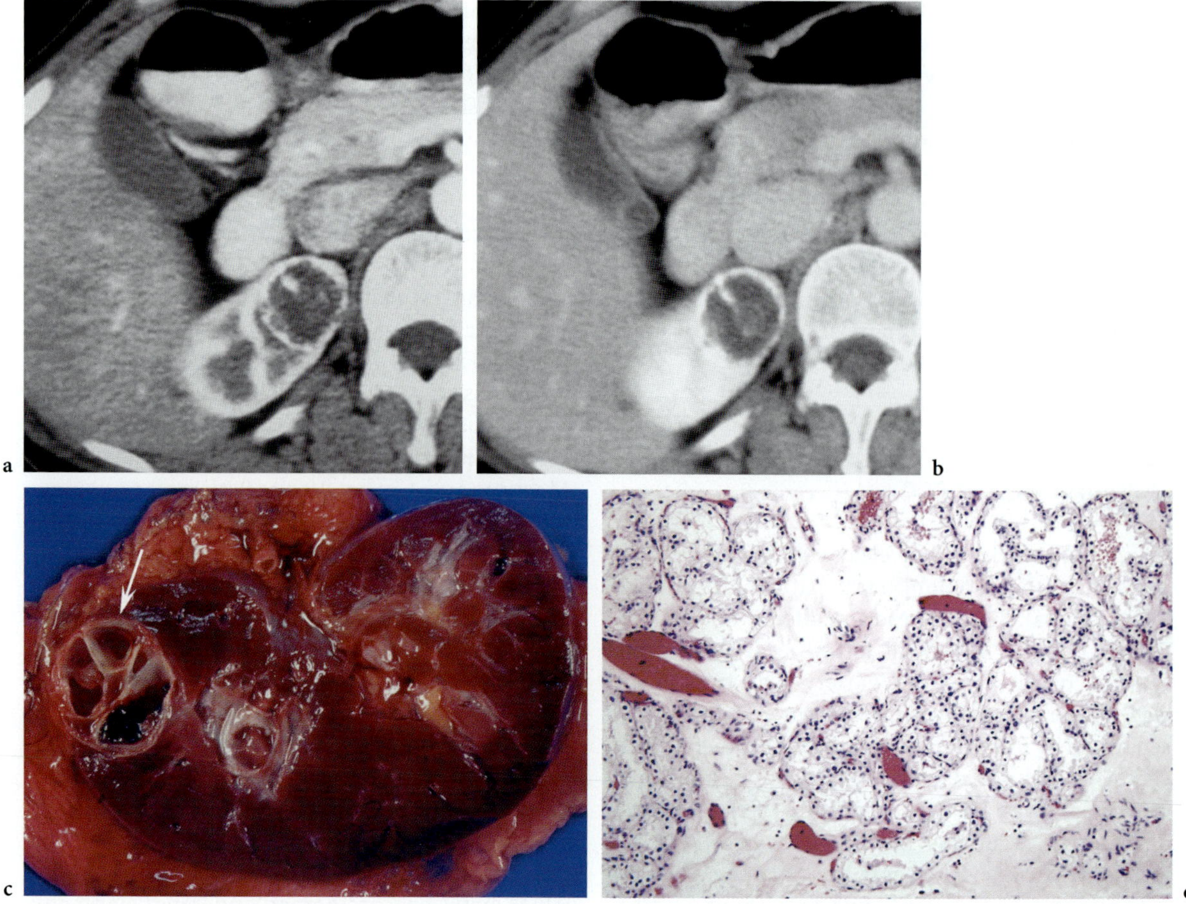

Fig. 14.10a-d. Multilocular cystic renal cell carcinoma with extensive calcification in a 56-year-old woman. Axial contrast-enhanced CT scans in **a** corticomedullary and **b** nephrographic phases show a hypodense mass with peripheral rim calcification. There is no definite enhancing portion within the mass. **c** Gross specimen shows well-circumscribed tumor with multicystic appearance (*arrow*). Note the absence of any expansile component to the tumor. **d** Microscopic examination shows small nests of clear cells within the fibrous tissue. This tumor has osseous metaplasia (Hematoxylin and eosin stain; original magnification, ×200).

14.4
Various Manifestations of RCC

14.4.1
Small RCC

Renal cell carcinomas are usually large, averaging 7–8 cm in diameter at diagnosis. With recent improved imaging techniques, RCCs smaller than 3 cm in diameter are discovered frequently. Their early detection is extremely important for therapy and prognosis but has opened new diagnostic issues including differential diagnosis, surgical or non-surgical management, and imaging follow-up. Small RCCs can be either solitary or multiple, synchronous, or metachronous.

YAMASHITA et al. (1992) correlated the radiologic and pathologic findings of 36 patients with small RCCs (≤3 cm in diameter). Tumors were discovered incidentally or by mass surveys with US. Of the 36 tumors, 24 were of solid (alveolar) architecture, five were of papillary architecture, three were of tubular architecture, and four were of multilocular cystic architecture. Cell arrangement was closely correlated with radiologic appearance, especially with regard to tumor vascularity and echogenicity. Histologically homogeneous tumors of solid architecture were hypoechoic on US and hypervascular on angiography and contrast-enhanced CT. Tumors of papillary, tubular, and multilocular cystic architecture were hyperechoic on US and hypovascular on angiography. There was no correlation of cell differentiation and cell architecture with echogenicity or tumor vascularity. Tumors with hemorrhage showed marked hyperdensity at CT. A tumor capsule was observed in 69%. This appeared as a rim on US or angiography.

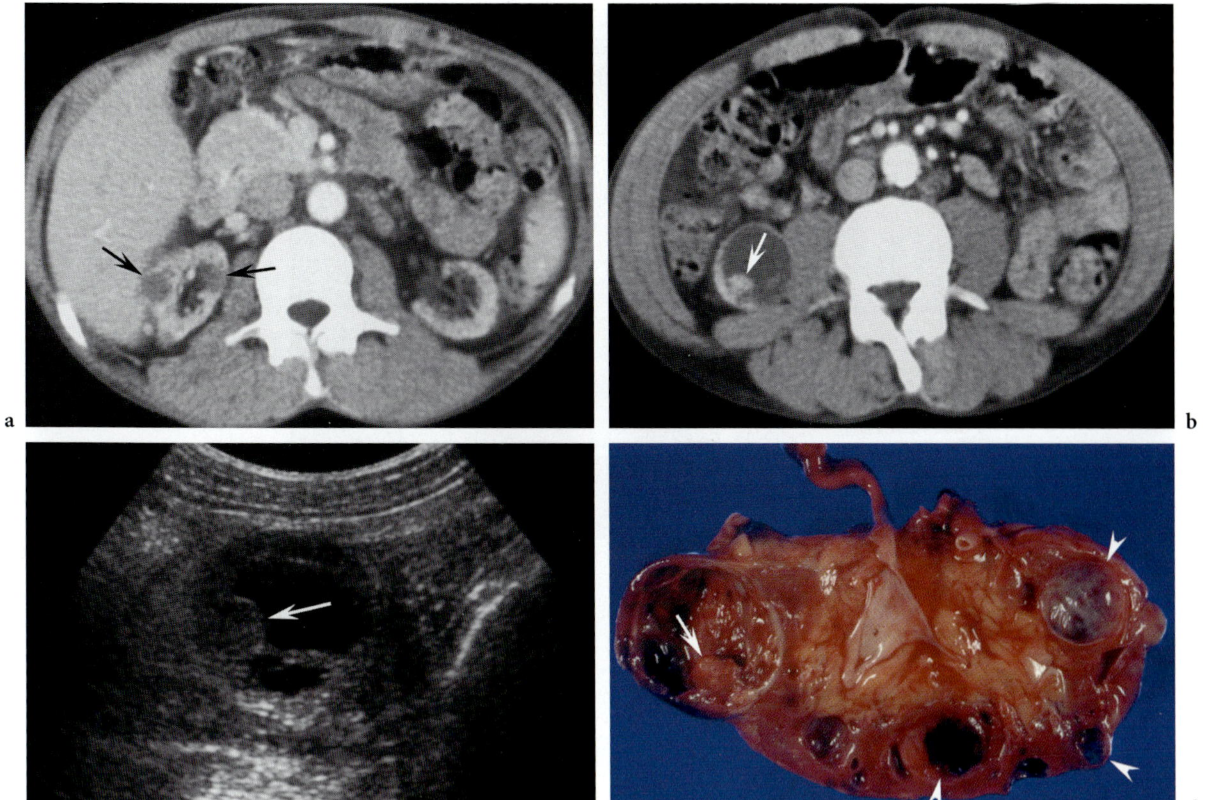

Fig. 14.11a-d. Renal cell carcinoma arising in a 41-year-old man with acquired cystic kidney disease and chronic renal failure. Axial contrast-enhanced CT scans in corticomedullary phase show **a** multiple acquired renal cysts (*arrows*) and **b** an enhancing nodule (*arrow*) within a cyst. **c** Transverse ultrasound image shows an echogenic nodule (*arrow*) within a cyst. Color Doppler study showed hypervascular arterial flows at a nodule within a cyst (not shown). **d** Gross specimen shows the tumor (*arrow*) arising within a preexisting cyst. There are multiple cysts (*arrowheads*) with hemorrhage and degeneration.

The difference in attenuation of the renal medulla and that of the masses was statistically significantly greater during the nephrographic phase. False-positive results occurred only on corticomedullary-phase scans because of the lack of enhancement of the renal medulla. Nephrographic-phase scans allow greater lesion detection and better characterization of small renal masses than corticomedullary-phase scans (Fig. 14.12). Nephrographic-phase scans should be obtained when only monophasic scanning is used to detect small renal masses (Szolar et al. 1997).

14.4.2
Calcifications in RCC

Calcification and ossification typically occur within necrotic zones and are demonstrated in 10–15% of RCCs (Fukuoka et al. 1987). Radiographically, calcified renal masses are found in 4–11% of all renal masses (Daniel et al. 1972; Kikkawa et al. 1969). Renal cell carcinoma is the most common of these and 7–18% of RCC show radiographic calcification (Patterson et al. 1987). Ring-like peripheral calcification may be more frequent in RCC (Kikkawa et al. 1969; Krieger et al. 1979). Kim et al. (2002) reported that calcification in RCC was noted in 11% of cases with conventional RCC, 32% with papillary RCC and 38% with chromophobe RCC. Calcification is more common in papillary and chromophobe RCC (Fig. 14.13). They concluded that the prognosis of calcified RCC is favorable.

Calcification in a solid renal mass has traditionally been considered to indicate a malignant process; however, calcifications can be seen in benign as well as malignant cystic renal masses (Daniel et al. 1972). The majority of renal cysts encountered in daily radiologic practice represent uncomplicated cysts and are easy to diagnose; however, differentiating between benign complicated cysts and those requiring surgical intervention may be difficult and

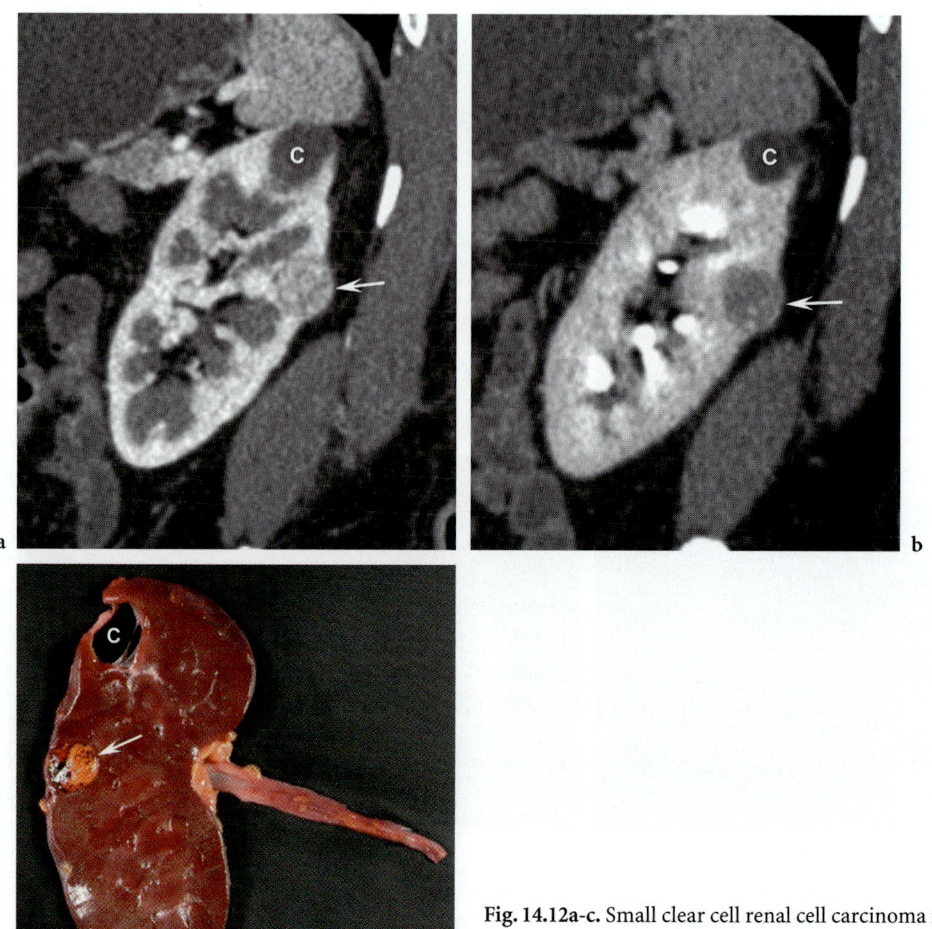

Fig. 14.12a-c. Small clear cell renal cell carcinoma in a 44-year-old man. Sagittal reconstruction contrast-enhanced CT scan with **a** corticomedullary and **b** nephrographic phases showing a 1.2 cm-sized mass (*arrow*) in left kidney. Nephrographic phase scan enables greater lesion detection and better characterization of small renal mass than corticomedullary phase scan. **c** Gross specimen shows a small, well-defined mass in left kidney (*arrow*). *C* cyst

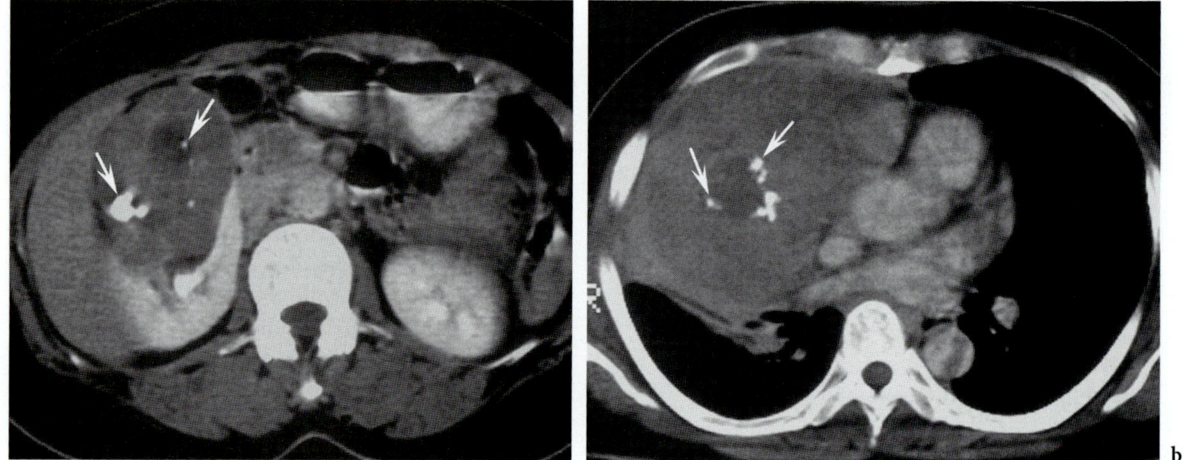

Fig. 14.13a,b. Chromophobe renal cell carcinoma in a 54-year-old woman with mediastinal metastasis. **a** Axial contrast-enhanced abdominal CT scan shows heterogeneous right renal mass with calcifications (*arrows*). **b** Axial contrast-enhanced chest CT scan shows another similar mass with calcifications (*arrows*) in right mediastinum.

can lead to differences in opinion between radiologists and clinicians (BOSNIAK 1986; BOSNIAK 1991; BOSNIAK 1997a). The presence of calcification may influence the decision to surgically explore or follow up a lesion.

Calcification in a cystic renal mass is not as important in diagnosis as is the presence of associated enhancing soft tissue elements. Cystic lesions that show considerable calcification – even thick and nodular calcification – but no evidence of tissue enhancement at CT (category IIF lesions) can be managed with follow-up CT examinations to monitor their stability. Lesions that show associated soft tissue enhancement of the wall or septa (category III lesions) in most instances must be evaluated surgically, although many of them will prove to be benign (ISRAEL and BOSNIAK 2003).

14.4.3
RCC with Fatty Component

In the most common type of RCC (clear cell carcinoma), the cells frequently contain lipid, which contributes to the histologic appearance (HELENON et al. 1993; STROTZER et al. 1993; CASTOLDI et al. 1995; ROY et al. 1998). Other malignant fat-containing renal tumors have been described, such as granular cell RCC with macrophage infiltration, atypical Wilms tumor, oncocytoma, hepatocellular carcinoma, and liposarcomas (PARVEY et al. 1981; CURRY et al. 1990; SHINOZAKI et al. 2001). Benign lesions, such as AML or lipoma, also contain fat. Identification of lipid in a renal mass may result in an erroneous diagnosis of AML (Fig. 14.14; ROY et al.1998). In urine cytology, intracellular lipid has been used to distinguish RCCs from other masses. With MR imaging, T1-weighted images show fat as increased signal; however, MR imaging evidence of lipid can best be demonstrated as signal drop-off on opposed-phase images compared with in-phase images or on water-saturated T1-weighted images (OUTWATER et al. 1997).

Fat occurs within RCCs in several ways: lipid-producing necrosis within a large RCC; intratumoral bone metaplasia with fatty marrow elements and calcification within a small RCC; and entrapment of perirenal or sinus fat by large irregular RCCs. Fat-containing RCC must be considered in cases of fat-containing renal tumors, even though the presence of intratumoral fat is characteristic of AML. A dedicated CT scanning protocol and strict diagnostic criteria are mandatory for accurate diagnosis. Malignancy should be suspected on the basis of these criteria: presence of intratumoral calcifications; large, irregular tumor invading the perirenal or sinus fat; large necrotic tumor with small foci of fat; and association with nonfatty lymph nodes or venous invasion (HELENON et al. 1997).

Metastasis from RCCs should be included in the differential diagnosis when one observes fatty density in a nodule or mass at extrarenal sites, especially in patients with a past history of clear cell carcinoma (Fig. 14.15; MURAM and AISEN 2003).

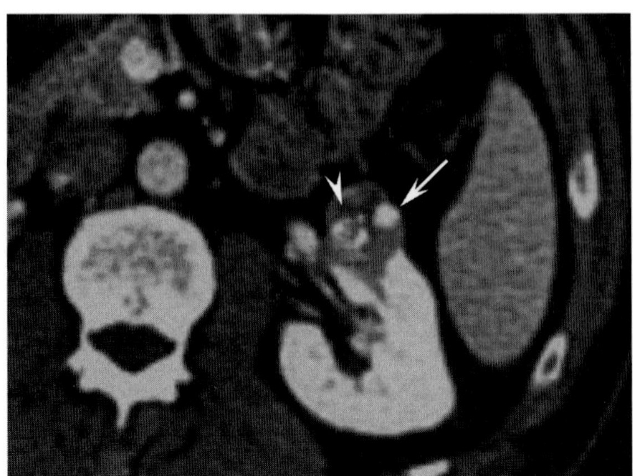

Fig. 14.14. Renal cell carcinoma with a fatty component mimicking angiomyolipoma in a 60-year-old woman. Axial contrast-enhanced CT scan in nephrogram phase shows a expansile mass in left kidney with fatty component (*arrowhead*) and enhancing nodular portions (*arrow*).

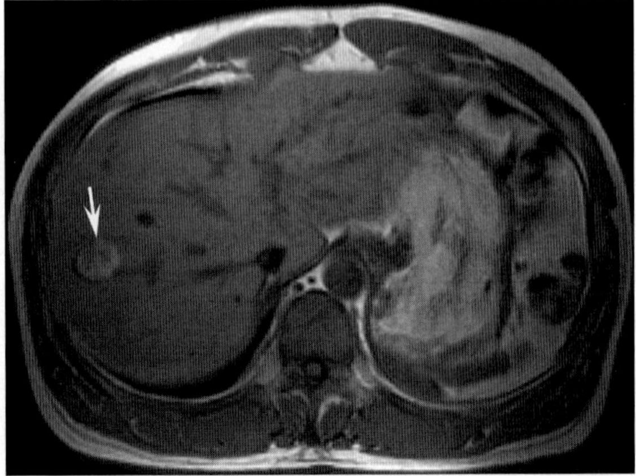

Fig. 14.15. Fatty hepatic metastasis from renal cell carcinoma in a 73-year-old man. Axial T1-weighted MR image of liver shows a high signal intensity mass (*arrow*). Ultrasound-guided needle biopsy confirms the hepatic metastasis from clear cell renal cell carcinoma.

14.4.4
Multiple or Bilateral RCC

Multicentricity in the same kidney occurs in approximately 4% of patients, and bilaterality is seen in 0.5–3.0% (Jacobs et al. 1980). The pathologic criteria for the distinction of multicentricity from intrarenal or contrarenal metastases have not been established, but a significant difference in the morphology of various tumors in the same or opposite kidneys favors multifocality (Fig. 14.16). Among multifocal cases, 75% of lesions are synchronous; the remainder are asynchronous (Zincke and Swanson 1982). Multicentricity and bilaterality are often associated with familial and associated conditions such as von Hippel-Lindau disease (Fig. 14.17).

14.4.5
RCC Associated with Hereditary Disease

Hereditary renal cancer syndromes can lead to multiple bilateral kidney tumors that occur at a younger age than do nonhereditary renal cancers. Imaging plays an important role in the diagnosis and management of these syndromes.

14.4.5.1
Von Hippel-Lindau Disease

Renal cell carcinoma occurs in 38–55% of patients with von Hippel-Lindau syndrome (Solomon and Schwartz 1988). Lesions tend to be bilateral and

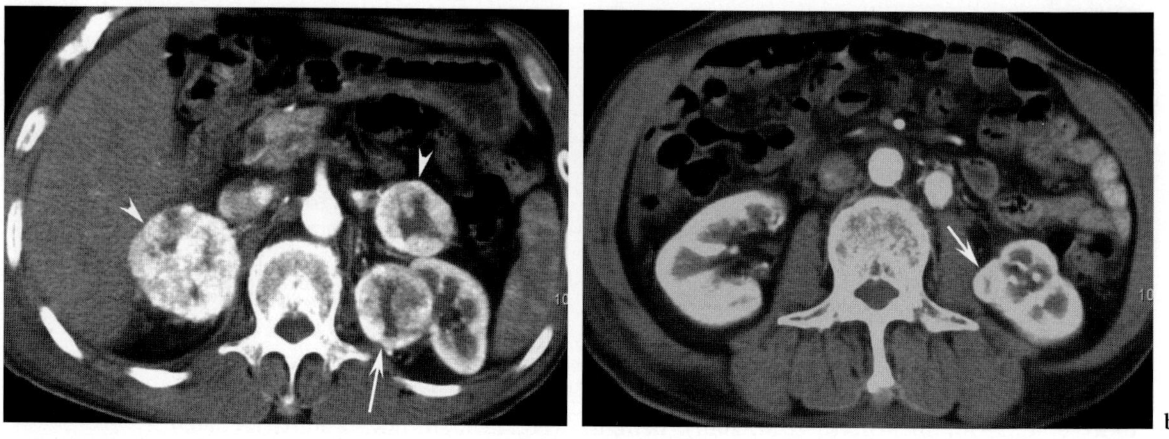

Fig. 14.16a,b. Multiple renal cell carcinomas with bilateral adrenal metastases in a 56-year-old woman. **a, b** Axial contrast-enhanced CT scans in corticomedullary phase show hypervascular expansile masses in left kidney (*arrows*) and both adrenal glands (*arrowheads*).

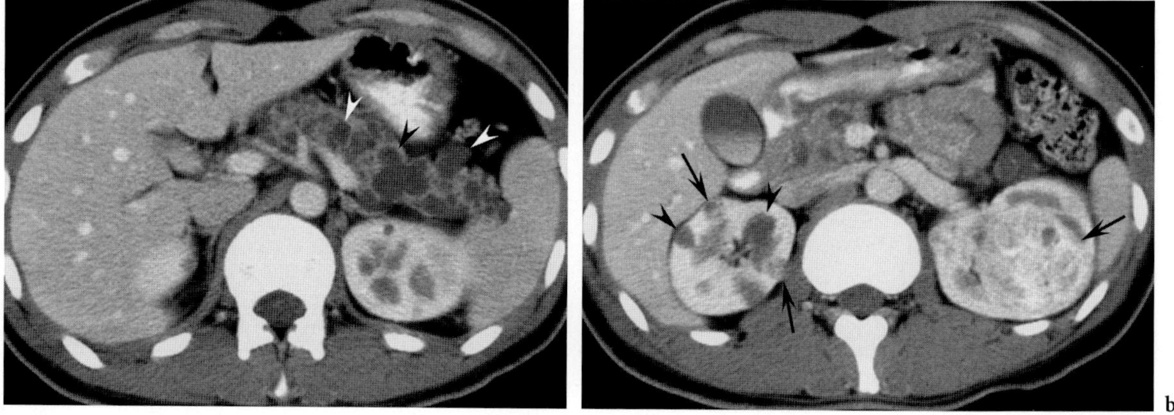

Fig. 14.17a,b. Multiple renal cell carcinomas in a 68-year-old man with von Hippel-Lindau disease. **a** Axial contrast-enhanced CT scan shows numerous cysts (*arrowheads*) in pancreas. **b** Axial contrast-enhanced CT scan shows multiple enhancing solid tumors (*arrows*) and multiple cysts (*arrowheads*) in both kidneys.

multicentric, are often associated with cysts, and occur at an earlier age than sporadic RCC. As many as one-third of patients with von Hippel-Lindau disease die of RCC. Papillary and solid tumor nodules are seen intracystically and typical clear cell RCCs may ultimately develop.

The hallmark of VHL disease in the kidney is bilateral cystic and solid renal neoplasms. The lesions run the gamut from simple cysts to complex cysts with solid enhancing septa or masses to almost entirely solid renal neoplasms. The key features are that the process is bilateral, occurs at a young age, and is associated with other manifestations of VHL disease (Fig. 14.17; MELMON and ROSEN 1964; GLENN et al. 1997). The cells lining the cysts, as well as the cells within tumors, have a clear cell appearance. Many of these lesions are below the resolution of imaging. Microscopic inspection of gross normal tissue reveals that approximately 600 microscopic tumorlets may be found in each kidney at pathologic examination (POSTON et al. 1995; WALTHER et al. 1995). Fortunately, only a few of these grow to become clinically important. On CT, the solid parts of the tumors enhance briskly (50–200 HU) after intravenous administration of contrast material. This is likely related to the increased levels of vascular endothelial growth factor and other angiogenic factors produced by these tumors. Renal cancers associated with VHL disease will eventually metastasize if left untreated (CHOYKE et al. 2003).

14.4.5.2
Tuberous Sclerosis

A increased risk of RCC is also seen in patients with tuberous sclerosis (TS). On average, patients with TS develop RCC in the fourth decade, with some cases occurring in childhood. Other renal lesions associated with this disorder include AMLs and cysts (BJORNSSON et al. 1996).

In most cases, renal lesions can be correctly characterized as cysts or AMLs on the basis of absence of enhancement (cysts) or the presence of hypodense fat (AMLs). Nonfatty AMLs, however, are difficult to differentiate from renal cancers and occur in over one-third of cases of TS. Typically, such lesions are hyperdense compared with surrounding renal parenchyma on unenhanced CT scans and are uniform in density despite their large size (LEMAITRE et al. 1997); however, definitive characterization requires biopsy. An alternative to biopsy is close follow-up, because AMLs characteristically grow very slowly, whereas malignancies tend to exhibit accelerated growth (LEMAITRE et al. 1995). The presence of calcification should also suggest a malignancy, because calcifications are unusual in AMLs. Most AMLs and renal cancers show dramatic enhancement after contrast material administration, so this is not a point of differentiation.

14.4.6
RCC with Varicocele

Varicoceles are the most frequently encountered masses of the spermatic cord. They may either be idiopathic, likely resulting from incompetent valves within the testicular veins, or develop secondary to an abdominal mass (Fig. 14.18; typically RCC) that compresses or invades the renal veins or inferior vena cava (BOSTWICK et al. 1997). An abdominal mass should always be suspected when an older man presents with a new varicocele (WOODWARD et al. 2003).

14.5
Conclusion

There are various unusual manifestations of RCCs. Sometimes they mimic other benign or malignant renal tumors or inflammation. Familiarity with these radiologic features of unusual RCCs can help ensure correct diagnosis and proper management.

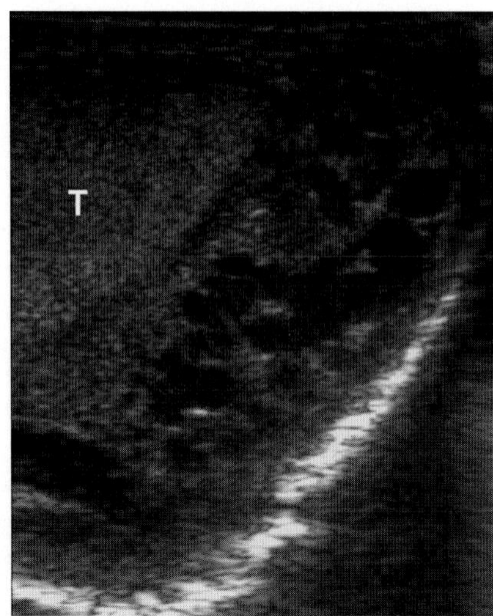
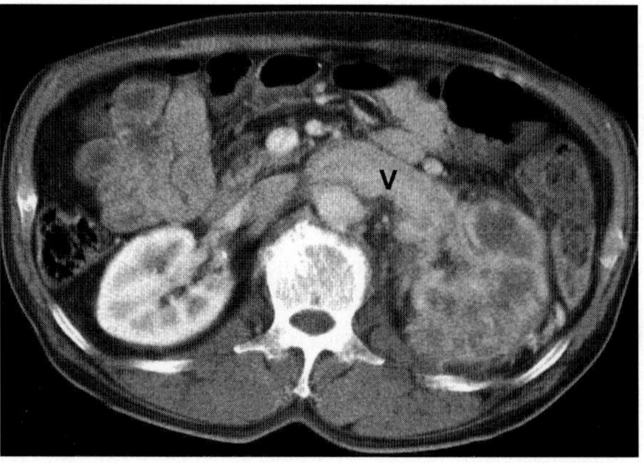

Fig. 14.18a,b. Renal cell carcinoma associated with varicocele in a 70-year-old man. **a** Sagittal ultrasound image of the left testis shows multiple, serpiginous, hypoechoic spaces around the testis (*T*). **b** Axial contrast-enhanced CT scan in corticomedullary phase shows diffuse infiltrative mass in left kidney with invasion of left renal vein (*V*).

References

Ambos MA, Bosniak MA, Madayag MA et al. (1977) Infiltrating neoplasms of the kidney. Am J Roentgenol 129:859–864

Bjornsson J, Short MP, Kwiatkowski DJ et al. (1996) Tuberous sclerosis-assocated renal cell carcinoma. Clinical, pathological, and genetic features. Am J Pathol 149:1201–1208

Bosniak MA (1986) The current radiological approach to renal cysts. Radiology 158:1–10

Bosniak MA (1991) Difficulties in classifying cystic lesions of the kidney. Urol Radiol 13:91–93

Bosniak MA (1997a) Diagnosis and management of patients with complicated cystic lesions of the kidney. Am J Roentgenol 169:819–821

Bosniak MA (1997b) The use of the Bosniak classification system for renal cysts and cystic tumors. J Urol 157:1852–1853

Bosnib SM (1999) Risk and prognosis in renal neoplasm: a pathologist's prospective. Urol Clin North Am 26:643–660

Bostwick DG (1997) Spermatic cord and testicular adnexa. In: Bostwick DG, Eble JN (eds) Urologic surgical pathology. Mosby, St. Louis, pp 647–674

Brinker DA, Amin MB, de Peralta-Venturina M et al. (2000) Extensively necrotic cystic renal cell carcinoma: a clinico-pathologic study with comparison to other cytic and necrotic renal cancers. Am J Surg Pathol 24:988–995

Castoldi MC, Dellafiore L, Renne G et al. (1995) CT demonstration of liquid intratumoral fat layering in a necrotic renal cell carcinoma. Abdom Imaging 20:483–485

Cheuk W, Lo ES, Chan AK et al. (2002) Atypical epithelial proliferations in acquired renal cystic disease harbor cytogenetic aberration. Hum Pathol 33:761–765

Cho KR, Park CM, Chung HH et al. (2002) Spiral CT findings of chromophobe renal cell carcinoma: correlation with pathologic features and prognosis. J Korean Radiol Soc 46:57–62

Choyke PL, Glenn GM, Walther MM et al. (2003) Hereditary renal cancers. Radiology 226:33–46

Curry NS, Schabel SI, Garvin AJ et al. (1990) Intratumoral fat in a renal oncocytoma mimicking angiomyolipoma. Am J Roentgenol 154:307–308

Daniel WW Jr, Hartman GW, Witten DM et al. (1972) Calcified renal masses. A review of ten years experience at the Mayo Clinic. Radiology 103:503–508

Davidson AJ, Choyke PL, Hartman DS et al. (1995) Renal medullary carcinoma associated with sickle cell trait: radiologic findings. Radiology 195:83–85

Davis CJ, Mostofi FK, Sesterhenn IA (1995) Renal medullary carcinoma: the seventh sickle nephropathy. Am J Surg Pathol 19:1–11

Dimopoulos MA, Logothetis CJ, Markowitz A et al. (1993) Collecting duct carcinoma of the kidney. Br J Urol 71:388–391

Eble JN, Bosnib SM (1998) Extensively cystic renal neoplasm: cystic nephroma, cystic partially differentiated nephroblastoma, multilocular cystic renal cell carcinoma and cystic hamartoma of the renal pelvis. Semin Diagn Pathol 15:2–20

Eble JN, Sauter G, Epstein JI et al. (2004) World Health Organization classification of tumours: pathology and genetics of tumours of the urinary system and male genital organs. IARC Press, Lyons

Fukuoka T, Honda M, Namiki M et al. (1987) Renal cell carcinoma with heterotopic bone formation. Case report and review of the Japanese liteature. Urol Int 42:458–460

Fukuya T, Honda H, Goto K et al. (1996) Computed tomographic findings of Bellini duct carcinoma of the kidney. J Comput Assist Tomogr 20:399–403

Glenn GM, Gnarra JR, Choyke PL et al. (1997) The molecular genetics of renal cell carcinoma. In: Raghaven D, Scher HI, Lange PH (eds) Principles and practice of genitourinary oncology. Lippincott-Raven, Philadelphia, pp 85–97

Gregoire JR, Torres VE, Holley KE et al. (1987) Renal epithelial hyperplastic and neoplastic proliferation in autosomal dominant polycystic kidney disease. Am J Kidney Dis 9:27–38

Hartman DS, Davis CJ Jr, Johns T et al. (1986) Cystic renal cell carcinoma. Urol 28:199–216

Hartman DS, Davidson AJ, Davis CJ et al. (1988) Infiltrative renal lesions: CT–sonographic–pathologic correlation. Am J Roentgenol 150:1061–1064

Helenon O, Chretien Y, Paraf F et al.(1993) Renal cell carcinoma containing fat: demonstration with CT. Radiology 188:429–430

Helenon O, Merran S, Paraf F et al. (1997) Unusual fat-containing tumors of the kidney: a diagnostic dilemma. Radiographics 17:129–144

Herts BR, Coll DM, Novick AC et al. (2002) Enhancement characteristics of papillary renal neoplasms revealed on triphasic helical CT of the kidneys. Am J Roentgenol 178:367–372

Hughson MD, Buchwald D, Fox M (1986) Renal neoplasia and acquired cystic kidney disease in patients receiving long-term dialysis. Arch Pathol Lab Med 110:592–601

Ishigawa I, Saito Y, Shikura N et al. (1990) Ten-year prospective study on the development of renal cell carcinoma in dialysis patients. Am J Kidney Dis 16:452–458

Israel GM, Bosniak MA (2003) Calcification in cystic renal masses: Is it important in diagnosis? Radiology 226:47–52

Jacobs SC, Berg SI, Lawson RK (1980) Synchronous bilateral renal cell carcinoma: total surgical excision. Cancer 46:2341–2345

Kikkawa K, Lasser EC (1969) "Ring-like" or "rim-like" calcification in renal cell carcinoma. Am J Roentgenol Radium Ther Nucl Med 107:737–742

Kim JC, Kim KH, Lee JW (2000) CT and US findings of multilocular cystic renal cell carcinoma. Korean J Radiol 1:104–109

Kim JK, Kim TK, Ahn HJ et al. (2002) Differentiation of subtypes of renal cell carcinoma on helical CT scans. Am J Roentgenol 178:1499–1506

Koga S, Nishikido M, Inuzuka S et al. (2000) An evaluation of Bosniak's radiological classification of cystic renal masses. BJU Int 86:607–609

Krieger JN, Sniderman KW, Seligson GR et al. (1979) Calcified renal cell carcinoma: a clinical, radiographic and pathologic study. J Urol 121:575–580

Kumar S, Cederbaum AI, Pletka PG (1980) Renal cell carcinoma in polycystic kidneys: case report and review of literature. J Urol 124:708–709

Lemaitre L, Robert Y, Dubrulle F et al. (1995) Renal angiomyolipoma: growth followed up with CT and/or US. Radiology 197:598–602

Lemaitre L, Claudon M, Dubrulle F et al. (1997) Imaging of angiomyolipomas. Semin Ultrasound CT MR 18:100–114

London NJ, Messions N, Kinder RB et al. (1989) A prospective study of the value of conventional CT, dynamic CT, ultrasonography and arteriography for staging renal carcinoma. Br J Urol 64:209–217

Matas AJ, Simmons RI, Kjellstrand CM et al. (1975) Increased incidence of malignancy during chronic renal failure. Lancet 1:883–885

Matson MA, Cohen EP (1990) Acquired cystic kidney disease: occurrence, prevalence, and renal cancers. Medicine 69:217–226

Mehanna D, Abu-Zidan FM, Rao S (2004) Liver metastasis in renal chondrosarcoma. Singapore Med J 45:183–185

Melmon KL, Rosen SW (1964) Lindau's disease. Am J Med 36:595–617

Murad T, Komaiko W, Oyasu R et al. (1991) Multilocular cystic renal cell carcinoma. Am J Clin Pathol 95:633–637

Muram TM, Aisen A (2003) Fatty metastatic lesions in 2 patients with renal clear-cell carcinoma. J Comput Assist Tomogr 27:869–870

Murphy WM, Grignon DJ, Perlman EJ (2004) Tumors of the kidney, bladder, and related urinary structures. Armed Forces Institute of Pathology Atlas of Tumor Pathology, Fourth Series , Washington, DC

Onishi T, Ohishi Y, Iizuka N et al. (1996) Clinicopathological study on patients with chromophobe cell renal carcinoma. Nippon Hinyokika Gakkai Zasshi 87:1167–1174

Onishi T, Oishi Y, Goto H et al. (2002) Histological features of hypovascular or avascular renal cell carcinoma: the experience at four university hospitals. Int J Clin Oncol 7:159–164

Outwater EK, Bhatia M, Siegelman ES et al. (1997) Lipid in renal clear cell carcinoma: detection on opposed-phase gradient-echo MR images. Radiology 205:103–107

Parvey LS, Warner RM, Callihan TR et al. (1981) CT demonstration of fat tissue in malignant renal neoplasms: atypical Wilms' tumors. J Comput Assist Tomogr 5:851–854

Patterson J, Lohr D, Briscoe C et al. (1987) Calcified renal masses. Urology 29:353–356

Peralta-Venturina M de, Moch H, Amin M et al. (2001) Sarcomatoid differentiation in renal cell carcinoma: a study of 101 cases. Am J Surg Pathol 25:275–284

Pickhardt PJ, Lonergan GJ, Davis CJ et al. (2000) Infiltrative renal lesions: radiologic–pathologic correlation. Radiographics 20:215–243

Pickhardt PJ, Siegel CL, McLarney JK (2001) Collecting duct carcinoma of the kidney: Are imaging findings suggestive of the diagnosis? Am J Roentgenol 176:627–633

Poston CD, Jaffe GS, Lubensky IA et al. (1995) Characterization of the renal pathology of a familial form of renal cell carcinoma associated with von Hippel-Lindau disease: clinical and molecular genetic implications. J Urol 153:22–26

Press GA, McClennan BL, Melson GL et al. (1984) Papillary renal cell carcinoma: CT and sonographic evaluation. Am J Roentgenol. 143:1005–1009

Reuter VE, Presti JC Jr. (2000) Contemporary approach to the classification of renal epithelial tumors. Semin Oncol 27:124–137

Roy C, Tuchmann C, Linder V et al. (1998) Renal cell carcinoma with a fatty component mimicking angiomyolipoma on CT. Br J Radiol 71:977–979

Shinozaki K, Yoshinitsu K, Honda H et al. (2001) Metastatic adrenal tumor from clear-cell renal cell carcinoma: a pitfall of chemical shift MR imaging. Abdom Imaging 26:439–442

Solomon D, Schwartz A (1988) Renal pathology in von Hippel-Lindau disease. Hum Pathol 19:1012–1029

Srigley JR, Eble JN (1998) Collecting duct carcinoma of the kidney. Semin Diagn Pathol 15:54–67

Storkel S, Eble JN, Adlakha K et al. (1997) Classification of renal cell carcinoma: Workgroup No. 1. Union Internationale Contre le Cancer (UICC) and the American Joint Committee on Cancer (AJCC). Cancer 80:987–989

Strotzer M, Lehner KB, Becker K (1993) Detection of fat in a renal cell carcinoma mimicking angiomyolipoma. Radiology 188:427–428

Swartz MA, Karth J, Schneider DT et al. (2002) Renal medullary carcinoma; clinical, pathologic, immunohistochemical, and genetic analysis with pathogenetic implications. Urology 60:1083–1089

Szolar DH, Kammerhuber F, Altziebler S et al. (1997) Multiphasic helical CT of the kidney: increased conspicuity for detection and characterization of small (<3 cm) renal masses. Radiology 202:211–217

Takase K, Takahashi S, Tazawa S et al. (1994) Renal cell carcinoma associated with chronic renal failure: evaluation with sonographic angiography. Radiology 192:787–792

Takebayashi S, Hidai H, Chiba T et al. (1999) Using helical CT to evaluate renal cell carcinoma in patients undergoing hemodialysis: value of early enhanced images. Am J Roentgenol 172:429–433

Thoenes W, Storkel S, Rumpelt HJ (1988) Chromophobe cell renal carcinoma and its variant: a report on 32 cases. J Pathol 155:277–287

Walther MM, Lubensky IA, Venzon D et al. (1995) Prevalence of microscopic lesions in grossly normal renal parenchyma from patients with von Hippel-Lindau disease, sporadic renal cell carcinoma and no renal disease: clinical implications. J Urol 154:2010–2014

Weyman PJ, McClennan BL, Stabley RJ et al. (1980) Comparison of computed tomography and angiography in the evaluation of renal cell carcinoma. Radiology 137:417–424

Woodward PJ, Schwab CM, Sesterhenn IA (2003) From the archives of the AFIP: extratesticular scrotal masses: radiologic–pathologic correlation. Radiographics 23:215–240

Yamashita Y, Takahashi M, Watanabe O et al. (1992) Small renal cell carcinoma: pathologic and radiologic correlation. Radiology 184:493–498

Yamashita Y, Watanabe O, Miyazaki T et al. (1994) Cystic renal cell carcinoma. Imaging findings with pathologic correlation. Acta Radiol 35:19–24

Yamashita Y, Miyazaki T, Ishii A et al. (1995) Multilocular cystic renal cell carcinoma presenting as a solid mass: radiologic evaluation. Abdom Imaging 20:164–168

Zagoria RJ, Wolfman NT, Karstaedt N et al. (1990) CT features of renal cell carcinoma with emphasis on relation to tumor size. Invest Radiol 25:261–266

Zincke H, Swanson SK (1982) Bilateral renal cell carcinoma: influence of synchronous and asynchronous occurrence on patient survival. J Urol 128:913–915

15 Hereditary Renal Cancer

Toshiyuki Miyazaki and Mutsumasa Takahashi

CONTENTS

T. Miyazaki, MD
Chairman, Department of Radiology, Arao City Hospital, 2600
Arao, Arao city 864-0041, Japan
M. Takahashi, MD
Emeritus Professor, Department of Radiology, Kumamoto
University, International Imaging Center, 1-2-23 Kuhonji,
Kumamoto city 862-0976, Japan

15.1 Introduction

Renal cancer is diagnosed in over 30,000 Americans each year, accounting for approximately 12,000 deaths annually. Smoking, obesity, and occupational exposure have been implicated in the development of renal cancers but, in general, their cause remains obscure (Moyad 2001). Although hereditary renal cancer makes up only about 4% of the total number of cases, this percentage is expected to increase as a more complete understanding of the genetic causes of cancer is elucidated (Gago-Dominguez et al. 2001).

Increasing knowledge of hereditary renal cancer syndromes has provided insights into the mechanisms of cancer development in the general population and has assisted efforts to prevent and treat renal cancers. These cancers include von Hippel-Lindau disease, hereditary papillary renal cancer, hereditary leiomyoma renal cell carcinoma, Birt-Hogg-Dubé syndrome, hereditary renal oncocytoma, familial renal oncocytoma, medullary carcinoma of kidney, and tuberous sclerosis (Table 15.1; Choyke at al. 2003). The most common cell type in renal cancer is the clear cell carcinoma, followed by papillary (types 1 and 2), chromophobe carcinoma, and oncocytoma (Amin et al. 2002). Medullary carcinoma and duct of Bellini cancers are rare. Over the past 5 years, hereditary renal cancer syndromes have been associated with one or more of these cancer cell types.

Many of the genes responsible for these syndromes have been discovered and research is underway to explain the molecular pathways that guide tumor development. A more complete picture of the mechanisms underlying the development of tumors of varying cell types is emerging.

Hereditary cancers are typically multifocal and bilateral, and the radiologist is often the first to raise the possibility of a hereditary cause for a particular renal cancer (Table 15.2). It is therefore important to be familiar with the expanding list of diseases known to predispose to renal cancers.

Table 15.1. Hereditary renal cancers in adults. *CNS* central nervous system, *HGF* hepatocyte growth factor. (With permission from CHOYKE et al. 2003)

Syndrome	Gene, "gene name," (gene product)	Frequency of cancer (%)	Predominant renal tumor type	Other renal tumor types	Associated abnormalities
von Hippel-Lindau disease	3p26, "VHL," (pVHL)	28–45	Clear cell	Cysts	CNS hemangioblastomas, retinal angiomas, pancreatic cysts, neuroendocrine tumors of the pancreas, pheochromocytoma
Hereditary papillary renal cancer	7q34, "c-MET," (HGF receptor)	19	Papillary type 1	None	None
Hereditary leiomyoma renal cell carcinoma	1q42-43, "FH," (fumarate hydratase)	15–30	Papillary type 2	None	Cutaneous and uterine leiomyomas
Birt-Hogg-Dubé syndrome	17p11.2, "BHD," (folliculin)	8–15	Chromophobe, oncocytic neoplasm	Clear cell, papillary, oncocytoma	Fibrofolliculomas, lung cysts, pneumothoraces
Familial renal oncocytoma	Unknown	Unknown	Oncocytoma	None	Renal dysfunction
Medullary carcinoma of kidney	11p	Unknown	Medullary carcinoma	None	Sickle cell trait
Tuberous sclerosis	9q34 "TSC1," (hamartin) 16p13 "TSC2," (tuberin)	1–2	Clear cell	Cysts, angiomyolipoma, papillary, chromophobe, oncocytoma	CNS tubers, angiofibromas of skin, cardiac rhabdomyomas

15.2
Histologic Subtypes of Renal Cancer

Before considering the individual hereditary renal cancer syndromes, it is important to review the characteristics of the different cell types of renal cancer. Renal cancers can be subclassified into a variety of cell types (Fig. 15.1; STORKEL et al. 1997).

Clear cell carcinomas are the most frequent type of renal cancer, accounting for approximately 75% of renal cancers. The term "clear cell carcinoma" encompasses the clear cell variant, the granular cell variant, and mixed cell types. The high glycogen content within the cytoplasm of clear cell cancer cells accounts for their lucent appearance on conventional histologic stains. When glycogen is less abundant, the cytoplasm is darker and the cells are termed "granular." A delicate but rich and permeable vascular supply is often seen throughout these tumors, although regions of necrosis, fibrosis, or hemorrhage are avascular or hypovascular. Clear cell carcinomas are thought to arise from the proximal tubular epithelium of the kidney.

The second leading type of renal cancer is termed "papillary," or sometimes "chromophil," renal cancer, and accounts for 10–15% of all renal cancers. There are two subtypes of papillary renal cell carcinoma, types 1 and 2, which are distinguished by tumor architecture and cellular morphology. Both types share a common papillary structure: a fibrovascular core with tumor cells lining the surface of each papilla (Fig. 15.1; KOVACS et al. 1997). Type 1, or basophilic renal cancer, usually is considered clinically low grade and has a favorable prognosis. This tumor is composed of fronds of fibrovascular papillary and tubular structures covered by cells with scanty cytoplasm and small oval nuclei. Foamy macrophages, which are thought to represent a host immune response, are often present within the interstitium, and psammoma bodies also are frequently present. Despite the apparent vascularity on histology, type 1 papillary renal tumors typically enhance poorly on CT or during renal angiography. Type 2 papillary tumors, or eosinophilic renal cancers, bear a superficial resemblance to type 1 tumors in that the basic frond-like architecture is present but they may not be related at a biologic level. Type 2 papillary renal cancers consist of papillae covered by large cells with abundant eosinophilic cytoplasm and large nuclei with prominent nucleoli. Type 2 papillary tumors often are more clinically aggressive than type 1 papillary tumors and can enhance more intensely. Papillary tumors also are thought to arise from the proximal tubular epithelium.

Table 15.2. Summary of six patients with renal cell carcinoma in von Hippel-Lindau disease. *ML* multilocular, *UL* unilocular, *CNS* central nervous system, *ND* not detected

Case no./ age (years)/ gender	Pathologic findings	Structure	Size (cm)	CNS	Non-CNS
1/71/F	Right, ML cystic	Cystic	5×4×4.5	ND	Pancreas cysts
	UL cystic	Tubular	ø1.3		
	UL cystic	Tubular	ø1.2		
	Solid	Tubular	ø1.0		
	Left, ML cystic	Tubular	3.5×3×3		
	ML cystic	Tubular	ø2.0		
	Solid	Tubular	ø3.0		
2/65/F	Right, ML cystic	Alveolar	ø4.5	ND	Pancreas cysts
	Solid	Alveolar	ø3.0		Renal cysts, bilateral
	Left, solid	Alveolar	ø3.5		
	Solid	Alveolar	ø2.0		
3/60/M	Right, ML cystic	Tubular	8×7×7	ND	Pancreas cysts
	Left, ML cystic	Tubular	5×5×4		Renal cysts, bilateral
					Adrenal tumor, right
4/47/M	Right, solid	Cystic	ø2.3	Hemangioblastoma (lumbar)	Pancreas cysts
	Left, ML cystic	Cystic	5×5×4		Renal cysts, bilateral
	ML cystic	Cystic	ø3.2		
	ML cystic	Cystic	ø2.5		
5/36/M	Right, solid	Alveolar	ø5.0	Acoustic neurinoma, left	ND
	Solid	Papillary	ø5.0		
	Solid	Papillary	ø1.5		
	Left, ML cystic	Alveolar	ø8.0		
	Solid	Tubular	ø0.8		
6/22/M	Right, solid	Alveolar > tubular	ø2.0	Hemangioblastoma (cervical, lumbar)	Renal cysts, bilateral
	Solid	Alveolar > tubular	ø1.3		
	Solid	Alveolar > tubular	ø0.9		
	Left, solid	Alveolar > tubular	ø1.5		
	Solid	Alveolar > tubular	ø0.16		

The chromophobe carcinoma, so-named because of its resistance to staining with typical histologic stains such as hematoxylin and eosin, is the third most common type of renal cancer, accounting for about 5% of renal tumors. Chromophobe carcinoma can be stained with Hale's colloidal iron, which yields a homogeneous blue cytoplasmic stain (NAGASHIMA 2000). In routine histologic sections the cytoplasm tends to condense near the cell membrane producing a halo around the nucleus. The cytoplasm is rich in mitochondria much as in oncocytoma (ERLANDSON et al. 1997). Oncocytoma itself is considered a benign renal neoplasm; however, this categorization has been called into question by the resemblance of oncocytoma to chromophobe carcinoma and by reports of "metastasizing" oncocytomas (AMIN et al. 1997b; NOGUCHI et al. 1995; WARFEL and EBLE 1982). Oncocytomas are comprised of cells with abundant eosinophilic cytoplasm filled with mitochondria which cause the brown color on gross pathology. When they are numerous the term "oncocytosis" is used and can be seen in patients with chromophobe carcinomas (WARFEL and EBLE 1982). Chromophobe carcinomas and oncocytomas are thought to arise from intercalated cells in the distal tubules.

Collecting duct carcinoma includes the medullary carcinoma of kidney associated with sickle cell trait and duct of Bellini tumors. Medullary carcinoma is characterized histologically by irregular channels lined by highly atypical epithelium that sometimes have a "hobnail" appearance. The channels are found in an inflamed desmoplastic stroma (FIGENSHAU et al. 1998; DAVIDSON et al. 1995). Both medullary renal cancer and duct of Bellini tumors are clinically aggressive neoplasms. Medullary carcinoma and its variants arise from the collecting ducts, which are histologically and embryologically distinct from the tubular epithelium.

15.3
von Hippel-Lindau Disease

15.3.1
Clinical Features

von Hippel-Lindau disease (VHL) is a multisystem autosomal dominant hereditary disorder characterized by the formation of hemangioblastomas in the

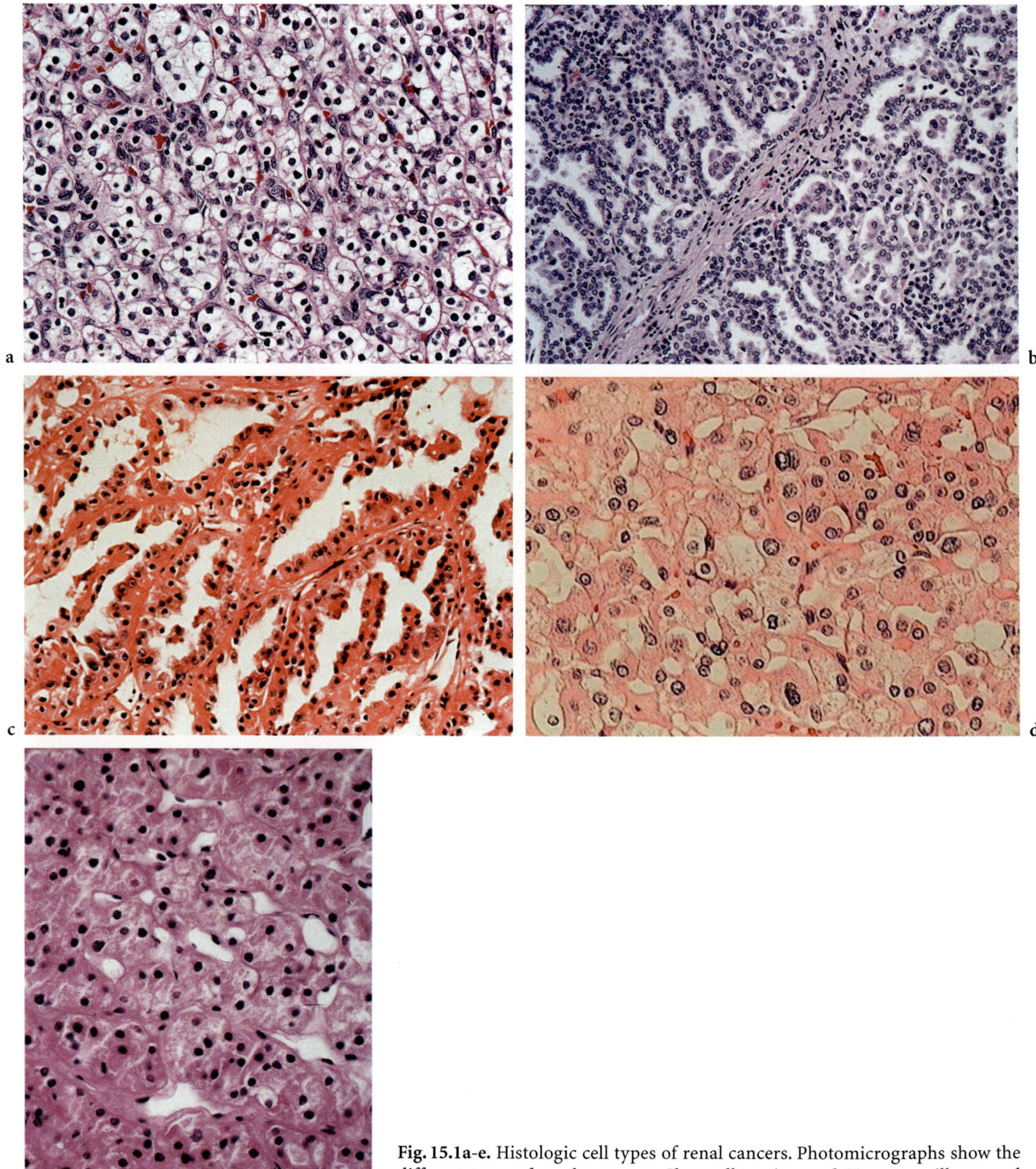

Fig. 15.1a-e. Histologic cell types of renal cancers. Photomicrographs show the different types of renal cancers. **a** Clear cell carcinoma. **b** Type 1 papillary renal cancer. **c** Type 2 papillary renal cancer. **d** Chromophobe carcinoma. **e** Oncocytoma (Hematoxylin and eosin stain; original magnification, ×100).

spine and posterior fossa, retinal angiomas, pheochromocytomas, pancreatic cysts, cystadenomas and renal neuroendocrine tumors, epididymal and broad ligament cystadenomas, and renal cysts and tumors. The prevalence of the disease in Europe and the North America is one in 36,000–40,000 (NEUMANN and WIESTLER 1991).

Cerebellar and spinal hemangioblastomas can cause neurologic deficits and symptoms such as ataxia, paraplegia, sensory loss, and dysequilibrium. Spinal lesions can lead to secondary syringomyelia. Endolymphatic sac tumors are tumors that develop in the labyrinth of the inner ear and can lead to hearing loss and dysequilibrium. Although these tumors do not metastasize, they can be locally aggressive and may lead to complete deafness.

The pancreas is most commonly affected by cysts that are classified histologically as serous cystadenomas. These can range in severity from single isolated cystic lesions or clusters of cysts to complete replacement of the pancreatic parenchyma with cysts. Occasionally, severe pancreatic cystic disease will cause exocrine insufficiency requiring pancreatic enzyme replacement. Large cysts can lead to partial bowel obstruction, pain, and early satiety. The cysts can be drained and sclerosed. Pancreatic neuroendocrine tumors are solid enhancing lesions occurring in fewer than 8% of patients with VHL disease (LIBUTTI et al. 1998). Pancreatic neuroendocrine tumors are often found with pheochromocytomas and, thus, may be genetically linked; however, each can be found without the other (LIBUTTI et al. 1998; ZBAR 2000). Pheochromocytomas can be asymptomatic or "silent" when small but gradually produce levels of catecholamines sufficient to cause symptoms such as tachycardia, hypertension, and profuse sweating (WALTHER et al. 1999) and can be life threatening if not identified and treated prior to stressful events such as surgery or childbirth.

von Hippel-Lindau disease gives rise to a variety of renal cystic lesions ranging from pure cysts to mixed solid and cystic masses (Fig. 15.2), and to purely solid clear cell carcinomas (Fig. 15.3) of the kidney.

15.3.2
Genetics

The VHL gene is considered an important housekeeping or tumor suppressor gene that in its normal state functions to prevent the development of renal cancers. Mutations or inactivation of the VHL gene are found in over 60% of sporadic clear cell renal carcinomas indicating that it is one of the crucial genes in the development of clear cell carcinoma of the kidney (HAMANO et al. 2002; HERMAN et al. 1994).

A tumor suppressor gene normally functions to decrease the chance of developing cancer. When a tumor suppressor gene is mutated and the resulting protein product is abnormal, the affected cells are at increased risk of malignancy. Tumor development requires that both copies of the gene become mutated or deleted. Unlike other diseases in which more than one genetic locus has been implicated, VHL seems to

be caused by mutations at a single gene locus, 3p25 (short arm of third chromosome).

The gene was first discovered in 1993 (LATIF et al. 1993). Subsequently, it was demonstrated that the VHL gene codes for a protein, pVHL. One of the normal roles of pVHL is to assist in the degradation of an intracellular growth factor known as hypoxia inducible factor-α (HIFα; KAELIN et al. 1998). HIFα is an important regulator of metabolism and is dependent on the oxygen tension within a cell. Normally, HIFα is produced when the cell is exposed to hypoxic conditions. Once normal oxygen tension is restored, HIFα is quickly degraded in a process mediated by pVHL.

A variety of mutations of the VHL gene have been discovered including complete and partial deletions, single missense mutations, and frame shift mutations. Patients suspected of the disease can now be tested for VHL with a simple blood sample. DNA from peripheral white cells is used to check for recorded mutations in VHL. The test is 99% accurate for the diagnosis of VHL (STOLLE et al. 1998).

15.3.3
Imaging and Management

Renal lesions are a common manifestation of VHL. Between 60 and 70% of patients develop cysts in the kidney and about 40% develop radiologically evident renal cancers. The normal-appearing tissue of a kidney from a patient with VHL contains hundreds of small tumorlets scattered throughout the parenchyma, invisible to the naked eye (Fig. 15.4; POSTON et al. 1995). That only a few of many tumors grow to become apparent on CT is one of the unusual features of VHL. Bilateral tumors can take many forms in VHL. They can appear as cysts, cystic renal cancers, and solid renal cancers (Fig. 15.5; CHOYKE et al. 1995; MIYAZAKI et al. 2000). The cell lining of even a simple renal cyst in VHL contains clear cells similar in appearance to those found within clear cell carcinomas. Cysts can regress or grow. The solid components of mixed lesions tend to grow over time, whereas the cystic areas remain unchanged or regress. Solid lesions tend to grow progressively (CHOYKE et al. 1992). Occasionally, heavily calcified or hemorrhagic cystic disease is seen. Both are usually associated with less aggressive forms of renal cancer, but this is not universally true.

Renal cancers in VHL tend to be well differentiated or Fuhrman grades I–II when they are under 3 cm in diameter. Only one report of a metastatic

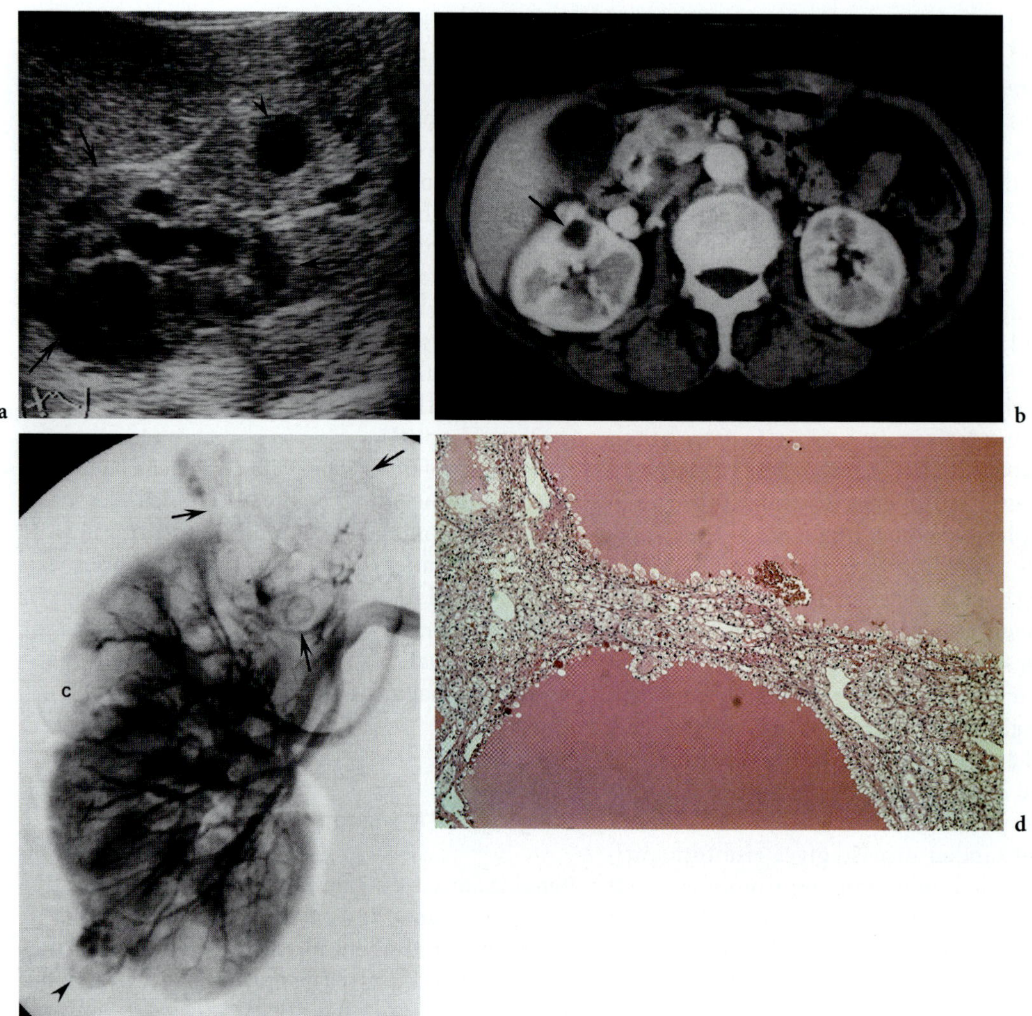

Fig. 15.2a-d. Unilocular and multilocular cystic renal cell carcinomas in a 71-year-old woman. **a** Oblique US image shows an anechoic mass 1.3 cm in diameter in the middle portion of the right kidney (*arrowhead*). Wall irregularity or the solid component is not visualized. A large multilocular cystic renal cell carcinoma is also seen in the upper portion (*arrows*). **b** Minimal wall irregularity is suspected on axial contrast-enhanced CT scan through the unilocular cystic lesion (*arrow*). **c** Anteroposterior projection of selective renal angiography of the right kidney demonstrates an avascular area of unilocular cystic renal cell carcinoma in the middle portion (*c*). A hypovascular multilocular cystic renal cell carcinoma is present in the upper pole (*arrows*) and a small hypovascular solid renal cell carcinoma is in the lower pole (*arrowhead*). Nephrectomy of the right kidney was performed. **d** Photomicrograph of the unilocular cystic lesion reveals an atypical hyperplastic layer, suggesting cystic renal cell carcinoma (hematoxylin and eosin stain; original magnification, ×25).

renal tumor less than 3 cm in diameter (2.5 cm) has appeared in the literature (TURNER et al. 2001). As a consequence, it is generally believed that treatment should be reserved for patients with larger lesions, 3 cm in diameter or greater. This strategy has been successful in preserving renal function while avoiding metastatic disease (HERRING et al. 2001).

Renal cancers are typically detected and measured on serial contrast-enhanced CT scans (Fig. 15.5). Using multidetector CT, unenhanced images through the liver and kidneys are first obtained with 5-mm collimation. An intravenous bolus of 130 ml of a nonionic iodinated contrast agent can be administered at 3 ml/s and 2.5-mm-thick sections (reconstructed at 5-mm intervals) are obtained during the arterial phase (approximately 25 s) and during the venous phase (approximately 80 s). The unenhanced scans are useful for judging whether a lesion is actually enhancing and are of particular use when a hemorrhagic cyst is present. Arterial phase images are useful for detecting pancreatic neuroendocrine tumors (found in approximately 10–15% of

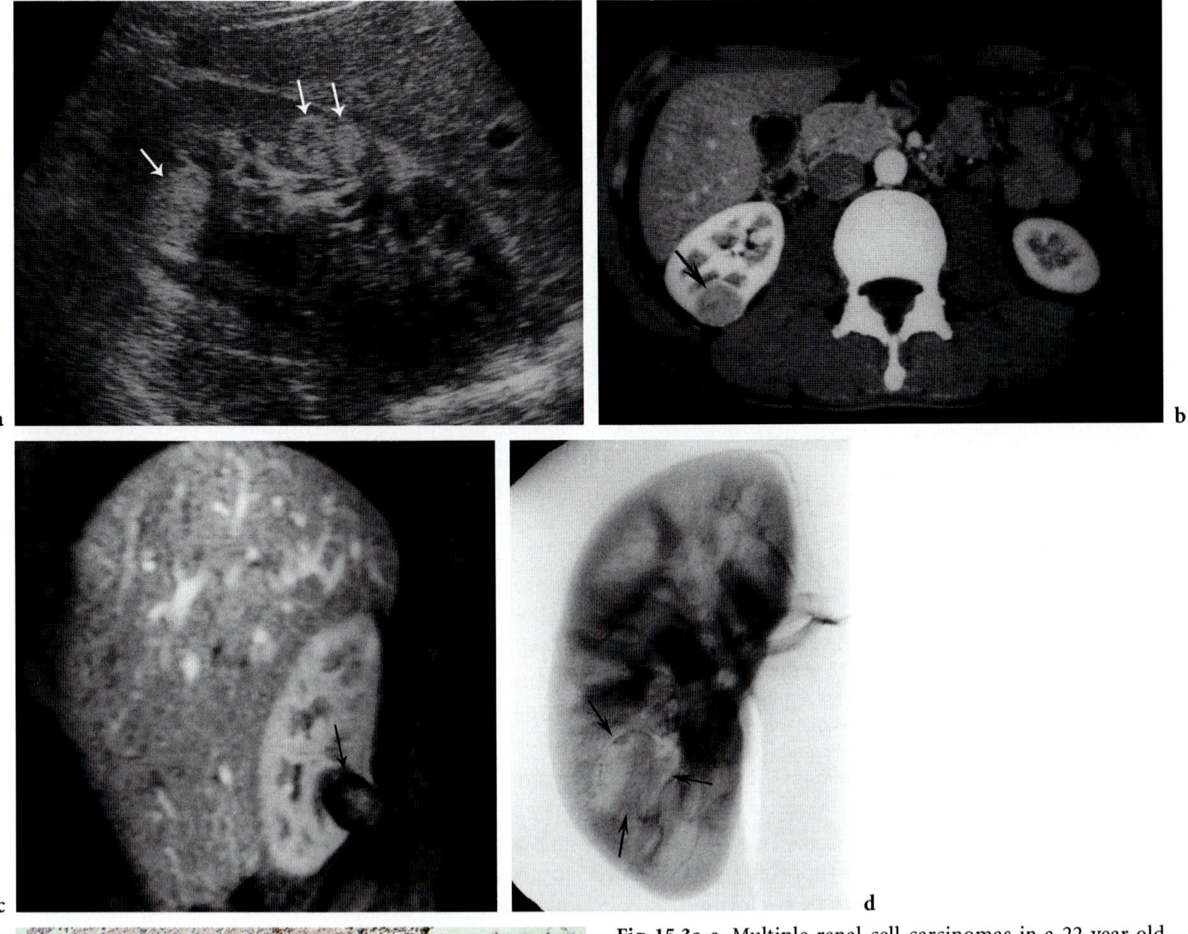

Fig. 15.3a-e. Multiple renal cell carcinomas in a 22-year-old man. **a** Longitudinal US image reveals three hyperechoic masses in the right kidney, less than 2 cm in diameter (*arrows*). **b** Axial dynamic contrast-enhanced CT scan through the largest tumor demonstrates slight parenchymal enhancement (*arrow*); however, its surrounding rim is not visualized. **c** Parasagittal dynamic contrast-enhanced T1-weighted MR image reveals mild enhancement of the tumor and surrounding hypointense rim clearly (*arrow*). **d** Anteroposterior projection of selective renal angiography of the right kidney demonstrates a hypovascular lesion (*arrows*). Nephrectomy of the right kidney was performed. **e** Photomicrograph of the largest tumor shows a renal cell carcinoma composed of clear cells (clear cell carcinoma) in an alveolar configuration. Microcystic changes with hemorrhage are also seen (*arrows*; hematoxylin and eosin stain; original magnification, ×25).

VHL patients), which enhance intensely only on the arterial phase, whereas the venous phase is the most important phase for evaluating the kidneys. The adrenals are seen equally well on all three phases.

Three-dimensional CT angiography and reconstruction can also be performed as clinically necessary before surgery. A three-dimensional model of the kidney can be created to assist the surgeon in identifying lesions for removal.

Serial CT imaging is recommended for patients with VHL, even if they have minimal or no renal disease. The lifetime risk of renal cancer is high in VHL and the key to preserving renal function and preventing metastatic disease is careful monitoring of the patient (GLENN et al. 1997). Patients with minimal disease can be scanned at 1- to 2-year intervals, whereas patients with active renal tumors need to be seen more frequently (every 6–12 months). In patients

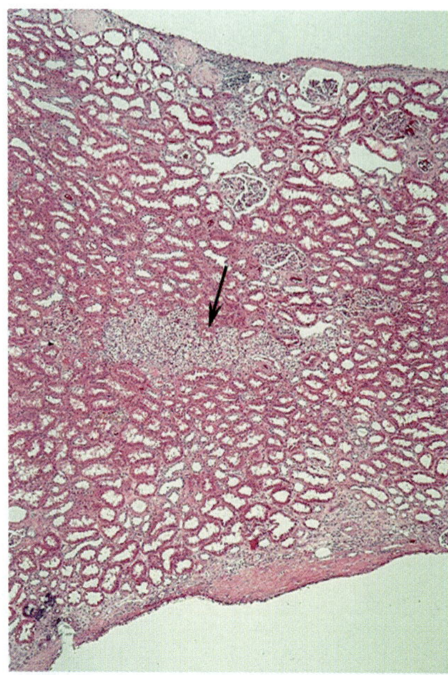

Fig. 15.4. von Hippel-Lindau disease in a 32-year-old man. Photomicrograph shows clear cell tumorlet in the renal parenchyma. Note that there is a tiny focus of tumor within the renal parenchyma (*arrow*). Hundreds of these lesions are found in the kidneys of patients with VHL (Hematoxylin and eosin stain; original magnification, ×25). (With permission from CHOYKE et al. 2003)

with lesions of borderline size (approximately 3 cm) even more frequent studies may be performed.

Tumor growth is not always linear and predictable, and for this reason the record of past CT is not necessarily predictive for any given lesion. Computed tomography is the preferred method of screening because it is relatively less expensive than MR imaging and the CT appearance of renal masses is

well understood. Magnetic resonance imaging with gadolinium chelate administration is a viable alternative in patients with poor renal function, those wishing to avoid ionizing radiation, or with severe allergy to iodinated contrast media. Magnetic resonance imaging should be performed with a torso array coil and fat suppression. If possible, the lesion should be imaged before and after contrast using the same parameters (Ho et al. 2002). Ultrasound is less accurate than other techniques for detecting and characterizing renal masses in VHL and should not be relied on exclusively (JAMIS-DOW et al. 1996).

The standard method of treatment of renal tumors in VHL is nephron-sparing surgery (HERRING et al. 2001). In this procedure, the surgeon enucleates visible tumors and cysts on the renal surface. Deeper lesions are detected using intraoperative ultrasound (Fig. 15.6; CHOYKE et al. 2001). The purpose of the nephron-sparing approach is to remove the relevant lesions while maximally preserving renal parenchyma. Of course, there is a limit to the number of procedures that can be performed on a single kidney and "completion nephrectomies" are sometimes necessary. If the patient is diagnosed too late for nephron-sparing approaches, total nephrectomy may be necessary.

Recently, radiofrequency ablation and cryotherapy have been used because they are comparatively minimally invasive methods for treating small renal cancers in VHL and other hereditary renal masses (WOOD et al. 2002; PAVLOVICH et al. 2002; GERVAIS et al. 2000). For lesions positioned close to the bowel, laparoscopically guided radiofrequency ablation or cryotherapy can be performed (Fig. 15.7; CHEN et al. 2000; PAUTLER et al. 2001; REMER et al. 2000).

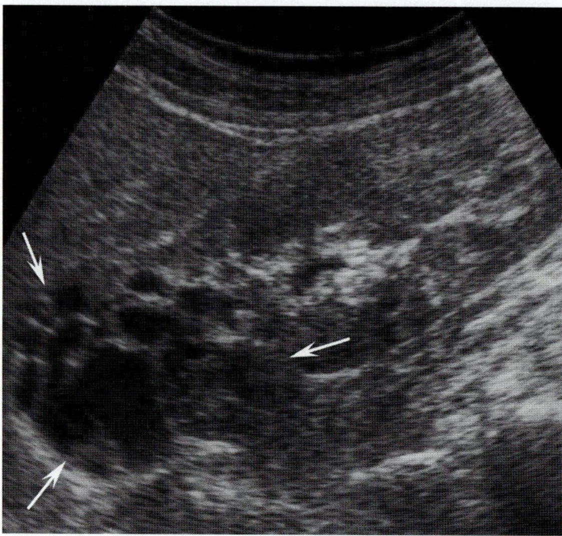

a

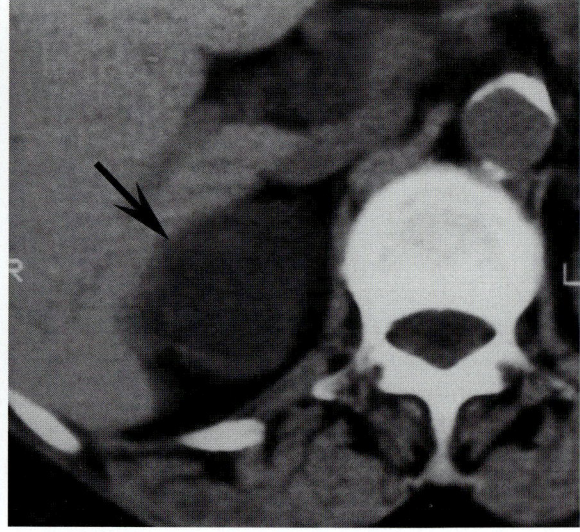

b

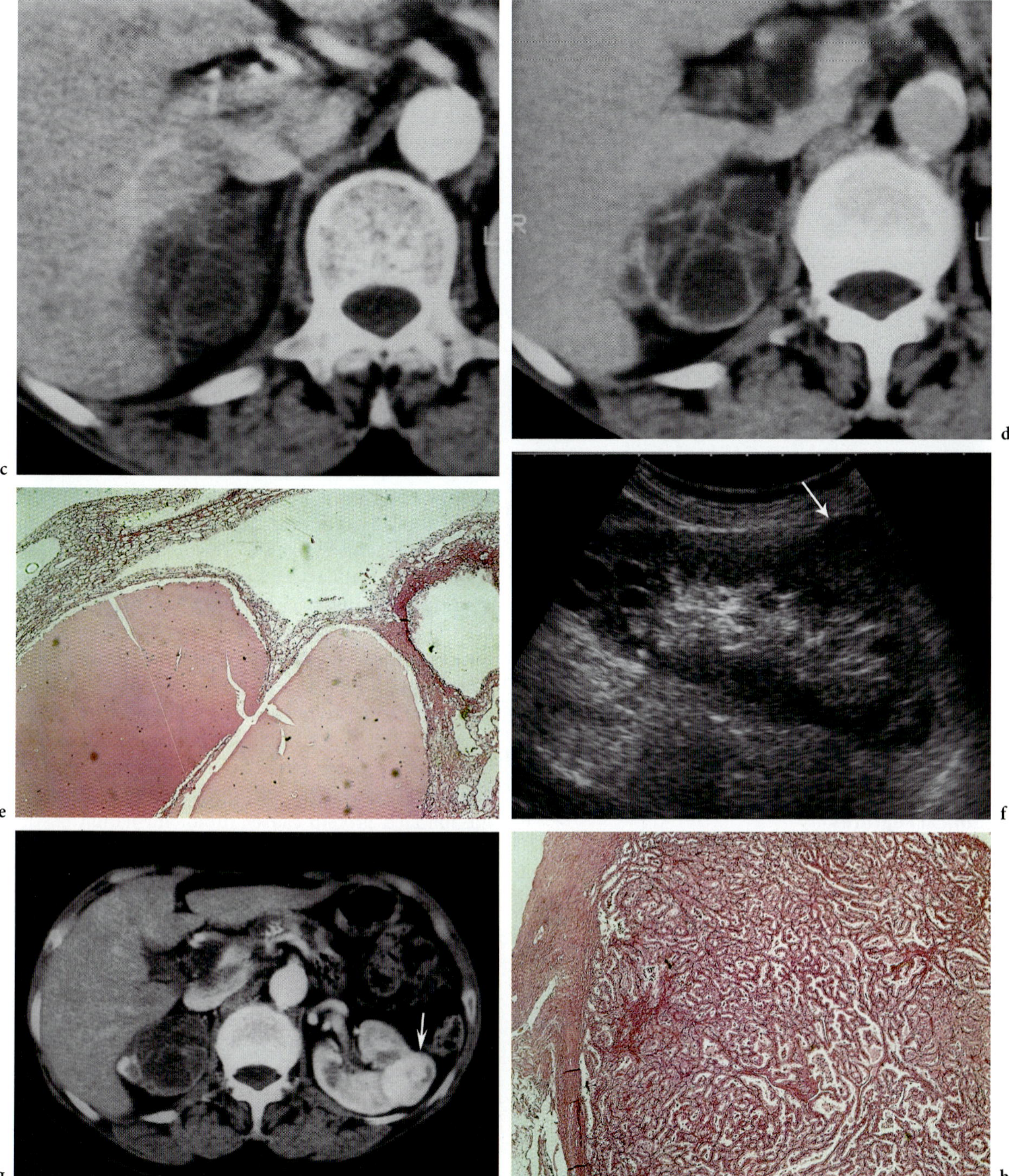

Fig. 15.5a-h. Multilocular cystic renal cell carcinoma and solid renal cell carcinoma in a 65-year-old woman. **a** Longitudinal US image reveals a multilocular mass in the right kidney, approximately 4 cm in diameter (*arrows*). Axial **b** unenhanced and **c, d** dynamic contrast-enhanced CT scans through the tumor (*arrow*) demonstrate slight enhancement and wall irregularity in the septa; however, there is no definite enhancement in the tumor parenchyma. Partial nephrectomy of the right kidney was performed. **e** Photomicrograph of the multilocular cystic tumor reveals an atypical hyperplastic layer, suggesting cystic clear cell renal carcinoma (hematoxylin and eosin stain; original magnification, ×25). **f** Longitudinal US image reveals a hypoechoic solid mass in the left kidney, approximately 3 cm in diameter (*arrow*). **g** Axial contrast-enhanced CT scan through the left renal tumor demonstrates mild enhancement (*arrow*); however, its surrounding rim is not visualized. Partial nephrectomy of the left kidney was performed. **h** Photomicrograph of the solid tumor shows a clear cell renal carcinoma with an alveolar configuration. Microcystic changes with hemorrhage are also seen (*arrows*; hematoxylin and eosin stain; original magnification, ×25).

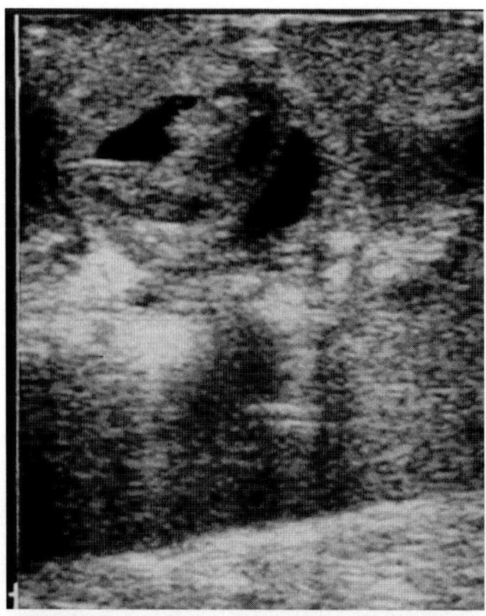

Fig. 15.6. Renal mass in a 31-year-old woman with von Hippel-Lindau disease. Intraoperative US image shows the mixed solid and cystic lesion of the kidney. Note that the mass is below the surface of the kidney and is not visible to the surgeon. Intraoperative ultrasound assists the surgeon by demonstrating the parenchyma below the surface. (With permission from CHOYKE et al. 2003)

15.4
Hereditary Papillary Renal Cancer

15.4.1
Clinical Features

Hereditary papillary renal cancer (HPRC) is an autosomal-dominant hereditary condition in which the kidneys develop multiple, bilateral type 1 papillary renal cancers. No other extrarenal manifestations have been reported in this syndrome. Sporadic type 1 papillary renal tumors have a better prognosis than other cell types, so it is not surprising that the tumors associated with HPRC tend to be slow growing and rarely cause death (AMIN et al. 1997a). Because of the favorable prognosis of HPRC, the patient may not come to medical attention and the disease often is not diagnosed until the patient is middle aged, unlike patients with VHL who are often diagnosed in their teens and twenties.

15.4.2
Genetics

The gene responsible for HPRC has been found at 7q31.3 and is known as the c-MET proto-oncogene (INOUE et al. 1998). This gene was first described in 1984 but was only recently linked to renal cancer (SCHMIDT et al. 1998). Unlike VHL, where it is thought that a mutation leads to lower levels of the VHL protein, c-MET seems to be over expressed in type 1 papillary tumors. The gene codes for a transmembrane tyrosine kinase, which acts as a receptor for hepatocyte growth factor. The mutations associated with HPRC are found on the extracellular portion of the transmembrane protein where hepatocyte growth factor interacts with the receptor. The mechanism by which the mutated protein causes tumor formation is still unknown. Interestingly, alterations in the hepatocyte growth factor receptor have also been found in VHL-related tumors. Moreover, there is some evidence that

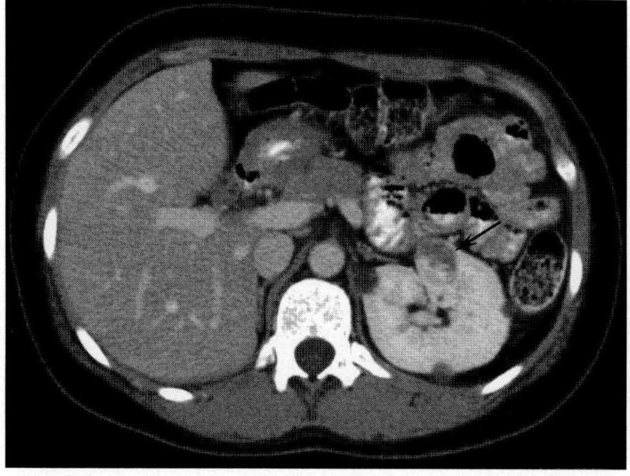
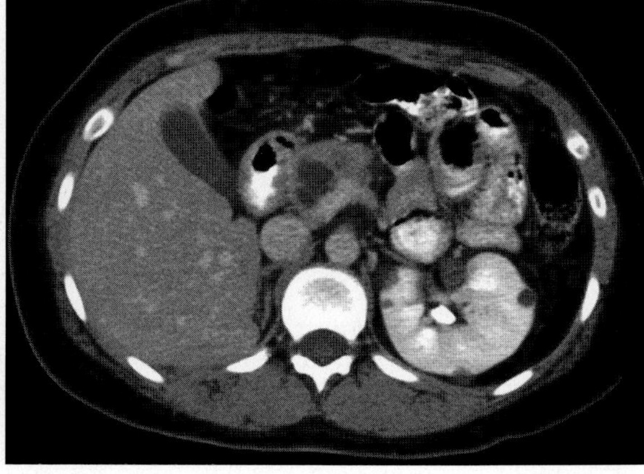

Fig. 15.7a,b. von Hippel-Lindau disease in a 44-year-old man successfully treated with laparoscopic assisted radiofrequency ablation. **a** Axial contrast-enhanced pretreatment CT scan shows a solid lesion (*arrow*) in the left kidney. **b** Axial contrast-enhanced CT scan 6 months after treatment shows that the lesion has become nonenhancing and smaller after radiofrequency ablation. Cystic disease is also present in the head of the pancreas. (With permission from CHOYKE et al. 2003)

sporadic papillary renal tumors found in the general population that have c-MET alterations are more biologically aggressive (KOOCHEKPOUR et al. 1999).

15.4.3
Imaging and Management

Unlike clear cell carcinomas of VHL that are highly vascular on contrast-enhanced CT, the lesions of HPRC tend to be hypovascular (Fig. 15.8). Indeed, if density measurements are not obtained carefully, some lesions may be mistaken for cysts (SCHMIDT et al. 1998; CHOYKE et al. 1997). The change in enhancement before and after intravenous contrast media can be as little as 10–15 HU. This places a premium on obtaining scans of high quality using the same technique (kilovolt, peak; milliamp; slice thickness; field of view; and so forth) both before and after contrast media administration. Precontrast CT is used, as with VHL, as well as postcontrast helical CT in the arterial and venous phases. Enhancement on MR imaging after gadolinium chelate administration is often only modest (15–20% over baseline; Ho et al. 2002; CHOYKE et al. 1997). Renal US can be misleading because the lesions are often isoechoic when less than 3 cm in diameter. Ultrasound should not be used to monitor patients with HPRC (CHOYKE et al. 1997).

Hereditary papillary renal cancer should be considered in a patient with two or more poorly enhancing renal masses. Renal cystic disease is not usually a feature of the disease, but incidental cysts can occur in HPRC. If the patient has a family history of renal cancer, and particularly if the cell type is papillary type 1, the presumptive diagnosis of HPRC can be made. The diagnosis can be confirmed with genetic testing of peripheral blood.

Treatment of HPRC renal tumors is similar to VHL. It is generally believed that surgery can be delayed until one of the tumors reaches 3 cm in diameter and that renal-preserving surgery should be attempted whenever feasible. If a tumor greater than 3 cm is found, every attempt should be made to perform a nephron-sparing procedure. If that is not possible, however, nephrectomy may be necessary. Alternatively, minimally invasive radiofrequency ablation or cryoablation may be suitable in some patients. In general, the prognosis for HPRC is considered excellent and many patients live normal lives with this condition. The radiologist, however, should be alert to the possibility of HPRC when multiple or bilateral hypodense solid renal tumors are seen.

15.5
Hereditary Leiomyoma Renal Cell Carcinoma

15.5.1
Clinical Features

Hereditary leiomyoma renal cell carcinoma (HLRCC) is an autosomal-dominant genodermato-

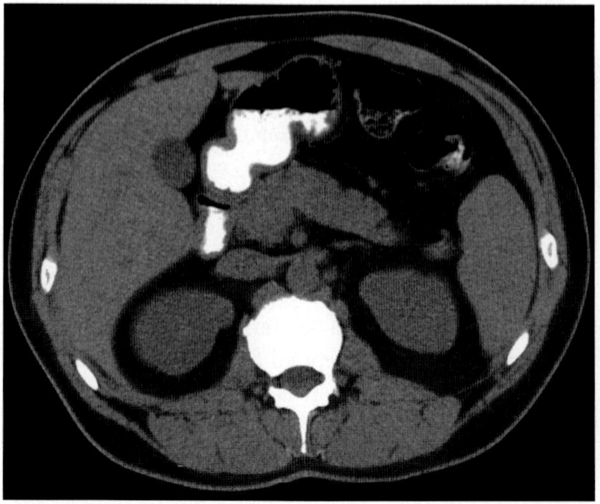
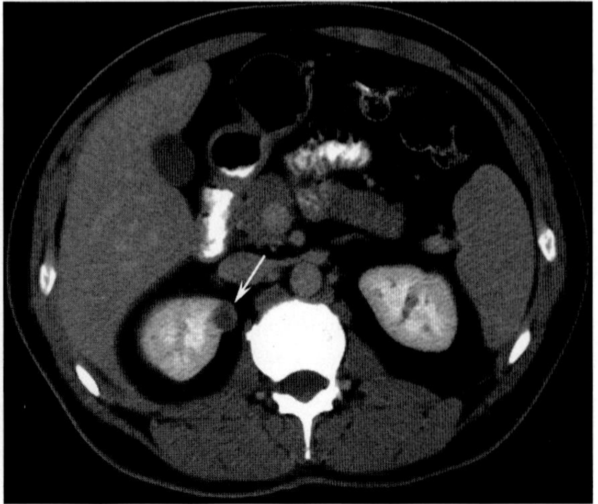

Fig. 15.8a,b. Hereditary papillary renal cancer in a 28-year-old man. Axial **a** unenhanced and **b** contrast-enhanced CT scans demonstrate a poorly enhancing mass (*arrow*) in the right kidney. This lesion increased in density by only 12 HU after intravenous contrast. Minimally enhancing solid tumors are typical of the tumors found in hereditary papillary renal cancer. (With permission from CHOYKE et al. 2003)

sis. The syndrome, originally described in Finland among families with hereditary uterine leiomyoma, has now been seen throughout Europe and North America. The association of cutaneous and uterine leiomyomas is known as Reed syndrome, but the association with renal tumors is only recent (LAUNONEN et al. 2001). The hallmarks of HLRCC are (a) cutaneous leiomyomas over the trunk and extremities and more rarely the face; (b) uterine fibroids at an early age (<30 years); and (c) type 2 papillary renal tumors.

15.5.2
Genetics

The gene for HLRCC is found on the first chromosome 1q42.3-q43 and is known as the fumarate hydratase gene. Interestingly, this enzyme is a critical component in the Krebs tricarboxylic acid cycle, but its role in causing renal tumors is unknown. Fumarate hydratase likely acts as a tumor suppressor because fumarate hydratase enzyme activity is low or absent in tumors found in HLRCC (TOMLINSON et al. 2002).

Type 2 papillary renal cancers are found in about 17% of individuals with HLRCC and can be clinically aggressive (Figs. 15.9, 15.10). Metastases are seen in over half of cases even with relatively small primary tumors. The HLRCC renal tumors differ from the other hereditary renal cancer syndromes in several important ways. Histologically, they appear to be type 2 papillary tumors except for the occasional collecting duct renal cancer.

15.5.3
Imaging and Management

The renal tumors in HLRCC are usually solitary and unilateral as opposed to the other syndromes in which the tumors are usually multiple and bilateral. The tumors are also substantially more aggressive with Fuhrman nuclear grades III or IV in all reported cases and have a tendency to metastasize even when small (Figs. 15.9, 15.10). In contrast, the tumors associated with VHL and HPRC are typically only Fuhrman nuclear grades I or II and rarely metastasize when less than 3 cm in diameter. It is particularly important to differentiate HLRCC from HPRC. Watchful waiting is adequate for HPRC, but treatment is urgent in patients with HLRCC. Tumors should be removed when they are first seen.

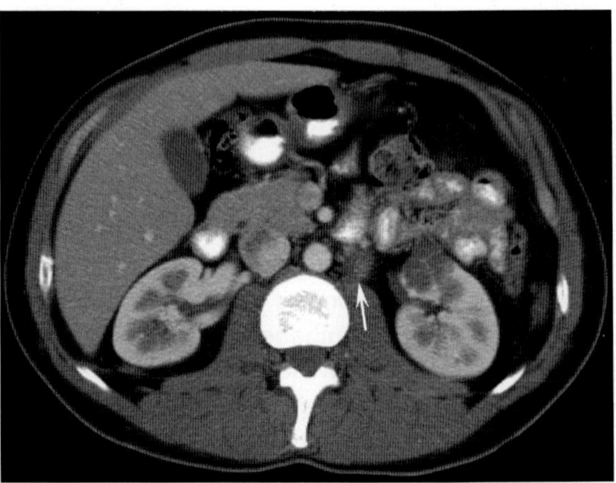

Fig. 15.9. Hereditary leiomyoma renal cell carcinoma in a 34-year-old woman. Axial contrast-enhanced CT scan at the level of kidneys shows that a small mass (3 cm) is present in the middle portion of the left kidney. It is poorly enhancing, typical of papillary renal cancer; however, in addition, there is a metastatic lymphadenopathy (*arrow*) adjacent to the aorta. This proved to be a papillary type 2 renal cancer. The renal lesion was not visible on ultrasound. (With permission from CHOYKE et al. 2003)

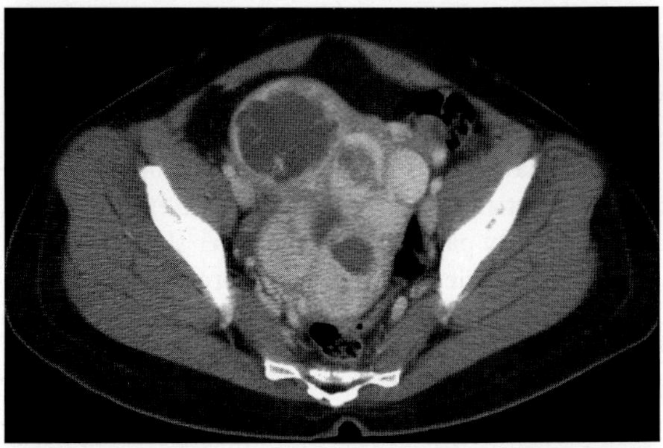

Fig. 15.10. Hereditary leiomyoma renal cell carcinoma in a 32-year-old woman. Axial contrast-enhanced CT scan of the pelvis demonstrates multiple enhancing leiomyomas within the uterus. (With permission from CHOYKE et al. 2003)

Uterine fibroids occur in over 90% of women with HLRCC. Most of these women also have skin leiomyomas. Almost half the women with HLRCC require a hysterectomy by the age of 30 years (Figs. 15.9, 15.10). In addition to screening for renal cancer, patients should be screened for uterine leiomyomas and leiomyosarcomas. It is thought that this entity has a high frequency of transformation to malignant leiomyosarcoma within the uterus, but imaging criteria for these transformations are lacking. Although the cutaneous leiomyomas do not degenerate into malignancies in general, a few cases of cutaneous leiomyosarcomas have been reported (TOMLINSON et al. 2002). The cutaneous manifestations become more prominent with age: they are hardly noticeable when the patients are young but can become a cosmetic issue by the patient's fifth decade.

Computed tomography is used to screen for HLRCC renal cancers and to assess the status of the uterus. Interestingly, although the tumors tend to be hypovascular like type 1 papillary tumors, they are much more lethal. Careful screening for metastatic disease should be performed. Magnetic resonance imaging and ultrasound are suitable substitutes when contrast-enhanced CT is not available. Magnetic resonance imaging of the uterus is particularly helpful in detecting and characterizing uterine leiomyomas.

15.6
Birt-Hogg-Dubé Syndrome

15.6.1
Clinical Features

Birt-Hogg-Dubé syndrome (BHD), an autosomal-dominant disorder, was originally described as a dermatologic disorder characterized by fibrofolliculomas (growths in the hair follicles) of the face and trunk (BIRT et al. 1977). Later it became clear that there were other markers for the disease including pulmonary cysts and renal tumors (ROTH et al. 1993; NICKERSON et al. 2002). The pulmonary cysts vary in severity and size from one or two small, scattered cysts to severe cystic disease complicated by spontaneous pneumothoraces, which may be refractory to conventional pleurodesis. Between 15 and 30% of patients with BHD develop renal cancers. The renal tumors seen in BHD are commonly, but not always, chromophobe carcinomas or oncocytomas. Both clear cell and papillary tumors have also been seen in BHD (PAVLOVICH et al. 2002). Approximately 34% of the tumors are characterized as chromophobe carcinomas and about 50% are hybrid chromophobe oncocytomas; the remainder are oncocytoma (5%), clear cell carcinoma (9%), and papillary renal cancer (2%; PAVLOVICH et al. 2002). A higher rate of colonic polyps have been observed in some families, but the risk for colon cancer has not been clearly defined (KHOO et al. 2002; ZBAR et al. 2002).

15.6.2
Genetics

The gene for BHD is located at 17p11.2 and codes for a protein named folliculin (NICKERSON et al. 2002; KHOO et al. 2002). Little is known of the mechanism of tumor formation or the function of folliculin. It is thought that this gene acts as a tumor suppressor and as a structural protein in the lung where it may form a component of the cytoskeletal network. This might explain the tendency of BHD patients to develop lungs cysts. The Hornstein-Knickenberg syndrome overlaps BHD and is now considered to be part of BHD (SCHULZ and HARTSCHUH 1999). Birt-Hogg-Dubé syndrome differs from other forms of hereditary renal cancer in that it produces a variety of cell types of renal cancer, with chromophobe cancers, and their variants predominant. The chromophobe tumors and oncocytomas also arise from the distal renal tubules, in contrast to VHL and HPRC-related tumors which arise from the proximal tubules (NICKERSON et al. 2002).

15.6.3
Imaging and Management

The imaging of BHD should always include scans of the lungs and abdomen (Fig. 15.11). The pulmonary cysts are generally found in the lower lobes and vary in size and number from a few to many. Pneumothoraces may be seen despite the absence of symptoms. Although severe cystic disease is present in some individuals, the patients do not usually become oxygen dependent. This differs from the cystic lung disease found in lymphangioleiomyomatosis associated with tuberous sclerosis. The chromophobe or mixed-cell types typically demonstrate moderate uniform enhancement on CT, unlike VHL-associated tumors, which typically have cystic components.

Birt-Hogg-Dubé syndrome is managed similarly to VHL. Tumors are generally observed until they reach 2–3 cm diameter, whereupon nephron-sparing surgery is performed. Chromophobe carcinomas tend to be highly enhancing and are relatively homogeneous in appearance. Radiofrequency ablation or cryotherapy also can be considered, although there is little information available on their utility.

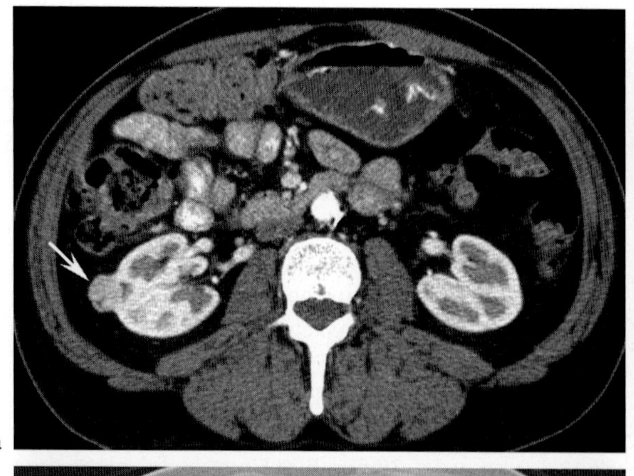

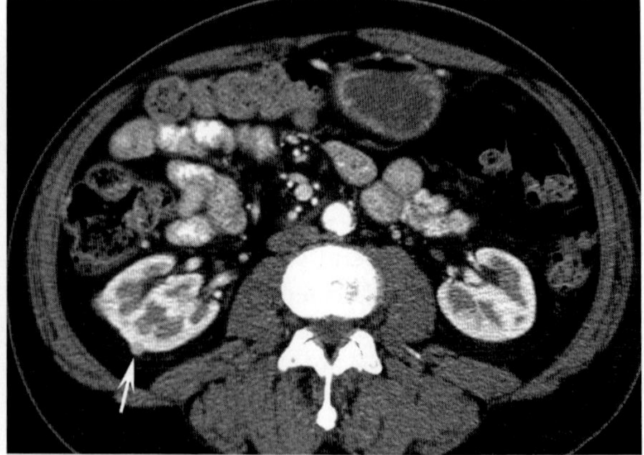

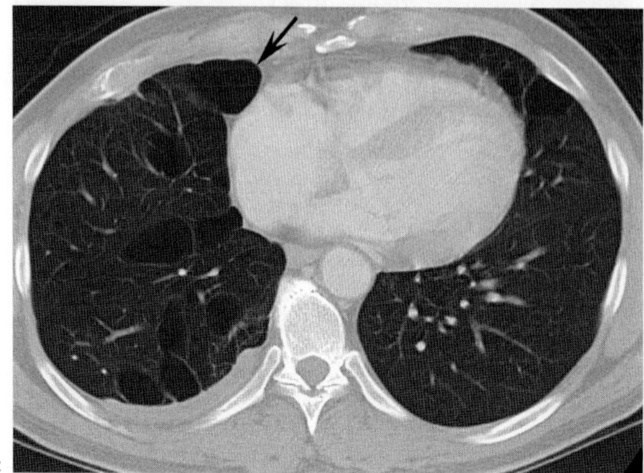

Fig. 15.11a-c. Birt-Hogg-Dubé syndrome in a 38-year-old man. **a** Axial contrast-enhanced CT scan demonstrates an enhancing mass (*arrow*) in the right kidney typical of a chromophobe carcinoma. **b** An additional smaller lesion (*arrow*) is present in the lower pole. **c** Axial CT scan of the chest shows multiple cysts and a loculated pneumothorax (*arrow*). This patient had experienced multiple pneumothoraces as a consequence of cystic lung disease. (With permission from CHOYKE et al. 2003)

15.7
Familial Renal Oncocytoma

15.7.1
Clinical Features

Familial renal oncocytoma (FRO) is an incompletely characterized condition in which affected individuals develop renal oncocytomas (ERLANDSON et al. 1997). The term "familial" is used instead of "hereditary" to indicate that a clear hereditary pattern has not yet been established. Five families with a hereditary predisposition to renal oncocytomas were first described by WEIRICH et al. (1998). Some families had extensive bilateral disease and compromised renal function (WARFEL and EBLE 1982). Other families had mild manifestations of FRO. There may be some overlap with BHD, because several families initially thought to have FRO proved to have features of BHD. Renal dysfunction without extensive neoplastic disease was also noted in some family members.

15.7.2
Genetics

The prevalence of this entity is unknown and no genetic locus has yet been identified.

15.7.3
Imaging and Management

The diagnosis is based on the identification of multiple oncocytomas in one or more family members. On imaging, the lesions are indistinguishable from malignant renal cancers and must be treated as if they were renal cancers (Fig. 15.12; DAVIDSON et al. 1993). When oncocytomas are extensive and confluent the term "renal oncocytosis" can be applied (WARFEL and EBLE 1982). Because renal function is frequently compromised, these patients are often scanned with MR imaging using gadolinium contrast agents. Lifelong monitoring with imaging studies is recommended, although compliance is often

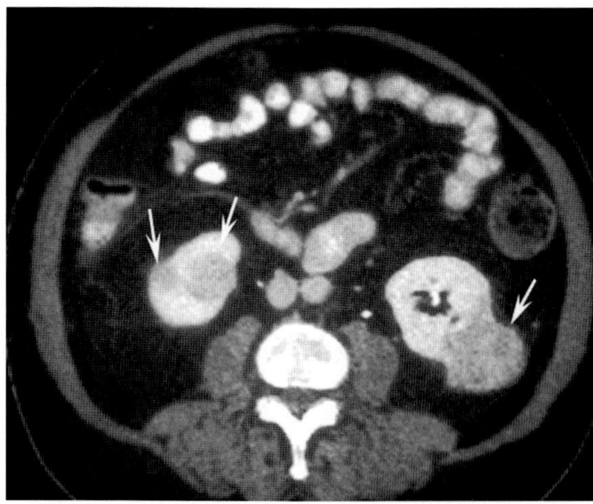

Fig. 15.12. Hereditary renal oncocytoma in a 58-year-old man. Axial contrast-enhanced CT scan shows bilateral renal oncocytomas (*arrows*). Note that the lesions are homogeneously enhancing. Stellate central scars, seen commonly in sporadic oncocytomas, are unusual in this condition. (With permission from Choyke et al. 2003)

less than ideal, as the patient may perceive the risk of disease as low.

15.8
Medullary Carcinoma of Kidney

15.8.1
Clinical Features

Medullary carcinoma of the kidney is a rare and aggressive neoplasm that develops in young patients of African ancestry (age range 11–39 years) with sickle cell trait (Davis et al. 1995). This has led some observers to comment that the renal tumors may be a secondary complication of sickle cell trait (Ataga and Orringer 2000). This seems doubtful because the sickle cell trait produces only mild symptoms and the youth of the patients (median age about 20 years) makes it unlikely to be the result of a chronic process. The rate of renal tumor development even among people with sickle cell trait is low. Approximately 1 in 12 Africans have HbAS (sickle cell trait) and relatively few reports of medullary carcinoma of the kidney have been published (Ashley-Koch et al. 2000). The risk of developing medullary carcinoma of the kidney even in the presence of sickle cell trait is negligible.

17.8.2
Genetics

The sickle cell gene is located at 11p15.

17.8.3
Imaging and Management

Tumors at presentation tend to be large and are often metastatic. The tumor is generally advanced by the time it is discovered and the median survival from the time of diagnosis is only 15 weeks (Pickhardt 1998). Surgery seems to be only palliative.

The tumors are generally large, central, and heterogeneous in character. There is often evidence of adenopathy or pulmonary metastases. These tumors should be evaluated with MR imaging or CT before surgery to provide accurate clinical staging (nodal and inferior vena cava involvement). Systemic therapies are recommended but do little to modify the course of the illness.

15.9
Tuberous Sclerosis

15.9.1
Clinical Features

Tuberous sclerosis (TS) is a genetic disease characterized by hamartomas in the skin, brain, and viscera. Although not technically considered a cancer syndrome, TS is associated with an increased risk of renal malignancy. Tuberous sclerosis has a prevalence in the population of approximately 1:10,000. The most common manifestations of TS in the kidneys are cysts and angiomyolipomas. Approximately one-third of angiomyolipomas may not contain fat visible on CT and are difficult to differentiate from cancer. Most often the mass is a non-fatty angiomyolipoma. Approximately 1–2% of patients with TS develop renal cancer, which is substantially higher than the expected rate of renal cancer in the general population (Bjornsson et al. 1996; Chan et al. 1983).

15.9.2
Genetics

There is a complex relationship between renal cancer and TS. As mentioned, renal cancers are found more frequently in patients with TS than in the general population. They have also been associated with mutations in both TSC1 and TSC2, the two gene loci associated with TS (BJORNSSON et al. 1996; ROBERTSON et al. 1996).

Supportive evidence comes from the animal model of TS, the Eker rat, which has an insertional mutation in the rat TSC2 gene. The Eker rat develops tumors (adenomas and carcinomas) and cysts in the kidney (EKER et al. 1981).

15.9.3
Imaging and Management

Occasionally, renal cancers are the presenting sign of TS (KULKARNI et al. 2000). Multifocal renal cancer has been found in siblings from a single family with TSC1 (SAMPSON et al. 1995). Features indicating an association with renal cancer include a striking female predominance (81% female vs 70% male predominance for sporadic renal cancers), median age of only 28 years (vs sixth and seventh decades for sporadic renal cancers), multifocality, and bilaterality (43%; EKER et al. 1981; TORRES et al. 1997).

A variety of cell types of renal cancer have been reported in humans with TS including clear cell (most common), papillary, and chromophobe carcinomas (HIDAI et al. 1997; PECCATORI et al. 1997). Oncocytomas have also been reported with increased frequency in TS (JIMENEZ et al. 2001). The origins of some renal tumors associated with TS are not completely clear: some lesions may actually be malignant epithelioid angiomyolipomas, which can mimic renal cancers (PEA et al. 1998).

15.10
Translocation of Chromosome 3

A number of families have been found in which part of the short arm of chromosome 3 has been translocated to another chromosome (AMIN et al. 1997a; WALTHER et al. 1999). These balanced translocations predispose the patient to the development of clear cell carcinoma of the kidney. Because the gene responsible for VHL is also located on chromosome 3, it was originally assumed that the translocation was a subset of VHL; however, patients with chromosome 3 translocation do not have other stigmata of VHL and the VHL portion of the short arm of chromosome 3 is often intact (BODMER et al. 1998; COHEN et al. 1979).

Translocation of chromosome 3 can result in a clear cell predominant form of hereditary renal cancer. Unlike the other syndromes, which require a careful analysis of the genes for mutations, this abnormality can be detected on a karyotype of peripheral white blood cells.

15.11
Familial Renal Cancer

Not all families with tendencies to develop renal cancers are explained by the syndromes described previously. As a result, the term "familial renal cancer" is used to characterize patients with apparent genetic predisposition to renal cancer in whom the exact gene involved has not yet been determined. As more is learned about the origins of hereditary renal cancer and more patients receive specific diagnoses, this category is diminishing.

15.12
Conclusion

Over the past 5 years there have been dramatic developments in the understanding of hereditary renal cancers. von Hippel-Lindau disease is now understood to be associated with clear cell carcinoma, and other associations have also become known: hereditary papillary renal cancer is associated with type 1 papillary renal cancer, and hereditary leiomyoma renal cell carcinoma with type 2 papillary renal cancer. Birt-Hogg-Dubé syndrome and familial renal oncocytoma are associated with chromophobe carcinoma and oncocytomas, although other histologic tumor types have been found in Birt-Hogg-Dubé syndrome. Medullary carcinoma of kidney is associated with the sickle cell trait.

Although the genes associated with these tumors have been discovered, the exact mechanisms by which they cause renal cancer remain to be elucidated. It is quite likely that other genes also are involved in this process. Using VHL disease as an example, research is now underway on using mutant pVHL or excess HIF for diagnostic and therapeutic purposes. Understanding the mechanisms that lead to cancer may open new avenues of opportunity for drug development. This improved knowledge of the biogenetic pathways used to form tumors will affect the development of new therapeutic techniques for treating both hereditary and nonhereditary forms of renal cancer.

Acknowledgements

The authors extend sincere thanks to Dr. PETER L. CHOYKE for informative cases and advice, and to Dr. YASUYUKI YAMASHITA for advice regarding the dynamic study using multidetector CT.

References

Amin MB, Corless CL, Renshaw AA, Tickoo SK, Kubus I, Schultz DS (1997) Papillary (chromophil) renal cell carcinoma: histomorphologic characteristics and evaluation of conventional pathologic prognostic parameters in 62 cases. Am J Surg Pathol 2l:62l–635

Amin MB, Crotty TB, Tickoo SK, Farrow GM (1997) Renal oncocytoma: a reappraisal of morphologic features with clinicopathologic findings in 80 cases. Am J Surg Pathol 2l:1–12

Amin MB, Tamboli P, Javidan J Stricker H, de-Peralta Ventunna M, Deshpande A et al. (2002) Prognostic impact of histologic subtyping of adult renal epithelial neoplasms: an experience of 405 cases. Am J Surg Pathol 26:281–291

Ashley-Koch A, Yang Q, Olney RS (2000) Sickle hemoglobin (HbS) allele and sickle cell disease: a HuGE review. Am J Epidemiol 151:839–845

Ataga KI, Orringer EP (2000) Renal abnormalities in sickle cell disease. Am J Hematol 63:205–211

Birt AR, Hogg GR, Dube WJ (1977) Hereditary multiple fibrofolliculomas with trichodiscomas and acrochordons. Arch Dermatol 13 1674–1677

Bjornsson J, Short MP, Kwiatkowski DJ, Henske EP (1996) Tuberous sclerosis-associated renal cell carcinoma: clinical, pathological, and genetic features. Am J Pathol 149:1201–1208

Bodmer D, Eleveld MJ, Ligtenberg MJ, Weterman MA, Janssen BA, Smeets DF et al. (1998) An alternative route for multistep tumorigenesis in a novel case of hereditary renal cell cancer and a t(2;3)(q35;q21) chromosome translocation. Am J Hum Genet 62:1475–1483

Chan HS, Daneman A, Gribbin M, Martin DJ (1983) Renal cell carcinoma in the first two decades of life. Pediatr Radiol 13:324–328

Chen RN, Novick AC, Gill IS (2000) Laparoscopic cryoablation of renal masses. Urol Clin North Am 27:813–820

Choyke PL, Glenn GM, Walther MM, Zbar B, Weiss GH, Alexander RB et al. (1992) The natural history of renal lesions in von Hippel-Lindau disease: a serial CT study in 28 patients. Am J Roentgenol 159:1229–1234

Choyke PL, Glenn GM, Walther MM, Patronas NJ, Linehan WM, Zbar B (1995) von Hippel-Lindau disease: genetic, clinical, and imaging features. Radiology 194:629–642

Choyke PL, Watther MM, Glenn GM, Wagner JR, Venzon DJ, Lubensky IA et al. (1997) Imaging features of hereditary papillary renal cancers. J Comput Assist Tomogr 21:737–741

Choyke PL, Pavlovich CP, Daryanani KD, Hewitt SM, Linehan WM, Walther MM (2001) Intraoperative ultrasound during renal parenchymal sparing surgery for hereditary renal cancers: a 10-year experience. J Urol 165:397–400

Choyke PL, Glenn GM, Walther MM, Zbar B, Linehan WM (2003) Hereditary renal cancers. Radiology 226:33–46

Cohen AJ, Li FP, Berg S, Marchetto DJ, Tsai S, Jacobs SC et al. (1979) Hereditary renal-cell carcinoma associated with a chromosomal translocation. N Engl J Med 301:592–595

Davidson AJ, Hayes WS, Hartman DS, McCarthy CJ, Davis CJ Jr (1993) Renal oncocytoma and carcinoma: failure of differentiation with CT. Radiology 186:693–696

Davidson AJ, Choyke PL, Hartman DS, Davis CJ Jr (1995) Renal medullary carcinoma associated with sickle cell trait: radiologic findings. Radiology 195:83–85

Davis CJ Jr, Mostofi FK, Sesterhenn IA (1995) Renal medullary carcinoma: the seventh sickle cell nephropathy. Am J Surg Pathol 19:1–11

Eker R, Mossige J, Johannessen JV, Aars H (1981) Hereditary renal adenomas and adenocarcinomas in rats. Diagn Histopathol 4:99–110

Erlandson RA, Shek TW, Reuter VE (1997) Diagnostic significance of mitochondria in four types of renal epithelial neoplasms: an ultrastructural study of 60 tumors. Ultrastruct Pathol 21:409–417

Figenshau RS, Basler JW, Ritter JH, Siegel CL, Simon JA, Dierks SM (1998) Renal medullary carcinoma. J Urol 159:711–713

Gago-Dominguez M, Yuan JM, Castelao JE, Ross RK, Yu MC (2001) Family history and risk of renal cell carcinoma. Cancer Epidemiol Biomarkers Prev 10:1001–1004

Gervais DA, McGovem FJ, Wood BJ, Goldberg SN, McDougal WS, Mueller PR (2000) Radio-frequency ablation of renal cell carcinoma: early clinical experience. Radiology 217:665–721

Glenn GM, Gnarra JR, Choyke PL, Walther MM, Zbar B, Linehan WM (1997) The molecular genetics of renal cell carcinoma. In: Raghaven D, Scher Hl, Lange PH (eds) Principles and practice of genitourinary oncology. Lippincott-Raven, Philadelphia, pp 85–97

Hamano K, Esumi M, Igarashi H, Chino K, Mochida J, Ishida A, Okada K (2002) Biallelic inactivation of the von Hippel-Lindau tumor suppressor gene in sporadic renal cell carcinoma. Urology 167:713–771

Herman JG, Latif F, Weng Y, Lerman MI, Zbar B, Liu S et al. (1994) Silencing of the VHL tumor-suppressor gene by DNA methylation in renal carcinoma. Proc Natl Acad Sci USA 91:9700–9704

Herring JC, Enquist EG, Chemoff A, Linehan WM, Choyke PL, Walther MM (2001) Parenchymal sparing surgery in patients with hereditary renal cell carcinoma: 10-year experience. J Urol 165:777–781

Ho VB, Allen SF, Hood MN, Choyke PL (2002) Renal masses: quantitative assessment of enhancement with dynamic MR imaging. Radiology 224:695–700

Hidai H, Chiba T, Takagi Y, Taki A, Nagashima Y, Kuroko K (1997) Bilateral chromophobe cell renal carcinoma in tuberous sclerosis complex. Int J Urol 4:86–89

Inoue K, Karashima T, Chikazawa M, Iiyama T, Yoshikawa C, Funhata M et al. (1998) Overexpression of c-met protooncogene associated with chromophilic renal cell carcinoma with papillary growth. Virchows Arch 433:511–515

Jamis-Dow CA, Choyke PL, Jennings SB, Linehan WM, Thakore KN, Walther MM (1996) Small (≤3 cm) renal masses: detection with CT versus US and pathologic correlation. Radiology 198:785–788

Jimenez RE, Eble JN, Reuter VE, Epstein JI, Folpe AL, Peralta-Venturina M de et al. (2001) Concurrent angiomyolipoma and renal cell neoplasia: a study of 36 cases. Mod Pathol 14:157–163

Kaelin WG, Iliopoulos O, Lonergan KM, Ohh M (1998) Functions of the von Hippel-Lindau tumour suppressor protein. J Intern Med 243:535–539

Khoo SK, Giraud S, Kahnoski K, Chen J, Motorna O, Nickolov R et al. (2002) Clinical and genetic studies of Birt-Hogg-Dubé syndrome. J Med Genet 39:906–912

Koochekpour S, Jeffers M, Wang PH, Gong C, Taylor GA, Roessler LM et al. (1999) The von Hippel-Lindau tumor suppressor gene inhibits hepatocyte growth factor/scatter factor-induced invasion and branching morphogenesis in renal carcinoma cells. Mol Cell Biol 19:5902–5912

Kovacs G, Akhtar M, Beckwith BJ, Bugert P, Cooper CS, Delahunt B et al. (1997) The Heidelberg classification of renal cell tumors. J Pathol 183:131–133

Kulkarni S, Uddar M, Deshpande SG, Vaid S, Wadia RS (2000) Renal cell carcinoma as significant manifestation of tuberous sclerosis complex. J Assoc Physicians India 48:351–353

Latif F, Tory K, Gnarra J, Yao M, Duh FM, Orcutt ML et al. (1993) Identification of the von Hippel-Lindau disease tumor suppressor gene. Science 260:1317–1320

Launonen V, Vierimaa O, Kiuru M, Isola J, Roth S, Pukkala E et al. (2001) Inherited susceptibility to uterine leiomyomas and renal cell cancer. Proc Natl Acad Sci USA 98:3387–3392

Libutti SK, Choyke PL, Bartlett DL et al. (1998) Pancreatic neuroendocrine tumors associated with von-Hippel Lindau disease: diagnostic and management recommendations. Surgery 124:1153–1159

Miyazaki T, Yamashita Y, Yoshimatsu S, Tsuchigame T, Takahashi M (2000) Renal cell carcinomas in von Hippel-Lindau disease; tumor detection and management. Comput Med Imaging Graph 24:105–113

Moyad MA (2001) Review of potential risk factors for kidney (renal cell) cancer. Semin Urol Oncol 19:280–293

Nagashima Y (2000) Chromophobe renal cell carcinoma: clinical, pathological and molecular biological aspects. Pathol Int 50:872–878

Neumann HP, Wiestler OD (1991) Clustering of features of von Hippel-Lindau syndrome: evidence for a complex genetic locus. Lancet 337:1052–1054

Nickerson ML, Warren MB, Toro JR, Matrosova V, Glenn G, Tuner ML et al. (2002) Mutations in a novel gene lead to kidney tumors, lung wall defects and benign tumors of the hair follicle in patients with Birt-Hogg-Dubé syndrome. Cancer Cell 2:157–164

Noguchi S, Nagashima Y, Shuin T, Kubota Y, Kitamura H, Yao M et al. (1995) Renal oncocytoma containing "chromophobe" cells. Int J Urol 2:279–280

Pautler SE, Pavlovich CP, Mikityansky I, Drachenberg DE, Choyke PL, Linehan WM et al. (2001) Retroperitoneoscopic-guided radiofrequency ablation of renal tumors. Can J Urol 8:1330–1333

Pavlovich CP, Walther MM, Eyler RA, Hewitt SM, Zbar B, Lineman WM et al. (2002) Renal tumors in the Birt-Hogg-Dubé syndrome. Am J Surg Pathol 26:1542–1552

Pea M, Bonetti F, Martignoni G, Henske EP, Manfrin E, Colato C et al. (1998) Apparent renal cell carcinomas in tuberous sclerosis are heterogeneous: the identification of malignant epithelioid angiomyolipoma. Am J Surg Pathol 22:180–187

Peccatori I, Pitingolo F, Battini G, Meroni M, Giordano F, Guarino M et al. (1997) Pulmonary lymphoangioleiomyomatosis of tuberous sclerosis? Nephron Dial Transplant 12:2740–2743

Pickhardt PJ (1998) Renal medullary carcinoma: an aggressive neoplasm in patients with sickle cell trait. Abdom Imaging 23:531–532

Poston CD, Jaffe GS, Lubensky IA, Solomon D, Zbar B, Solomon D, Linehan WM et al. (1995) Characterization of the renal pathology of a familial form, of renal cell carcinoma associated with von Hippel-Lindau disease: clinical and molecular genetic implications. J Urol 153:22–26

Remer EM, Weinberg EJ, Oto A, O'Malley CM, Gill IS (2000) MR imaging of the kidneys after laparoscopic cryoablation. Am J Roentgenol 174:635–640

Robertson FM, Cendron M, Klauber GT, Harris BH (1996) Renal cell carcinoma in association with tuberous sclerosis in children. J Pediatr Surg 31:729–730

Roth JS, Rabinowitz AD, Benson M, Grossman ME (1993) Bilateral renal cell carcinoma in the Birt-Hogg-Dubé syndrome. J Am Acad Dermatol 29:1055–1056

Sampson JR, Patel A, Mee AD (1995) Multifocal renal cell carcinoma in sibs from a chromosome 9 linked (TSC1) tuberous sclerosis family. J Med Genet 31:843–850

Schmidt L, Junker K, Weirich G, Glenn G, Choyke P, Lubensky I et al. (1998) Two North American families with hereditary papillary renal carcinoma and identical novel mutations in the MET proto-oncogene. Cancer Res 58:1719–1722

Schulz T, Hartschuh W (1999) Birt-Hogg-Dubé syndrome and Hornstein-Knickenberg syndrome are the same: different sectioning technique as the cause of different histology. J Cutan Pathol 26:55–61

Stolle C, Glenn G, Zbar, B, Humphrey JS, Choyke P, Walther M et al. (1998) Improved detection of germline mutations in the von Hippel-Lindau disease tumor suppressor gene. Hum Mutat 12:417–423

Storkel S, Eble JN, Adlakha K, Amin M, Blute ML, Bostwick DG et al. (1997) Classification of renal cell carcinoma: Workgroup No. 1. Union Internationale Contre le Cancer (UICC) and the American Joint Committee on Cancer (AJCC). Cancer 80:987–989

Tomlinson IP, Alam NA, Rowan AJ, Barclay E, Jaeger EE, Kelsell D et al. (2002) Germline mutations in FH predispose to dominantly inherited uterine fibroids, skin leiomyomata and papillary renal cell cancer. Nat Genet 30:406–410

Torres VE, Zincle H, King BK, Bjornson J (1997) Renal manifestations of tuberous sclerosis complex. Contrib Nephrol 122:64–75

Turner KJ, Huson SM, Moore N, Britton BJ, Cranston D (2001) von Hippel-Lindau disease: renal tumors less than 3 cm can metastasize. J Urol 165:1207

Walther MM, Keiser HR, Linehan WM (1999) Pheochromocytoma: evaluation, diagnosis and treatment. World J Urol 17:35–39

Warfel KA, Eble JN (1982) Renal oncocytomatosis. J Urol 127:179–180

Weirich G, Glenn G, Junker K, Merino M, Strokel S, Lubensky I et al. (1998) Familial renal oncocytoma: clinicopathological study of 5 families. J Urol 160:335–340

Wood BJ, Ramkaransingh JR, Fojo T, Walther MM, Libutti SK (2002) Percutaneous tumor ablation with radiofrequency. Cancer 94:443–451

Zbar B (2000) Inherited epithelial tumors of the kidney: old and new diseases. Semin Cancer Biol 10:313–318

Zbar B, Alvord WG, Glenn G, Turner M, Pavlovich CP, Schmidt L et al. (2002) Risk of renal and colonic neoplasms and spontaneous pneumothorax in the Birt-Hogg-Dubé syndrome. Cancer Epidemiol Biomarkers Prev 11:393–400

16 Extraosseous Metastases and Local Recurrence

ALI GUERMAZI, IMAN EL-HARIRY, and YVES MIAUX

CONTENTS

A. GUERMAZI, MD
Senior Radiologist, Scientific Director, Oncology Services,
Department of Radiology Services, Synarc Inc., 575 Market
Street, 17th Floor, San Francisco, CA 94105, USA
I. EL-HARIRY, MD, PhD
Senior Director, Oncology Clinical Development and Medical
Affairs, Glaxo Smith Kline R&D, Greenford Road, Greenford,
Middlesex UB6 0HE, England, UK
Y. MIAUX, MD, MSc
Senior Vice President, Radiology Services, Synarc Inc., 575
Market Street, 17th Floor, San Francisco, CA 94105, USA

16.1 Introduction

Renal cell cancer metastasizes in approximately 33% of patients (FLANIGAN et al. 2003; RUSSO 2003) and recurs locally in about 5% (SCATARIGE et al. 2001a). Accurate detection of recurrent disease provides key prognostic information and assists the oncologist in making treatment decisions involving surgery or immunotherapy (MOTZER et al. 1996). Common sites of metastases include the lung, mediastinum, bones, brain, and liver. Less common sites include the contralateral kidney, the adrenal gland, pancreas, mesentery, and abdominal wall. Several reports detail the capacity of renal carcinoma to appear almost anywhere in the body (FLANIGAN et al. 2003; JANZEN et al. 2003; THRASHER and PAULSON 1993). More than one organ is often involved in the metastatic process (FLANIGAN et al. 2003). Metastases may be found at diagnosis or at some interval after nephrectomy (FLANIGAN et al. 2003; ITANO et al. 2000). Indeed, approximately 20–50% of patients with renal cell carcinoma (RCC) eventually develop metastatic disease after nephrectomy (FLANIGAN et al. 2003; ITANO et al. 2000; JANZEN et al. 2003). A shorter interval between nephrectomy and the development of metastases is associated with a poorer prognosis. Patients with metastatic RCC face a dismal prognosis, with a median survival time of only 6–12 months and a 2-year survival rate of 10–20%. Recent advances in biologic response modifier therapy have given hope to the small percentage of patients who respond to this therapy (FLANIGAN et al. 2003), and has rekindled interest in cytoreductive nephrectomy as an integral part of the management of these patients (FLANIGAN and YONOVER 2001; FLANIGAN et al. 2003).

The purpose of this chapter is to illustrate both typical and less typical US, CT, and MR imaging appearances of metastases and local recurrence from renal cancers. The emphasis is on spiral CT, which is considered the ideal modality for conducting postoperative surveillance in patients at risk of recurrent or metastatic disease (SCATARIGE et al. 2001a). Of importance for the reader, bone metastases will be discussed in Chap. 17.

16.2
Clinical Features and Pathophysiology

Metastatic dissemination is unpredictable and occurs via lymphatic and hematogenous routes (SCATARIGE et al. 2001a). Retrograde collateral flow via the lumbar veins into the vertebral plexus of Batson appears to be particularly important in metastasis to the axial skeleton and the meninges (ARKLESS 1965), as well as to the head and neck (SOM et al. 1987). Local recurrence is associated with incomplete resection of the primary tumor, positive surgical margins, and regional lymph node metastasis (RABINOVITCH et al. 1994).

The most important determinant in predicting local recurrence or distant metastasis is the surgical stage of RCC. Large tumors that invade locally or propagate as venous tumor thrombus have higher rates of distant metastasis. Other factors that may influence prognosis include regional lymph node metastases, a high Fuhrman grade on histopathology, and spindled (sarcomatoid) tumor architecture (CHAE et al. 2005; JANZEN et al. 2003; JOHNSEN and HELLSTEN 1997; SAIDI et al. 1998).

Distant metastases or local recurrence usually occur within the first 6 years after surgery (RABINOVITCH et al. 1994; SAIDI et al. 1998). Late metastasis is a distinctive clinical aspect of renal cancer, and can be observed in as many as 11% of patients surviving 10 years or more after surgery (NEWMARK et al. 1994). The most frequent sites for late metastases are lung, pancreas, bone, skeletal muscle, and bowel (NEWMARK et al. 1994; SAITOH et al. 1982).

Spontaneous regression of metastases from renal cancer is now well documented. This rare event, reported in less than 1% of the patients, may effect one (GUTHBJARTSSON and GISLASON 1995) or multiple (OMLAND and FOSSA 1989) locations, but is usually not permanent (MIGNON and MESUROLLE 2003). Spontaneous regression of metastases is most commonly seen following nephrectomy but has been reported after irradiation of the primary tumor, embolization with or without nephrectomy (LOKICH 1997), following infusion of recombinant interleukin-2 (MIZUO et al. 1990), or after radiofrequency ablation of the primary tumor (SANCHEZ-ORTIZ et al. 2003). It most commonly involves pulmonary

metastases followed by skeletal, soft tissue, brain, and liver metastases (GUTHBJARTSSON and GISLASON, 1995; HAMMAD et al. 2003; OMLAND and FOSSA 1989). The mechanism is unknown, but the evidence seems to favor an immunologic basis (GUTHBJARTSSON and GISLASON 1995; OMLAND and FOSSA 1989).

Local recurrences and distant metastases are usually highly vascular, like the primary tumor; therefore, arterial-phase scanning is essential for maximizing lesion conspicuity. To facilitate detection of vascular liver metastases, the abdomen and pelvis are scanned first, from the diaphragm to the symphysis pubis, during the arterial phase of enhancement. Next, the chest is imaged from the lung apices through the liver and remaining kidney. Because these patients, as well as those with familial renal carcinoma or von Hippel-Lindau disease, are at increased risk for additional renal primary carcinomas, the remaining kidney must be carefully scrutinized on each follow-up CT (SCATARIGE et al. 2001a). The venous phase is also important since some metastatic nodules or masses are difficult, if not impossible, to discern within the hypervascular cortex at arterial phase, and appear as hypodense nodules at the venous phase (MIGNON and MESUROLLE 2003). Retroperitoneal anatomy is significantly modified after nephrectomy (Fig. 16.1). Indeed, the small bowel and colon may migrate into the nephrectomy fossa. For CT scanning, a good oral opacification of the bowel is mandatory to differentiate nonopacified bowel from local recurrence (SCATARIGE et al. 2001a).

Hypervascular metastases are not specific to kidney cancer metastases and may be seen in metastases from thyroid cancer, neuroendocrine tumors, hepatocarcinoma, and pheochromocytoma (MIGNON and MESUROLLE 2003).

16.3
Thoracic Metastases

16.3.1
Lung and Endobronchus

The reported incidence of lung metastases ranges from 3 to 16% (JANZEN et al. 2003). Pulmonary metastases occur in 29–60% of patients with distant disease (JANZEN et al. 2003; MOTZER et al. 1996). The latency period can be as long as 25 years (SHIONO et al. 2004). Most lung metastases are asymptomatic, at least early in their history, indicating the use of chest CT rather than chest radiographs for follow-up

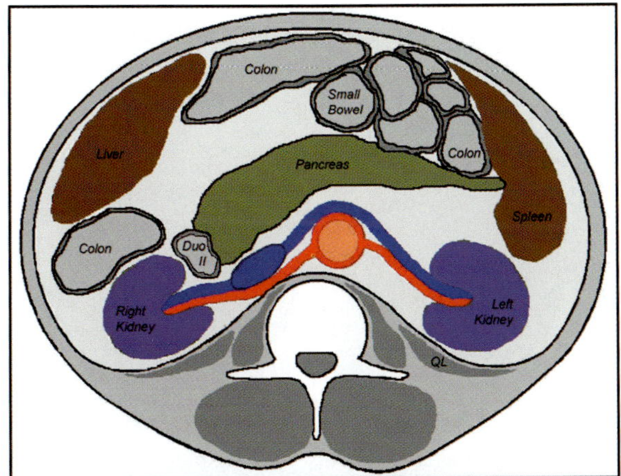

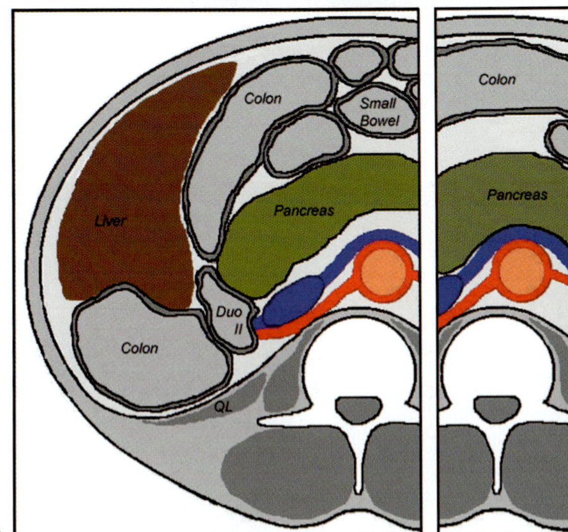

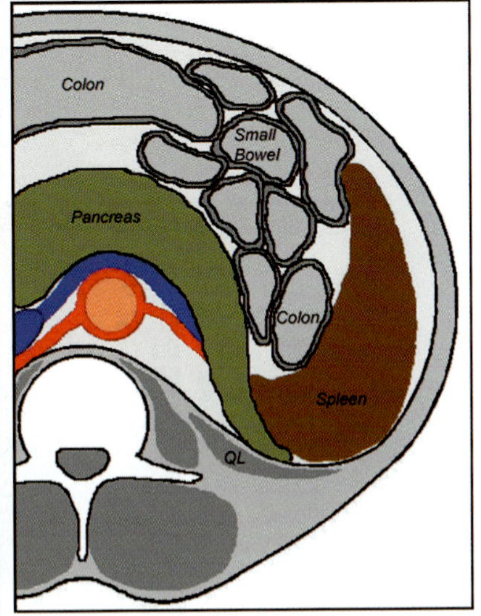

Fig. 16.1a-c. Normal and surgically altered retroperitoneum. **a** Normal retroperitoneum. **b** After right nephrectomy, the right colon and right hepatic lobe occupy the renal fossa. Second portion of duodenum and pancreatic head may assume more posterolateral position. **c** After left nephrectomy, pancreatic tail assumes a more posterior position, approaching quadratus lumborum. Spleen shifts posteromedially. Caudal to pancreas, proximal jejunum and descending colon fill left renal fossa. *Duo II* second portion of duodenum, *QL* quadratus lumborum. (Modified from Scatarige et al. 2001)

after nephrectomy, because chest CT is more sensitive and more likely to display metastases earlier (Saidi et al. 1998). The lung is the most common site of single metastases (Johnsen and Hellsten 1997). Also, patients with lung-only metastases have better survival rates compared with patients with metastases at other sites (Flanigan and Yonover 2001; Russo 2003); therefore, an aggressive surgical approach that aims to remove all neoplastic growth is believed to benefit these patients (Janzen et al. 2003; Johnsen and Hellsten 1997), and repeat metastasectomies are warranted (Shiono et al. 2004). Incomplete resection of renal carcinoma pulmonary metastases is associated with a poor prognosis, with a 5-year survival rate of 22.1% compared with 41.5% in patients with complete resection (Shiono et al. 2004). The lung is also the most common site for spontaneous regression of metastases from renal cancer (Lokich 1997; Mizuo et al. 1990; Omland and Fossa 1989; Sanchez-Ortiz et al. 2003).

Computed tomography is considered the state-of-the-art technology for assessing pulmonary involvement (Lim and Carter 1993). Pulmonary metastases appear as one or multiple, well-defined, rounded or oval, solid nodules or masses, of variable size (Fig. 16.2; Badoual et al. 2002; Chae et al. 2005; Mignon and Mesurolle 2003). Small nodules may be missed on radiographs (Fig. 16.3; Lim and Carter 1993). They are usually bilateral and peripherally located, predominantly in the inferior lobes. Numerous pulmonary metastases confined to one lobe have been reported that were initially confused radiologically with lobar pneumonia (Toye et al. 1990). The hypervascularity of renal metastases to the lung is demonstrated with the large masses (Mignon and Mesurolle 2003), and may lead to hemorrhage (Scatarige et al. 2001a). Atypical presentations are the involvement of the interstitial lymphatics leading to a nonspecific carcinomatous lymphangitis (Fig. 16.4; Scatarige et al. 2001a),

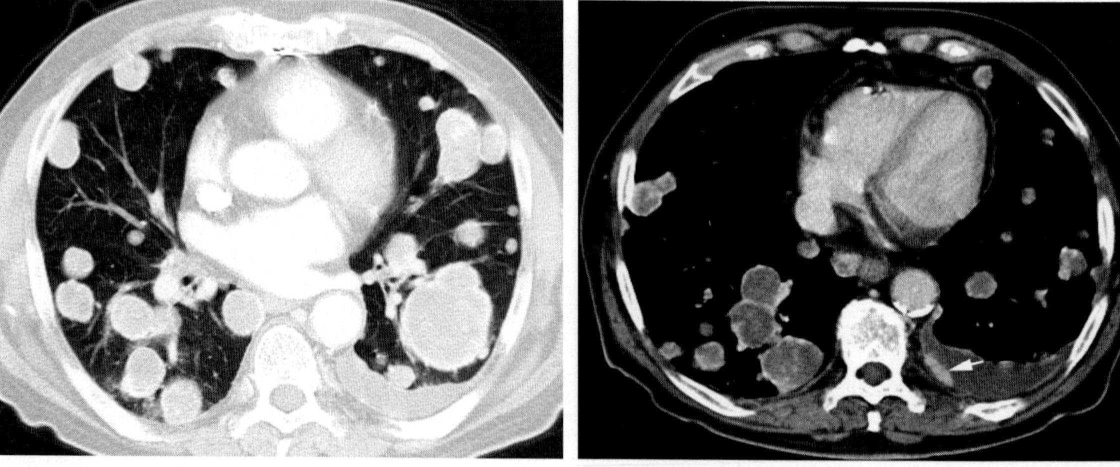

Fig. 16.2a,b. Lung and pleural metastases in a 67-year-old man who underwent nephrectomy for renal cell carcinoma. **a** Axial CT scan shows several bilateral rounded and oval pulmonary nodules of different sizes. **b** Axial contrast-enhanced CT scan of the chest shows that the pulmonary lesions are enhancing peripherally. It also shows a strongly enhanced left pleural-based lesion (*arrow*) associated with left pleural effusion.

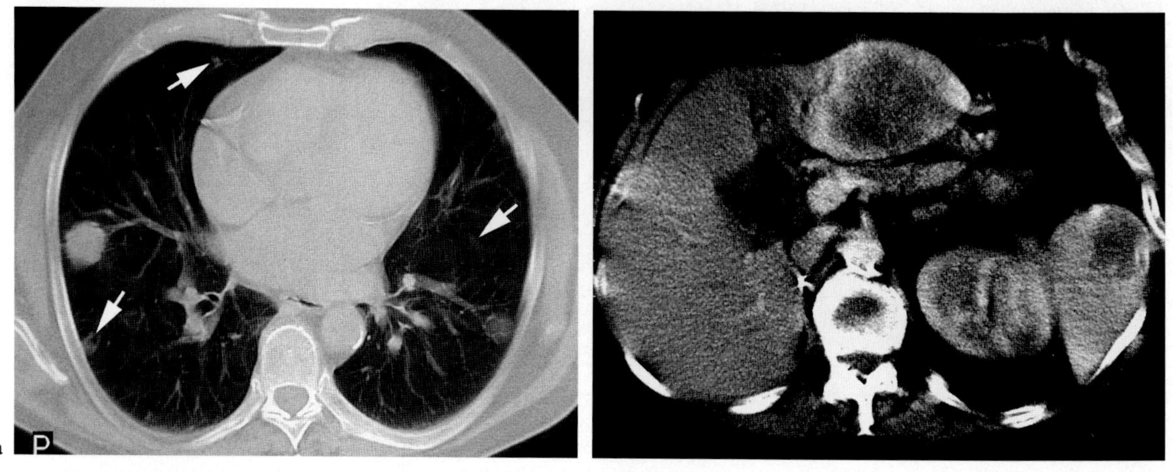

Fig. 16.3a,b. Lung, liver, and spleen metastases in a 66-year-old man who underwent right nephrectomy for renal cell carcinoma. **a** Axial CT scan shows bilateral rounded pulmonary nodules of different sizes. The small peripheral nodules (*arrows*) were not seen on a conventional radiograph. **b** Axial contrast-enhanced CT scan of the abdomen shows large lesions in left hepatic lobe and spleen with peripheral enhancement and central necrosis.

or the coexistence of pulmonary cystic lesions (Fig. 16.5), micronodules, and recurrent pneumothoraces leading to some confusion with Langerhans cell histiocytosis (ESSADKI et al. 1998). Solitary pulmonary nodules are rare and still challenging since conventional imaging modalities, including radiograph, CT, and MR imaging, cannot reveal the exact nature of the lesion. Histological biopsy is often required to establish a definite diagnosis and may detect benign diseases such as hematoma, fibrosis, hamartoma, calcified nodules (CHANG et al. 2003), and intrapulmonary lymph node (KOLOSSEUS et al. 1995). 18F-fluoro-2-deoxyglucose positron emission tomography (FDG-PET) has been shown to be a sen-

sitive, specific, and accurate modality to differentiate radiologically indeterminate solitary pulmonary lesions in patients with RCC (CHANG et al. 2003).

Endobronchial metastases can be detected incidentally or on imaging or bronchoscopy in patients presenting with hemoptysis or atelectasis (BARTHWAL et al. 2003; MERINE and FISHMAN 1988).

16.3.2
Pleura

Metastases to the pleura are considered exceptionally rare (GRINIATSOS et al. 2003). Metastases to the

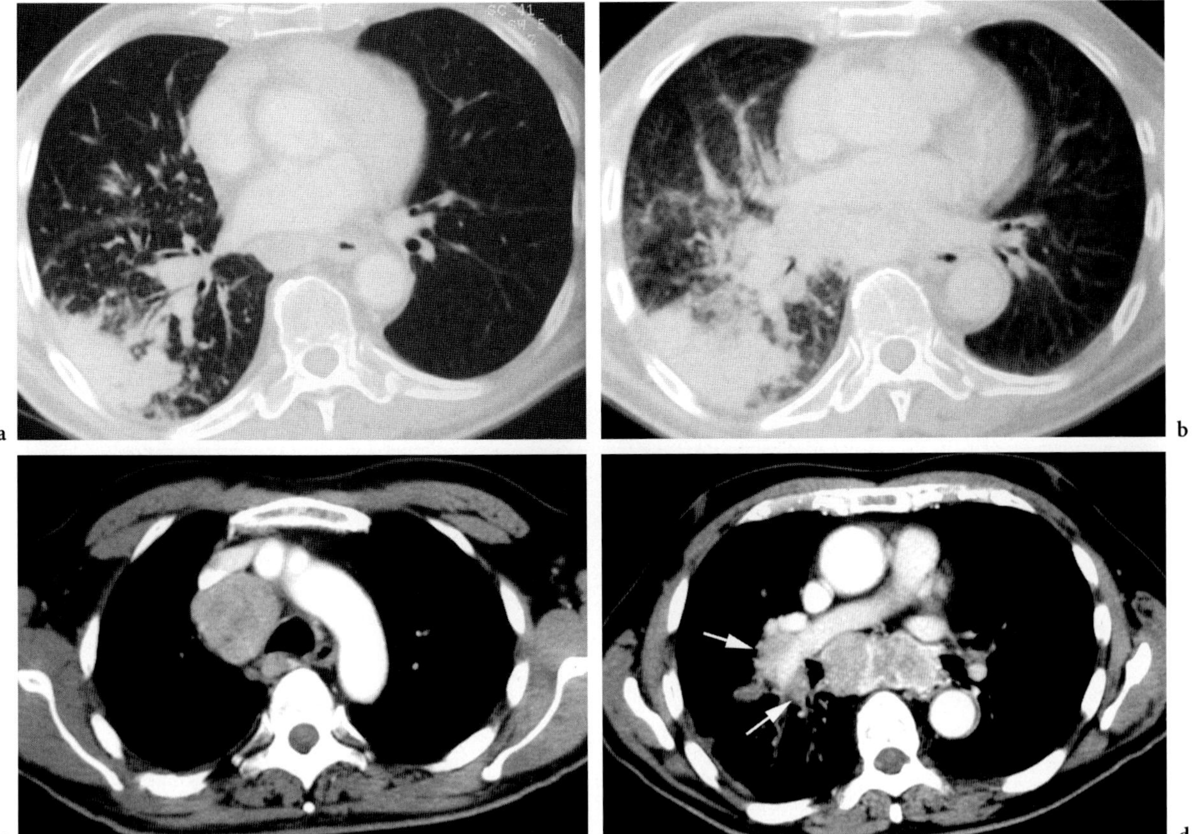

Fig. 16.4a-d. Pulmonary lymphangitic carcinomatosis and mediastinal lymph node metastases in a 48-year-old man who underwent nephrectomy for renal cell carcinoma. **a** Axial CT scan shows right inferior lobe with ill-defined parenchymal consolidation surrounded by thickened nodular, interlobular septa forming polygonal arcades, indicating an interstitial lymphangitic disease. There is also a mild enlargement of the right hilar lymph nodes. **b** Two-month follow-up axial CT scan shows worsening of the pulmonary consolidation, interstitial disease, and right hilar lymph nodes. **c,d** Axial contrast-enhanced CT scans show enhancement at different intensities of enlarged (**c**) right lateral tracheal, (**d**) subcarinal and right hilar (*arrows*) lymph nodes.

pleura are usually associated with lung metastases and spread via arteries (Ohgou et al. 1998). Metastases to the pleura without metastases to the lung are rare. This suggests that the pleural metastases may also spread via Batson's venous plexus (Ohgou et al. 1998). Pleural metastases were thought never to occur without involving other metastatic sites (Saitoh et al. 1982), but a few exclusively pleural metastases in RCC have been reported (Thoroddsen et al. 2002). The prognosis of pleural metastasis is poor and the majority of patients die within 6 months of diagnosis (Griniatsos et al. 2003). Spontaneous regression of pleural metastases has been reported (Lokich 1997; Thoroddsen et al. 2002).

Radiologically, CT is the best modality for the diagnosis of pleural metastases that may be associated with pleural-based solid masses and/or malignant effusion (Lokich 1997). Masses can be solitary or multiple (Fig. 16.6; Griniatsos et al. 2003). When

solitary, the mass may be large and associated, or not, with pleural effusion (Fig. 16.7; Griniatsos et al. 2003). In a case report with several pleural metastases, radiography showed abnormal shadows that were suspected as malignant mesothelioma. Computed tomography showed several enhanced pleural nodules (Fig. 16.8) and also hepatic metastases (Ohgou et al. 1998).

16.3.3
Heart and Pericardium

The reported incidence of metastases to the heart and pericardium from RCC is about 4% (Carroll et al. 1994). Clinically, they are usually silent (Carroll et al. 1994; Cheng 2003), although they may present with dyspnea and lower-extremity edema if the right cavities are involved (Carroll

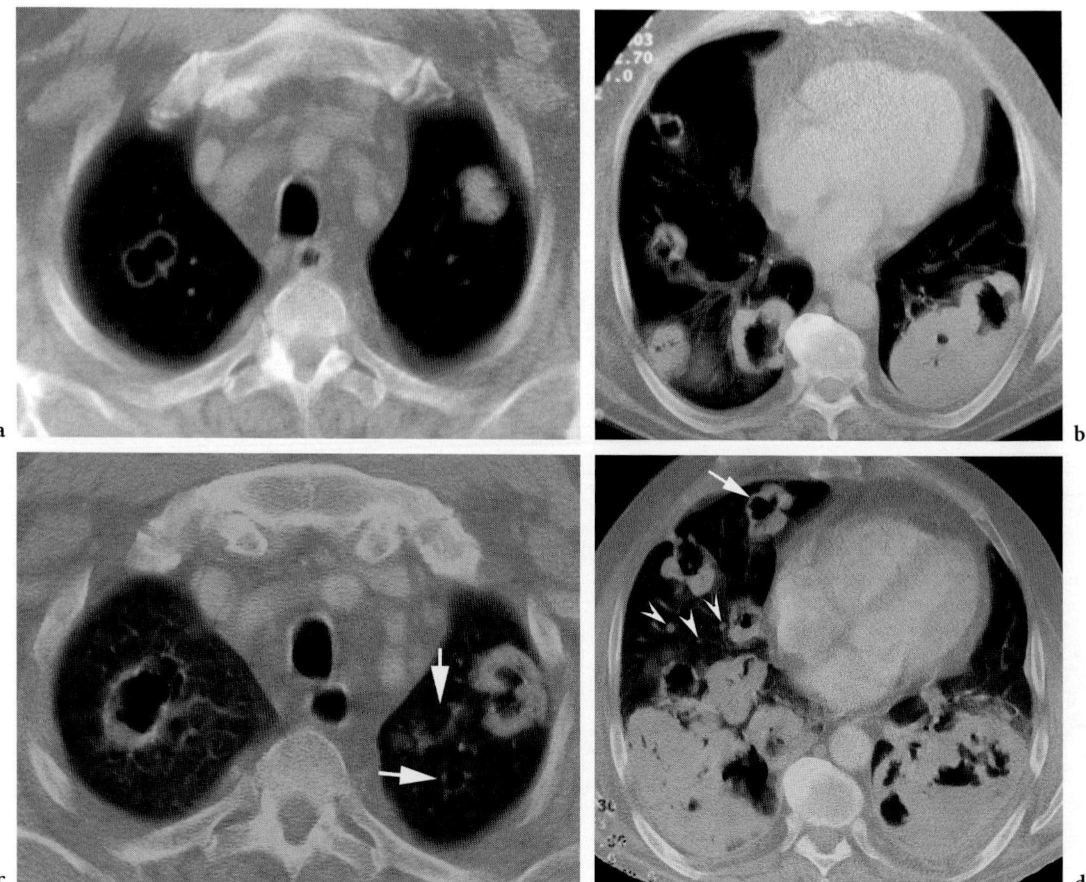

Fig. 16.5a-d. Mixed nodular and cystic lung metastases in a 67-year-old woman who underwent nephrectomy for renal cell carcinoma. **a** Axial CT scan of the upper chest shows a left solid oval pulmonary nodule and a right cystic lung nodule showing a thin and smooth wall. **b** Axial CT scan of the lower chest shows several bilateral excavated lung nodules. The left posterior mass is probably secondary to several confluent nodules. **c, d** Five-month follow-up axial CT scans at the same levels as a and b show enlargement of both solid and cystic nodular lesions. There are also new solid micronodules (*arrowheads*) and cystic nodules (*arrows*).

et al. 1994; SANTO-TOMAS et al. 1998), and syncope or signs of pulmonary vascular congestion if the left cavities are involved (SAFI et al. 2003). In the majority of cases, RCC invades the inferior vena cava and extends up the vena cava into the right atrium (Fig. 16.9; ALLEN et al. 1991). Cardiac metastases without extension to the vena cava are extremely rare (CHENG 2003; SAFI et al. 2003). In these very few cases, the primary tumor metastasizes to the heart systemically via hematogenous or lymphatic routes (SAFI et al. 2003).

It is important to differentiate muscular metastatic lesions to the heart (MAHNKEN and TACKE 2000) with right cardiac cavities involvement from an inferior vena cava tumoral thrombosis extension (ALLEN et al. 1991; CARROLL et al. 1994; SANTO-TOMAS et al. 1998).

Transthoracic, or better transesophageal, echocardiography is an important diagnostic tool for superior preoperative images of the tumor and its extensions (ALLEN et al. 1991). In the case of metastases invading the right ventricular myocardium without caval involvement, echocardiography shows a large mass within the right ventricle that spares the right atrium and inferior vena cava (CARROLL et al. 1994; CHENG 2003; SANTO-TOMAS et al. 1998). Left ventricular involvement may show the same appearance as right involvement, with a large mobile mass infiltrating the left ventricle (SAFI et al. 2003). Doppler may show partial or complete obstruction of the flow into the heart or within the cavity or outflow from the cavity (CARROLL et al. 1994; SAFI et al. 2003). Echocardiography, and less importantly CT, remain the most commonly used diagnostic modalities.

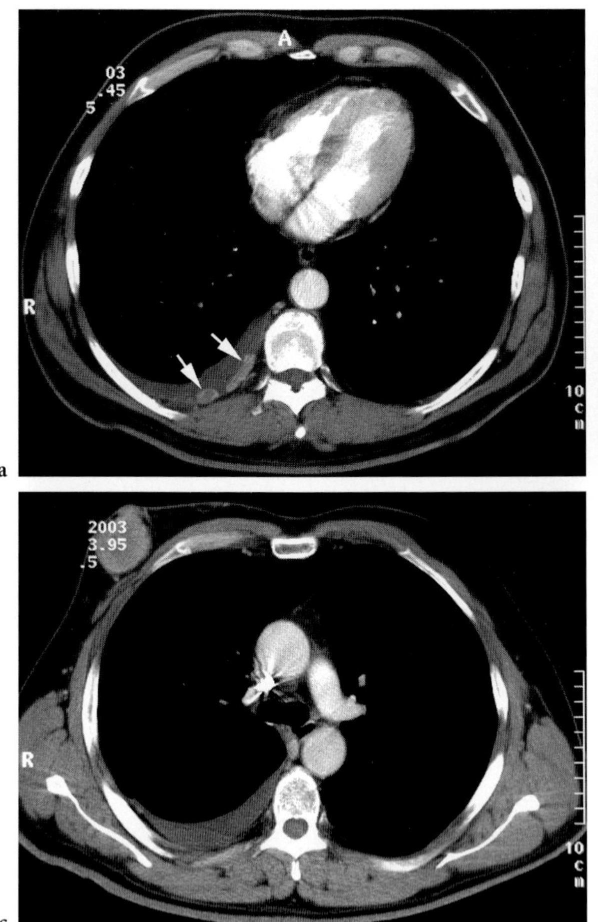

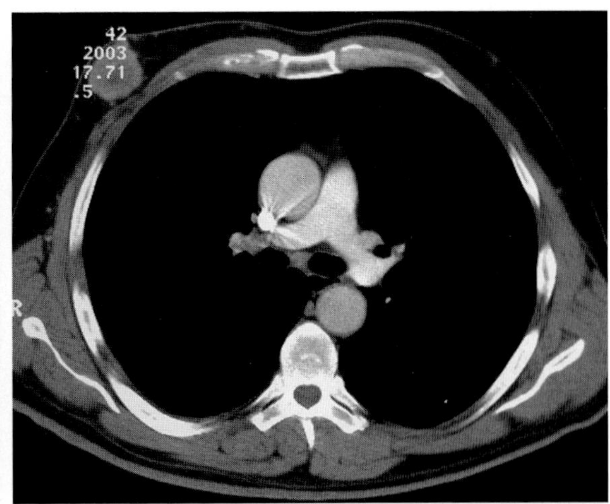

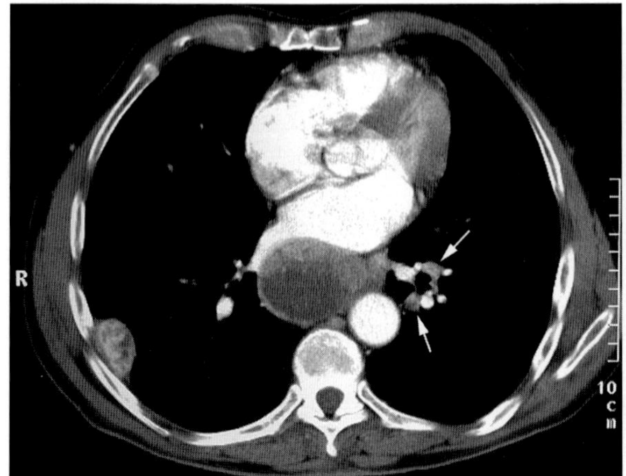

Fig. 16.6a-c. Pleural and breast metastases in a 61-year-old man who underwent nephrectomy for renal cell carcinoma. **a** Axial contrast-enhanced CT scan shows two right pleural-based enhancing masses (*arrows*) associated with ipsilateral pleural effusion. **b** Axial contrast-enhanced CT scan cephalad to **a** shows a well-defined moderately enhancing right breast mass with central necrosis. **c** Seven-week follow-up axial contrast-enhanced CT scan at the same level of **b** shows that the breast mass is increasing in size with more obvious cutaneous involvement. The right pleural effusion has also increased in size.

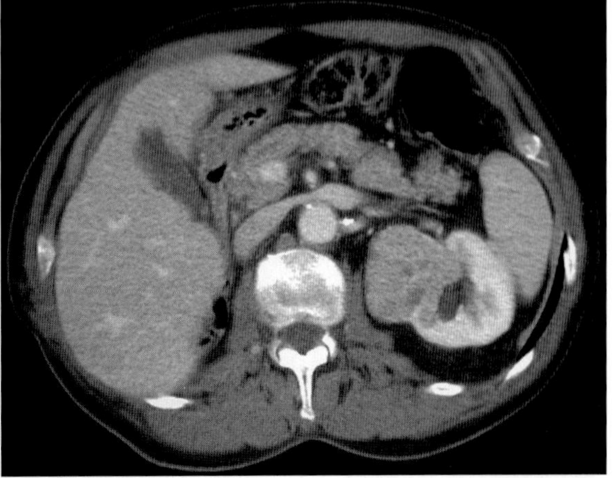

Fig. 16.7a,b. Pleural, nodal, and contralateral kidney metastases in a 70-year-old man who underwent right nephrectomy for renal cell carcinoma. **a** Axial contrast-enhanced CT scan shows a single right pleural-based lesion that enhances heterogeneously. There is a large, moderately enhancing subcarinal adenopathy with central necrosis and two small left hilar adenopathies (*arrows*). **b** Axial contrast-enhanced CT scan at the portal venous phase shows a moderately enhancing mass of the left kidney with areas of necrosis.

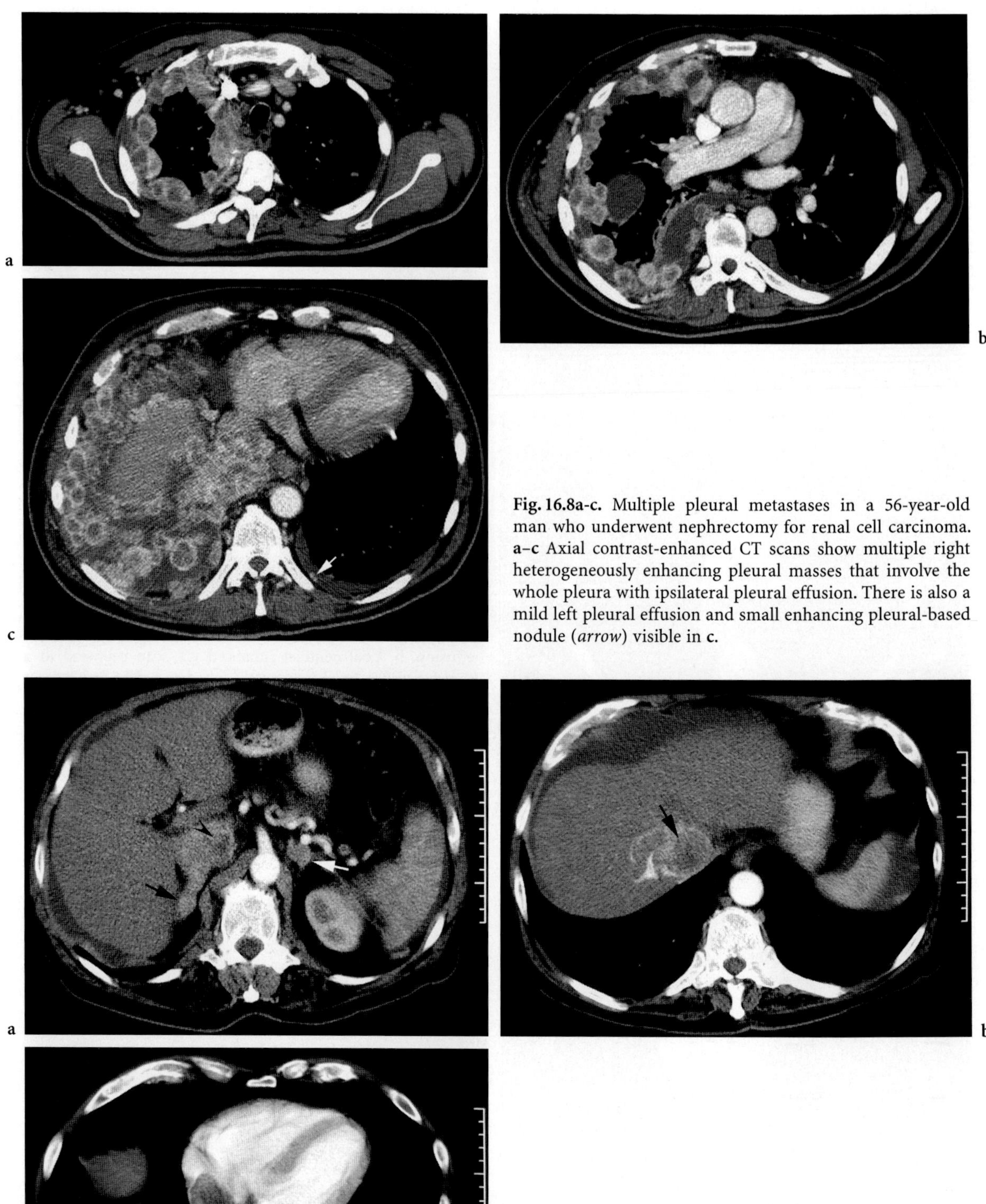

Fig. 16.8a-c. Multiple pleural metastases in a 56-year-old man who underwent nephrectomy for renal cell carcinoma. **a–c** Axial contrast-enhanced CT scans show multiple right heterogeneously enhancing pleural masses that involve the whole pleura with ipsilateral pleural effusion. There is also a mild left pleural effusion and small enhancing pleural-based nodule (*arrow*) visible in **c**.

Fig. 16.9a-c. Inferior vena cava tumoral thrombosis extension in a 72-year-old man who underwent right nephrectomy for renal cell carcinoma. Axial contrast-enhanced CT scans show **a** an inferior vena cava tumoral thrombus (*arrowhead*) that **b** extends up into the intrahepatic vena cava (*arrow*) and **c** right atrium (*arrow*). There is involvement of bilateral adrenal glands (*arrows*) seen in **a** and a mild ascites seen in **a** and **b**.

Recently, MR imaging has been shown to be superior to echocardiography not only in demonstrating a global view of cardiac anatomy involvement (i.e., pericardium, myocardium, or cardiac cavities) but also in providing a better preoperative assessment of anatomic relations of cardiac metastatic masses to their surrounding structures (SAFI et al. 2003).

16.3.4
Breast

Metastasis to the breast is unusual in RCC. The involvement is usually metachronous (PURSNER et al. 1997; VASSALLI et al. 2001). The latency period can be as long as 18 years. Clinically, metastases to the breast are asymptomatic with the lesion most commonly solitary and well circumscribed, located superficially in the upper quadrant of the breast (VASSALLI et al. 2001). Bilateral involvement has been reported once in a 14-year-old girl (PURSNER et al. 1997). Pain, tenderness, or discharge are rare. The overlying skin is rarely dimpled or adherent to the tumor (VASSALLI et al. 2001). Pathologically, the tumor may infiltrate in a pattern that mimics ductal carcinoma in situ (GUPTA et al. 2001). The prognosis is generally poor since breast involvement can be a signal of rapid widespread dissemination (GUPTA et al. 2001; VASSALLI et al. 2001).

Mammography and breast ultrasound may show a nodular mass. Because CT is routinely performed for the follow-up evaluation of patients after nephrectomy, it is important to look carefully at breast area since it may show a well-defined breast mass (Figs. 16.6, 16.10; PURSNER et al. 1997).

16.4
Abdominal and Pelvic Metastases

16.4.1
Liver

Liver metastases have been reported in 1–7% of cases (JANZEN et al. 2003). Metastasis to the liver seems to be associated with a particularly poor prognosis (FLANIGAN et al. 2001; RAPTOPOULOS et al. 2001)

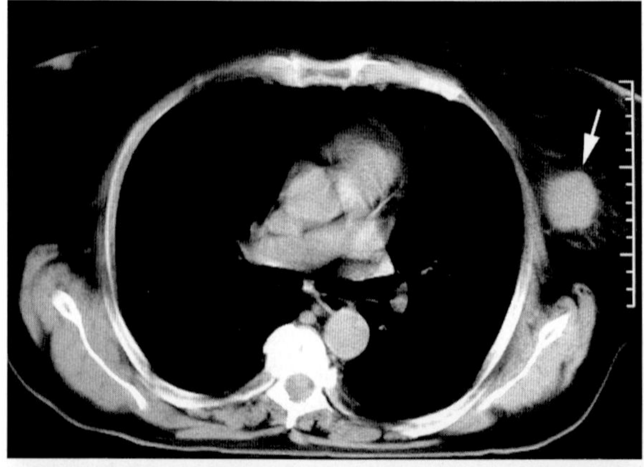

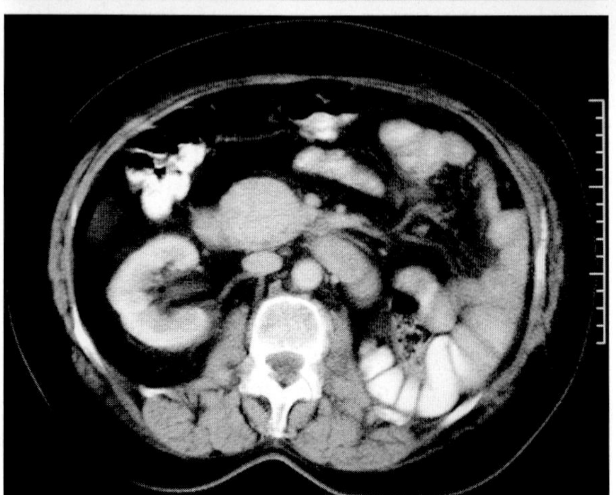

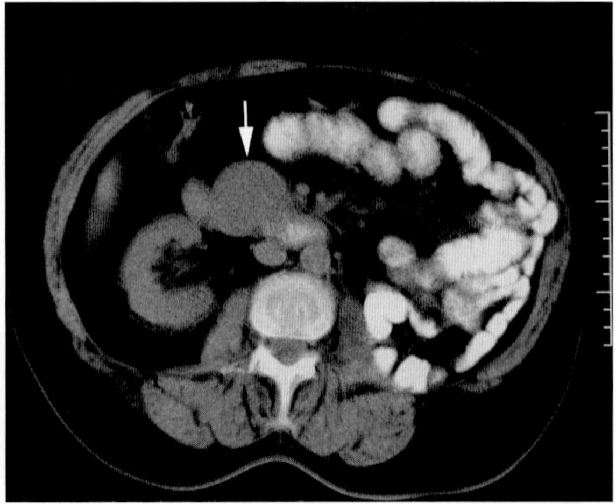

Fig. 16.10a-c. Breast and duodenal metastases in a 69-year-old woman who underwent left nephrectomy for renal cell carcinoma. a Axial contrast-enhanced CT scan of the chest shows a well-defined enhancing mass of the left breast (*arrow*) with infiltration of adjacent tissue. b Axial unenhanced CT scan of the abdomen discloses a rounded mass in the wall of the third duodenum (*arrow*) which enhances strongly and homogeneously (c) after contrast injection.

because of its association with widely disseminated disease (JANZEN et al. 2003). Solitary metastasis to the liver is reported to occur in 5.4% of all cases with metastasis, but improved survival with surgery is anecdotal (JANZEN et al. 2003; SAITOH et al. 1982). Spontaneous regression of liver metastases from renal cancer has been reported (RITCHIE et al. 1988; WYCZOLKOWSKI et al. 2001).

On ultrasound (US), liver metastases from RCC are usually hypoechoic (CHAE et al. 2005). On CT, they are suggestive when highly vascular, like the primary tumor (Fig. 16.11). Because the hypervascular hepatic lesion may become isodense or nearly isodense on contrast-enhanced CT, unenhanced CT should be performed and may show hypodense lesions if conventional CT scan is used (Fig. 16.12; BRESSLER et al. 1987). With spiral CT, arterial-phase scanning is essential for detecting vascular liver metastases which appear hyperdense (Fig. 16.13; MIGNON and MESUROLLE 2003; SCATARIGE et al. 2001a). In a study using multiphase contrast-enhanced spiral CT of 46 patients with liver metastases from RCC, the authors found that 10% of the hepatic lesions were missed in the portal-venous phase; all were smaller than 2 cm and most were seen in the enhanced scans and arterial phase. They concluded that the combination of unenhanced, arterial phase, and portal-venous phase should be used in the initial evaluation of patients with metastatic RCC for improved lesion detection and characterization. For subsequent follow-up monitoring of treatment, the combination of unenhanced and portal-venous phase is preferred. The delayed phase does not contribute significantly to lesion detection (RAPTOPOULOS et al. 2001). Liver metastases vary in size (Figs. 16.14, 16.15). Because most hepatic metastases are large, they may have central necrotic areas which appear hypodense after contrast administration (Figs. 16.16, 16.17; CHAE et al. 2005; FEDERLE et al. 1981). Occasionally, these lesions are calcified (FEDERLE et al. 1981), contain fat (MURAM and AISEN 2003), or spontaneously rupture (Fig. 16.18) with intraperitoneal hemorrhage (MURAKAMI et al. 2000).

16.4.2
Adrenal Gland

The incidence of adrenal metastases varies from 4.3 to 13.0% (O'BRIEN and LYNCH 1987; SAGALOWSKY and MOLBERG 1999; SAITOH et al. 1982; SIEMER et al. 2004). Metastases may involve the ipsilateral adrenal

gland if it has been spared during surgery (Fig. 16.14; SAITOH et al. 1982) and less frequently the contralateral adrenal gland (Fig. 16.19; HASEGAWA et al. 1988; SAITOH et al. 1982). Bilateral involvement of the adrenal gland is possible (Fig. 16.20; DUGGAN et al. 1987; SELLI et al. 1987; SIEMER et al. 2004; YU et al. 1992) as well as tumoral hemorrhage of the remaining adrenal gland (MIGNON and MESUROLLE 2003). Isolated involvement of the contralateral adrenal gland is possible but rare and is always hematogenous (MIGNON et al. 1999). Adrenal metastases may be synchronous (LAU et al. 2003; SELLI et al. 1987; VESPASIANI et al. 1990) or metachronous (HASEGAWA et al. 1988; LAU et al. 2003; MIGNON et al. 1999). The latency period after surgical removal of the primary renal tumor can be as long as 19 years for bilateral involvement (DUGGAN et al. 1987) and 28 years for contralateral involvement (HUISMAN and SANDS 1991). It is known that the risk of ipsilateral adrenal metastasis correlates to the large advanced T-stage tumors of the upper pole. On the other hand, predisposing factors for contralateral involvement are unknown (MESUROLLE et al. 1997; SIEMER et al. 2004). An aggressive surgical approach is justified with a solitary adrenal metastasis since it carries a better prognosis and prolongs patient survival (LAU et al. 2003; MIGNON et al. 1999).

Adrenal involvement is usually detectable preoperatively on CT (Fig. 16.21), MR imaging, or angiography (O'BRIEN and LYNCH 1987; SELLI et al. 1987; SIEMER et al. 2004). Computed tomography is very sensitive and has an excellent positive predictive value for detecting adrenal involvement (MIGNON et al. 1999). It shows a homogeneous or heterogeneous enhancing nodule or mass of varying sizes within the adrenal gland (MESUROLLE et al. 1997; MIGNON et al. 1999). Differential diagnosis may be difficult with adrenal adenoma. Chemical-shift MR imaging may help. If there is no change of signal from the adrenal lesion between in-phase and out-of-phase sequences, the lesion is a metastasis. It is an adrenal adenoma if the signal intensity decreases between the two sequences (MIGNON et al. 1999). Computed tomography may be a less expensive and more widely available diagnostic alternative. A difference of 10 HU in density between unenhanced and contrast-enhanced images has a sensitivity of 75% and specificity around 100% (MIGNON et al. 1999). In any case, the hypervascularity of the nodule on CT, MR imaging, or angiography demonstrated by the early and intensive contrast enhancement points to a metastatic nodule from RCC (MIGNON et al. 1999). If doubts persist, CT-guided fine-needle-aspiration

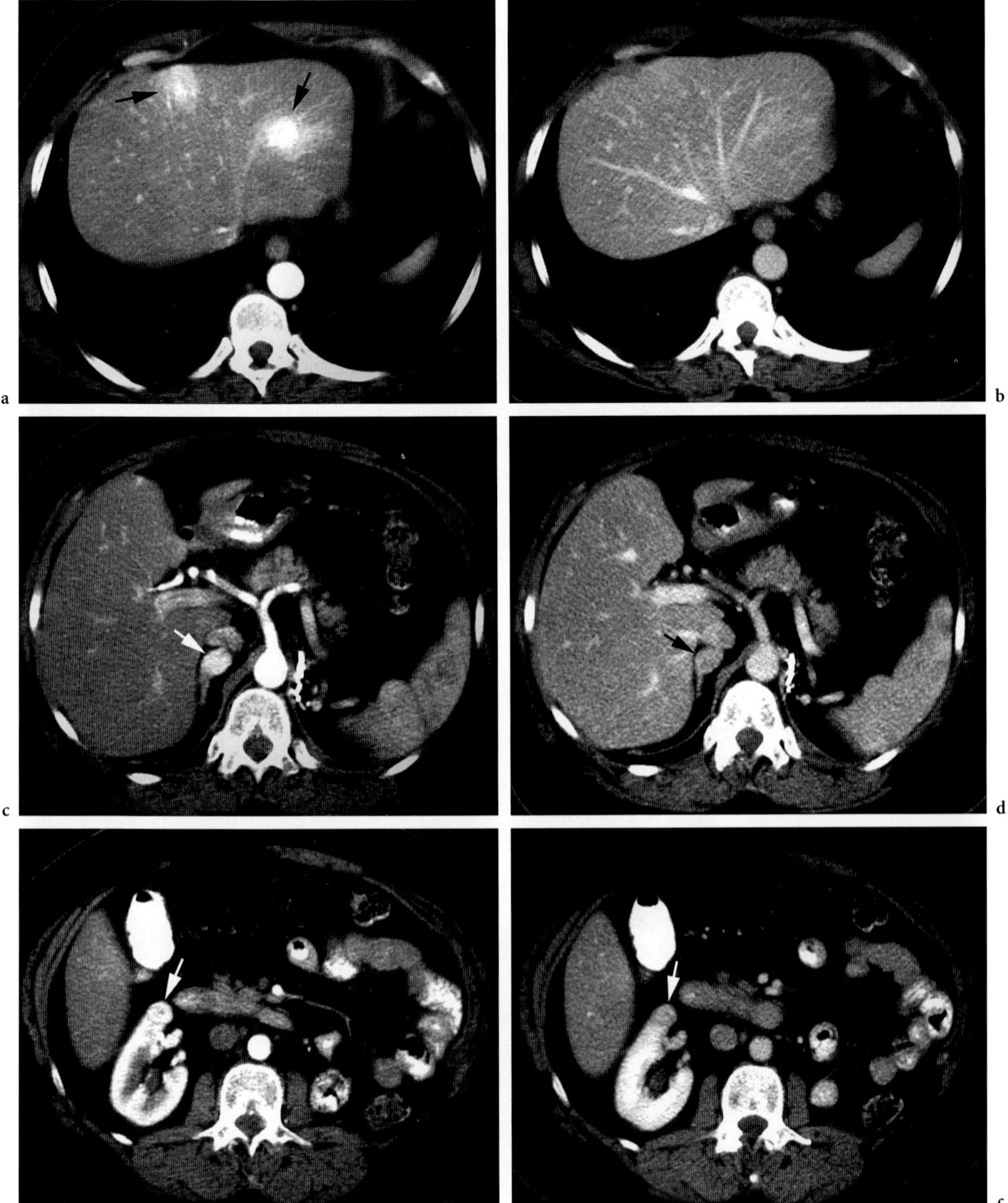

Fig. 16.11a-f. Liver and contralateral adrenal and kidney metastases in a 48-year-old man who underwent left nephrectomy for renal cell carcinoma. Axial contrast-enhanced CT scans show strongly enhancing hepatic metastases (*arrows*, **a**) at the arterial phase, which are **b** invisible at the portal venous phase. Right adrenal metastasis (*arrow*) is also strongly enhancing at **c** the arterial phase but **d** still visible at portal venous phase because of its nodular shape. Conversely, the right kidney metastasis (*arrow*) is difficult to see **e** at arterial phase because it has the same density as the normal renal parenchyma. It is better detected at **f** portal venous phase because it is hypodense (*arrow*) compared with the renal parenchyma.

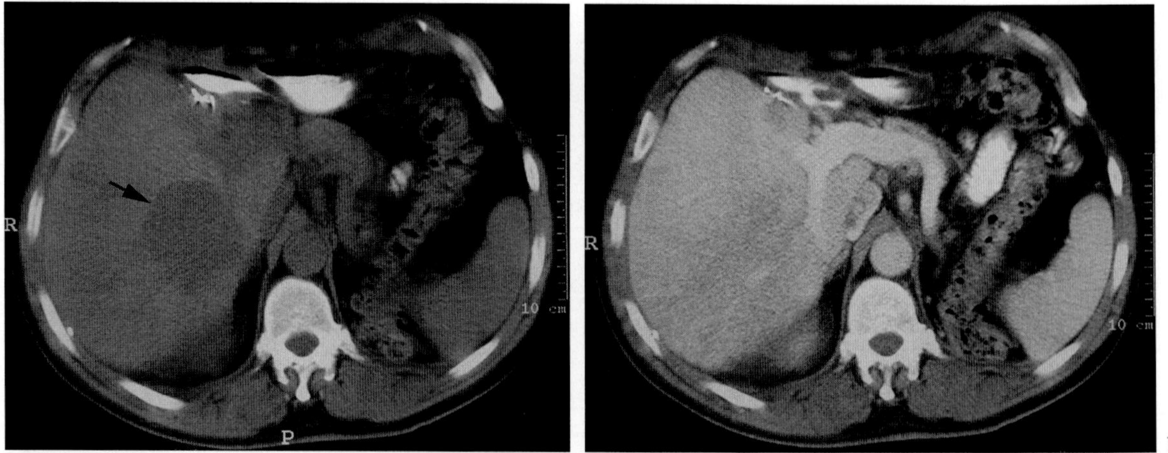

Fig. 16.12a,b. Liver metastasis in a 51-year-old man who underwent left nephrectomy for renal cell carcinoma. **a** Axial unenhanced conventional CT scan shows a large, round hypodense mass lesion in the liver (*arrow*) which is barely detectable (**b**) after contrast injection.

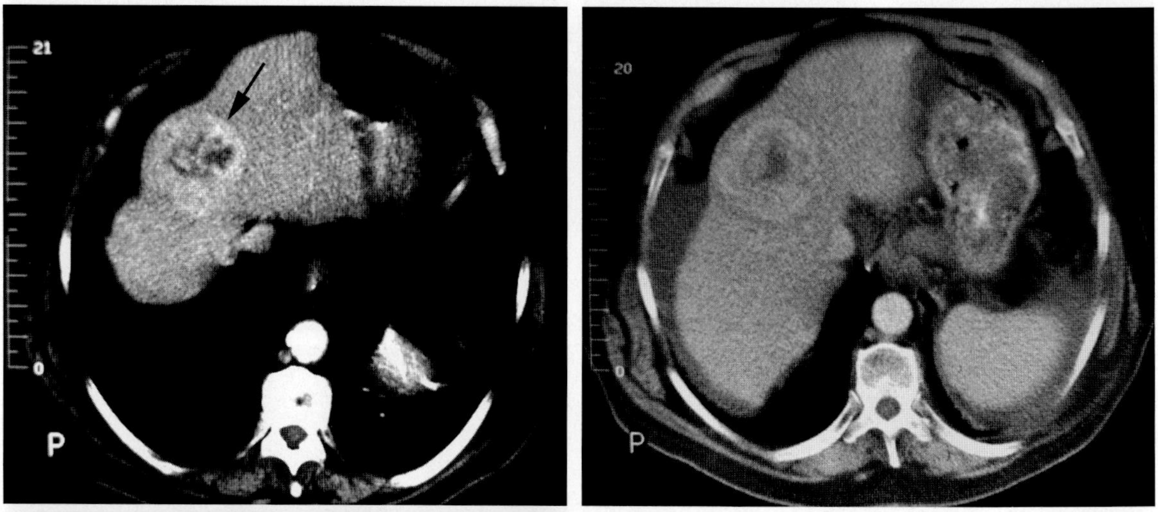

Fig. 16.13a-c. Liver metastasis and local recurrence in a 71-year-old man who underwent left nephrectomy for renal cell carcinoma. Axial contrast-enhanced CT scans show a strongly enhancing heterogeneous hepatic mass (*arrow*) with central necrosis **a** at the arterial phase which is less conspicuous **b** at the portal venous phase. There is also an ascites. **c** Axial contrast-enhanced CT scan at portal venous phase at the level of the kidneys shows an enhancing heterogeneous mass (*arrows*) with central necrosis occupying the left kidney fossa and probably invading the psoas muscle.

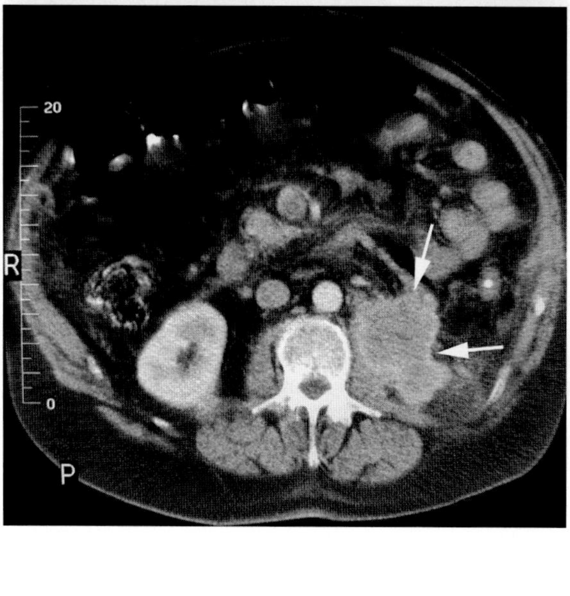

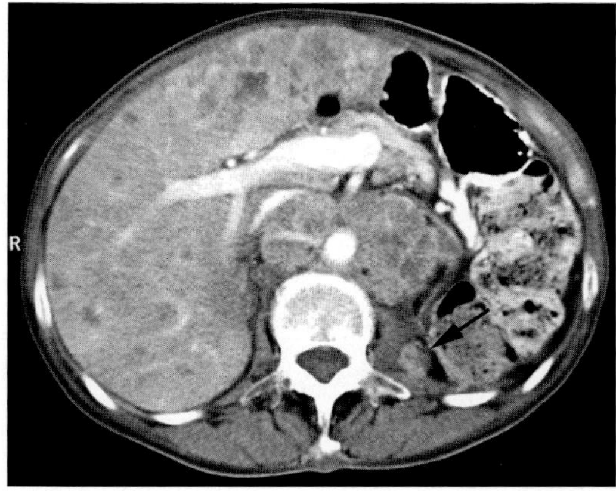

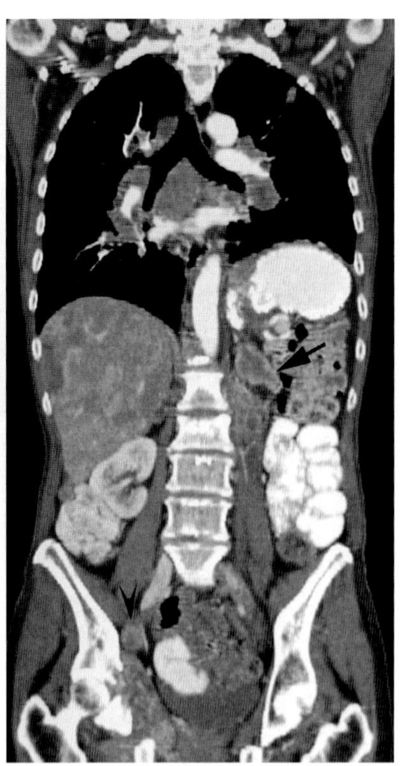

Fig. 16.14a,b. Small liver metastases with local recurrence and ipsilateral adrenal gland, bone, lung, and diffuse lymph node metastases in a 60-year-old woman who underwent left nephrectomy for renal cell carcinoma. **a** Axial contrast-enhanced CT scan shows multiple, small heterogeneous hypodense liver lesions with very thin peripheral enhancement. There is also a small heterogeneous enhancing mass in the left renal fossa invading the psoas muscle (*arrow*) and large heterogeneous enhancing retroperitoneal para-aortic adenopathies. **b** Coronal two-dimensional CT reconstruction of whole body confirms the earlier lesions and also shows heterogeneous, enhancing ipsilateral, left adrenal gland (*arrow*) mass, large mediastinal adenopathies, left pulmonary nodule, obturator lymph node enlargement (*arrowhead*), and large heterogeneously enhancing mass destroying the right acetabulum, and superior and inferior pubis rami.

biopsy is a simple, safe, and reliable method for the diagnosis of RCC metastases to the adrenal gland. It should be performed after biological diagnostic exclusion of pheochromocytoma, especially in patients with blood hypertension (MESUROLLE et al. 1997; MIGNON et al. 1999).

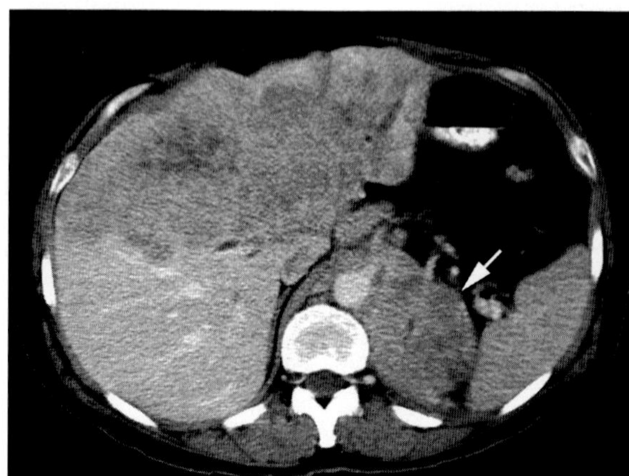

Fig. 16.15. Large liver and adrenal metastases in a 49-year-old man who underwent left radical nephrectomy for renal cell carcinoma. Axial contrast-enhanced CT scan shows a very large heterogeneous hepatic lesion with central necrosis and heterogeneously enhancing tumor in the left adrenal bed (*arrow*) which is invading the left diaphragm.

16.4.3
Spleen

Splenic metastases from RCC are extremely rare. They present a diagnostic dilemma since fine-needle aspiration of splenic tumors is often avoided because of possible hemorrhage (MCGREGOR et al. 2003). Involvement may be synchronous (MCGREGOR et al. 2003) or metachronous (TATSUTA et al. 2001). The latency period can be as long as 22 years (TATSUTA et al. 2001). Renal cell carcinoma may also occasionally secondarily involve the spleen by direct invasion (SUZUKI et al. 1982). Splenic metastasis is infrequently diagnosed clinically (MCGREGOR et al. 2003) because it is usually asymptomatic (TATSUTA et al. 2001). Splenectomy is usually the effective treatment because it is associated with complete resection of the tumor. The prognosis associated with splenic metastasis is favorable when there is only a solitary lesion (TATSUTA et al. 2001).

On US and CT, the appearance of spleen metastases varies. They may appear as a large complex heterogeneous mass in the spleen containing both solid and fluid components (Figs. 16.3, 16.22, 16.23; MCGREGOR et al. 2003; TATSUTA et al. 2001). Other appearances include diffuse splenomegaly or small nodules (TATSUTA et al. 2001).

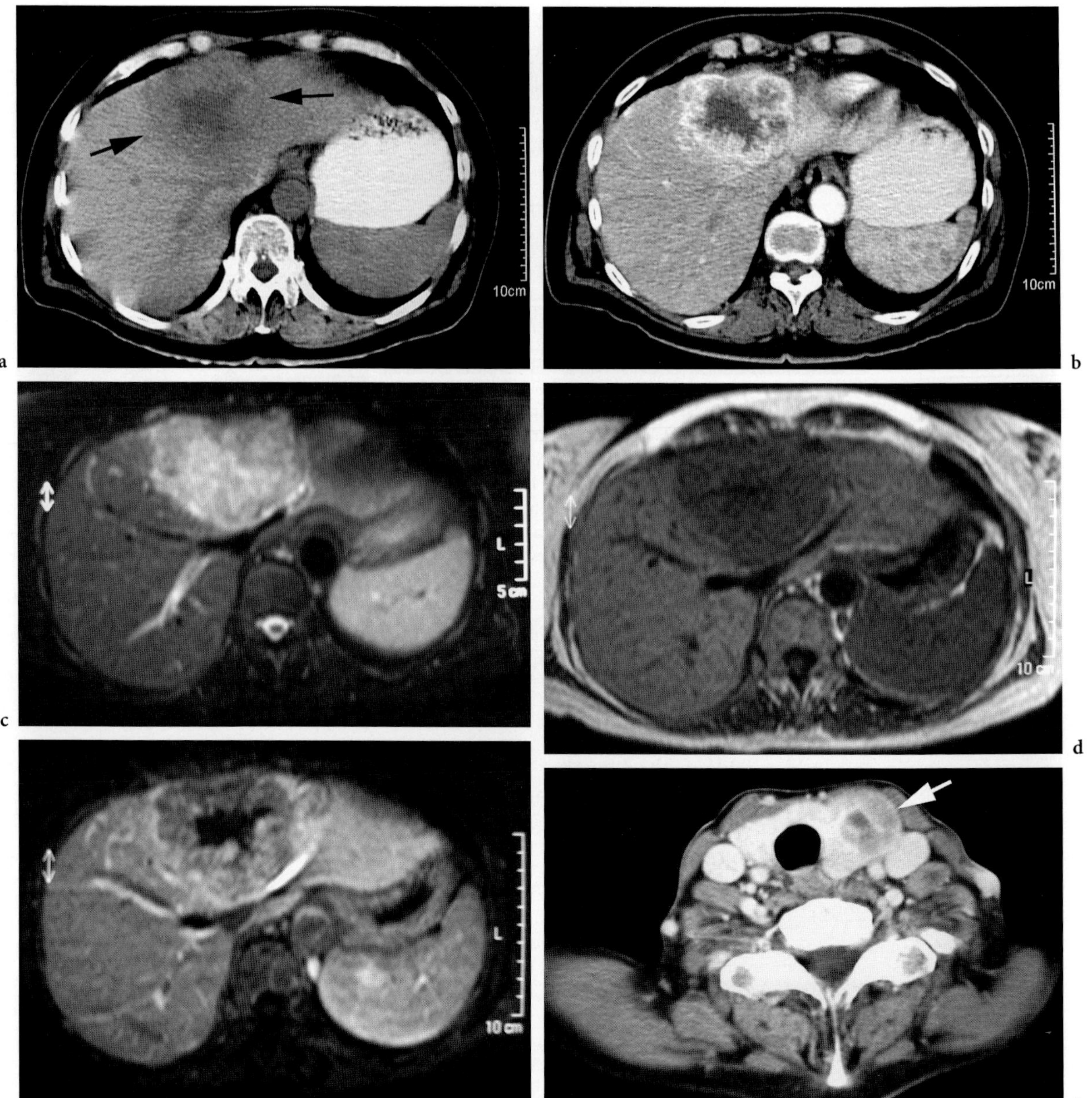

Fig. 16.16a-f. Liver and thyroid metastases in a 69-year-old woman who underwent left nephrectomy for renal cell carcinoma. **a** Axial unenhanced CT scan shows an ill-defined large hypodense hepatic lesion with central necrosis (*arrows*). **b** This lesion strongly heterogeneously enhances after contrast injection and its contours are more conspicuous and its central necrosis is more obvious. This lesion is hyperintense on **c** axial turbo spin T2-weighted MR image and hypointense on **d** fast-field-echo T1-weighted MR image. The tumoral enhancement is less obvious on **e** contrast-enhanced fast-field-echo T1-weighted MR image than on CT. **f** Axial contrast-enhanced CT of the neck shows large heterogeneous nodule of the left thyroid lobe (*arrow*).

16.4.4
Pancreas

Renal cell carcinoma metastases to the pancreas are uncommon and count for only 1–3% of cases (GHAVAMIAN et al. 2000). Nevertheless, RCC is the most commonly reported primary tumor metas-

tasizing to the pancreas (GHAVAMIAN et al. 2000; KLEIN et al. 1998). They may be synchronous (ZHAO et al. 1997) or occur several years after nephrectomy (DOUSSET et al. 1995; KLEIN et al. 1998) with a latency period as long as 32 years (BASSI et al. 2003). The pancreas may be the sole site of RCC metastases (CHAO et al. 2002). Clinically, patients are often

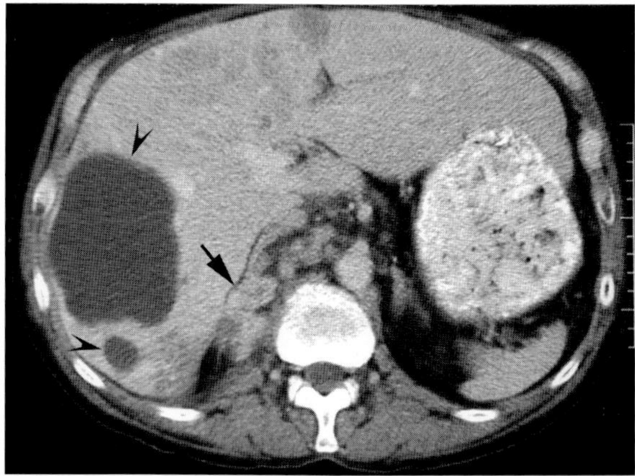

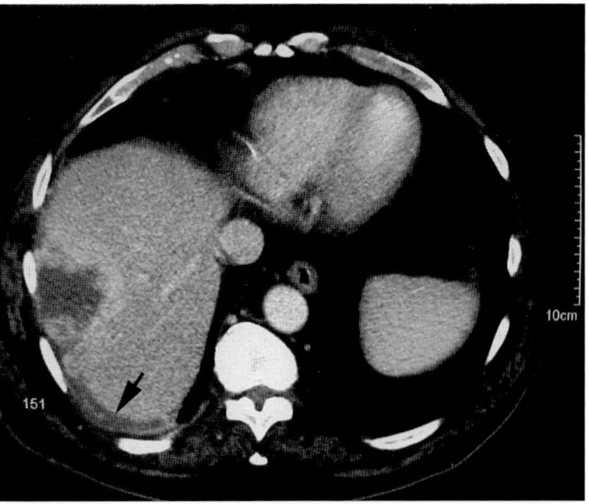

Fig. 16.17. Liver and adrenal metastases in a 59-year-old man who underwent right radical nephrectomy for renal cell carcinoma. Axial contrast-enhanced CT scan shows two well-defined water-density hepatic lesions of different sizes corresponding to cystic metastases (*arrowheads*). There are several other slightly hypodense solid mass liver metastases. There is also a heterogeneously enhancing tumor in the right adrenal bed (*arrow*).

Fig. 16.18. Spontaneous rupture of liver metastasis in a 65-year-old man who underwent nephrectomy for renal cell carcinoma. Axial contrast-enhanced CT scan shows a subcapsular hypodense lesion with slightly peripheral enhancement that spontaneously ruptured with hepatic subcapsular effusion (*arrow*).

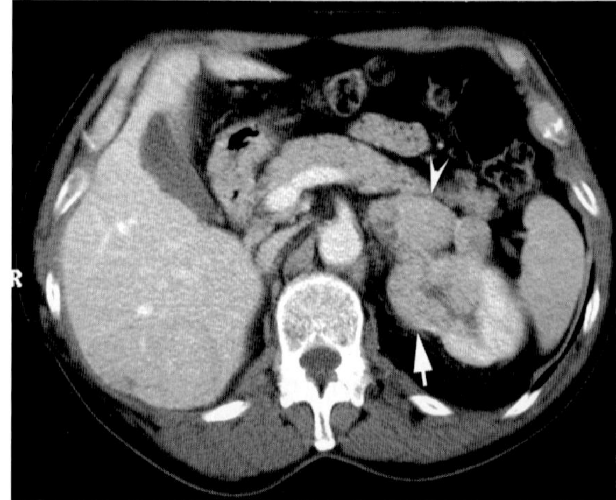

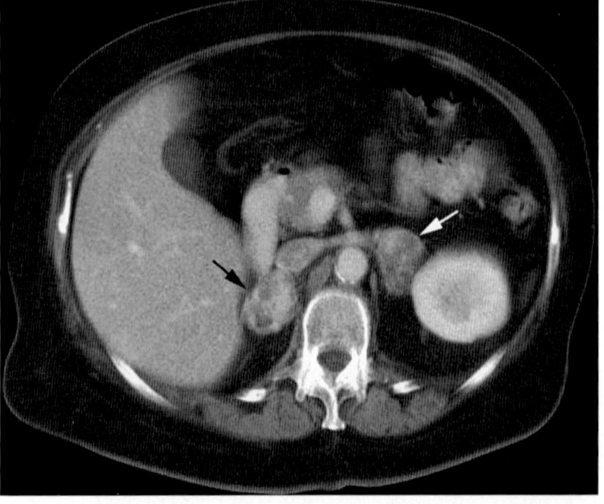

Fig. 16.19. Contralateral adrenal and kidney metastases in a 70-year-old man who underwent right nephrectomy for renal cell carcinoma. Axial contrast-enhanced CT scan at portal venous phase shows heterogeneously enhancing masses of the left adrenal gland (*arrowhead*) and left kidney (*arrow*).

Fig. 16.20. Bilateral adrenal metastases in a 67-year-old man who underwent right nephrectomy for renal cell carcinoma. Axial contrast-enhanced CT scan at portal venous phase shows heterogeneously enhancing masses of both adrenal glands (*arrows*).

asymptomatic (BASSI et al. 2003; GHAVAMIAN et al. 2000). Clinical abnormalities may include palpable abdominal mass, gastrointestinal bleeding, abdominal pain, bile duct obstruction, steatorrhea, and weight loss (GHAVAMIAN et al. 2000; KASSABIAN et al. 2000). In solitary pancreatic involvement, surgical resection can improve the likelihood of patient survival (ANDOH et al. 2004; GHAVAMIAN et al. 2000; GIULINI et al. 2003; KASSABIAN et al. 2000; MARUSCH et al. 2001). Spontaneous regression of pancreatic metastasis has been reported (ALTSCHULER and RAY 1998). The prognosis of pancreatic metastasis from RCC is much better than that of primary pancreatic adenocarcinoma (DOUSSET et al. 1995;

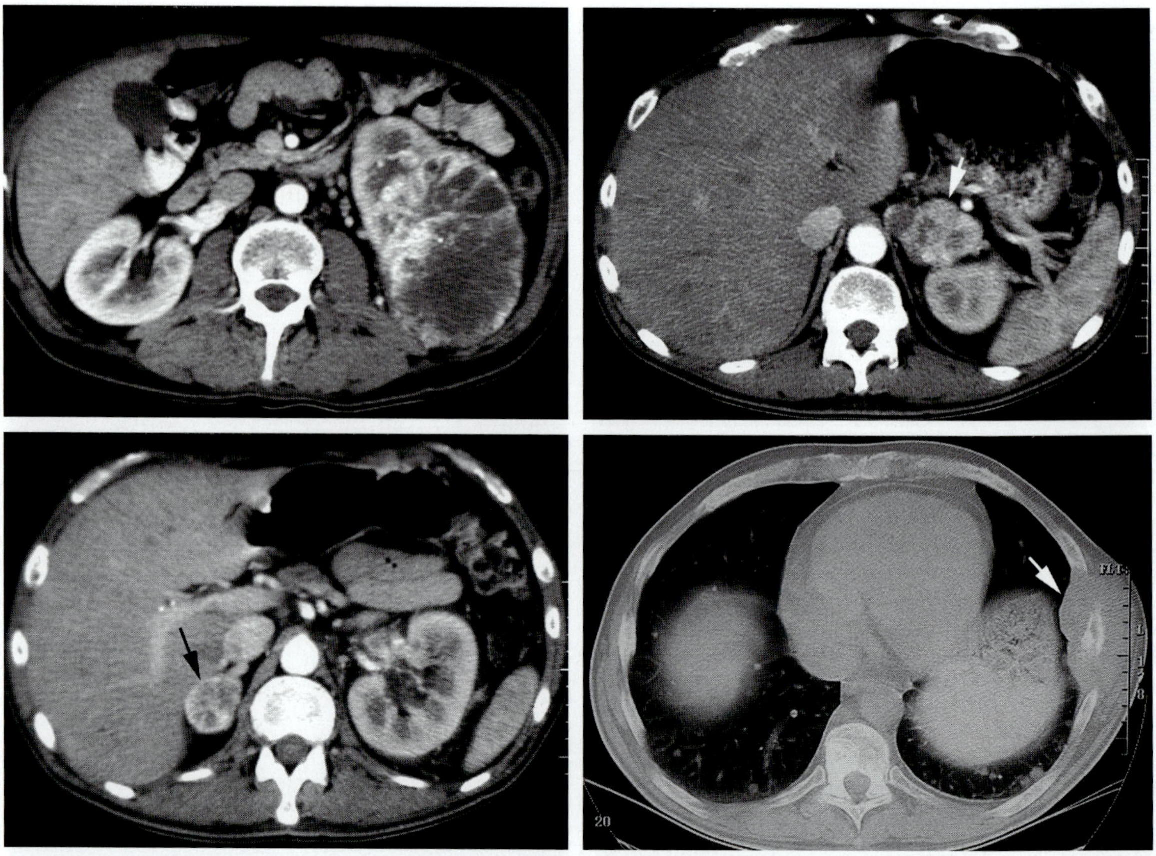

Fig. 16.21a-d. Bilateral adrenal, chest wall, and lung metastases diagnosed preoperatively in a 41-year-old man with renal cell carcinoma. **a** Axial contrast-enhanced CT scan shows heterogeneously enhancing large posterior left renal mass corresponding to the renal cell carcinoma. Axial contrast-enhanced CT scans show heterogeneously enhancing masses of the left (*arrow*, **b**) and right (*arrow*, **c**) adrenal glands. **d** Axial CT scan of the chest shows a large lytic mass involving the left lateral chest wall (*arrow*) and several bilateral small pulmonary nodules.

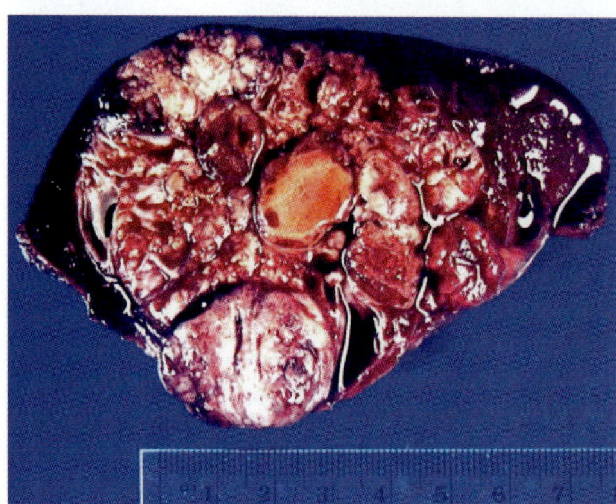

Fig. 16.22. Spleen metastasis in a 65-year-old man with synchronous renal cell carcinoma of the left kidney. Gross specimen shows massive replacement of the splenic parenchyma by metastatic tumor. There are multiple nodules fusing together to form a tumor mass occupying approximately 70% of the splenic parenchyma. Microscopic features of this splenic tumor are of a metastatic papillary carcinoma, identical to the histologic appearance of the primary renal cell carcinoma, chromophil (papillary) type (not shown). (Image courtesy of D.H. McGregor)

GHAVAMIAN et al. 2000; KLEIN et al. 1998; RIVOIRE and VOIGLIO 1996).

On imaging, pancreatic metastases may be solitary or multiple, and usually appear as well-defined soft tissue masses (GHAVAMIAN et al. 2000; KLEIN et al. 1998). Ultrasound and CT are reliable and highly specific (BASSI et al. 2003). On US or endoscopic US (DOUSSET et al. 1995), pancreatic metastases may be hypoechoic (KASSABIAN et al. 2000; RIVOIRE and VOIGLIO 1996; STRIJK 1989), or hyperechoic (RYPENS et al. 1992) due to their hypervascularity. On unenhanced CT, lesions are usually isodense to the pancreatic parenchyma (ALTSCHULER and RAY 1998; NG et al. 1999), and are rarely reported as mixed isodense and hypodense (STRIJK 1989). Calcifications may occur but are very rare (KLEIN et al. 1998). Spiral CT with its optimization of vascular phases is particularly efficient in demonstrating these hypervascular pancreatic lesions (KLEIN et al. 1998; GHAVAMIAN et al. 2000; KASSABIAN et

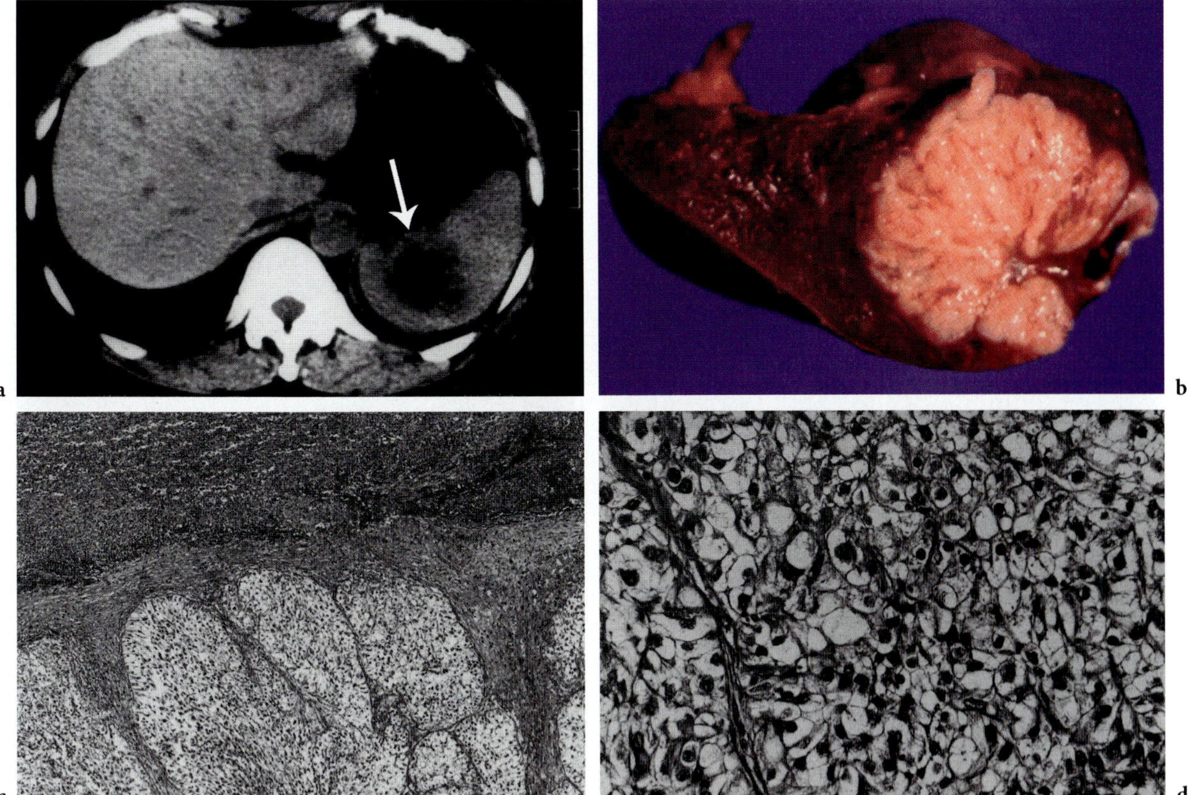

Fig. 16.23a-d. Spleen metastasis in a 69-year-man who underwent left nephrectomy for renal cell carcinoma 17 months previously. **a** Axial unenhanced CT scan shows an ill-defined heterogeneous hypodense mass of 6×6 cm in the spleen (*arrow*). **b** Gross specimen shows a milky-white tumor in the upper half of the spleen, 6 cm in diameter, that did not invade the capsule. Photomicrographs confirm a clear cell carcinoma in the spleen (hematoxylin and eosin stain; original magnification, **c** ×15, **d** ×75). (With permission from TATSUTA et al. 2001)

al. 2000; SCATARIGE et al. 2001a; HERNANDEZ et al. 2003), which can also be seen on angiography (ANDOH et al. 2004; KASSABIAN et al. 2000; STRIJK 1989; ZHAO et al. 1997) and on early contrast-enhanced MR imaging (KELEKIS et al. 1996). This is unlike primary pancreatic adenocarcinoma which is usually hypovascular and does not enhance after contrast administration (GHAVAMIAN et al. 2000; SCATARIGE et al. 2001a). This hypervascular effect is pronounced in early phases (i.e., arterial and portal) of enhancement (Fig. 16.24; GHAVAMIAN et al. 2000; NG et al. 1999). Such metastases may not be appreciated in the delayed phase or on unenhanced CT, especially if they are small (NG et al. 1999). Smaller lesions tend to be homogeneous and enhance uniformly, whereas larger masses usually contain internal ischemic or necrotic components that appear as central hypodense areas (Figs. 16.25, 16.26; BASSI et al. 2003; GHAVAMIAN et al. 2000; KASSABIAN et al. 2000; SCATARIGE et al. 2001b). In this respect the

radiological appearance of pancreatic metastases from RCC resembles the appearance of primary RCC (GHAVAMIAN et al. 2000; KLEIN et al. 1998).

16.4.5
Contralateral Kidney

Contralateral kidney metastases are rare accounting for approximately 1–2% of cases (JANZEN et al. 2003). There is still debate on whether tumors that occur in the contralateral kidney after radical or partial nephrectomy represent de novo malignancy or metastasis (JANZEN et al. 2003). The synchronous appearance of a single nodule or mass with the primary cancer suggests a possible second contralateral kidney cancer (MIGNON and MESUROLLE 2003). On the other hand, multiplicity of the lesions in the contralateral kidney or the synchronous appearance of these lesions with other organ metastases indi-

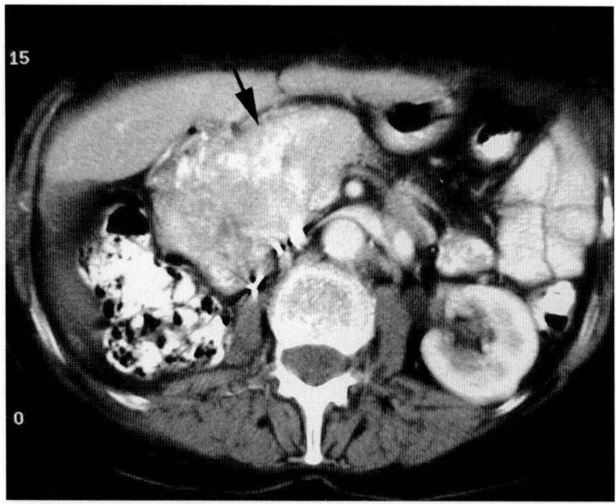

Fig. 16.24. Pancreatic metastasis in a 71-year-old man who underwent right nephrectomy for renal cell carcinoma. Axial contrast-enhanced CT scan at arterial phase shows heterogeneously enhancing very large mass of the head and body of the pancreas (*arrow*).

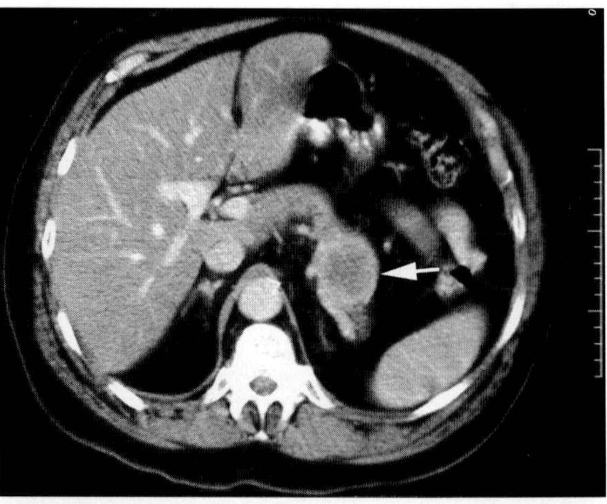

Fig. 16.25. Pancreatic metastasis in a 62-year-old man who underwent right nephrectomy for renal cell carcinoma. Axial contrast-enhanced CT scan at portal venous phase shows heterogeneously enhancing mass in the tail of the pancreas (*arrow*).

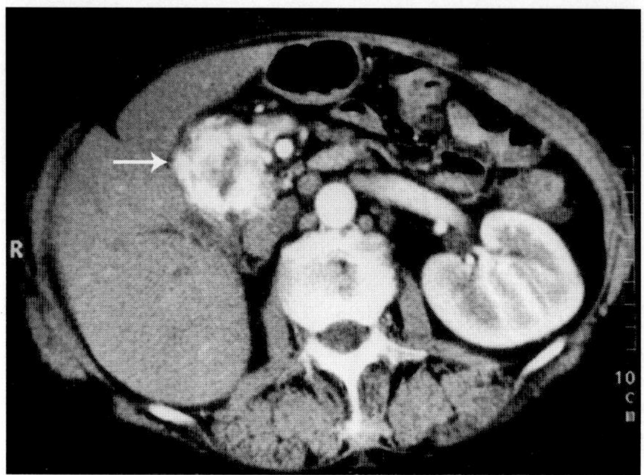

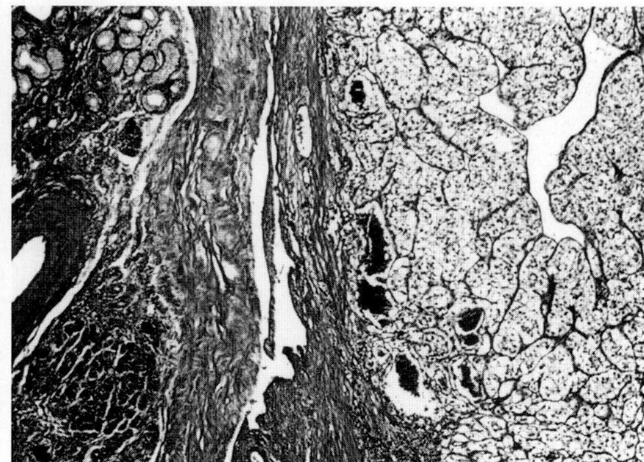

Fig. 16.26a,b. Pancreatic metastasis in a 73-year-old woman with renal cell carcinoma. **a** Axial contrast-enhanced CT scan shows large enhancing mass of the head of the pancreas (*arrow*) with central hypodense areas corresponding to necrosis. **b** Photomicrograph shows metastatic cells that are very glycogen rich like the clear cell primary renal tumor (hematoxylin and eosin stain). (Image courtesy of G. Butturini and C. Bassi)

cates metastases (Mignon and Mesurolle, 2003; Scatarige et al. 2001a).

On imaging, contralateral kidney metastases are usually hypoechoic on US and show a strongly enhancing mass on CT. The enhancement may be homogeneous (Chae et al. 2005) or heterogeneous with central necrosis (Fig. 16.27; Scatarige et al. 2001a).

16.4.6
Gallbladder

The gallbladder is only very rarely the site of RCC metastases (Furukawa et al. 1997; Limani et al.

2003; Stattaus et al. 1999). They are usually asymptomatic (Furukawa et al. 1997; Nagler et al. 1994), and usually metachronous (Furukawa et al. 1997) with a latency period as long as 27 years (Aoki et al. 2002). If possible, surgical resection should be performed, as it can provide a better chance of survival (Furukawa et al. 1997; Limani et al. 2003).

Ultrasound may show a polypoid mass in the gallbladder (Furukawa et al. 1997). Color Doppler US may show abundant pulsatile blood flow signal intensity within the mass. Spiral CT at the arterial phase may demonstrate an enhancing polypoid mass in the gallbladder (Fig. 16.28). The density of the lesion is usually higher than that of the

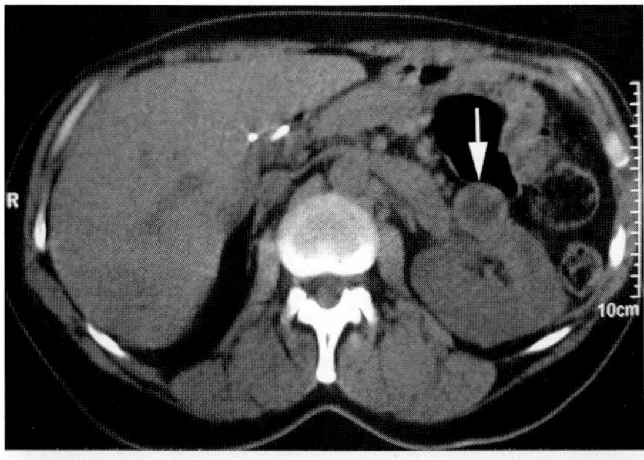
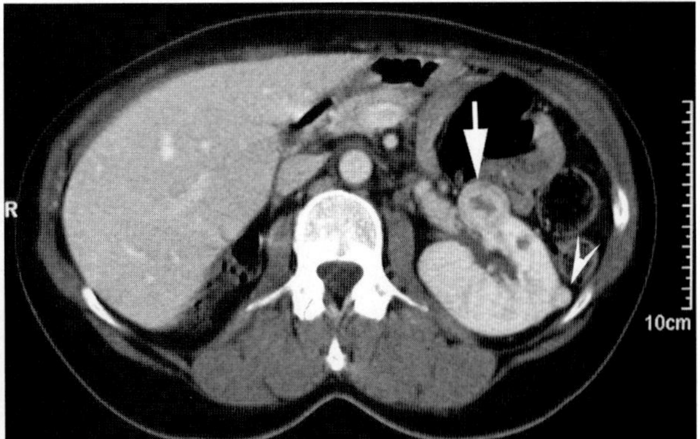
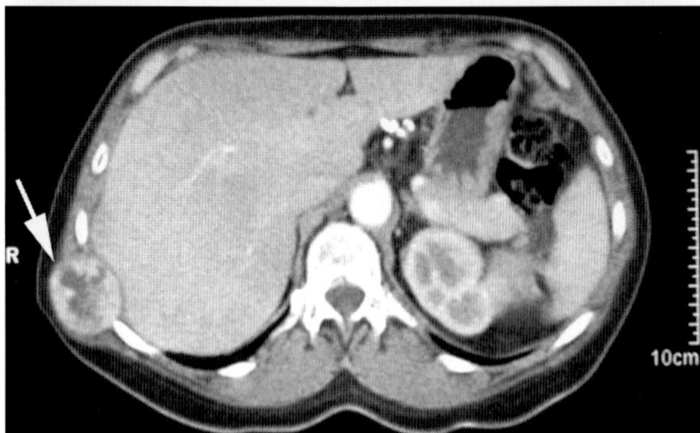

Fig. 16.27a-c. Contralateral kidney and chest wall metastases in a 54-year-old woman who underwent right nephrectomy for renal cell carcinoma. **a** Axial unenhanced CT scan shows heterogeneous anterior mass of the left kidney (*arrow*) with central necrosis. **b** Axial contrast-enhanced CT scan at the same level as **a** shows a heterogeneous enhancement of the anterior mass (*arrow*) and a subcapsular, homogeneously enhancing small nodule (*arrowhead*) that induces a posterior bulge in the capsule. There is also a small benign renal cyst. **c** Axial contrast-enhanced CT scan cephalad to **b** shows a heterogeneous enhancing mass (*arrow*) involving the right posterolateral chest wall.

liver parenchyma (Furukawa et al. 1997). Imaging studies are often futile for differentiating between primary and secondary tumors of the gallbladder (Limani et al. 2003). Primary tumors often coexist with gallstones. A polypoid lesion in an acalculous gallbladder is more consistent with metastasis than primary tumor (Limani et al. 2003) especially in case of hypervascularity on imaging studies (Aoki et al. 2002; Furukawa et al. 1997).

16.4.7
Peritoneum

Intraperitoneal metastatic spread of RCC involving the mesentery and omentum is very uncommon, and is identified in only 1% of patients with metastases at autopsy (Tartar et al. 1991). These widespread diffuse intraperitoneal metastases may be present synchronously to the RCC (Tartar et al. 1991) or may represent advanced recurrence (Scatarige et al. 2001a). Intraperitoneal spread of RCC can occur by one of two mechanisms. Firstly, RCC may break through the renal capsule, the anterior renal fascia, and the apposed posterior parietal peritoneum to spread along the peritoneal surfaces. In the second mechanism, embolic hematogenous metastases

reach the omentum, mesentery, or other peritoneal organs with subsequent intraperitoneal spread. Abdominal complaints are the dominant clinical symptoms. Other presentations include abdominal distension due to ascites, early satiety, anorexia, and weight loss (Tartar et al. 1991).

Ultrasound may show cake-like omental thickening and ascites (Tartar et al. 1991). A barium enema may show narrowed bowel segments with an appearance consistent with serosal implants (Tartar et al. 1991). Computed tomography shows patterns of peritoneal carcinomatosis (Fig. 16.29; Scatarige et al. 2001a) which include extensive ascites, widespread omental infiltration (omental cake), and peritoneal soft tissue implants, as well as retroperitoneal metastases (Tartar et al. 1991). It may also show soft tissue masses in the cul-de-sac consisting of "drop" metastases (Tartar et al. 1991).

16.4.8
Esophagus, Stomach, and Duodenum

Esophageal metastases are very uncommon, especially when esophageal involvement is isolated. Clinically, they may be associated with progressive dysphagia. Resection of the esophageal metastasis is an option

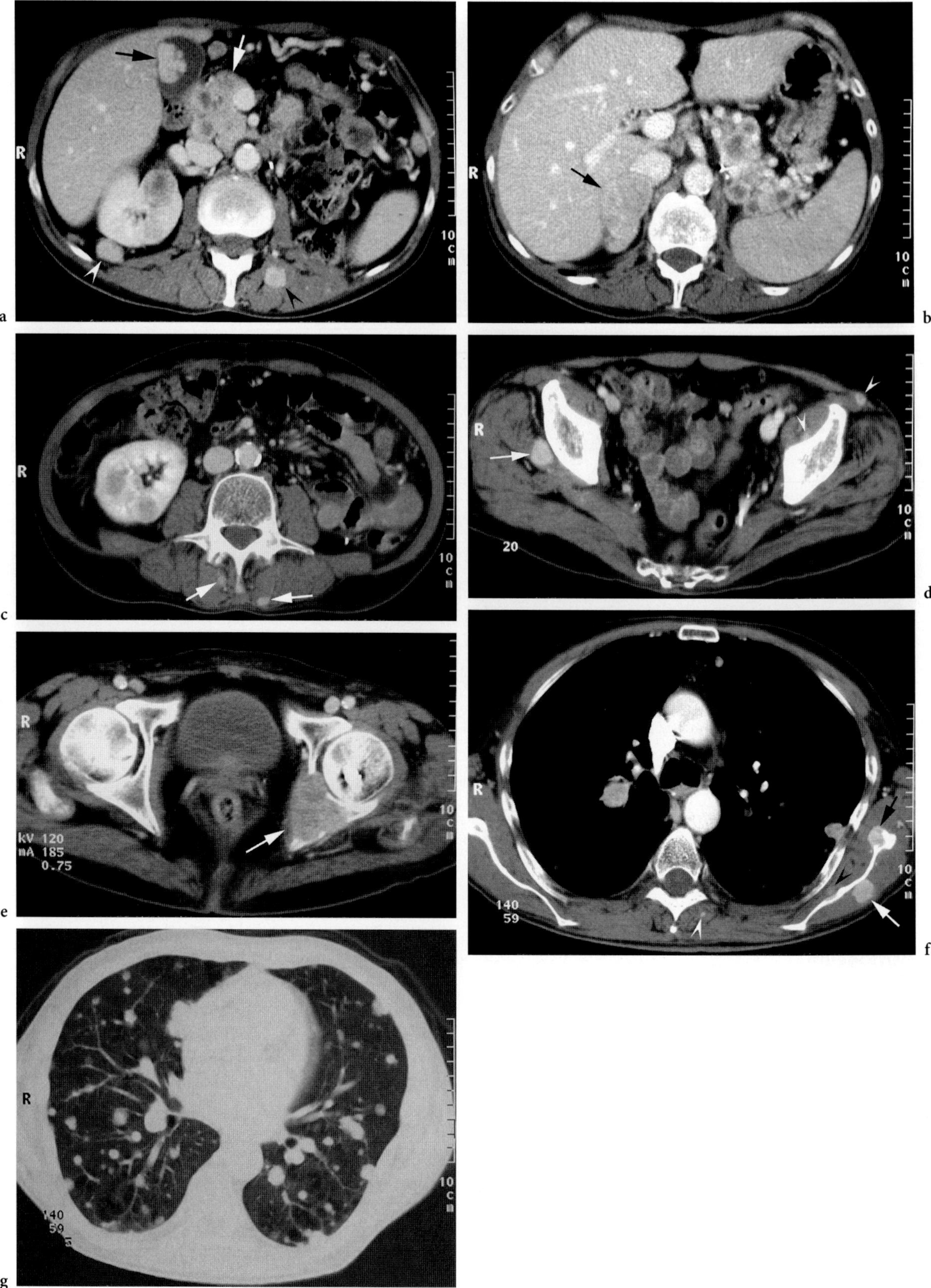

Fig. 16.28a-g. Gallbladder, contralateral kidney and adrenal gland, muscle, lung, and bone metastases in a 54-year-old man who underwent left nephrectomy for renal cell carcinoma. **a** Axial contrast-enhanced CT scan shows an enhancing heterogeneous polypoid mass in the gallbladder (*black arrow*). It also shows multiple heterogeneous enhancing masses at the head of the pancreas (*white arrow*) and anterior right kidney, a solid enhancing right posterior perirenal mass (*white arrowhead*), and an enhancing mass in the left erector spinae muscle (*black arrowhead*). **b** Axial contrast-enhanced CT scan cephalad to **a** shows multiple enhancing mixed round and annular masses in the body and tail of the pancreas. There is a large enhancing mass in the contralateral adrenal gland (*arrow*). **c** Axial contrast-enhanced CT scan at portal venous phase and caudad to **a** shows multiple hypodense lesions of varying sizes in the lower pole of the right kidneys. There are bilateral enhancing nodular lesions involving longissimus dorsi muscles (*arrows*). **d** Axial contrast-enhanced CT scan of the pelvis shows multiple nodular enhancing lesions involving right gluteus minimus (*arrow*) and left iliopsoas muscles (*arrowheads*). **e** Axial contrast-enhanced CT scan shows an enhancing destructive mass of the left acetabulum (*arrow*). **f** Axial contrast-enhanced CT scan of the chest shows multiple enhancing nodular lesions of varying sizes involving the left erector spinae (*white arrowhead*), infraspinatus (*white arrow*), and subscapularis (*black arrowhead*) muscles. There is also a enhancing destructive bone lesion of the left scapula (*black arrow*). **g** Axial CT scan of the chest at lung window shows several bilateral pulmonary nodules of varying sizes.

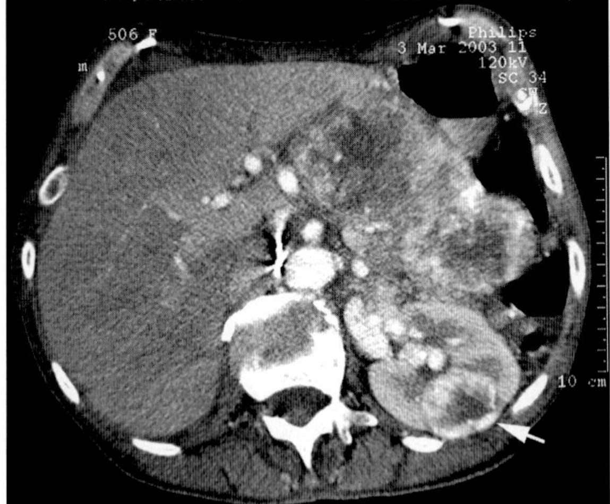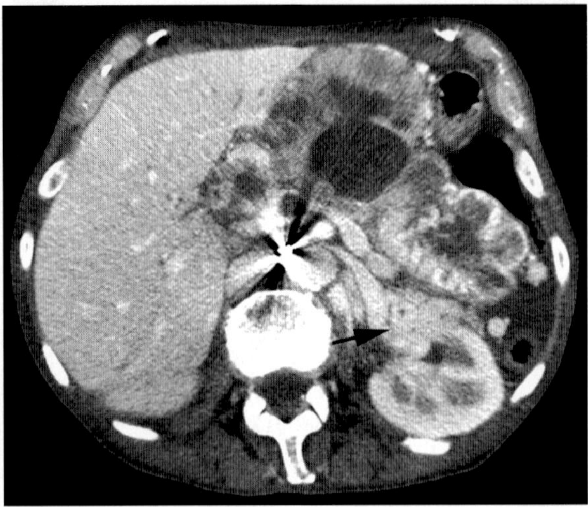

a b

Fig. 16.29a,b. Peritoneal carcinomatosis and contralateral kidney metastases in a 80-year-old woman who underwent right nephrectomy for renal cell carcinoma. **a, b** Axial contrast-enhanced CT scans show extensive widespread heterogeneous peritoneal infiltration with solid and cystic components associated with ascites. There are also heterogeneous enhancing masses of the left kidney of **a** posterior (*arrow*) and **b** anterior (*arrow*) locations.

when isolated, but its presence should be considered an adverse prognostic factor. Esophagography shows an esophageal tumor. Endoscopy may also show the tumor and also allows histological diagnostic biopsies (Monteros-Sanchez et al. 2004).

Stomach metastases from RCC are very rare. They may be synchronous or more frequently metachronous. The latency period can be as long as 9 years (Odori et al. 1998). They are more commonly located in the body and fundus than in the antrum (Adams et al. 2003), and are more likely to be single than multiple (Adams et al. 2003). Clinically, they may be asymptomatic, or associated with hematemesis, anemia, melena, dyspepsia, and/or epigastric pain (Adams et al. 2003; Mascarenhas et al. 2001). Surgical resection is appropriate for isolated gastric metastases because prolonged survival

is possible (Mascarenhas et al. 2001). The typical endoscopic appearance is a submucosal nodule with apical depression or ulceration (Adams et al. 2003; Mascarenhas et al. 2001; Odori et al. 1998). Other appearances vary from polypoid lesion (Fig. 16.30) to small or larger ulcers, sometimes with elevated margins (Adams et al. 2003; Mascarenhas et al. 2001). Their appearance may be indistinguishable from that of gastric cancers (Adams et al. 2003). Endoscopy allows biopsies that are positive in more than 90% of the cases (Adams et al. 2003). Endoscopic US is sensitive and may typically show a relatively hypoechoic nodule lying in the submucosal layer (Odori et al. 1998). Computed tomography may show the tumor as a mass in the stomach.

Duodenal metastases are very rare. They may be synchronous (Yavascaoglu et al. 1999) or meta-

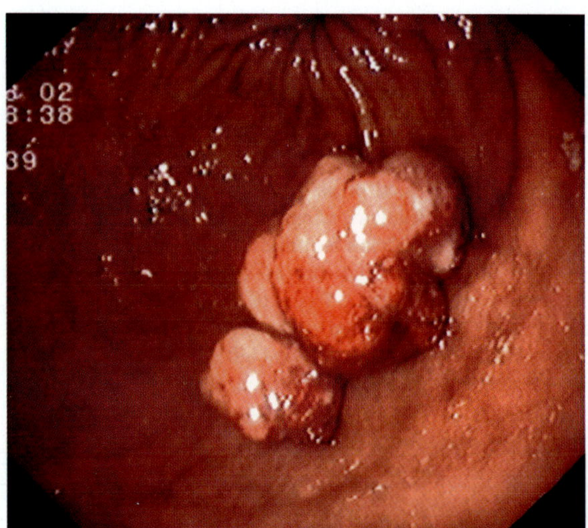

Fig. 16.30. Gastric metastases in a 64-year-old man with advanced renal cell cancer. Endoscopic view shows polypoid metastases in the body of the stomach. (With permission from ADAMS et al. 2003; image courtesy of I.C. Roberts-Thomson)

chronous with a latency period as long as 11 years (HASHIMOTO et al. 2001). They usually occur in patients with widespread nodal and visceral involvement, but may also be the only metastatic localization (HASHIMOTO et al. 2001). Clinically they may present with dyspepsia (LEE et al. 2002) or obstruction (THARAKAN et al. 1995), or mainly with gastrointestinal tract bleeding (HASHIMOTO et al. 2001; ROBERTSON and GERTLER 1990; YAVASCAOGLU et al. 1999). Duodenal metastases are most frequently located in the periampullary region, followed by the duodenal bulb (HASHIMOTO et al. 2001). Resection en bloc of a single duodenal metastasis may give a favorable prognosis (GASTACA MATEO et al. 1996; HASHIMOTO et al. 2001). Duodenoscopy shows a large and ulcerative protruding mass that may obstruct the duodenum and a biopsy can be performed during the procedure (HASHIMOTO et al. 2001; LEE et al. 2002). Angiography typically demonstrates a hypervascular tumor and is particularly useful for demonstrating small hypervascular lesions (Fig. 16.31; HASHIMOTO et al. 2001). Ultrasound may show a thickened duodenum wall (HASHIMOTO et al. 2001). Computed tomography may show circumferential wall thickening with high enhancement at the duodenum (HASHIMOTO et al. 2001; LEE et al. 2002), or a soft tissue enhancing mass at the pancreaticoduodenal region (YAVASCAOGLU et al. 1999). This tumor enhancement is also well seen at MR imaging (HASHIMOTO et al. 2001).

16.4.9
Intestine

Renal cell carcinoma metastasis to the intestine is thought to occur by dissemination through Batson's venous plexus (DIAZ-CANDAMIO et al. 2000). All segments of the small and large bowels may be involved by renal cancer metastasis.

Metastases in the small intestine are uncommon. Only 4% of RCC metastasize to the small intestine (YAVASCAOGLU et al. 1999). They are rarely synchronous and usually metachronous with latency period as long as 20 years (NOZAWA et al. 2003). These metastases usually show widespread nodal and visceral involvement (HASHIMOTO et al. 2001). Clinical presentation includes ileus, nausea, abdominal pain, loss of weight, gastrointestinal hemorrhage, intussusception, and/or perforation (NOZAWA et al. 2003; PAVLAKIS et al. 2004; SCATARIGE et al. 2001a). A hematogenous pathway through pulmonary circulation is considered to play a critical role in the cascade of multiple-step metastases from kidney to small intestine (NOZAWA et al. 2003). Histologically, almost all cases show clear cell metastatic RCC. Only one reported case included a sarcomatoid component in part of the primary tumor. These findings are consistent with the concept that sarcomatoid histology suggests high-grade malignancy and poor prognosis (NOZAWA et al. 2003). These metastases are classified as polypoid type (Fig. 16.32) in the majority of cases, or Borrmann-2 (Fig. 16.33) or Borrmann-3 type (localized or infiltrating tumor with ulcer, respectively; NOZAWA et al. 2003). Management should be aggressive since metastasectomy can extend patent survival (PAVLAKIS et al. 2004). Barium meal may show single or multiple tumors of varied sizes protruding into the lumen of the small intestine (NOZAWA et al. 2003). A CT scan may show single or multiple tumors protruding into the small intestine lumen (Fig. 16.34; PAVLAKIS et al. 2004).

Metastases to the colon from RCC are extremely rare. They may produce pain in the abdomen (LEE et al. 2002) or melena episodes (DIAZ-CANDAMIO et al. 2000) but may also be asymptomatic. They are often metachronous with a latency period as long as 8 years (DIAZ-CANDAMIO et al. 2000). Solitary colonic metastasis is possible and it is usually associated with better prognosis and long-term survival. Colonoscopy may reveal a polypoid, exophytic, and nodular mass in the colon, and may also permit biopsy (DIAZ-CANDAMIO et al. 2000; LEE et al. 2002). A barium enema study may show a filling defect at the colonic wall that mimics colonic adeno-

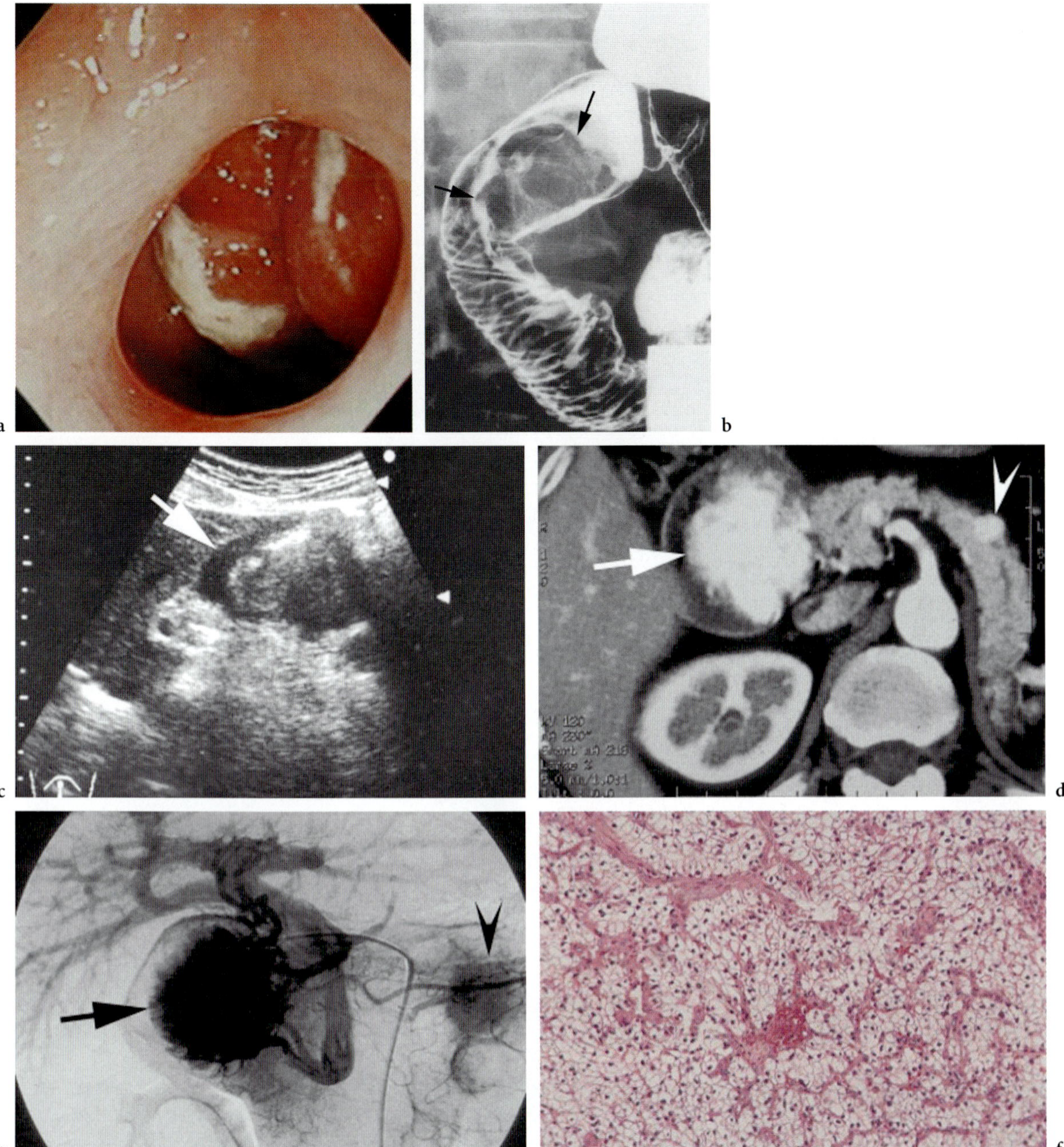

Fig. 16.31a-f. Concomitant duodenal and pancreatic metastases in a 68-year-old man who underwent left nephrectomy 11 years previously for renal cell carcinoma. This patient presented with dyspnea on exertion and severe anemia. **a** Upper gastrointestinal endoscopy reveals an ulcerated bleeding duodenal tumor. **b** Barium meal study of the duodenum discloses the presence of a large tumor of the duodenum bulb (*arrows*). **c** Longitudinal US image of the duodenum shows thickening of the wall of the duodenum (*arrow*) adjacent to the pancreas. **d** Axial contrast-enhanced CT scan shows a large enhanced mass of the duodenum (*arrow*) and a small enhanced nodule in the body of the pancreas (*arrowhead*). **e** Selective common hepatic angiography demonstrates hypervascular tumors in the duodenal wall (*arrow*) and body of the pancreas (*arrowhead*). **f** Photomicrograph of the resected duodenum and pancreas shows clear cell carcinoma compatible with metastasis from renal cell carcinoma (hematoxylin and eosin stain; original magnification, ×100). (With permission from HASHIMOTO et al. 2001)

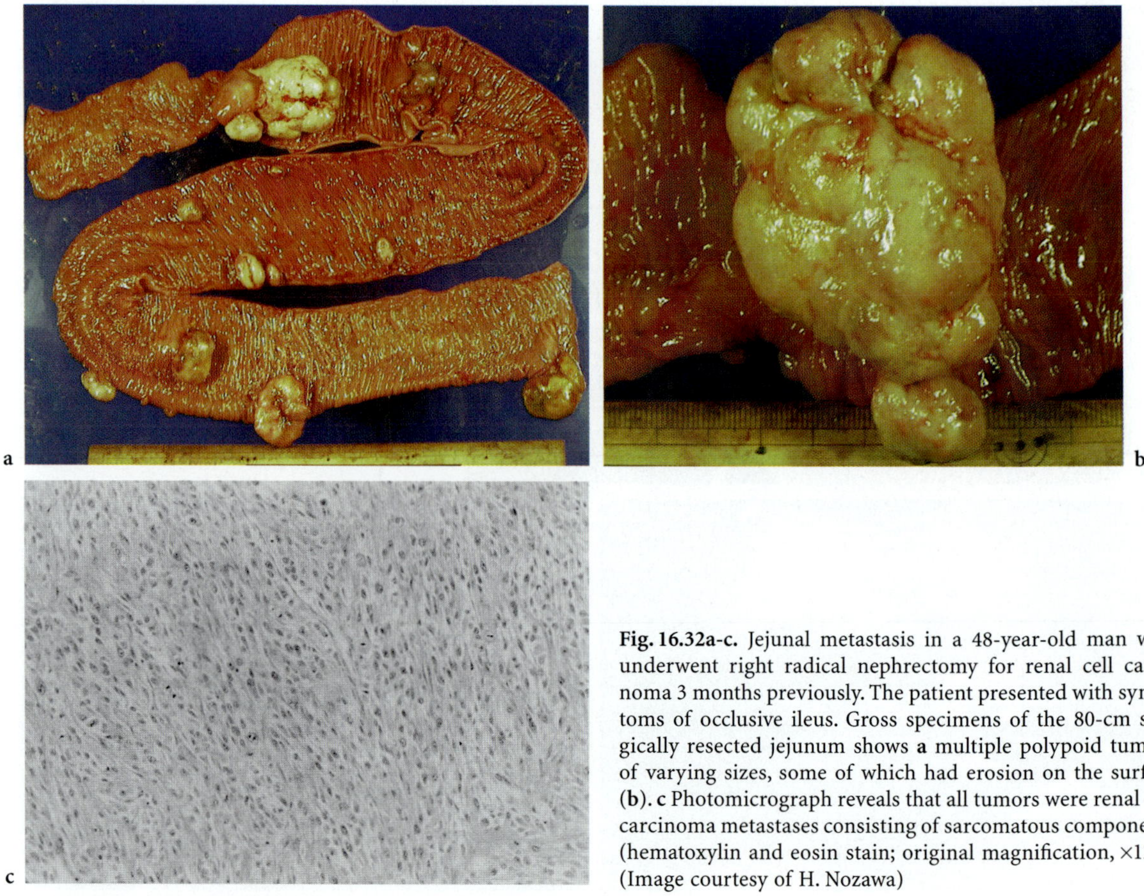

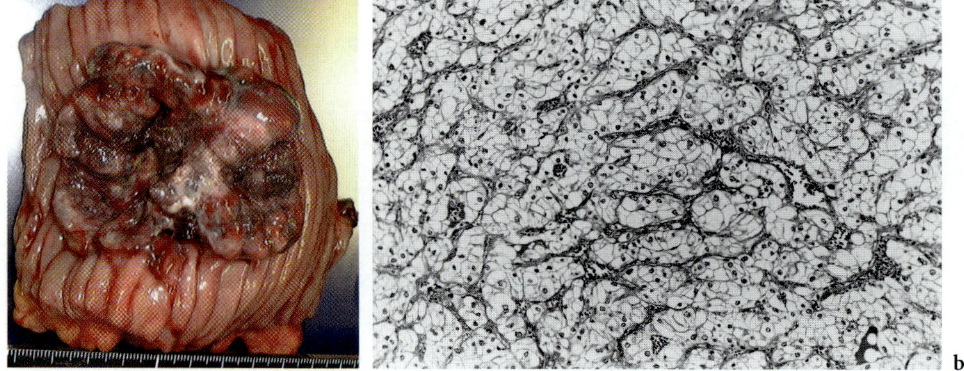

Fig. 16.32a-c. Jejunal metastasis in a 48-year-old man who underwent right radical nephrectomy for renal cell carcinoma 3 months previously. The patient presented with symptoms of occlusive ileus. Gross specimens of the 80-cm surgically resected jejunum shows **a** multiple polypoid tumors of varying sizes, some of which had erosion on the surface (**b**). **c** Photomicrograph reveals that all tumors were renal cell carcinoma metastases consisting of sarcomatous components (hematoxylin and eosin stain; original magnification, ×125). (Image courtesy of H. Nozawa)

Fig. 16.33a,b. Jejunal metastasis in a 62-year-old man who underwent left nephrectomy for renal cell carcinoma 6 years previously. The patient complained of tarry stools on 10 consecutive days and frequent episodes of shortness of breath. **a** Gross specimen of the surgically resected jejunum shows an ulcerating lesion surrounded by elevated borders typical of a Borrmann-2-like tumor. **b** Photomicrograph reveals clear cell type renal cell carcinoma metastasis (hematoxylin and eosin stain; original magnification, ×125). (Image courtesy of H. Nozawa)

carcinoma (Diaz-Candamio et al. 2000). Spiral CT, especially at arterial phase, may show an early and heavily enhancing irregular mass (Lee et al. 2002) or broad-based polypoid lesion (Diaz-Candamio et al. 2000) protruding into the lumen of the colon.

16.4.10
Genitourinary Tract

All sites in the genitourinary tract may be involved including ureter (Kamota et al. 2003; Lee et al. 1998),

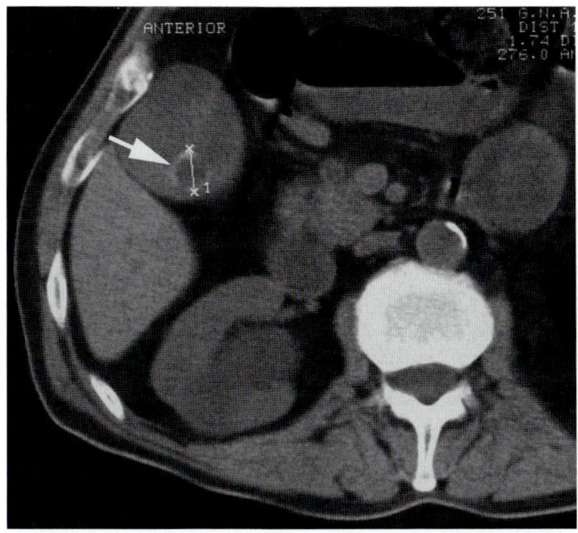

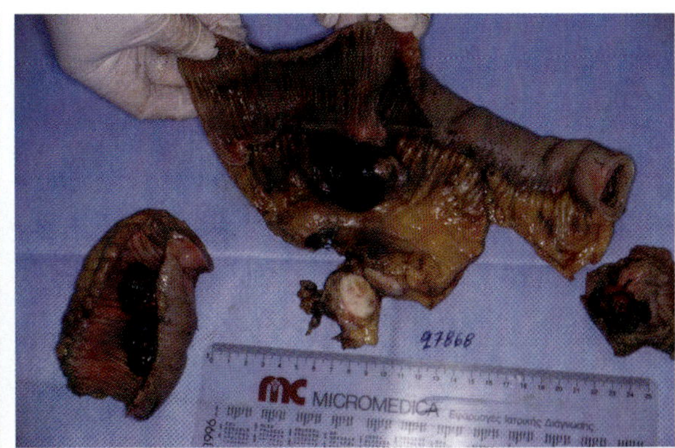

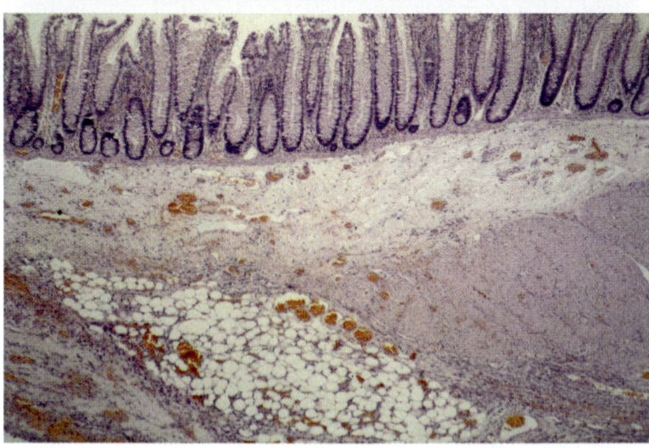

Fig. 16.34a-c. Ileal metastasis in a 65-year-old man who underwent left nephrectomy for renal cell carcinoma 2 years previously. The patient experienced vomiting, abdominal dilation secondary to intestinal obstruction, and melena. **a** Axial unenhanced CT scan shows a marked dilation of the small intestine and a lesion protruding into the lumen of the ileum (*arrow*). **b** Gross specimen shows the presence of multiple intra-luminal hemorrhagic lesions. **c** Photomicrograph shows the presence of metastatic renal cell carcinoma in the intestinal wall (hematoxylin eosin stain; original magnification, ×150). (With permission from Pavlakis et al. 2003; image courtesy of G.M. Sakorafas)

bladder (Kamota et al. 2003; Shiraishi et al. 2003), prostate (Mearini et al. 2004), urethra (Mearini et al. 2004), ovary (Insabato et al. 2003), vagina (Yokoyama et al. 1998), Bartholin glands (Leiman et al. 1986), testis (Calleja Escudero et al. 2004; Daniels and Schaeffer 1991; Nabi et al. 2001;), and penis (Daniels and Schaeffer 1991). The mechanism responsible for these metastases is still not entirely clear (Mearini et al. 2004).

Bladder metastasis from RCC is extremely rare with a frequency of 0.3–1.6% (Raviv et al. 2002; Saitoh et al. 1982; Shiraishi et al. 2003). The latency period can be as long as 12 years (Shiraishi et al. 2003). The mechanism is controversial. The localization of the bladder lesion around the ureteral orifice may argue in favor of endoluminal implantation of cancer cells (Shiraishi et al. 2003), a route that has been termed "drop metastasis" (Raviv et al. 2002). The prognosis is poor with most patients dying in the first year (Shiraishi et al. 2003). Nevertheless, a case has been reported with a 6-year survival after resection of bladder metastases. Clinically, patients usually present with painless hematuria (Raviv et al. 2002). A transurethral complete resection is usually possible, but this tumor may necessitate a partial cystectomy (Raviv et al. 2002; Shiraishi et al. 2003). Cystoscopy may show a solitary sessile, spherical tumor protruding into the bladder (Fig. 16.35; Kamota et al. 2003; Shiraishi et al. 2003). Computed tomography shows an enhanced mass within bladder wall (Shiraishi et al. 2003).

Prostate metastases from RCC are extremely rare with the exception of metastasis by direct extension from adjacent structures (Moudouni et al. 2001). Involvement may be synchronous or metachronous to the RCC (Yavascaoglu et al. 1999). In one case report, prostate metastasis appears as a well-defined heterogeneous hyperechoic nodule or mass located in one of the prostate lobes (Fig. 16.36; Mearini et al. 2004), but it can also appear as prostatic hypertrophy mimicking benign prostatic hyperplasia (Moudouni et al. 2001). A unique case of periprostatic metastasis presenting as a periprostatic mass displacing the prostate gland has been reported (Yavascaoglu et al. 1999).

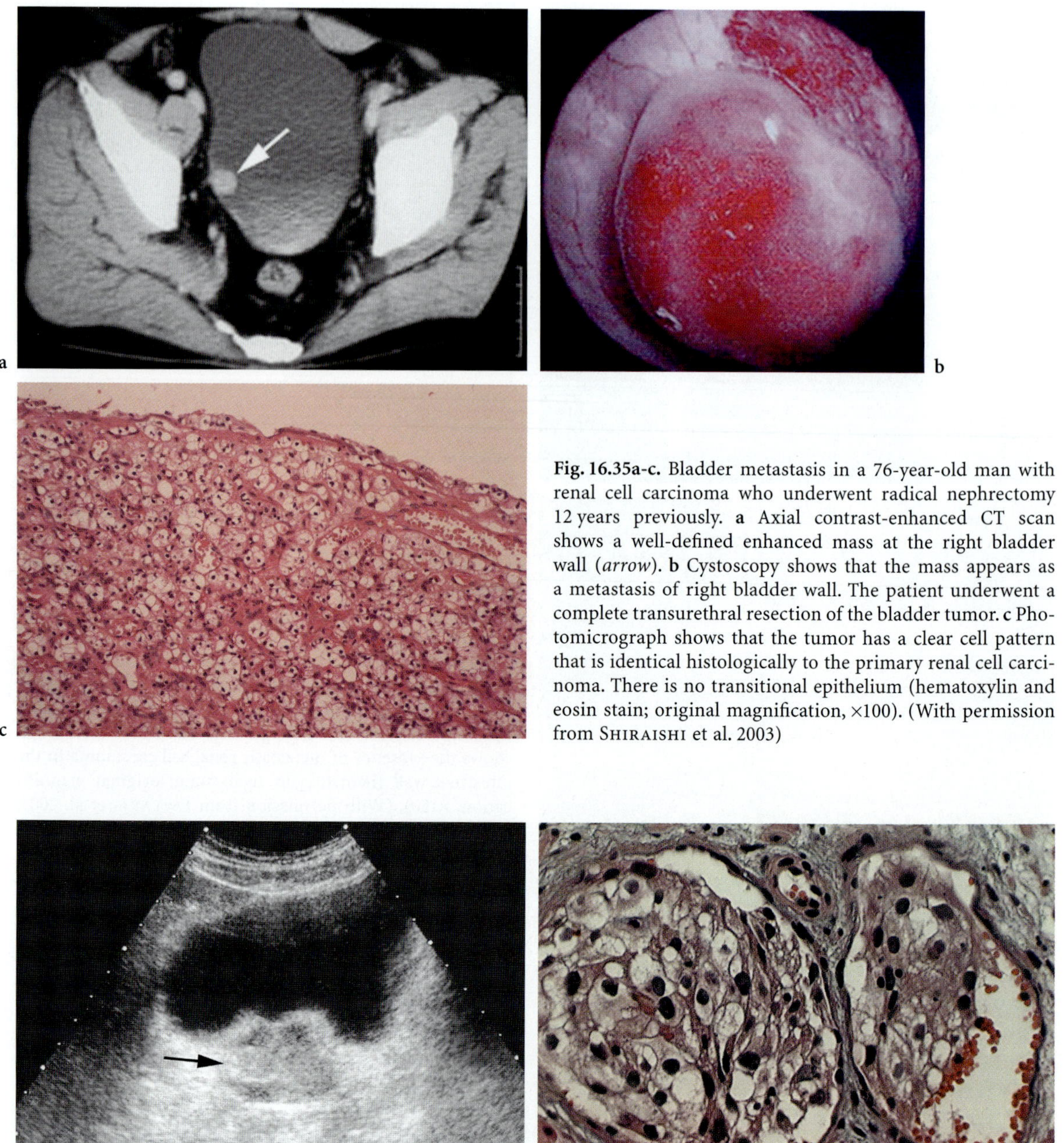

Fig. 16.35a-c. Bladder metastasis in a 76-year-old man with renal cell carcinoma who underwent radical nephrectomy 12 years previously. a Axial contrast-enhanced CT scan shows a well-defined enhanced mass at the right bladder wall (*arrow*). b Cystoscopy shows that the mass appears as a metastasis of right bladder wall. The patient underwent a complete transurethral resection of the bladder tumor. c Photomicrograph shows that the tumor has a clear cell pattern that is identical histologically to the primary renal cell carcinoma. There is no transitional epithelium (hematoxylin and eosin stain; original magnification, ×100). (With permission from SHIRAISHI et al. 2003)

Fig. 16.36a,b. Prostate metastasis in a 48-year-old man with renal papillary adenocarcinoma for which he underwent renal conservative surgery 46 months previously. a Transverse US image of the pelvis shows a well-defined mass in the right lobe of the prostate (*arrow*). b Fine-needle-aspiration biopsy of this mass shows metastatic renal papillary adenocarcinoma (hematoxylin and eosin stain; original magnification, ×200). (Image courtesy of L. Mearini)

Ovarian metastases from RCC are also very rare. The distinction of ovarian metastasis from an ovarian primary tumor can be difficult, especially when the ovarian metastasis is discovered first and mimics an ovarian clear cell carcinoma. The latency period can be as long as 11 years. On US and CT, they usually appear as a large, solid, or solid and cystic mass (Fig. 16.37), or as one or a few small nodules within a well-defined cystic mass (Fig. 16.38; INSABATO et al. 2003).

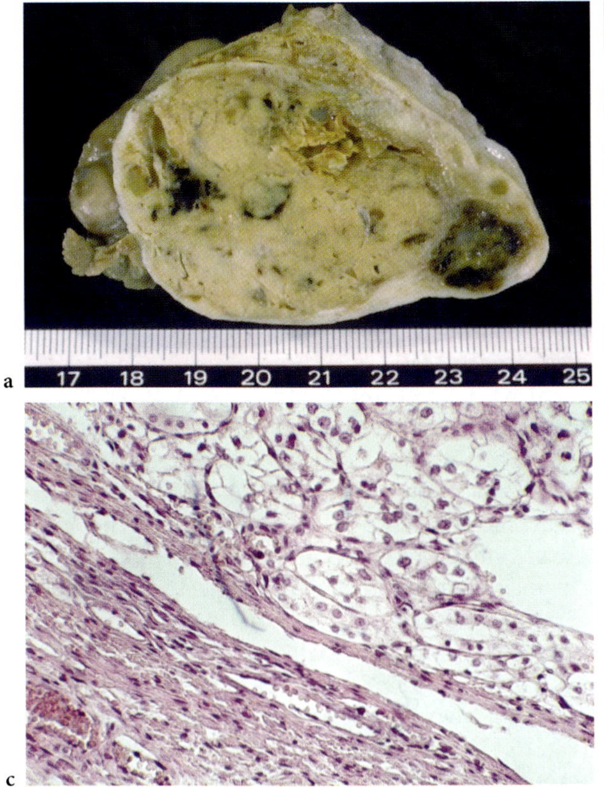

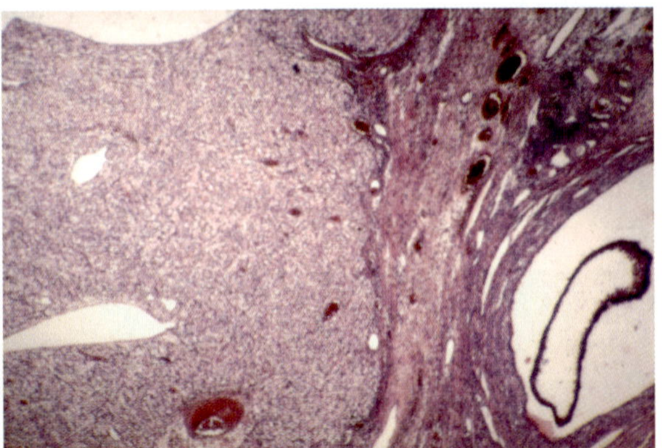

Fig. 16.37a-c. Ovarian metastasis in a 49-year-old woman which occurred 14 months after radical nephrectomy for renal cell carcinoma. a Macroscopic view of the right ovary shows a large ovarian mass with a yellowish cut surface and areas of necrosis and hemorrhage. b Photomicrograph shows the tumor cells with abundant pink cytoplasm and hyperchromatic nuclei with a focal glandular differentiation (hematoxylin and eosin stain; original magnification, ×400). c Photomicrograph shows neoplastic clear cell infiltrating the ovarian parenchyma (hematoxylin and eosin stain; original magnification, ×106). (Image courtesy of L. Insabato)

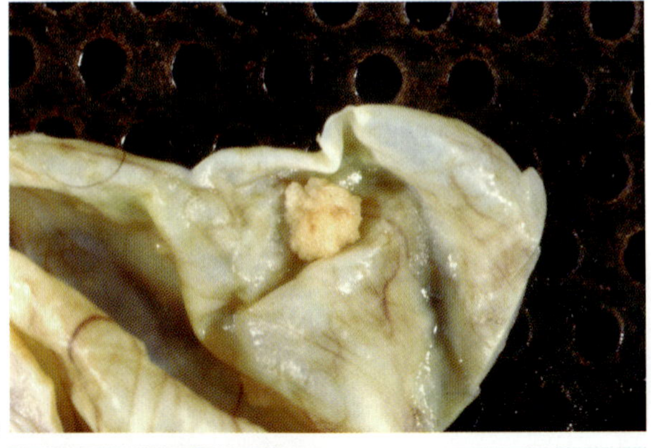

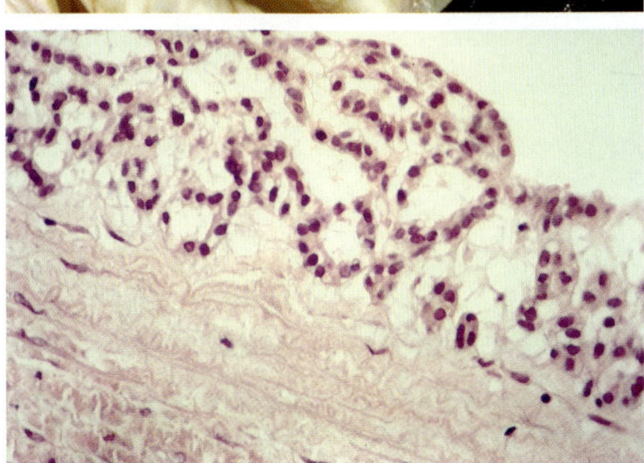

Fig. 16.38a-c. Ovarian cystic metastasis in a 17-year-old girl which occurred 2 years after radical nephrectomy for renal cell carcinoma. a Macroscopic view of the left ovary shows a metastatic small nodule on the ovarian cyst. b Photomicrograph shows papillary proliferation with pleomorphic and hyperchromatic nuclei (Hematoxylin and eosin stain; original magnification, ×106). c Photomicrograph of a different nodule shows a clear cell carcinoma with glandular pattern (Hematoxylin and eosin stain; original magnification, ×106). (Image courtesy of L. Insabato)

16.5
Lymph Node Metastases

The incidence of lymph node metastases in RCC varies from 14 to 30% (Johnsen and Hellsten 1997). The presence of regional lymph node metastases is an important predictor of multifocal distant metastases (Johnsen and Hellsten 1997) and hence carries a poor prognosis, with reported 5-year survival rates of 5–30% (Pantuck et al. 2003; Thrasher and Paulson 1993). The presence of regional lymph node metastases is associated with distant metastatic dissemination via the thoracic duct, mediasti-

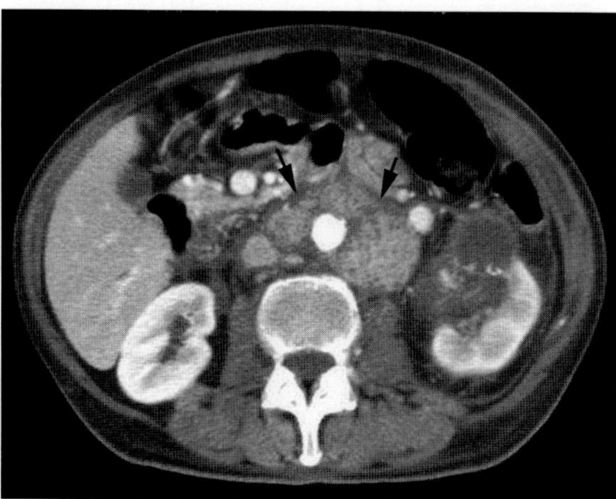

Fig. 16.39. Lymph node metastasis in 67-year-old woman synchronous with renal cell carcinoma. Axial contrast-enhanced CT scan shows large heterogeneous enhancing retroperitoneal and para-aortic lymph node mass (*arrows*) associated with a large heterogeneous hypodense anterior mass of the left kidney corresponding to cystic renal cell carcinoma.

nal lymph nodes, and the left subclavian lymph node (Mignon and Mesurolle 2003). The traditional view that RCC involving "locoregional" lymph nodes is potentially curable by classic radical nephrectomy has very little evidence to support it (Pantuck et al. 2003; Russo 2003). Moreover, it is now known that regional lymph node metastasis confers immunotherapy resistance and a graver prognosis than pulmonary metastasis (Russo 2003).

Lymph nodes close to the renal vascular pedicle are the most frequently involved (Scatarige et al. 2001a). Para-aortic and retroperitoneal lymph nodes are also frequently involved (Figs. 16.3, 16.39, 16.40). In a large series by Saitoh et al. (1982), para-aortic and retroperitoneal lymph nodes were involved in 24–35% of patients. More advanced patterns of recurrence include mesenteric lymphadenopathy (Scatarige et al. 2001a). In fact, lymph nodes at any site may be involved (Fig. 16.41): neck and clavicle; hilus of lungs (Fig. 16.42); pancreas; hilus of liver; stomach (Fig. 16.43); axilla; and inguinal region (Saitoh et al. 1982; Savas et al. 1998; Yamashita et al. 2000). Involvement of mediastinal lymph nodes (Fig. 16.44) may result from retrograde extension through thoracic duct tributaries (Tartar et al. 1991), may be isolated (Merine and Fishman 1988; Yamashita et al. 2000), and may present as an anterior mass leading to confusion with more common tumors such as thymus, thyroid, or germ cell neoplasms, and lymphomas (Koc et al. 1999; Mattana et al. 1996).

Computed tomography is the examination of choice and shows that metastatic nodes may enhance (Fig. 16.45), particularly if the primary tumor is very

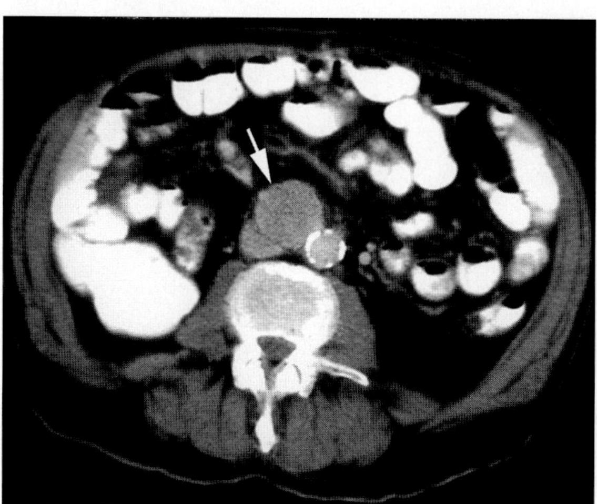
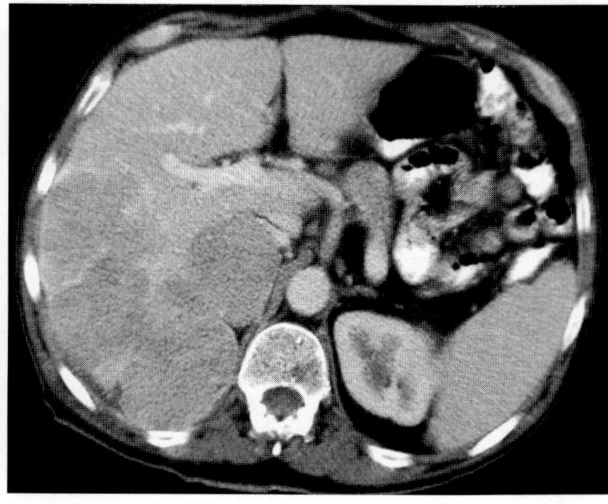

a

b

Fig. 16.40a,b. Lymph node and liver metastases in 73-year-old man who underwent right nephrectomy for renal cell carcinoma. a Axial contrast-enhanced CT scan shows interaortocaval lymph node enlargement (*arrow*). b Axial contrast-enhanced CT scan cephalad to a shows large confluent, slightly hypodense hepatic masses.

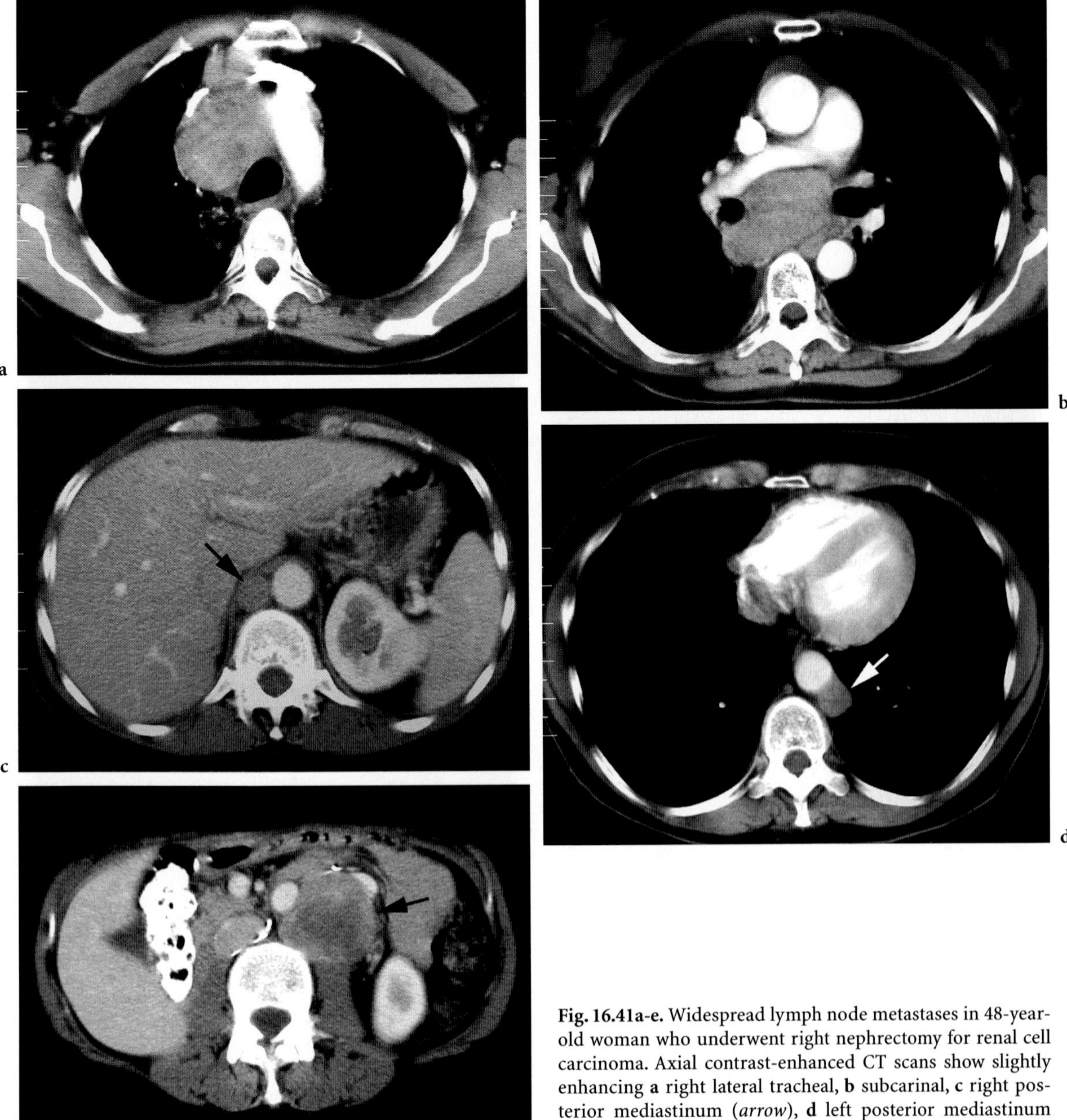

Fig. 16.41a-e. Widespread lymph node metastases in 48-year-old woman who underwent right nephrectomy for renal cell carcinoma. Axial contrast-enhanced CT scans show slightly enhancing **a** right lateral tracheal, **b** subcarinal, **c** right posterior mediastinum (*arrow*), **d** left posterior mediastinum (*arrow*), and **e** para-aortic (*arrow*) lymph node masses.

vascular (YAMASHITA et al. 2000). Nevertheless, in a study aiming to assess the predictive value of CT for the diagnosis of regional lymph node metastases, STUDER et al. (1990) showed the enlargement of regional lymph nodes frequently may be caused by inflammatory changes, especially in the presence of tumor necrosis. They concluded that the radiological finding should not be interpreted as metastatic disease, unless it has been proved cytologically by fine-needle aspiration.

16.6
Central Nervous System Metastases

16.6.1
Brain

The reported incidence of brain metastasis is 2%. Only 2–10% of patients with a recurrence of RCC developed brain metastases (JANZEN et al. 2003; NUSSBAUM et al. 1996; SEAMAN et al. 1995). Brain metastases are gen-

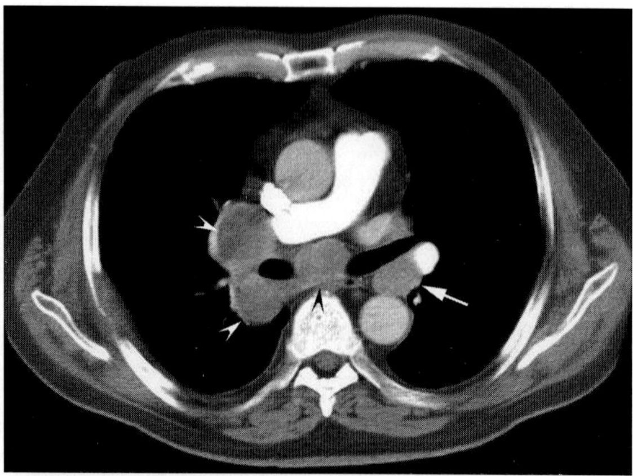

Fig. 16.42. Lymph node metastases in a 72-year-old man who underwent nephrectomy for renal cell carcinoma. Axial contrast-enhanced CT scan shows enlargement of right hilar bronchopulmonary (*white arrowheads*), subcarinal (*black arrowhead*), and para-aortic (*arrow*) lymph nodes.

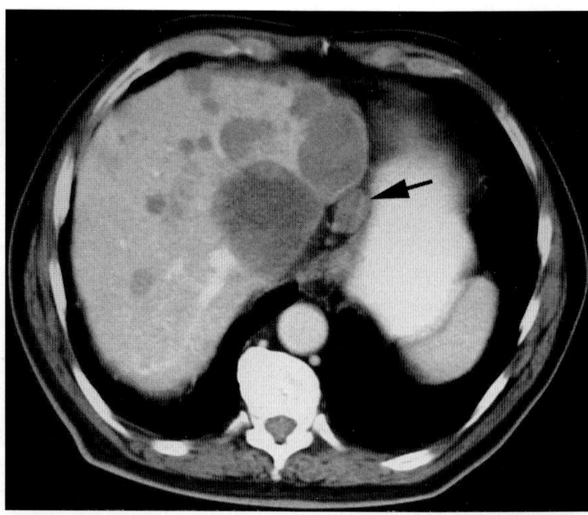

Fig. 16.43. Lymph node and liver metastases in 77-year-old man who underwent right nephrectomy for renal cell carcinoma. Axial contrast-enhanced CT scan shows enlargement of left gastric lymph node (*arrow*) and several hypodense liver masses of varying sizes.

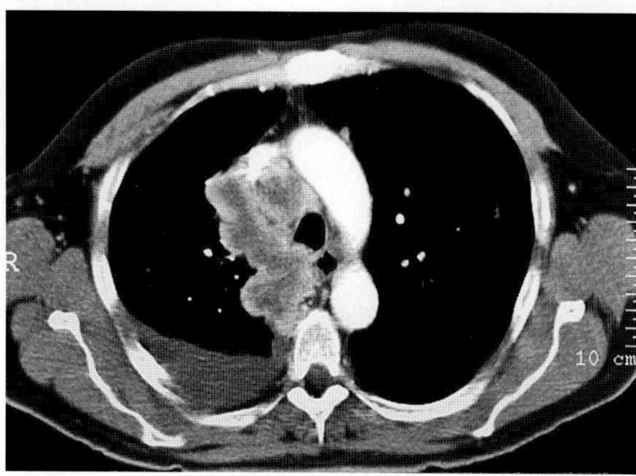

Fig. 16.44. Lymph node metastasis in a 63-year-old man who underwent nephrectomy for renal cell carcinoma. Axial contrast-enhanced CT scan shows large heterogeneous enhancing right mediastinal lymph node mass with mass effect on the trachea. There is also a right pleural effusion.

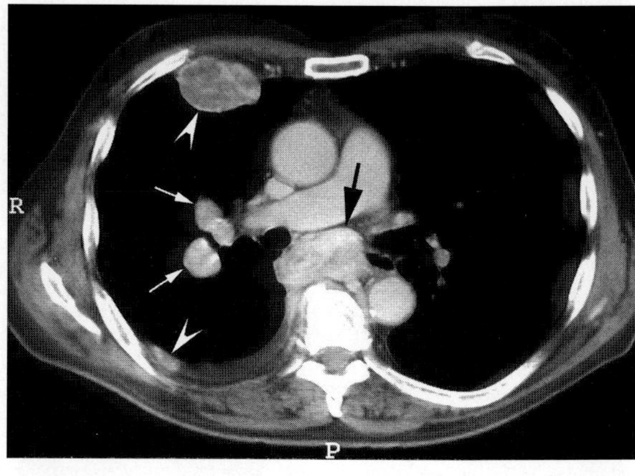

Fig. 16.45. Lymph node, lung, and pleural metastases in 76-year-old man who underwent nephrectomy for renal cell carcinoma. Axial contrast-enhanced CT scan shows strongly enhancing heterogeneous subcarinal lymphadenopathy (*black arrow*) and right pulmonary parahilar masses (*white arrows*). There are also two heterogeneously enhancing right pleural based masses (*arrowheads*) with pleural effusion.

erally believed to result from hematogenous spread of circulating tumor cells or frank tumor emboli. The sequence of events that initiates metastatic spread to the brain remains largely unknown (KLOS and O'NEILL 2004). The latency period is variable and can be as long as 18 years (RADLEY et al. 1993). The brain is rarely the sole site of metastasis (ISHIKAWA et al. 1990; JANZEN et al. 2003). Resection of a solitary metastasis is associated with a significantly improved survival, although the survival time is short (JANZEN et al. 2003). Spontaneous regression of cerebral metastases

is a very rare event that may involve the brain alone (GUTHBJARTSSON and GISLASON 1995) or in association with other metastatic locations (OMLAND and FOSSA 1989).

Clinically, brain metastases may present with focal or generalized symptoms. Headache is the most common symptom. Other symptoms include focal weakness, mental change, seizure, gait ataxia, sensory disturbance, and/or speech problems (KLOS and O'NEILL, 2004; MARSHALL et al. 1990). Unusual but characteristic clinical syndromes have been described in patients with brain metastases, including sagittal sinus occlusion, subdural effusion, miliary metastases that produce a progressive confusional state, and diabetes insipidus (KLOS and O'NEILL 2004; YOKOYAMA et al. 1998;). Asymptomatic brain lesions are often seen in patients with metastatic RCC (SAIDI et al. 1998; SEAMAN et al. 1995). This is especially true in the modern imaging era when more asymptomatic lesions are found with the aid of CT and MR imaging (KLOS and O'NEILL 2004; SEAMAN et al. 1995).

Surgical excision remains an important therapy for selected patients with large brain tumors. The best outcome after surgical resection is achieved in patients with a solitary, surgically accessible tumor and in patients without systemic disease (HOSHI et al. 2002; VLEEMING et al. 1994). Whole-brain radiotherapy (WBRT) is another therapeutic alternative and is usually recommended for patients with multiple brain metastases (KLOS and O'NEILL 2004). Gamma-knife radiosurgery is an effective noninvasive modality of treatment. It is a stereotactically guided high-precision irradiation method focusing ionizing radiation within the target volume in a single-dose application. The metastases from kidney cancers are ideal targets because of their spherical shape and sharp margins. Gamma-knife radiosurgery offers high local control rate and improved quality of life and survival (HOSHI et al. 2002).

Magnetic resonance imaging is the imaging modality of choice for brain metastases because of its superior resolution over CT, especially in evaluating the posterior fossa (KLOS and O'NEILL 2004) and pituitary gland (UCHINO et al. 1996; YOKOYAMA et al. 1998). Magnetic resonance imaging can detect a lesion as small as 1.9 mm (KLOS and O'NEILL 2004). For emergency evaluation of patients and because it is widely accessible, CT is especially helpful when clinical deterioration is rapid (KLOS and O'NEILL 2004).

Typically, the lesions are multiple, at the gray-white junction, have relatively smooth margins, are nodular enhancing lesions, and are tightly focused while surrounded by abundant vasogenic edema (Fig. 16.46; DESTIAN et al. 1989; KLOS and O'NEILL 2004). Lesions are usually supratentorial but sometimes may be located in the posterior fossa (Fig. 16.47; UCHINO et al. 1996). Nussbaum et al. (1996) reported 56% of patients with single brain metastases and 44% with multiple locations. When a solitary lesion is found on CT, MR imaging should be performed before surgical treatment is planned. Not only is management different than with multiple metastases, but so is the prognosis (KLOS and

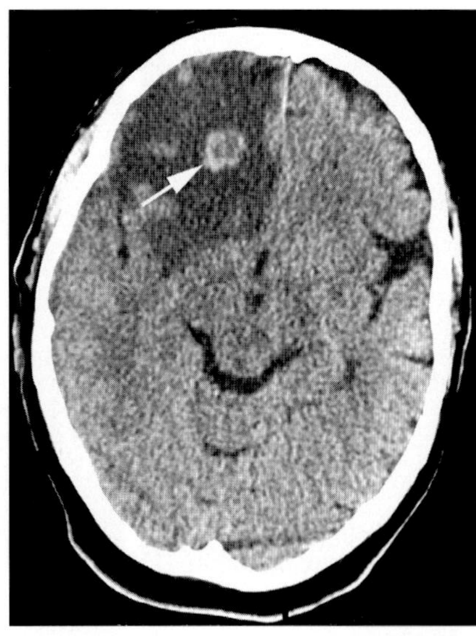

Fig. 16.46. Brain metastasis in a 74-year-old man who underwent nephrectomy for renal cell carcinoma. Axial contrast-enhanced CT scan shows a small right frontal annular lesion (*arrow*) at the gray–white junction surrounded by abundant vasogenic edema.

O'NEILL 2004). Lesions measuring less than 5 mm often have less surrounding edema (CHAE et al. 2005; KLOS and O'NEILL 2004). All lesions show enhancement, including homogeneous, nearly homogeneous, or ring enhancement (UCHINO et al. 1996). A cystic appearance is very rare (ISHIKAWA et al. 1990). Because of their hypervascularity, these lesions are sometimes hemorrhagic (DESTIAN et al. 1989; HODGSON et al. 1994; KLOS and O'NEILL 2004). Intracranial brain metastases are typically intraaxial. Uncommon locations include extraaxial locations (Fig. 16.48), as reported in a 4-year-old boy with two large extraaxial brain metastases from clear cell sarcoma of the kidney (PARK et al. 1997), and the choroid plexus with unilateral (Fig. 16.49) or exceedingly rarely bilateral involvement (HILLARD et al. 2003). The pituitary gland may also be involved (DJIMI et al. 2003; KOSHIYAMA et al. 1992; UCHINO et al. 1996; YOKOYAMA et al. 1998).

Recently developed imaging techniques, such as MR spectroscopy, SPECT technology, and increased contrast dose with delayed imaging, and the latest imaging techniques utilizing transfer of magnetization, dynamic contrast-enhanced MR imaging (Fig. 16.50), and PET, may offer improved diagnostic utility, but further studies are needed to identify whether these modalities will provide an appropriate and cost-effective advantage over current imaging techniques (KLOS and O'NEILL 2004; KREMER et al. 2003).

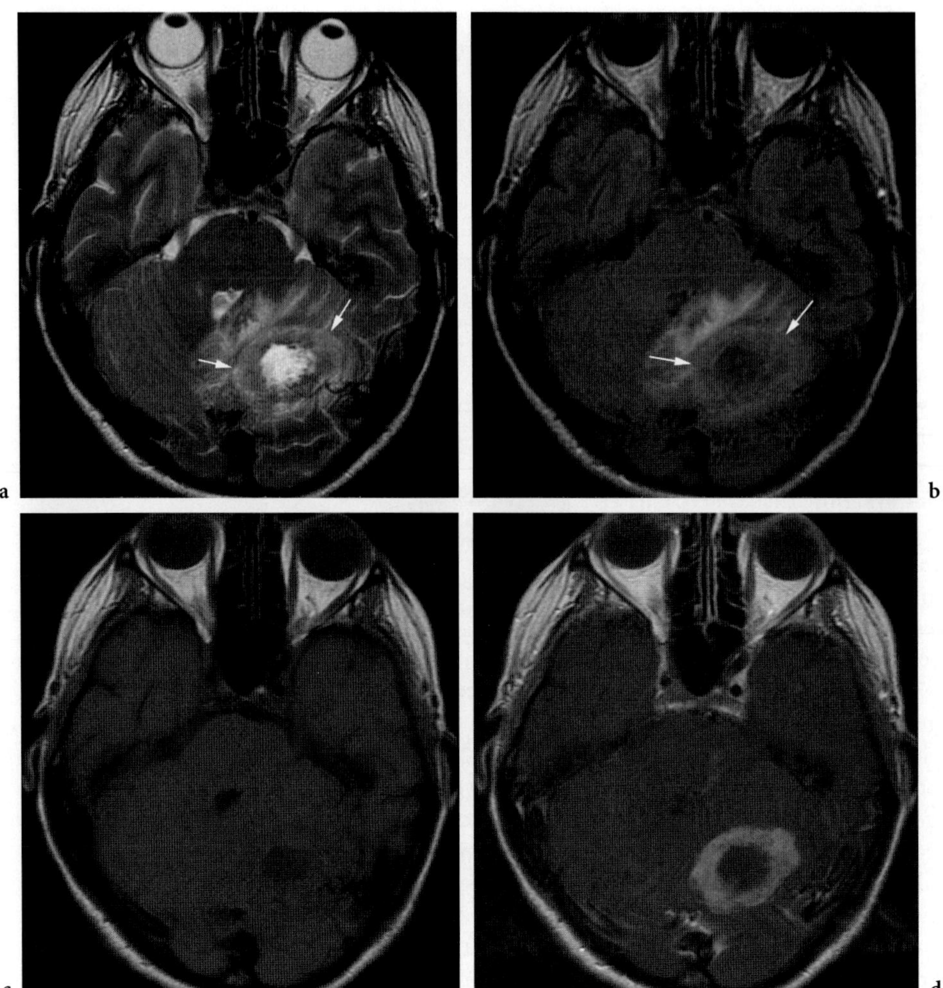

Fig. 16.47a-d. Unique cerebellar metastasis in a 46-year-old woman treated for renal cell carcinoma. Axial **a** T2-weighted and **b** fluid-attenuated inversion recovery (FLAIR) MR images show a large left cerebellar lobe lesion which has a slightly hyperintense thick peripheral ring (*arrow*) and is surrounded by hyperintense vasogenic edema with mass effect on the fourth ventricle. The frank central hyperintensity on T2-weighted and hypointensity on FLAIR images corresponds to necrosis. **c** Axial unenhanced T1-weighted MR image shows that the ring and edema are difficult to discern. Only the hypointense necrosis and mass effect on the fourth ventricle are obvious. **d** Axial contrast-enhanced T1-weighted MR image demonstrates a characteristic strong ring enhancement of the lesion. (Image courtesy of F. Lafitte)

16.6.2
Spinal Cord, Cauda Equina, and Epidural Space

Intramedullary spinal cord metastases are very rare and make up only 4–8.5% of central nervous system metastases. Clinical symptoms include progressive pain, autonomic dysfunction, and/or neurological deficits, e.g., Brown-Sequard syndrome (FAKIH et al. 2001; SCHIJNS et al. 2000). There is a rapid progression of neurological deficits and treatment is urgent (SCHIJNS et al. 2000). Occasionally, patients present first with symptoms from spinal cord metastases that precede the detection of the primary RCC

(FAKIH et al. 2001; SCHIJNS et al. 2000). On the other hand, most reported cases are associated with brain metastases. Treatment options include surgery as well as radiotherapy with or without chemotherapy (FAKIH et al. 2001). Magnetic resonance imaging is very sensitive for the detection of intramedullary metastases. The MR imaging characteristics of intramedullary metastases are the presence of peritumoral edema and contrast enhancement of the lesion. T2-weighted sequences principally show hyperintensity due to edema, and when normal may exclude intramedullary metastasis. Administration of contrast improves sensitivity and makes the MR

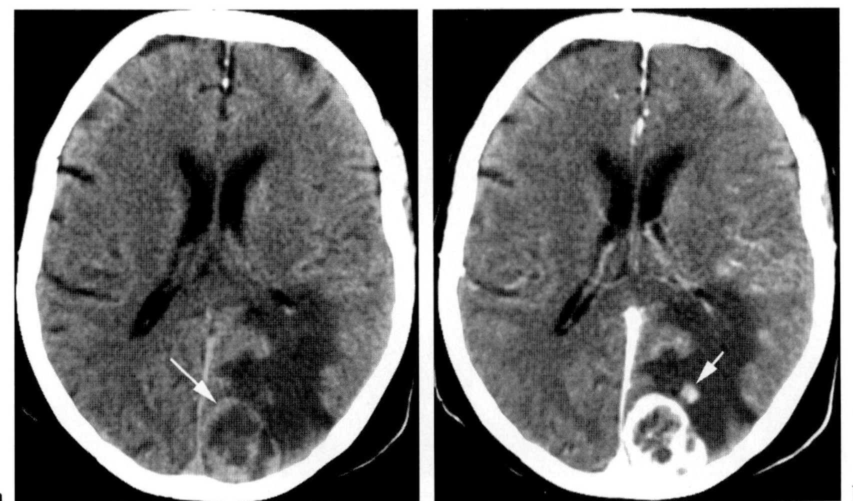

Fig. 16.48a,b. Brain metastases in 72-year-old man who underwent left nephrectomy for renal cell carcinoma. **a** Axial unenhanced CT scan shows a superficially located parasagittal left occipital heterogeneous large mass with broad base (*arrow*) near the vertex and surrounded by abundant vasogenic edema. **b** Axial contrast-enhanced CT scan at the same level shows the mass heterogeneously enhancing and also discloses an additional small rounded enhancing lesion (*arrow*) within the same vasogenic edema.

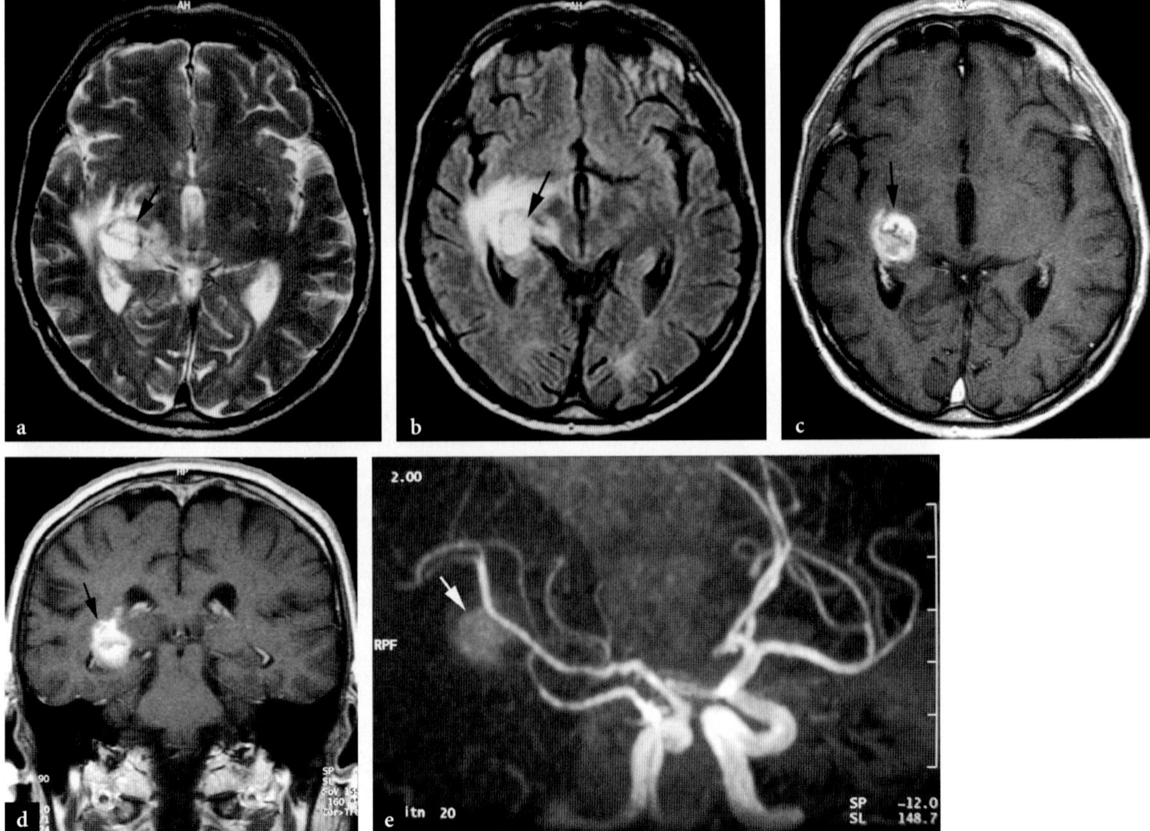

Fig. 16.49a-e. Brain metastases in a 72-year-old man who underwent nephrectomy for renal cell carcinoma. Axial **a** T2-weighted and **b** FLAIR MR images show a hyperintense round lesion within the right trigone (*arrow*) and surrounded by a vasogenic edema. **c** Axial and **d** coronal contrast-enhanced T1-weighted MR images demonstrate a heterogeneously enhancing mass of the choroid plexus of the trigone (*arrow*). **e** Cerebral MR angiogram reveals tumor blush in region of the right trigone (*arrow*).

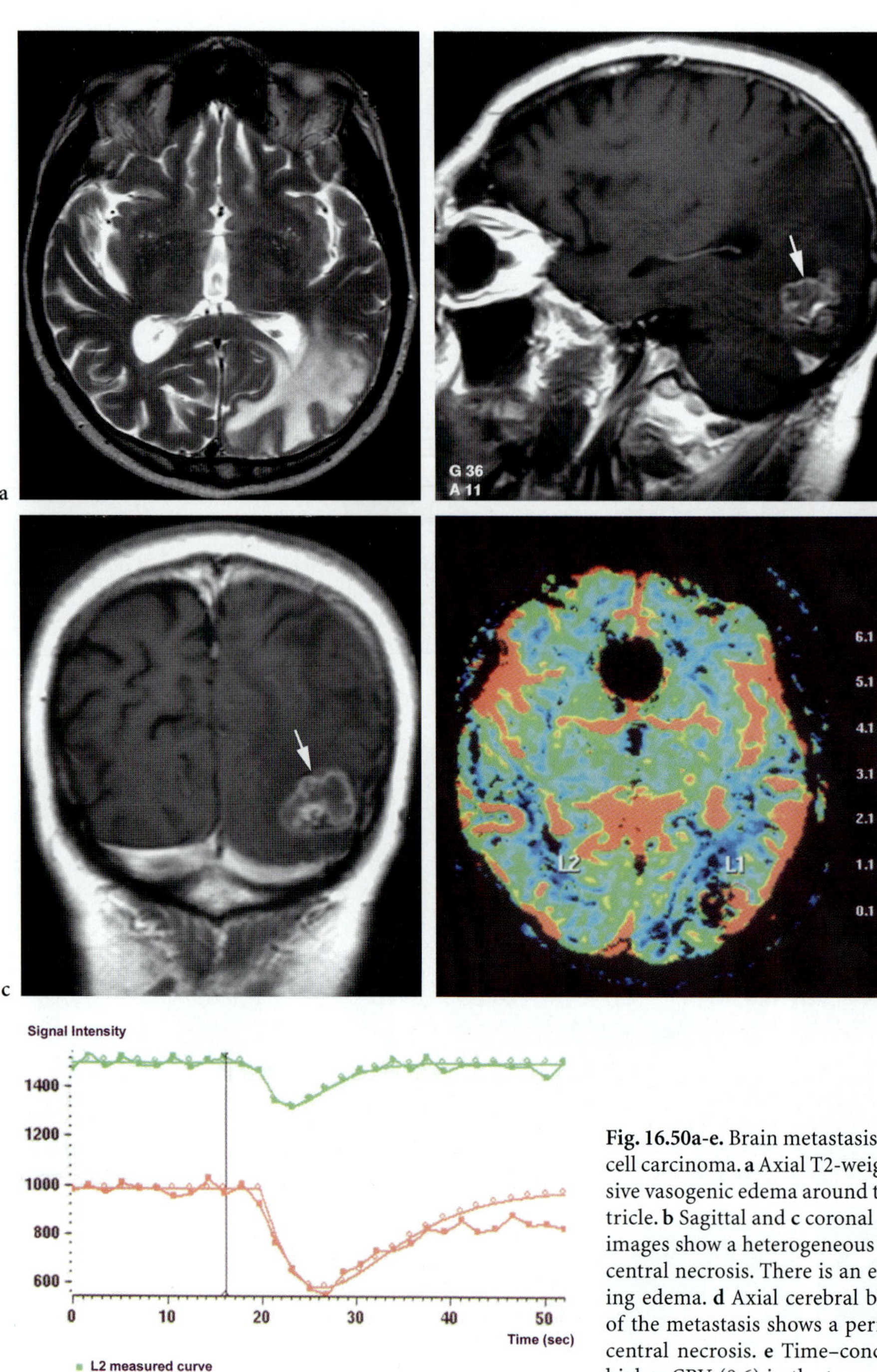

Fig. 16.50a-e. Brain metastasis in a 68-year-old man with renal cell carcinoma. **a** Axial T2-weighted MR image shows an extensive vasogenic edema around the trigone of the left lateral ventricle. **b** Sagittal and **c** coronal contrast-enhanced T1-weighted images show a heterogeneous ring enhancement (*arrow*) with central necrosis. There is an extensive hypointense surrounding edema. **d** Axial cerebral blood volume (CBV) map image of the metastasis shows a peripheral hypervascular ring with central necrosis. **e** Time–concentration curves show a much higher CBV (8.6) in the tumor than in the contralateral white matter [1.3, maximum relative CBV (rCBVmax) of 6.61]. (Image courtesy of S. Grand)

imaging more specific in distinguishing between edema and the tumor which is generally well circumscribed (Fig. 16.51; FAKIH et al. 2001; SCHIJNS et al. 2000).

Cauda equina metastases from renal cancer are exceedingly rare and only a few cases have been published (TAKADA et al. 2003; MAXWELL et al. 1999). Clinical symptoms include characteristic cramping pain provoked by light percussion on the lumbar spine, becoming severe when sleeping in the flexion or sitting position (TAKADA et al. 2003), or lower back pain radiating to both legs without sensorial or motor deficit (MAXWELL et al. 1999). Magnetic resonance imaging is a useful and sensi-

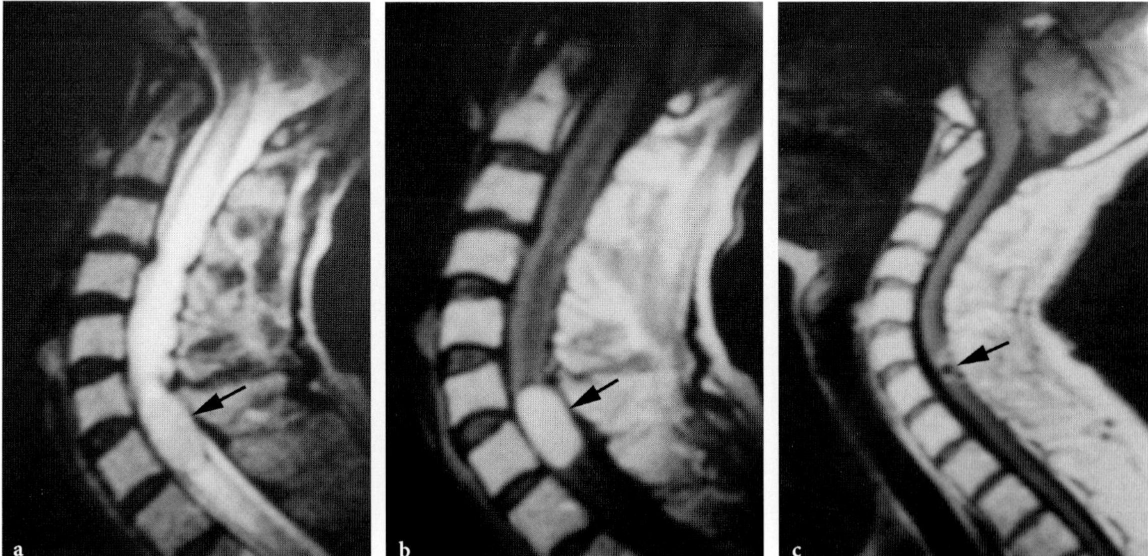

Fig. 16.51a-c. Spinal cord metastasis as a first manifestation of renal cell carcinoma in a 70-year-old woman who developed Brown-Sequard syndrome within 6 weeks. **a** Sagittal T2-weighted MR image of the cervical spine demonstrates a solitary lesion (*arrow*) at the level of C7 isointense to the spinal cord, but slightly bulging its contours. The hyperintense areas above and below the lesion correspond to edema. **b** Sagittal contrast-enhanced T1-weighted MR image displays a clear enhancement of the well-demarcated intramedullary lesion (*arrow*). The edema is now hypointense but less so than the cerebrospinal fluid. **c** Sagittal contrast-enhanced T1-weighted MR image obtained 6 weeks after surgery shows surgical sequela at the site of the tumor (*arrow*), which has been completely removed, and the complete disappearance of edema. (Image courtesy of O.E.M. Schijns)

tive but less specific tool for detecting cauda equine intradural metastases. It shows various appearance patterns and intensities, because the lesion may contain necrotic tissues and/or old hemorrhage. Administration of contrast media is mandatory to improve tumor conspicuity (Fig. 16.52; Takada et al. 2003).

Metastasis to the epidural space is relatively uncommon but has been described in several cancers including kidney cancer (Trufflandier et al. 2002). Although suspicion of epidural involvement is based on progressive pain with axial or radicular distribution, early symptoms are often nonspecific. Imaging diagnosis of epidural compression is clinically important because early treatment of spinal epidural metastasis improves patient survival and function (Fig. 16.53). A complete study of the spine with MR imaging has been shown to be highly sensitive and specific for detection of epidural metastases and incomparable for the diagnosis of cord compression (Kim et al. 2000). A case report using PET/CT in an asymptomatic patient showed promising results in the diagnosis of epidural involvement; however, the place of PET/CT in the management of epidural involvement has yet to be defined (Fig. 16.54; Jadvar et al. 2004).

16.7
Head and Neck Metastases

Metastases of RCC to the head and neck region are rare; however, RCC is one of the most common infra-clavicular primary tumors to metastasize to the nose and paranasal sinuses (Janzen et al. 2003; Navarro et al. 2000; Simo et al. 2000). These metastases are usually vascular and may either precede the diagnosis of the primary renal neoplasm or occur many years after treatment of the primary tumor (Som et al. 1987). Individual case reports suggest that surgical resection of solitary distant metastases can improve survival (Janzen et al. 2003; Navarro et al. 2000).

16.7.1
Parotid Gland

Renal cell carcinoma metastasizing to the parotid gland is extremely rare (Adil et al. 1999). Parotid metastasis may be the first clinical sign of the RCC (Coppa and Oszczakiewicz 1990; Park and Hlivko 2002). The most common presenting complaint is parotid mass; pain and tenderness occur

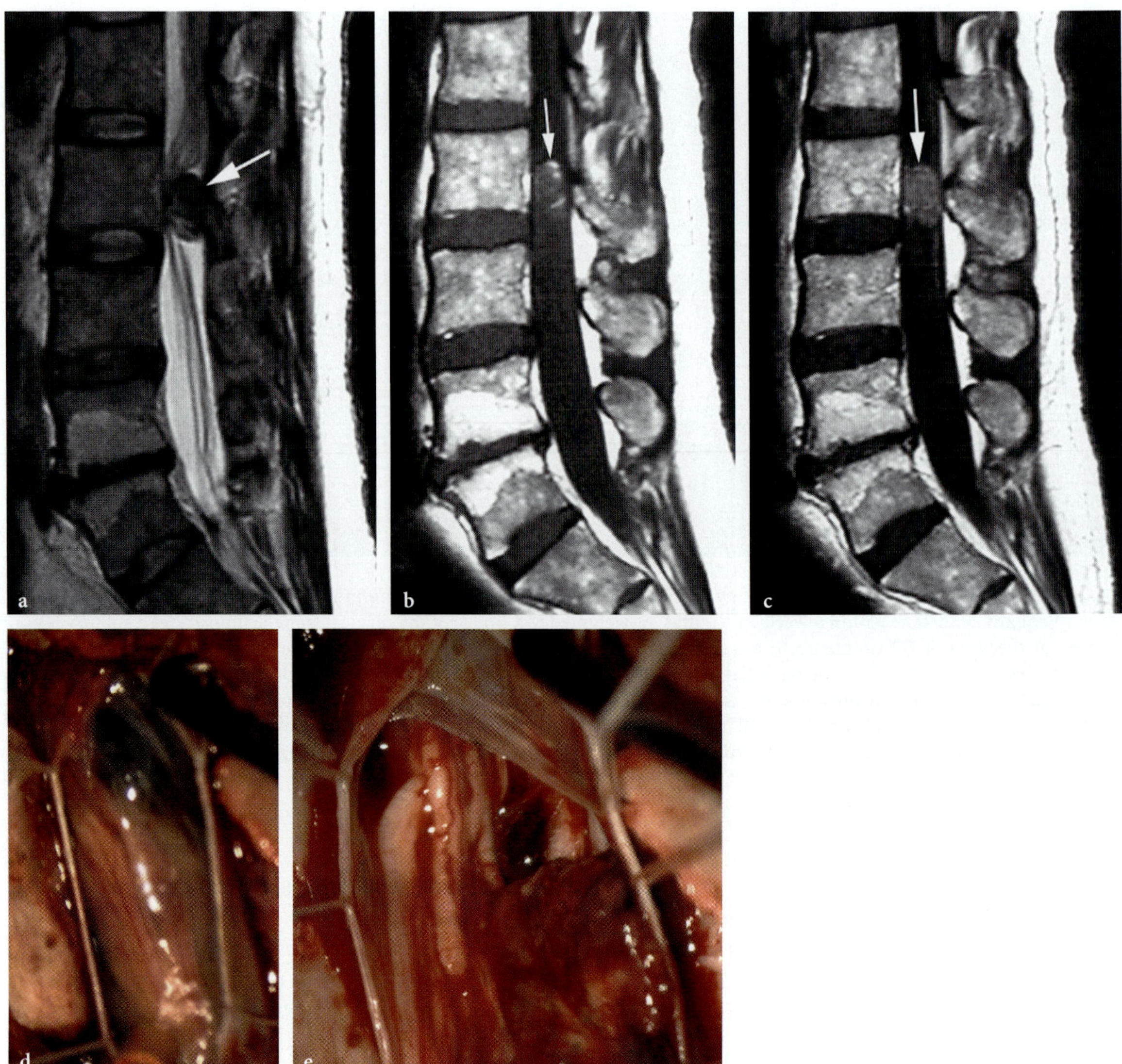

Fig. 16.52a-e. Cauda equina intradural metastasis from renal cell carcinoma in a 61-year-old man with a 10-month history of worsening lower back pain that radiated to both legs. **a** Sagittal spin-echo T2-weighted MR image shows intradural hypointense lesion (*arrow*) involving the cauda equina at the level of L2. **b** Sagittal unenhanced T1-weighted MR image shows small heterogeneous hyperintense areas within the ill-defined tumoral lesion (*arrow*). **c** Sagittal contrast-enhanced T1-weighted MR image shows a slight but homogeneous enhancement of the lesion (*arrow*) which appears more conspicuous. Intraoperative photographs **d** before and **e** after dural opening clearly show brown necrotic encapsulated tumor, which displays several nerves that run directly to the tumor. Macroscopically, the tumor contains old hemorrhagic and necrotic tissue corresponding to the imaging findings. (Image courtesy of M. Doita)

rarely (Park and Hlivko 2002). Usually, parotid metastasis presents as a solitary mass measuring 1.0–15.0 cm (Park and Hlivko 2002). Bilateral involvement of the parotids has been rarely reported and can be synchronous (Ravi et al. 1992) or metachronous (Li et al. 2001). Fine-needle-aspiration biopsy with immunohistochemical studies can provide crucial information, since the diagnosis of clear cell carcinoma of the parotid represents a challenge at the microscopic level as well (Som et al. 1987; Park

and Hlivko 2002). Parotidectomy with facial nerve preservation should be considered the therapy of choice for a solitary parotid metastasis (Park and Hlivko 2002).

Ultrasound shows a well-circumscribed hypoechoic mass at the parotid gland (Li et al. 2001). Computed tomography demonstrates homogeneous enhancement (Park and Hlivko 2002), or it may be heterogeneous due to central necrosis of the parotid mass (Li et al. 2001).

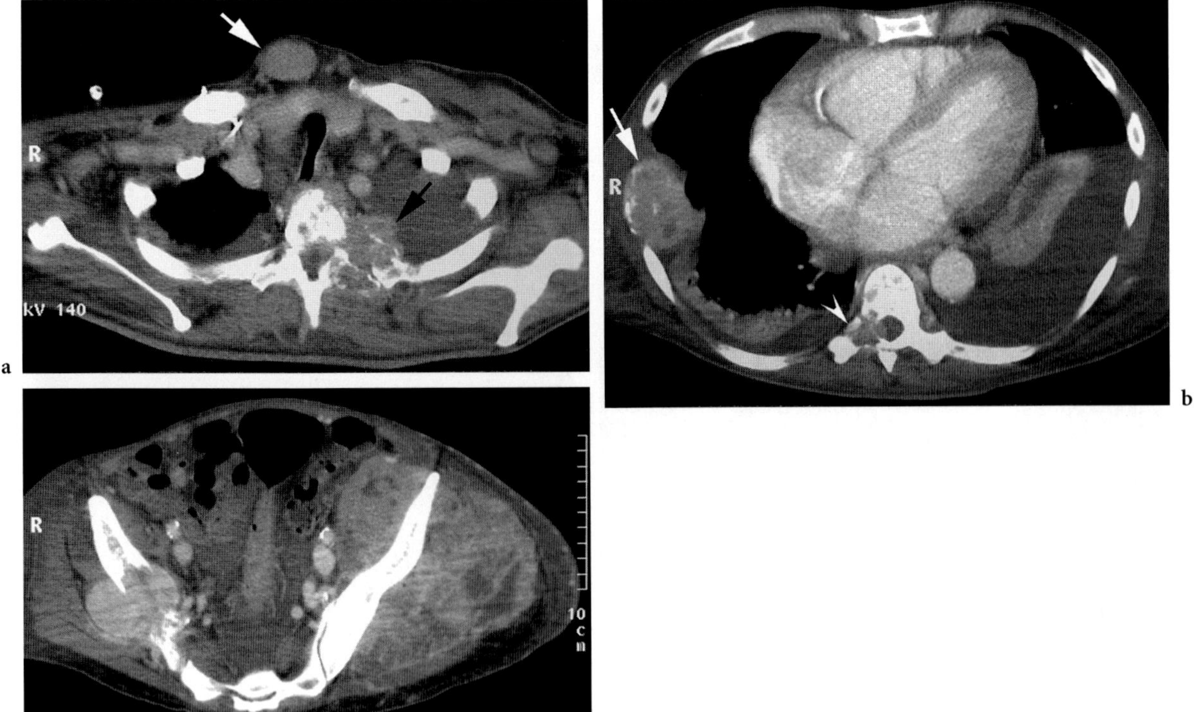

Fig. 16.53a-c. Epidural, chest wall, bone, and subcutaneous metastases in a 55-year-old man who underwent right nephrectomy for renal cell carcinoma. **a** Axial contrast-enhanced CT scan shows a large left paravertebral enhancing lytic lesion of upper thoracic vertebra (*black arrow*) which extends into the spinal canal with anterior and left epidural involvement and spinal cord compression. There is also an oval subcutaneous mass (*white arrow*) in front of the thyroid gland and bilateral pleural effusion. **b** Axial contrast-enhanced CT scan caudad to **a** shows a second lower thoracic right paravertebral lytic lesion (*arrowhead*) with extension to the spinal canal and right epidural involvement. There is a lateral chest wall heterogeneous mass (*arrow*) with rib lysis. **c** Axial contrast-enhanced CT scan of the pelvis shows large heterogeneous enhancing lytic masses involving both ilia.

16.7.2
Eye and Adnexa

Ocular metastases from RCC involve the iris, ciliary body, choroid, eyelid, orbit (HAIMOVICI et al. 1997; KINDERMANN et al. 1981; WARE et al. 1999), and extraocular muscles (SLAMOVITS and BURDE 1988). Ocular metastases may rarely be the initial presenting sign of RCC (HAIMOVICI et al. 1997).

Orbital metastasis from RCC is rare (KINDERMANN et al. 1981). Clinically, it is not specific and can appear like any other space-occupying lesion in the orbit with signs of exophthalmia, hyperemia of the conjunctiva, diplopia, or as a palpable mass (KINDERMANN et al. 1981; SCHMIDT et al. 1994). Among metastatic orbital carcinomas, RCC may be unique in producing pulsating exophthalmia due to its vascularity (KINDERMANN et al. 1981). In this respect, orbital metastasis from RCC can be confused with orbital hemangiomas (KINDERMANN et al. 1981). Because an orbital metastasis from renal carcinoma may pres-

ent as a well-circumscribed, pseudoencapsulated retrobulbar lesion, it can be confused with an orbital benign lesion (BERSANI et al. 1994). Ultrasound and CT usually show a well-delineated mass that is often hypervascular and separate from the globe (Fig. 16.55; KINDERMANN et al. 1981; SCHMIDT et al. 1994).

Choroidal metastases from RCC are uncommon. The choroidal involvement may be the sole or the initial manifestation of metastatic disease. Clinically, signs are variable (HAIMOVICI et al. 1997) and defective vision may be encountered (HAMMAD et al. 2003; SRINIVASAN and GRAY 2003). Choroidal metastases may cause diagnostic confusion with primary choroidal melanoma (KINDERMANN et al. 1981). The diagnostic efficacy of fine-needle-aspiration biopsy appears to be somewhat dependent on technical factors and the availability of an experienced cytopathologist (HAIMOVICI et al. 1997). Choroidal metastases respond well to external beam or proton irradiation (HAIMOVICI et al. 1997). They may also spontaneously regress after removal of the

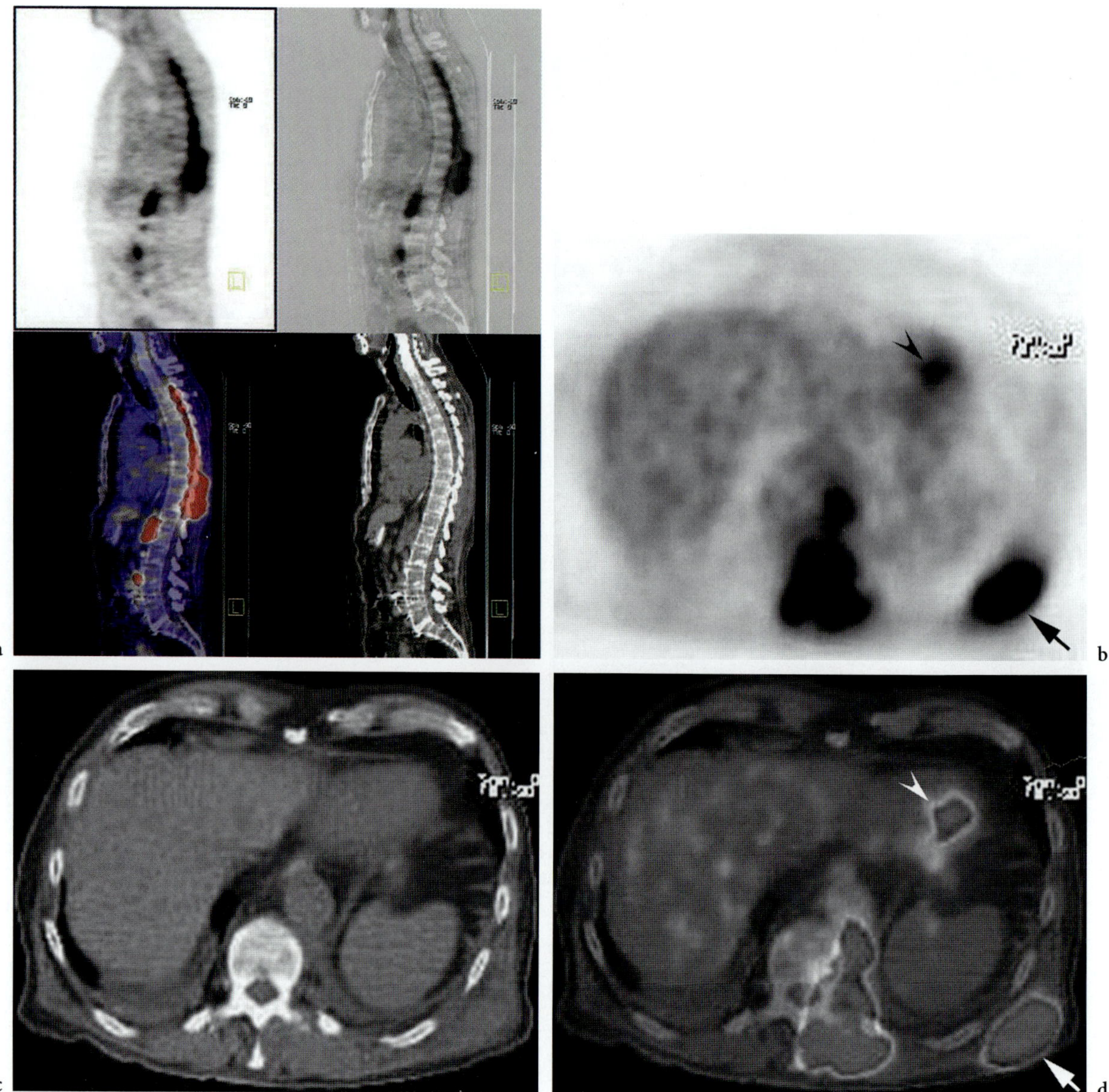

Fig. 16.54a-d. Epidural and muscle metastases in an 82-year-old man with a history of transitional cell carcinoma treated with left nephrectomy. **a** Sagittal PET/CT images demonstrate intense hypermetabolism along the distribution of the epidural space from T1 to T10 (*upper left panel:* FDG-PET alone; *upper right panel:* combined more PET and less CT; *lower left panel:* combined less PET and more CT; *lower right panel:* CT alone). Axial **b** PET, **c** CT, and **d** fused PET/CT images show the disease at the lower thoracic level, and also disclose disease in the left latissimus dorsi muscle (*arrow*). Note the normal anterior uptake of the heart (*arrowhead*). A subsequent MR imaging of the thoracic spine (not shown) confirmed the epidural disease without evidence for metastatic cord compression. (Image courtesy of H. Jadvar)

primary tumor (HAMMAD et al. 2003). The ophthalmoscopic, fluorescein angiographic, and US characteristics are diverse and nonspecific (HAIMOVICI et al. 1997). Examination of the fundus shows nonpigmented (HAIMOVICI et al. 1997) or lightly pigmented (i.e., discrete yellowish or reddish-orange) subretinal masses (SRINIVASAN and GRAY 2003). Fluorescein angiography shows variable fluorescein-staining tumors (HAIMOVICI et al. 1997). Ultrasound may show variable reflectivity, and a regular, or less frequently slightly irregular, internal structure (HAIMOVICI et al. 1997), and often a marked vascularity (Fig. 16.56; HAMMAD et al. 2003).

Metastases to the extraocular muscles are exceedingly rare. They may be bilateral. When they appear as the initial manifestation of metastatic RCC, the metastases can be difficult to distinguish from other pathologies common to the site. Imaging modalities,

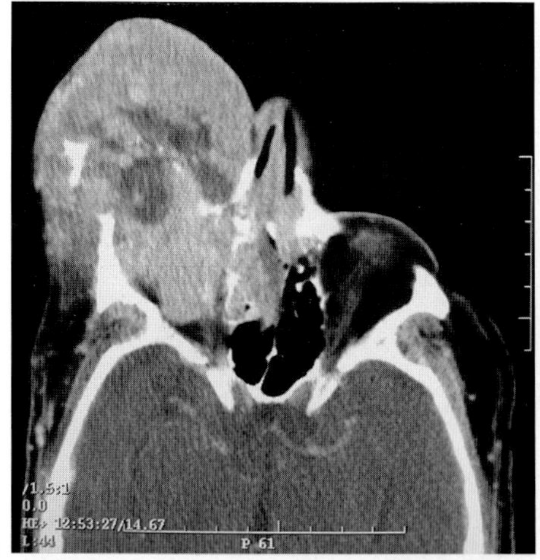

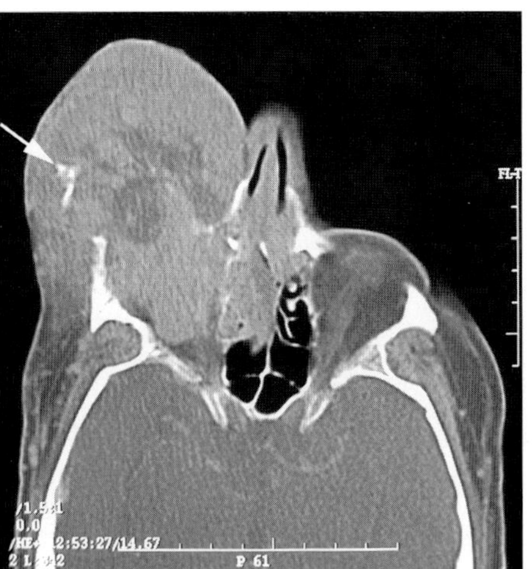

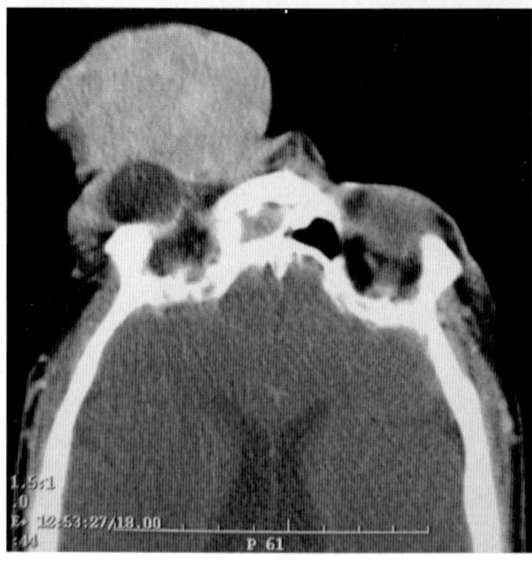

Fig. 16.55a-c. Orbital metastasis in a 58-year-old man with renal cell carcinoma. **a** Axial contrast-enhanced CT scan shows a large mass occupying the right orbit that enhances dramatically. There is central necrosis. This mass extends into the right nasal cavity and lateral mass of the ethmoid through bony destruction of the lateral wall of the right nasal cavity. **b** The same slice as **a** at bone window shows an involvement of the greater wing of sphenoidal bone and destruction of the frontal process of the zygomatic bone (*arrow*). **c** Axial contrast-enhanced CT scan cephalad to **a** shows marked right eye proptosis by the large mass.

such as US, CT, and MR imaging, may show bilateral diffuse enlargement of the extraocular muscles (Slamovits and Burde 1988).

Iris and conjunctival involvement are very rare. The involved iris appears fleshy and vascular and the conjunctival lesion appears as a highly vascular nodule. Iridocyclectomy and excision of the conjunctival nodule are considered the treatment of choice (Ware et al. 1999).

16.7.3
Nose and Sinuses

Metastases to the nose and paranasal sinuses are rare; however, RCC is the most frequent infraclavicular primary tumor to metastasize to the nose and paranasal sinuses. Clinically, it is seen as an intranasal mass causing nasal obstruction, recurrent epistaxis, facial pain, and induration (Simo et al. 2000; Szymanski et al. 2004). Orbital symptoms, such as diplopia and proptosis, are not rare.

An orbital mass may be seen and has been described once as the presenting symptom of a metastasis to the paranasal sinuses (Homer and Jones 1995). The final diagnosis usually depends on the clinical history and the histology of the lesion. This metastasis is assumed to have a very poor prognosis. Nevertheless, recent publications show that these tumors seem to respond to high-dose radiation and when solitary can be successfully treated surgically (Simo et al. 2000).

On imaging, appearances, although suggestive of malignancy, are usually nonspecific. Renal metastases to the sinusal cavities have an appearance similar to that of melanoma, extramedullary plasmacytoma, esthesioneuroblastoma, meningioma, other vascular metastases (i.e., thyroid, adrenal), lymphoma, and the primary malignant lesions (i.e., nasopharyngeal carcinoma, chordoma) at this site. The strong enhancement, soft tissue, and bone destruction, and lack of tumoral calcification, should suggest kidney cancer metastasis as the diagnosis (Som et al. 1987). Angiography usually shows a highly

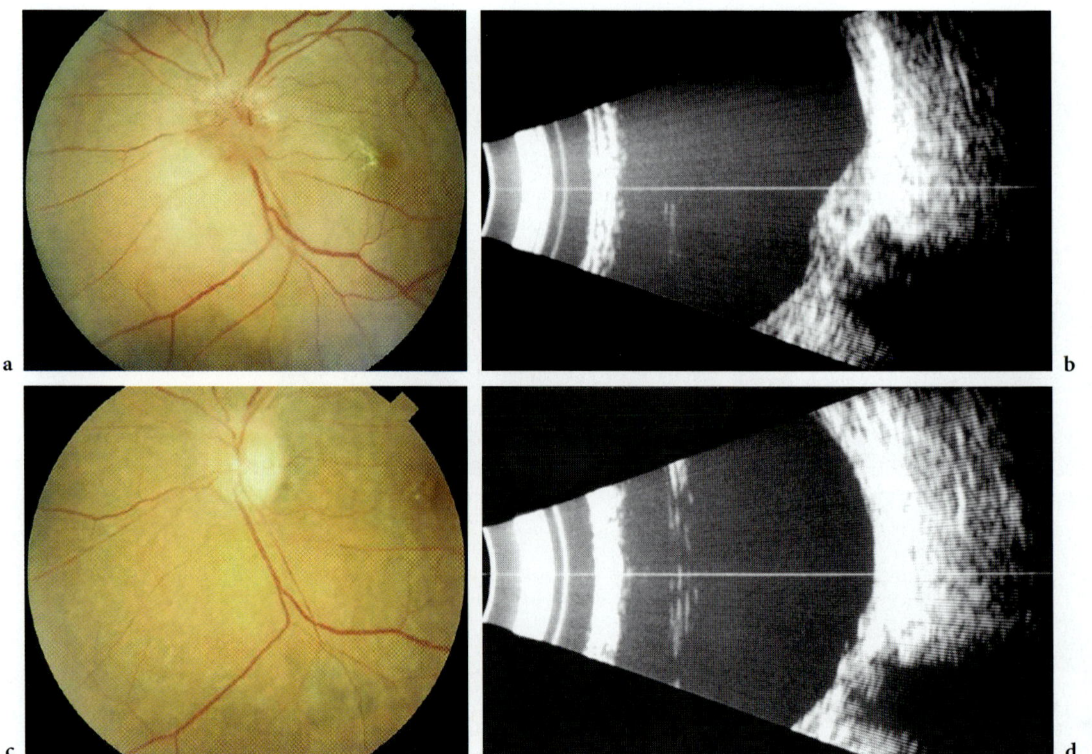

Fig. 16.56a-d. Spontaneous regression of choroidal metastasis in a 48-year-old woman 6 weeks after nephrectomy for renal cell carcinoma. **a** Fundus photograph of the left eye shows elevated choroidal lesion corresponding to the metastasis with swollen optic disc and adjacent exudative retinal detachment. **b** Longitudinal US image demonstrates choroidal lesion and retinal detachment. **c** Fundus photograph of the left eye performed 6 weeks after nephrectomy shows resolution of both optic disk swelling and retinal detachment. **d** Longitudinal US image performed at the same time shows no evidence of residual metastasis from renal cell carcinoma. (Image courtesy of W.A.J. van Heuven)

vascular mass. Computed tomography is thought to be the radiological investigation of choice in assessing the extent of metastatic lesions, especially to the bone. Magnetic resonance imaging is very helpful in precisely assessing tumoral extension, especially into the brain (Fig. 16.57), and in assessing residual disease after radiotherapy (Simo et al. 2000).

16.7.4
Tongue

Lingual metastasis is extremely rare, and no more than 20 cases have been reported in the literature (Tomita et al. 1998). Possible routes of metastasis to the tongue include the systemic circulation, the venous circulation, and the lymphatic circulation (Okabe et al. 1992). Metastasis to the tongue may be interpreted as a manifestation of widespread metastatic disease. Most of the tongue metastases are located in the basal region. This may be due to richer vascular supply, or to the relative immobility of this area (Okabe et al. 1992). Prognosis is poor, and treatment is mainly palliative.

Magnetic resonance imaging is the best imaging modality for the diagnosis and may demonstrate a mass within the tongue with enhancement after contrast intravenous administration (Tomita et al. 1998).

16.7.5
Thyroid Gland

The thyroid gland is the most common site in the head and neck of metastases from kidney cancers (Som et al. 1987), and RCC is the most common neoplasm to metastasize to the thyroid gland (Heffess et al. 2002). Nonetheless, RCC metastasis to the thyroid gland is a rare event, although it must be considered in the differential diagnosis of any thyroid gland clear cell neoplasm (Dal Fabbro et al. 1987; Giuffrida et al. 2003; Heffess et al. 2002). The tumor generally affects a single lobe as a solitary mass measuring 1.0–15.0 cm (Benoit et

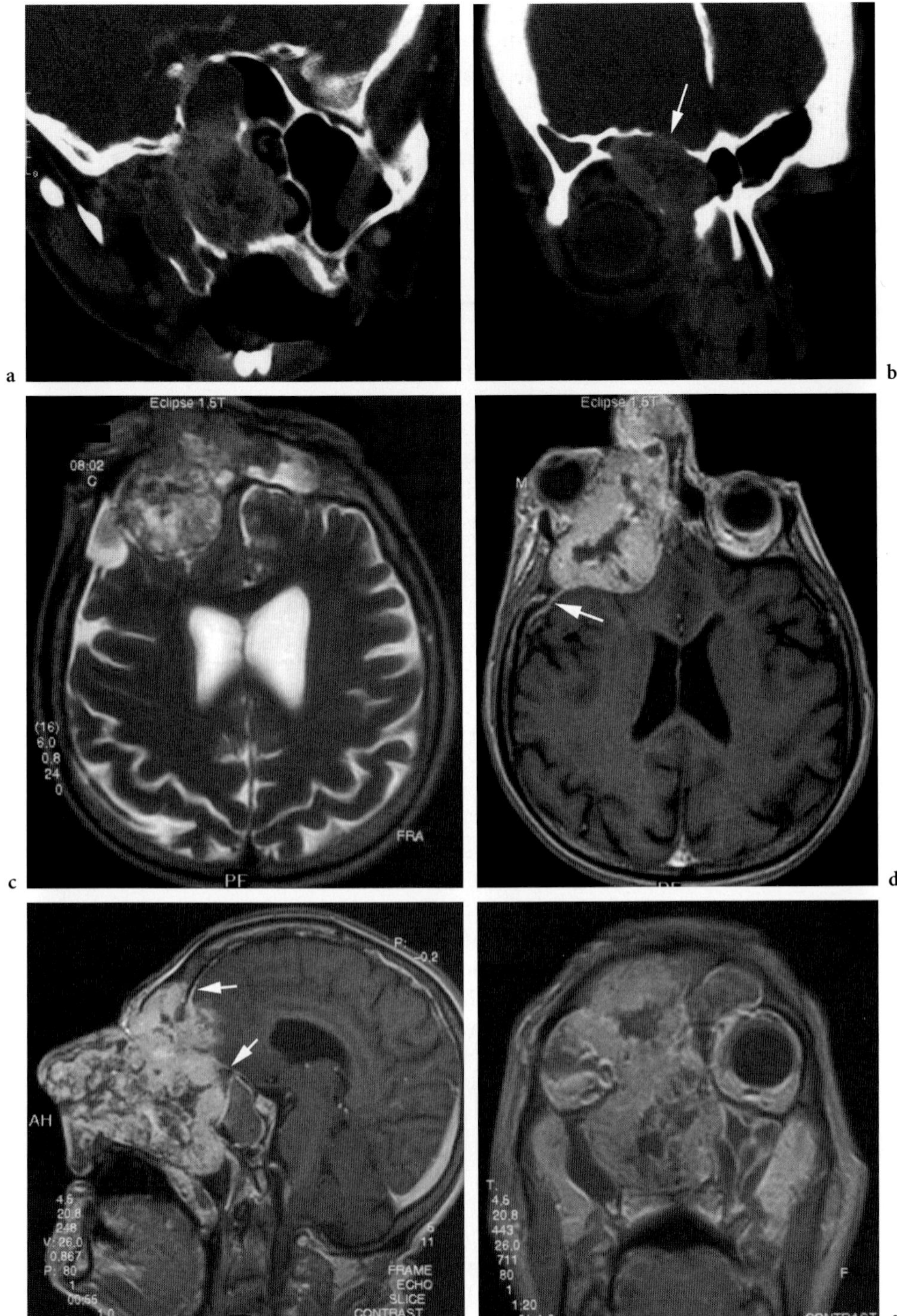

Fig. 16.57a-f. Nasal and paranasal sinus metastases in a 69-year-man concomitant to renal cell carcinoma of the left kidney. **a** Coronal oblique CT scan shows a large soft tissue mass occupying the right maxillary sinus, the right ethmoid cells, the sphenoidal sinus, and the lateral wall of the right nasal cavity, with extensive destruction of nasosinusal (bone) septum. **b** Coronal oblique CT scan anterior to **a** shows an extension of the tumoral mass into the right orbit and the frontal sinus with intracranial extension (*arrow*) through bony destruction of the upper wall of the frontal sinus. **c** Axial T2-weighted MR image shows the heterogeneous hyperintense mass, strongly enhancing after **d** contrast administration on axial T1-weighted image. There is central tumoral necrosis and marked right-eye proptosis. A dural tail enhancement (*arrow*) is also observed, probably due to meningeal involvement. **e** Sagittal and **f** coronal contrast-enhanced T1-weighted MR images demonstrate the extensive involvement of the nose and paranasal sinuses and confirms the meningeal involvement (*arrows*) as well. (Image courtesy of M. Szymanski)

al. 2004; Heffess et al. 2002; Hudson et al. 1991). Occasionally, the disease may be multifocal or bilateral (Heffess et al. 2002). A metastatic tumor in the thyroid could be the initial presentation of renal carcinoma (Benoit et al. 2004; Dal Fabbro et al. 1987; Heffess et al. 2002). Macroscopically, masses in the thyroid gland are well circumscribed, encapsulated, lobulated, and soft to partially necrotic (Heffess et al. 2002). The true metastatic nature of the tumor is recognized only after tumor sampling with pathological assessment; therefore, all patients with a solitary thyroid mass require a fine-needle-aspiration biopsy or a core-needle biopsy of the mass. Architectural, cytological, histological, histochemical, and immunohistochemical features are sufficiently distinctive to allow differentiation between primary neoplasm and metastatic RCC (Giuffrida et al. 2003; Heffess et al. 2002; May et al. 2003). Importantly, the differentiation between follicular carcinoma of the thyroid and metastasis is rendered possible by a combination of TTF-1, thyroglobulin, and CD 10 (Fig. 16.58; May et al. 2003), whereas clear cell carcinoma of the thyroid and metastasis can be distinguished by PAS staining (Dal Fabbro et al. 1987). Surgical treatment of a metastatic thyroid gland may prolong survival (Benoit et al. 2004; Heffess et al. 2002; May et al. 2003). This is particularly true with solitary metastases because of an unusually good prognosis (Heffess et al. 2002; May et al. 2003).

Imaging is not specific since both primary and secondary thyroid neoplasms have the same radiological appearance (Fig. 16.59). Ultrasound shows a heterogeneous hypoechoic mass. Radioiodine scintigraphy very often shows a "cold" nodule (Heffess et al. 2002).

16.8
Skeletal Muscle and Diaphragmatic Metastases

Skeletal muscle metastases from RCC are extremely rare (Schatteman et al. 2002); most are asymptomatic and occur in patients with advanced disease (Munk et al. 1992; Pretorius and Fishman 2000) but may occasionally be associated with pain (Pretorius and Fishman, 2000) or paraneoplastic syndrome such as erythrocytosis (Alimonti et al. 2003). They may be isolated (Scatarige et al. 2001a) or they may be the initial manifestation of the renal tumor, making the differentiation between

primary soft tissue tumor and renal metastasis difficult (Schatteman et al. 2002). The latency period can be as long as 16 years (Nabeyama et al. 2001). The erector spinae muscle is a favored site for skeletal muscle metastases (Fig. 16.28; Scatarige et al. 2001a), but other sites of involvement include deltoid (Fig. 16.60; Alimonti et al. 2003; Schatteman et al. 2002), gluteals (Fig. 16.28; Pretorius and Fishman 2000), trapezius (Munk et al. 1992), triceps brachii, biceps brachii, rectus abdominis (Fig. 16.61), and vastus lateralis (Nabeyama et al. 2001).

On imaging, renal metastases to the skeletal muscle tend to enhance uniformly (Scatarige et al. 2001a; Schatteman et al. 2002) and usually have regular contours (Pretorius and Fishman, 2000) or sometimes lobulated contours (Munk et al. 1992). Magnetic resonance imaging is the gold standard because of its superior intrinsic soft tissue contrast (Pretorius and Fishman 2000). Magnetic resonance imaging also accurately shows the boundaries of the metastasis with the surrounding normal tissues (Fig. 16.62; Schatteman et al. 2002). In general, the metastasis is hyperintense on T2-weighted images, hypointense on T1-weighted images, and enhances homogeneously after contrast administration (Munk et al. 1992). If hemorrhagic, the metastasis would appear slightly hyperintense on unenhanced T1-weighted images (Nabeyama et al. 2001). Magnetic resonance imaging has another advantage over CT with its ability to reveal changes suggestive of edema in the surrounding tissues, visible as a hyperintensity on T2-weighted images (Munk et al. 1992; Pretorius and Fishman 2000).

Diaphragmatic metastases are exceedingly rare. Ultrasound may occasionally show a diaphragmatic mass (Pilecki et al. 2002), but CT, and more efficiently MR imaging, accurately localizes the involvement to the diaphragm.

16.9
Cutaneous Metastases

Cutaneous metastases are rare and occasionally involve the initial surgical nephrectomy incision. Their incidence is reported to be 2.8% of which 20% were diagnosed at presentation. The majority of these lesions were multiple. None of the patients experienced a recurrence 10 or more years after initial surgery (Newmark et al. 1994). Cutaneous metastases to the nephrectomy scar respond favorably to surgical excision (Newmark et al. 1994).

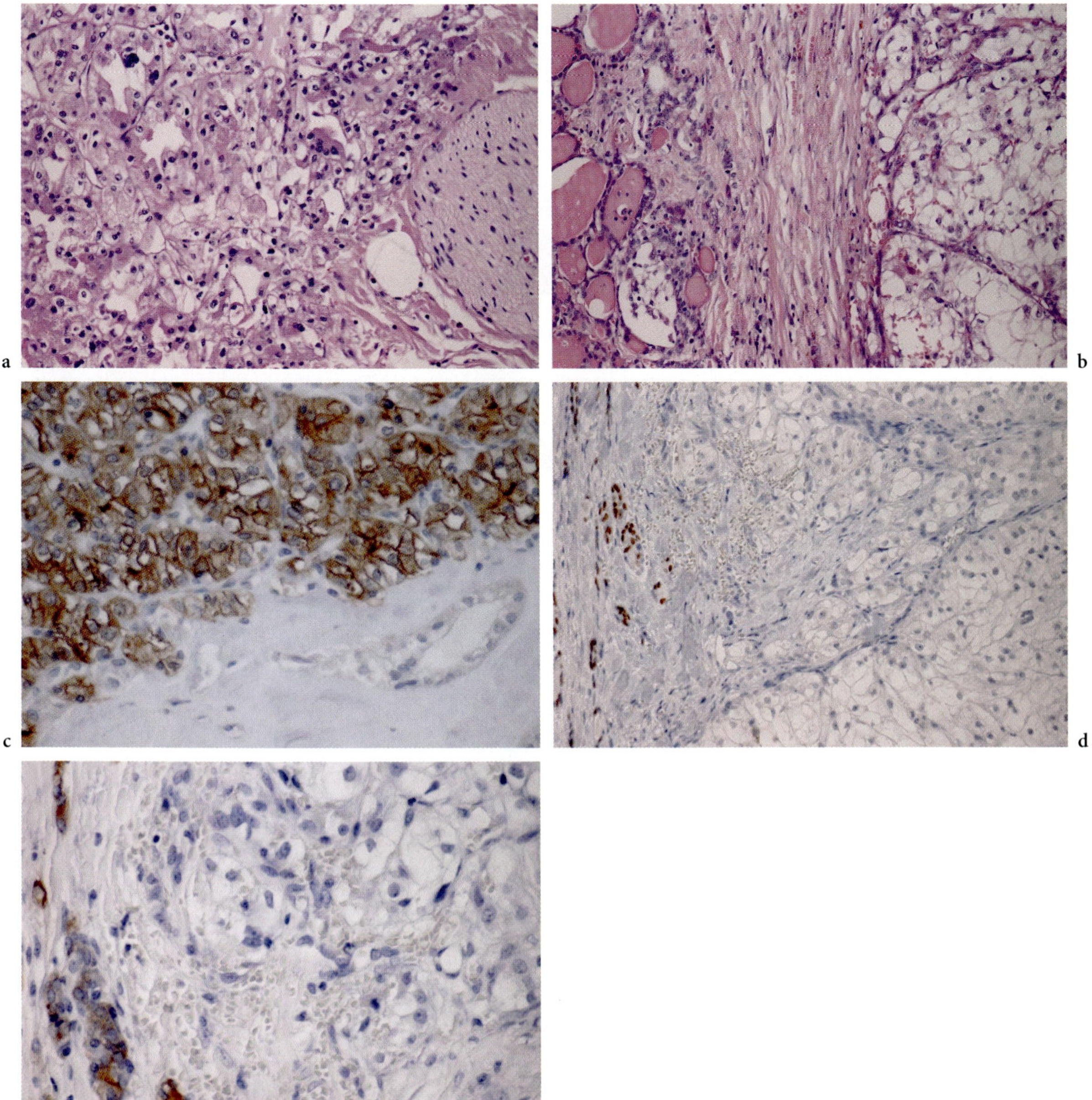

Fig. 16.58a-e. Thyroid metastasis in a 56-year-old man who underwent right nephrectomy for renal cell carcinoma 10 years previously. **a** Photomicrograph shows clear cell carcinoma of the right kidney (hematoxylin and eosin stain; original magnification, ×200). **b** Photomicrograph shows the thyroid metastasis with the same clear cell carcinoma histology (hematoxylin and eosin stain; original magnification, ×200). **c** Photomicrograph shows expression of CD10 by the thyroid metastasis (immunoperoxidase stain; original magnification, ×420). **d** Photomicrograph shows nuclear evidence of TTF-1 in the normal thyroid (*left side* of the slide) but not in the thyroid metastasis (immunoperoxidase stain; original magnification, ×200). **e** Photomicrograph shows expression of thyroglobulin in the residual normal thyroid tissue (*left side* of the slide) but not in the thyroid metastasis (immunoperoxidase stain; original magnification, ×420). (With permission from MAY et al. 2003)

The use of CT and MR imaging can greatly assist in delineating the extent of the lesion and planning surgical treatment (Fig. 16.63; NEWMARK et al. 1994). In a case report, contrast-enhanced CT showed a slightly heterogeneous nonenhancing extracavitary lesion. This lesion was heterogeneously hypointense on T1- and hyperintense on T2-weighted images (NEWMARK et al. 1994).

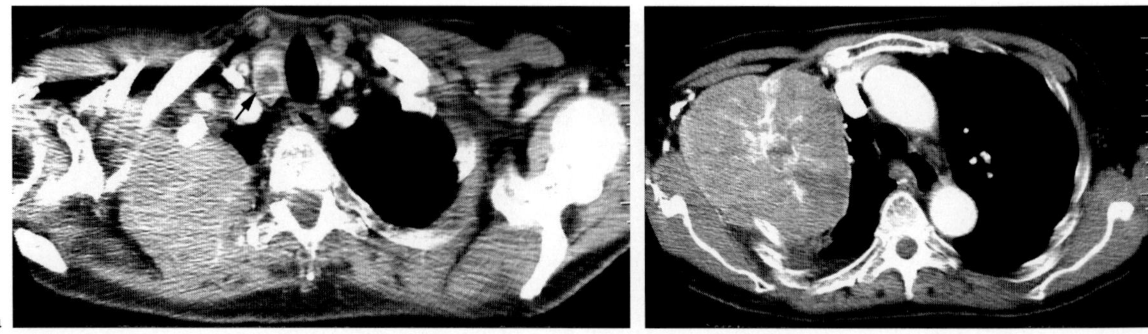

Fig. 16.59a,b. Thyroid and chest wall metastases in a 66-year-old woman who underwent left nephrectomy for renal cell carcinoma. **a** Axial contrast-enhanced CT scan shows a heterogeneously enhancing lesion of the right thyroid lobe (*arrow*) with central necrosis associated with a large right chest wall enhancing mass. This mass involves the right superior rib and is best seen on **b**.

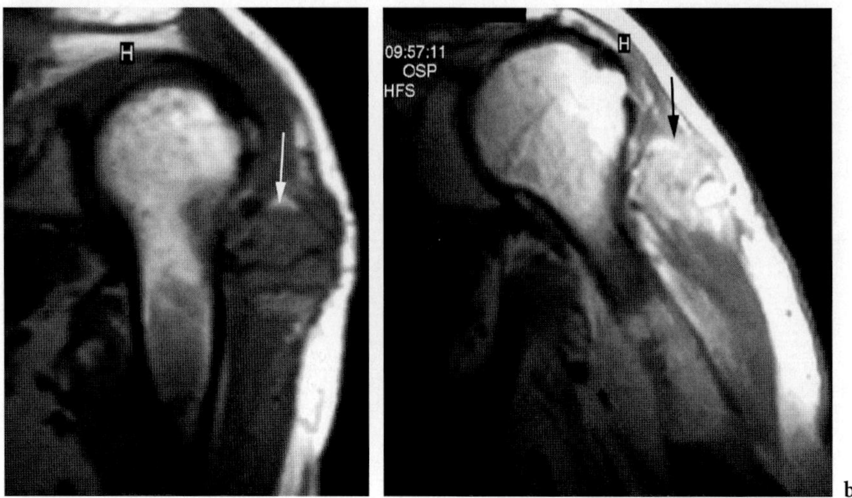

Fig. 16.60a,b. Muscle metastasis in a 63-year-old man with clear cell renal carcinoma 3 months after radical nephrectomy and who presented with deltoid swelling and paraneoplastic erythrocytosis. **a** Coronal unenhanced T1-weighted MR image shows an ill-defined and slightly hyperintense oval mass involving the left deltoid muscle (*arrow*). **b** Sagittal contrast-enhanced T1-weighted MR image shows strong enhancement of the mass (*arrow*). There is no adjacent involvement of the skin. (Image courtesy of A. ALIMONTI and S. TORMENTA)

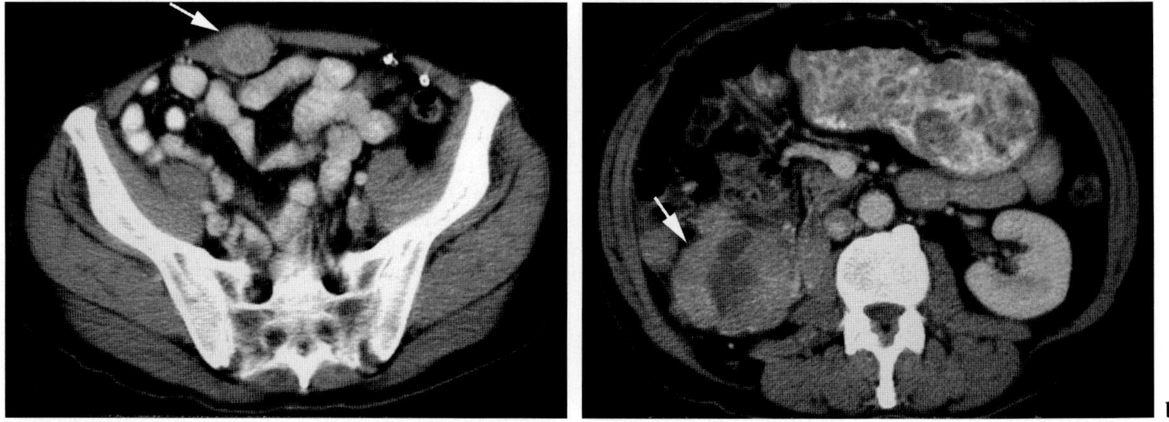

Fig. 16.61a,b. Muscle metastasis and local recurrence in a 59-year-old man who underwent right nephrectomy for renal cell carcinoma. **a** Axial contrast-enhanced CT demonstrates a homogeneously slightly enhancing mass to the right rectus abdominis muscle (*arrow*). **b** Axial contrast-enhanced CT scan cephalad to **a** shows a heterogeneously enhancing mass (*arrow*) in the right renal fossa.

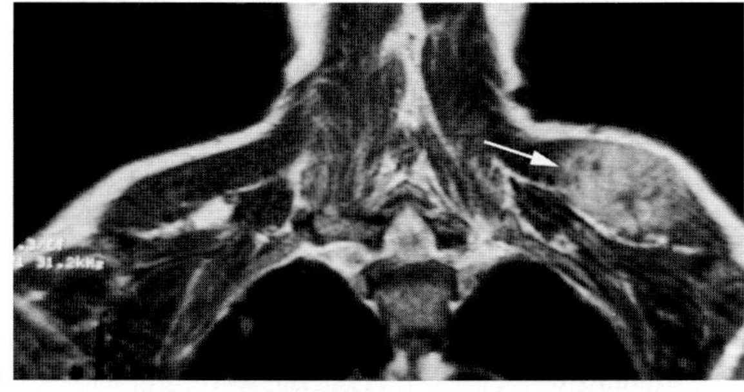 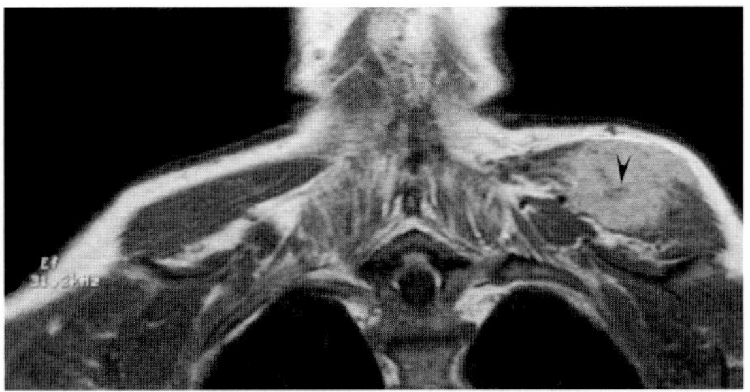

Fig. 16.62a,b. Muscle metastasis in a 63-year-old man with clear cell renal carcinoma 2 years after nephrectomy. **a** Coronal T2-weighted MR image shows well-defined and slightly heterogeneous hyperintense rounded mass involving the left deltoid muscle (*arrow*). **b** Coronal contrast-enhanced T1-weighted MR image shows a strong enhancement of the mass with central hypointensity corresponding to tumoral necrosis (*arrowhead*). There is no adjacent involvement of the skin. (Image courtesy of P. SCHATTEMAN)

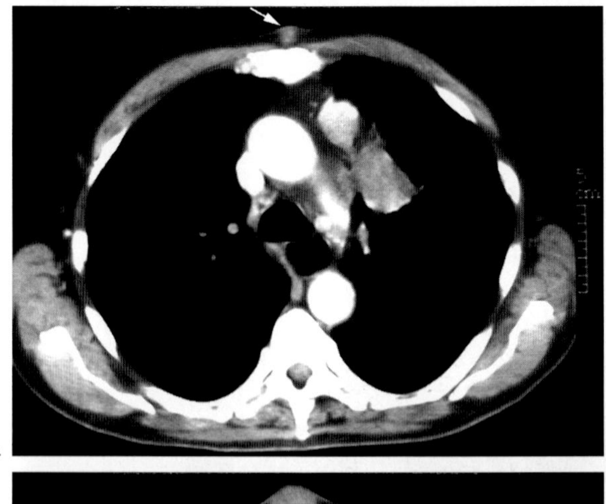 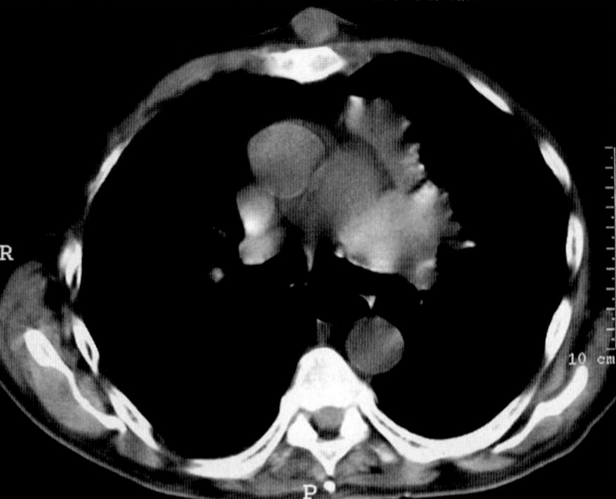

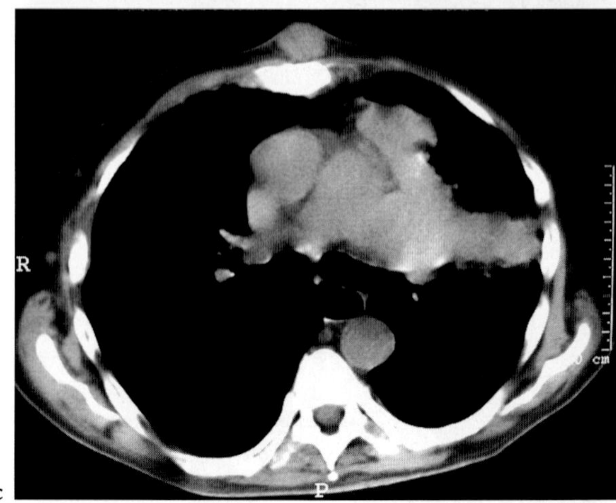

Fig. 16.63a-c. Subcutaneous and pulmonary metastases in a 67-year-old man who underwent left nephrectomy for renal cell carcinoma. **a** Axial contrast-enhanced CT scan shows a very small homogenous slightly enhancing mass (*arrow*) involving the subcutaneous tissue in front of the sternum. The scan also shows a left ill-defined pulmonary lesion. Both lesions are seen growing in follow-up CT **b** 2 months and **c** 4 months later.

16.10
Local Recurrence

Local recurrence of RCC in the renal fossa is an uncommon event following radical nephrectomy (ITANO et al. 2000; JANZEN et al. 2003), although the risk may be higher after partial nephrectomy

(JANZEN et al. 2003). Isolated late recurrence is rare with less than a 2% incidence at 5-year follow-up. It is controversial whether this entity is a remnant of microscopic disease or a form of metastatic disease (ITANO et al. 2000). The clinical disease-free interval is reported to be as long as 45 years after nephrectomy (TAPPER et al. 1997). An isolated recurrence of

302   A. Guermazi et al.

RCC in the renal bed may behave as a solitary metastasis and select patients may benefit from surgical resection (ITANO et al. 2000).

Recurrent renal carcinoma usually appears as an enhancing mass or nodule in the surgical site after nephrectomy (Figs. 16.13, 16.14; NAKADA et al. 2002; SCATARIGE et al. 2001a). The mass may be heterogeneous (TAPPER et al. 1997) with central necrosis (Fig. 16.61; CHAE et al. 2005). The recurrence often involves the quadratus lumborum and psoas muscles (Fig. 16.64). It can displace or invade nearby structures such as the spine. The adrenal bed may be involved in case of cephalic extent which can involve the ipsilateral adrenal gland if the latter was spared at the time of nephrectomy (SCATARIGE et al. 2001a; TAPPER et al. 1997). Locally recurrent renal carcinoma may directly invade the ascending or descending colon (SCATARIGE et al. 2001a). The recurrence may also extend posteriorly towards the surgical scar (Fig. 16.65; TAPPER et al. 1997). Following nephron-sparing surgery, local recurrence is suggested when an enhancing nodule develops in the wedge-shaped partial nephrectomy defect (SCATARIGE et al. 2001a).

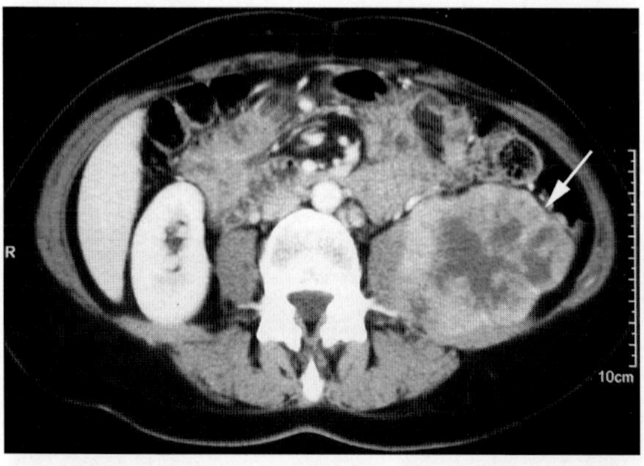

Fig. 16.64. Local recurrence in a 48-year-old woman who underwent left nephrectomy for renal cell carcinoma. Axial contrast-enhanced CT scan shows a large heterogeneously enhancing mass (*arrow*) with central necrosis of the left renal fossa and invading the left quadratus lumborum and psoas muscles.

16.11
Conclusion

Metastatic lesions from kidney cancer are seen in virtually every organ: the lung; pleura; pancreas; adrenal gland; liver; contralateral kidney; bone; lymph nodes; muscles; etc. These lesions can mas-

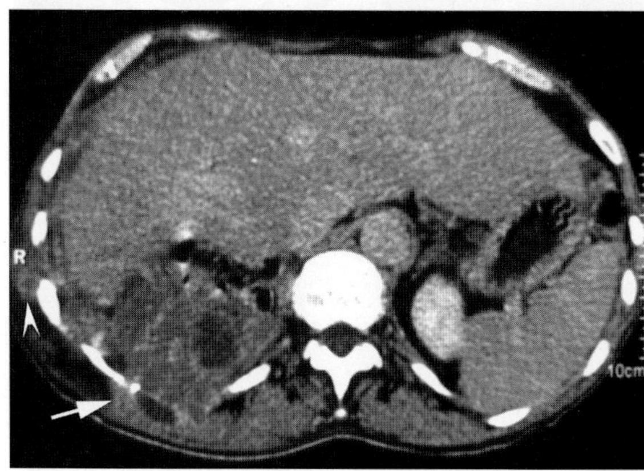

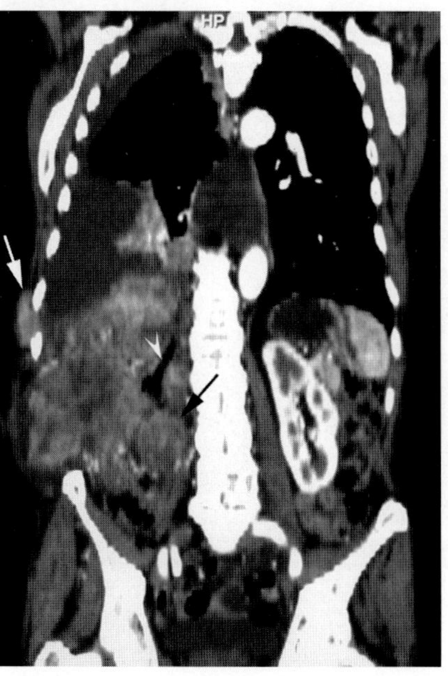

Fig. 16.65a,b. Local recurrence, chest wall, and pleural metastases in a 72-year-old man who underwent right nephrectomy for renal cell carcinoma. a Axial contrast-enhanced CT scan shows a large heterogeneously enhancing mass with central necrosis of the right renal fossa, extending posteriorly towards the surgical scar and invading the right latissimus dorsi muscle (*arrow*). It also shows a small heterogeneous mass of the lateral right chest wall (*arrowhead*). b Coronal contrast-enhanced two-dimensional CT reconstruction shows the large recurrent renal cell carcinoma mass that is locally and directly invading the ascending colon (*arrowhead*) and the right psoas muscle (*black arrow*). It also shows the right chest wall mass (*white arrow*) and important right pleural and pericardial effusions.

querade as another primary tumor. It is important to distinguish metastatic spread of RCC from primary tumors, as this knowledge is essential for the correct diagnosis and for determining the most effective treatment. Imaging studies are essential, as are histopathological examinations. Whole-body spiral CT is currently the method of choice for evaluating the postsurgical nephrectomy site for the presence of recurrent lesions and for detecting the usual anatomical sites of metastases. Like the primary tumor, metastatic lesions tend to be hypervascular and intravenous contrast administration is very useful. Other radiological modalities may be of interest when exploring particular organs, such as US for the liver and MR imaging for the brain and spine. Knowledge of the mechanisms, risk factors, and clinical timing of recurrent disease in surgically treated renal cancer aids the radiologist in understanding and detecting the patterns of recurrence observed on imaging.

Acknowledgements
We extend sincere thanks to Drs. A. Alimonti, C. Bassi, G. Butturini, M. Doita, S. Grand, M. Hashimoto, L. Insabato, H. Jadvar, F. Lafitte, M. May, D.H. McGregor, L. Mearini, H. Nozawa, I.C. Roberts-Thomson, G.M. Sakorafas, P. Schatteman, O.E.M. Schijns, K. Shiraishi, M. Szymanski, M. Tatsuta, S. Tormenta, and W.A.J. van Heuven for providing us with their excellent images.

References

Adams LA, Kaushik SP, Teo M, Roberts-Thomson IC (2003) Gastrointestinal: gastric metastases. J Gastroenterol Hepatol 18:343

Adil G, Murat D, Ayhan O, Ozgur TM, Ibrahim Y, Fuat PA, Rifki F (1999) Renal cell carcinoma metastasis to the parotid gland. BJU Int 83:861–862

Alimonti A, Cosimo S di, Maccallini V, Ferretti G, Pavese I, Satta F, Palma M di, Vecchione A (2003) A man with a deltoid swelling and paraneoplastic erythrocytosis: case report. Anticancer Res 23:5181–5184

Allen G, Klingman R, Ferraris VA, Fisher H, Harte F, Singh A (1991) Transesophageal echocardiography in the surgical management of renal cell carcinoma with intracardiac extension. J Cardiovasc Surg (Torino) 32:833–836

Altschuler EL, Ray A (1998) Spontaneous regression of a pancreatic metastasis of a renal cell carcinoma. Arch Fam Med 7:516–517

Andoh H, Kurokawa T, Yasui O, Shibata S, Sato T (2004) Resection of a solitary pancreatic metastasis from renal cell carcinoma with a gallbladder carcinoma: report of a case. Surg Today 34:272–275

Aoki T, Inoue K, Tsuchida A, Kasuya K, Kitamura K, Koyanagi Y, Shimizu T (2002) Gallbladder metastasis of renal cell carcinoma: report of two cases. Surg Today 32:89–92

Arkless R (1965) Renal carcinoma: how it metastasizes. Radiology 84:496–501

Badoual C, Tissier F, Lagorce-Pages C, Delcourt A, Vieillefond A (2002) Pulmonary metastases from a chromophobe renal cell carcinoma: 10 years' evolution. Histopathology 40:300–302

Barthwal MS, Chatterji RS, Jawed KZ (2003) Endobronchial metastases from renal cell carcinoma. J Assoc Physicians India 51:1027–1028

Bassi C, Butturini G, Falconi M, Sargenti M, Mantovani W, Pederzoli P (2003) High recurrence rate after atypical resection for pancreatic metastases from renal cell carcinoma. Br J Surg 90:555–559

Benoit L, Favoulet P, Arnould L, Margarot A, Franceschini C, Collin F, Fraisse J, Cuisenier J, Cougard P (2004) Metastatic renal cell carcinoma of the thyroid gland: about seven cases and review of the literature. Ann Chir 129:218–223

Bersani TA, Costello JJ Jr, Mango CA, Streeten BW (1994) Benign approach to a malignant orbital tumor: metastatic renal cell carcinoma. Ophthal Plast Reconstr Surg 10:42–44

Bressler EL, Alpern MB, Glazer GM, Francis IR, Ensminger WD (1987) Hypervascular hepatic metastases: CT evaluation. Radiology 162:49–51

Calleja Escudero J, Pascual Samaniego M, Martin Blanco S, Castro Olmedo C de, Gonzalo V, Fernandez del Busto E (2004) Intrascrotal metastasis in a renal cell carcinoma. Acta Urol Esp 28:311–313

Carroll JC, Quinn CC, Weitzel J, Sant GR (1994) Metastatic renal cell carcinoma to the right cardiac ventricle without contiguous vena caval involvement. J Urol 151:133–134

Chae EJ, Kim JK, Kim SH, Bae SJ, Cho KS (2005) Renal cell carcinoma: analysis of postoperative recurrence patterns. Radiology 234:189–196

Chang CH, Shiau YC, Shen YY, Kao A, Lin CC, Lee CC (2003) Differentiating solitary pulmonary metastases in patients with renal cell carcinomas by 18F-fluoro-2-deoxyglucose positron emission tomography: a preliminary report. Urol Int 71:306–309

Chao K, Hurley J, Neerhut G, Kiroff G (2002) Multiple pancreatic metastases from renal cell carcinoma. Aust NZ J Surg 72:310–312

Cheng AS (2003) Cardiac metastasis from a renal cell carcinoma. Int J Clin Pract 57:437–438

Coppa GF, Oszczakiewicz M (1990) Parotid gland metastasis from renal carcinoma. Int Surg 75:198–202

Dal Fabbro S, Monari G, Barbazza R (1987) A thyroid metastasis revealing an occult renal clear-cell carcinoma. Tumori 73:187–190

Daniels GF Jr, Schaeffer AJ (1991) Renal cell carcinoma involving penis and testis: unusual initial presentations of metastatic disease. Urology 37:369–373

Destian S, Sze G, Krol G, Zimmerman RD, Deck MD (1989) MR imaging of hemorrhagic intracranial neoplasms. Am J Roentgenol 152:137–144

Diaz-Candamio MJ, Pombo S, Pombo F (2000) Colonic metastasis from renal cell carcinoma: helical-CT demonstration. Eur Radiol 10:139–140

Djimi H, Donnio A, Ayeboua L, Vally P, Olindo S, Cabre P, Ventura E, Landau M, Richer R, Merle H (2003) Hypophysis metastasis of a hypernephroma tumor revealed by a chiasma syndrome. J Fr Ophtalmol 26:976–979

Dousset B, Andant C, Guimbaud R, Roseau G, Tulliez M, Gaudric M, Palazzo L, Chaussade S, Chapuis Y (1995) Late pancreatic metastasis from renal cell carcinoma diagnosed by endoscopic ultrasonography. Surgery 117:591–594

Duggan MA, Forestell CF, Hanley DA (1987) Adrenal metastases of renal-cell carcinoma 19 years after nephrectomy. Fine needle aspiration cytology of a case. Acta Cytol 31:512–516

Essadki O, Chartrand-Lefebvre C, Finet JF, Grenier P (1998) Cystic pulmonary metastasis simulating a diagnosis of histiocytosis X. J Radiol 79:886–888

Fakih M, Schiff D, Erlich R, Logan TF (2001) Intramedullary spinal cord metastasis (ISCM) in renal cell carcinoma: a series of six cases. Ann Oncol 12:1173–1177

Federle MP, Jeffrey RB Jr, Minagi H (1981) Case report. Calcified liver metastasis from renal cell carcinoma. J Comput Assist Tomogr 5:771–772

Flanigan RC, Yonover PM (2001) The role of radical nephrectomy in metastatic renal cell carcinoma. Semin Urol Oncol 19:98–102

Flanigan RC, Salmon SE, Blumenstein BA, Bearman SI, Roy V, McGrath PC, Caton JR Jr, Munshi N, Crawford ED (2001) Nephrectomy followed by interferon alfa-2b compared with interferon alfa-2b alone for metastatic renal-cell cancer. N Engl J Med 345:1655–1659

Flanigan RC, Campbell SC, Clark JI, Picken MM (2003) Metastatic renal cell carcinoma. Curr Treat Options Oncol 4:385–390

Furukawa H, Mizuguchi Y, Kanai Y, Mukai K (1997) Metastatic renal cell carcinoma to the gallbladder: color Doppler sonography and CT findings. Am J Roentgenol 169:1466–1467

Gastaca Mateo MA, Ortiz de Urbina Lopez J, Diaz Aguirregoitia J, Martinez Fernandez G, Campo Hiriart M, Echevarria Garcia-San Frechoso A (1996) Duodenal metastasis of renal cell adenocarcinoma. Rev Esp Enferm Dig 88:361–363

Ghavamian R, Klein KA, Stephens DH, Welch TJ, LeRoy AJ, Richardson RL, Burch PA, Zincke H (2000) Renal cell carcinoma metastatic to the pancreas: clinical and radiological features. Mayo Clin Proc 75:581–585

Giuffrida D, Ferrau F, Pappalardo A, Aiello RA, Bordonaro R, Cordio S, Giorgio CG, Squatrito S (2003) Metastasis to the thyroid gland: a case report and review of the literature. J Endocrinol Invest 26:560–563

Giulini SM, Portolani N, Bonardelli S, Baiocchi GL, Zampatti M, Coniglio A, Baronchelli C (2003) Distal pancreatic resection with splenic preservation for metastasis of renal carcinoma diagnosed 24 years later from the nephrectomy. Ann Ital Chir 74:93–96

Griniatsos J, Michail PO, Menenakos C, Hatzianastasiou D, Koufos C, Bastounis E (2003) Metastatic renal clear cell carcinoma mimicking stage IV lung cancer. Int Urol Nephrol 35:15–17

Gupta D, Merino MI, Farhood A, Middleton LP (2001) Metastases to breast simulating ductal carcinoma in situ: report of two cases and review of the literature. Ann Diagn Pathol 5:15–20

Guthbjartsson T, Gislason T (1995) Spontaneous regression of brain metastasis secondary to renal cell carcinoma. Scand J Urol Nephrol 29:215–217

Haimovici R, Gragoudas ES, Gregor Z, Pesavento RD, Mieler WF, Duker JS (1997) Choroidal metastases from renal cell carcinoma. Ophthalmology 104:1152–1158

Hammad AM, Paris GR, van Heuven WA, Thompson IM, Fitzsimmons TD (2003) Spontaneous regression of choroidal metastasis from renal cell carcinoma. Am J Ophthalmol 135:911–913

Hasegawa J, Okumura S, Abe H, Kanamori S, Yoshida K, Akimoto M (1988) Renal cell carcinoma with solitary contralateral adrenal metastasis. Urology 32:52–53

Hashimoto M, Miura Y, Matsuda M, Watanabe G (2001) Concomitant duodenal and pancreatic metastases from renal cell carcinoma: report of a case. Surg Today 31:180–183

Heffess CS, Wenig BM, Thompson LD (2002) Metastatic renal cell carcinoma to the thyroid gland: a clinicopathologic study of 36 cases. Cancer 95:1869–1878

Hernandez DJ, Kavoussi LR, Ellison LM (2003) Laparoscopic distal pancreatectomy for metastatic renal cell carcinoma. Urology 62:551

Hillard VH, Musunuru K, Hasan I, Zia S, Hirschfeld A (2003) Long-term management of bilateral metastases of renal cell carcinoma to the choroid plexus. Acta Neurochir (Wien) 145:793–797

Hodgson TJ, Howell SJ, Kean DM (1994) Case report: metastatic renal cell carcinoma presenting as intracerebral haemorrhage. Clin Radiol 49:213–214

Homer JJ, Jones NS (1995) Renal cell carcinoma presenting as a solitary paranasal sinus metastasis. J Laryngol Otol 109:986–989

Hoshi S, Jokura H, Nakamura H, Shintaku I, Ohyama C, Satoh M, Saito S, Fukuzaki A, Orikasa S, Yoshimoto T (2002) Gamma-knife radiosurgery for brain metastasis of renal cell carcinoma: results in 42 patients. Int J Urol 9:618–625; discussion 626; author reply 627

Hudson MA, Kavoussi LR, Catalona WJ (1991) Bilateral renal cell carcinoma with metastasis to thyroid. Urology 37:145–148

Huisman TK, Sands JP Jr (1991) Renal cell carcinoma with solitary metachronous contralateral adrenal metastasis. Experience with 2 cases and review of the literature. Urology 38:364–368

Insabato L, Rosa G de, Franco R, D'Onofrio V, Vizio D di (2003) Ovarian metastasis from renal cell carcinoma: a report of three cases. Int J Surg Pathol 11:309–312

Ishikawa J, Umezu K, Yamashita H, Maeda S (1990) Solitary brain metastasis from renal cell carcinoma 14 years after nephrectomy: a case report. Hinyokika Kiyo 36:1439–1441

Itano NB, Blute ML, Spotts B, Zincke H (2000) Outcome of isolated renal cell carcinoma fossa recurrence after nephrectomy. J Urol 164:322–325

Jadvar H, Cham D, Gamie S, Henderson RW (2004) Fusion positron emission tomography-computed tomography demonstration of epidural metastases. Clin Nucl Med 29:39–40

Janzen NK, Kim HL, Figlin RA, Belldegrun AS (2003) Surveillance after radical or partial nephrectomy for localized renal cell carcinoma and management of recurrent disease. Urol Clin North Am 30:843–852

Johnsen JA, Hellsten S (1997) Lymphatogenous spread of renal cell carcinoma: an autopsy study. J Urol 157:450–453

Kamota S, Harabayashi T, Suzuki S, Takeyama Y, Mitsui T, Mouri G, Hashimoto A, Nakamura M, Shinohara N, Nonomura K, Koyanagi T (2003) Ureteral and bladder metastases of renal cell carcinoma following synchronous renal cell carcinoma and bladder cancer; a case report. Nippon Hinyokika Gakkai Zasshi 94:705–708

Kassabian A, Stein J, Jabbour N, Parsa K, Skinner D, Parekh D, Cosenza C, Selby R (2000) Renal cell carcinoma metastatic to the pancreas: a single-institution series and review of the literature. Urology 56:211–215

Kelekis NL, Semelka RC, Siegelman ES (1996) MRI of pancreatic metastases from renal cancer. J Comput Assist Tomogr 20:249–253

Kim JK, Learch TJ, Colletti PM, Lee JW, Tran SD, Terk MR (2000) Diagnosis of vertebral metastasis, epidural metastasis, and malignant spinal cord compression: Are T1-weighted sagittal images sufficient? Magn Reson Imaging 18:819–824

Kindermann WR, Shields JA, Eiferman RA, Stephens RF, Hirsch SE (1981) Metastatic renal cell carcinoma to the eye and adnexae: a report of three cases and review of the literature. Ophthalmology 88:1347–1350

Klein KA, Stephens DH, Welch TJ (1998) CT characteristics of metastatic disease of the pancreas. Radiographics 18:369–378

Klos KJ, O'Neill BP (2004) Brain metastases. Neurologist 10:31–46

Koc M, Polat P, Erem T, Buyukavci M, Ozbey I, Gundogdu C, Suma S (1999) Quiz case of the month. Diagnosis: clear-cell renal cell carcinoma (RCC) with metastasis to lung, mediastinal and abdominal lymph nodes and bones. Eur Radiol 9:1935–1936

Kolosseus RC, Temes RT, Feddersen RM, Williamson M, Smith AY (1995) Intrapulmonary lymph nodes masquerading as renal cell carcinoma metastases. Urology 46:249–250

Koshiyama H, Ohgaki K, Hida S, Takasu K, Yumitori K, Shimatsu A, Koh T (1992) Metastatic renal cell carcinoma to the pituitary gland presenting with hypopituitarism. J Endocrinol Invest 15:677-681

Kremer S, Grand S, Berger F, Hoffmann D, Pasquier B, Remy C, Benabid AL, Bas JF (2003) Dynamic contrast-enhanced MRI: differentiating melanoma and renal carcinoma metastases from high-grade astrocytomas and other metastases. Neuroradiology 45:44–49

Lau WK, Zincke H, Lohse CM, Cheville JC, Weaver AL, Blute ML (2003) Contralateral adrenal metastasis of renal cell carcinoma: treatment, outcome and a review. BJU Int 91:775–779

Lee G, Sharma SD, Bullock KN (1998) An unusual case of renal cell carcinoma with two rare metastases. Scand J Urol Nephrol 32:239–240

Lee JG, Kim JS, Kim HJ, Kim ST, Yeon JE, Byun KS, Bak YT, Lee CH (2002) Simultaneous duodenal and colon masses as late presentation of metastatic renal cell carcinoma. Korean J Intern Med 17:143–146

Leiman G, Markowitz S, Veiga-Ferreira MM, Margolius KA (1986) Renal adenocarcinoma presenting with bilateral metastases to Bartholin's glands: primary diagnosis by aspiration cytology. Diagn Cytopathol 2:252–255

Li L, Friedrich RE, Schmelzle R, Donath K (2001) Metachronous bilateral metastases of renal cell carcinoma to the parotid region. J Oral Maxillofac Surg 59:434–438

Lim DJ, Carter MF (1993) Computerized tomography in the preoperative staging for pulmonary metastases in patients with renal cell carcinoma. J Urol 150:1112–1114

Limani K, Matos C, Hut F, Gelin M, Closset J (2003) Metastatic carcinoma of the gallbladder after a renal cell carcinoma. Acta Chir Belg 103:233–234

Lokich J (1997) Spontaneous regression of metastatic renal cancer. Case report and literature review. Am J Clin Oncol 20:416–418

Mahnken AH, Tacke J (2000) Myocardial heart metastasis in rapidly progressing renal cell carcinoma. Rofo 172:488–490

Marshall ME, Pearson T, Simpson W, Butler K, McRoberts W (1990) Low incidence of asymptomatic brain metastases in patients with renal cell carcinoma. Urology 36:300–302

Marusch F, Koch A, Dietrich F, Hoschke B, Gastinger I (2001) Singular late metastasis of renal cell carcinoma in the pancreas. An unusual pancreatic tumor. Zentralbl Chir 126:391–395

Mascarenhas B, Konety B, Rubin JT (2001) Recurrent metastatic renal cell carcinoma presenting as a bleeding gastric ulcer after a complete response to high-dose interleukin-2 treatment. Urology 57:168

Mattana J, Kurtz B, Miah A, Singhal PC (1996) Renal cell carcinoma presenting as a solitary anterior superior mediastinal mass. J Med 27:205–210

Maxwell M, Borges LF, Zervas NT (1999) Renal cell carcinoma: a rare source of cauda equina metastasis. Case report. J Neurosurg Spine 90:129–132

May M, Marusch F, Kaufmann O, Seehafer M, Helke C, Hoschke B, Gastinger I (2003) Solitary renal cell carcinoma metastasis to the thyroid gland: a paradigm of metastasectomy? Chirurg 74:768–774

McGregor DH, Wu Y, Weston AP, McAnaw MP, Bromfield C, Bhattatiry MM (2003) Metastatic renal cell carcinoma of spleen diagnosed by fine-needle aspiration. Am J Med Sci 326:51–54

Mearini L, Zucchi A, Pizzirusso G, Costantini E, Mearini E (2004) Renal papillary adenocarcinoma with unusual metastases: case report and review of the literature. Arch Ital Urol Androl 76:88–90

Merine D, Fishman EK (1988) Mediastinal adenopathy and endobronchial involvement in metastatic renal cell carcinoma. J Comput Tomogr 12:216–219

Mesurolle B, Mignon F, Travagli JP, Meingan P, Vanel D (1997) Late presentation of solitary contralateral adrenal metastasis of renal cell carcinoma. Eur Radiol 7:557–558

Mignon F, Mesurolle B (2003) Local recurrence and metastatic dissemination of renal cell carcinoma: clinical and imaging characteristics. J Radiol 84:275–284

Mignon F, Mesurolle B, Sissakian JF, Bruckert F, Guichoux F, Barre O, Chagnon S, Lacombe P (1999) Late solitary metastasis of a renal cancer to the contralateral adrenal gland. J Radiol 80:939–942

Mizuo T, Ohashi H, Tanizawa A, Okuno T (1990) Complete resolution of multiple pulmonary metastases of renal cell carcinoma following intravenous drip infusion of r-interleukin 2: a case report. Hinyokika Kiyo 36:931–935

Monteros-Sanchez AE de los, Medina-Franco H, Arista-Nasr J, Cortes-Gonzalez R (2004) Resection of an esophageal metastasis from a renal cell carcinoma. Hepatogastroenterology 51:163–164

Motzer RJ, Bander NH, Nanus DM (1996) Renal-cell carcinoma. N Engl J Med 335:865–875

Moudouni SM, En-Nia I, Rioux-Leclerq N, Manunta A, Guille F, Lobel B (2001) Prostatic metastasis of renal cell carcinoma. J Urol 165:190–191

Munk PL, Gock S, Gee R, Connell DG, Quenville NF (1992) Case report 708: Metastasis of renal cell carcinoma to skeletal muscle (right trapezius). Skeletal Radiol 21:56–59

Murakami R, Taniai N, Kumazaki T, Kobayashi Y, Ogura J, Ichikawa T (2000) Rupture of a hepatic metastasis from renal cell carcinoma. Clin Imaging 24:72–74

Muram TM, Aisen A (2003) Fatty metastatic lesions in 2 patients with renal clear-cell carcinoma. J Comput Assist Tomogr 27:869–870

Nabeyama R, Tanaka K, Matsuda S, Iwamoto Y (2001) Multiple intramuscular metastases 15 years after radical nephrectomy in a patient with stage IV renal cell carcinoma. J Orthop Sci 6:189–192

Nabi G, Gania MA, Sharma MC (2001) Solitary delayed contralateral testicular metastasis from renal cell carcinoma. Indian J Pathol Microbiol 44:487–488

Nagler J, McSherry CK, Miskovitz P (1994) Asymptomatic metachronous metastatic renal cell adenocarcinoma to the gallbladder. Report of a case and guidelines for evaluation of intraluminal polypoid gallbladder masses. Dig Dis Sci 39:2476–2479

Nakada SY, Johnson DB, Hahnfeld L, Jarrard DF (2002) Resection of isolated fossa recurrence of renal-cell carcinoma after nephrectomy using hand-assisted laparoscopy. J Endourol 16:687–688

Navarro F, Vicente J, Villanueva MJ, Sanchez A, Provencio M, Espana P (2000) Metastatic renal cell carcinoma to the head and neck area. Tumori 86:88–90

Newmark JR, Newmark GM, Epstein JI, Marshall FF (1994) Solitary late recurrence of renal cell carcinoma. Urology 43:725–728

Ng CS, Loyer EM, Iyer RB, David CL, DuBrow RA, Charnsangavej C (1999) Metastases to the pancreas from renal cell carcinoma: findings on three-phase contrast-enhanced helical CT. Am J Roentgenol 172:1555–1559

Nozawa H, Tsuchiya M, Kobayashi T, Morita H, Kobayashi I, Sakaguchi M, Mizutani T, Tajima A, Kishida Y, Yakumaru K, Kagami H, Sekikawa T (2003) Small intestinal metastasis from renal cell carcinoma exhibiting rare findings. Int J Clin Pract 57:329–331

Nussbaum ES, Djalilian HR, Cho KH, Hall WA (1996) Brain metastases. Histology, multiplicity, surgery, and survival. Cancer 78:1781–1788

O'Brien WM, Lynch JH (1987) Adrenal metastases by renal cell carcinoma. Incidence at nephrectomy. Urology 29:605–607

Odori T, Tsuboi Y, Katoh K, Yamada K, Morita K, Ohara A, Kuroiwa M, Sakamoto H, Sakata T (1998) A solitary hematogenous metastasis to the gastric wall from renal cell carcinoma four years after radical nephrectomy. J Clin Gastroenterol 26:153–154

Ohgou T, Okahara M, Kishimoto T (1998) Renal cell carcinoma with many transvenous pleural metastases. Nihon Kokyuki Gakkai Zasshi 36:369–373

Okabe Y, Ohoka H, Miwa T, Nagayama I, Furukawa M (1992) View from beneath: pathology in focus. Renal cell carcinoma metastasis to the tongue. J Laryngol Otol 106:282–284

Omland H, Fossa SD (1989) Spontaneous regression of cerebral and pulmonary metastases in renal cell carcinoma. Scand J Urol Nephrol 23:159–160

Pantuck AJ, Zisman A, Dorey F, Chao DH, Han KR, Said J, Gitlitz BJ, Figlin RA, Belldegrun AS (2003) Renal cell carcinoma with retroperitoneal lymph nodes: role of lymph node dissection. J Urol 169:2076–2083

Park DY, Kim YM, Chi JG (1997) Intracranial metastasis from clear cell sarcoma of the kidney: a case report. J Korean Med Sci 12:473–476

Park YW, Hlivko TJ (2002) Parotid gland metastasis from renal cell carcinoma. Laryngoscope 112:453–456

Pavlakis GM, Sakorafas GH, Anagnostopoulos GK (2004) Intestinal metastases from renal cell carcinoma: a rare cause of intestinal obstruction and bleeding. Mt Sinai J Med 71:127–130

Pilecki SE, Cieslinski K, Lasek WL, Purzycka-Jazdon AM, Lambrecht W (2002) Metastasis of renal carcinoma to the diaphragm. Wiad Lek 55:120–124

Pretorius ES, Fishman EK (2000) Helical CT of skeletal muscle metastases from primary carcinomas. Am J Roentgenol 174:401–404

Pursner M, Petchprapa C, Haller JO, Orentlicher RJ (1997) Renal carcinoma: bilateral breast metastases in a child. Pediatr Radiol 27:242–243

Rabinovitch RA, Zelefsky MJ, Gaynor JJ, Fuks Z (1994) Patterns of failure following surgical resection of renal cell carcinoma: implications for adjuvant local and systemic therapy. J Clin Oncol 12:206–212

Radley MG, McDonald JV, Pilcher WH, Wilbur DC (1993) Late solitary cerebral metastases from renal cell carcinoma: report of two cases. Surg Neurol 39:230–234

Raptopoulos VD, Blake SP, Weisinger K, Atkins MB, Keogan MT, Kruskal JB (2001) Multiphase contrast-enhanced helical CT of liver metastases from renal cell carcinoma. Eur Radiol 11:2504–2509

Ravi R, Tongaonkar HB, Kulkarni JN, Kamat MR (1992) Synchronous bilateral parotid metastases from renal cell carcinoma. A case report. Indian J Cancer 29:40–42

Raviv S, Eggener SE, Williams DH, Garnett JE, Pins MR, Smith ND (2002) Long-term survival after "drop metastases" of renal cell carcinoma to the bladder. Urology 60:697

Ritchie AW, Layfield LJ, deKernion JB (1988) Spontaneous regression of liver metastasis from renal carcinoma. J Urol 140:596–597

Rivoire M, Voiglio EJ (1996) Late pancreatic metastases from renal cell carcinoma. Surgery 119:240

Robertson GS, Gertler SL (1990) Late presentation of metastatic renal cell carcinoma as a bleeding ampullary mass. Gastrointest Endosc 36:304–306

Russo P (2003) Seeking the solution to the problem of metastatic renal carcinoma. Cancer 97:2941–2944

Rypens F, Van Gansbeke D, Lambilliotte JP, Van Regemorter G, Verhest A, Struyven J (1992) Pancreatic metastasis from renal cell carcinoma. Br J Radiol 65:547–548

Safi AM, Rachko M, Sadeghinia S, Zineldin A, Dong J, Stein RA (2003) Left ventricular intracavitary mass and pericarditis secondary to metastatic renal cell carcinoma: a case report. Angiology 54:495–498

Sagalowsky AI, Molberg K (1999) Solitary metastasis of renal cell carcinoma to the contralateral adrenal gland 22 years after nephrectomy. Urology 54:162

Saidi JA, Newhouse JH, Sawczuk IS (1998) Radiologic follow-up of patients with T1-3a,b,c or T4N+M0 renal cell carcinoma after radical nephrectomy. Urology 52:1000–1003

Saitoh H, Nakayama M, Nakamura K, Satoh T (1982) Distant metastasis of renal adenocarcinoma in nephrectomized cases. J Urol 127:1092–1095

Sanchez-Ortiz RF, Tannir N, Ahrar K, Wood CG (2003) Spontaneous regression of pulmonary metastases from renal cell carcinoma after radio frequency ablation of primary tumor: an in situ tumor vaccine? J Urol 170:178–179

Santo-Tomas M, Mahr NC, Robinson MJ, Agatston AS (1998) Metastatic renal cell carcinoma invading right ventricular myocardium without caval involvement. J Cardiovasc Surg (Torino) 39:811–812

Savas MC, Celik I, Benekli M, Gullu IH, Tekuzman G (1998) Renal cell carcinoma presenting as solitary cervical node metastasis compressing the brachial plexus. Nephron 79:107–108

Scatarige JC, Sheth S, Corl FM, Fishman EK (2001a) Patterns of recurrence in renal cell carcinoma: manifestations on helical CT. Am J Roentgenol 177:653–658

Scatarige JC, Horton KM, Sheth S, Fishman EK (2001b) Pancreatic parenchymal metastases: observations on helical CT. Am J Roentgenol 176:695–699

Schatteman P, Willemsen P, Vanderveken M, Lockefeer F, Vandebroek A (2002) Skeletal muscle metastasis from a conventional renal cell carcinoma, two years after nephrectomy: a case report. Acta Chir Belg 102:351–352

Schijns OE, Kurt E, Wessels P, Luijckx GJ, Beuls EA (2000) Intramedullary spinal cord metastasis as a first manifestation of a renal cell carcinoma: report of a case and review of the literature. Clin Neurol Neurosurg 102:249–254

Schmidt M, Schmidt T, Ugi I (1994) Orbital metastasis of kidney carcinoma. Klin Monatsbl Augenheilkd 205:40–43

Seaman EK, Ross S, Sawczuk IS (1995) High incidence of asymptomatic brain lesions in metastatic renal cell carcinoma. J Neurooncol 23:253–256

Selli C, Carini M, Barbanti G, Barbagli G, Turini D (1987) Simultaneous bilateral adrenal involvement by renal cell carcinoma: experience with 3 cases. J Urol 137:480–482

Shiono S, Yoshida J, Nishimura M, Nitadori J, Ishii G, Nishiwaki Y, Nagai K (2004) Late pulmonary metastasis of renal cell carcinoma resected 25 years after nephrectomy. Jpn J Clin Oncol 34:46–49

Shiraishi K, Mohri J, Inoue R, Kamiryo Y (2003) Metastatic renal cell carcinoma to the bladder 12 years after radical nephrectomy. Int J Urol 10:453–455

Siemer S, Lehmann J, Kamradt J, Loch T, Remberger K, Humke U, Ziegler M, Stockle M (2004) Adrenal metastases in 1635 patients with renal cell carcinoma: outcome and indication for adrenalectomy. J Urol 171:2155–2159

Simo R, Sykes AJ, Hargreaves SP, Axon PR, Birzgalis AR, Slevin NJ, Farrington WT (2000) Metastatic renal cell carcinoma to the nose and paranasal sinuses. Head Neck 22:722–727

Slamovits TL, Burde RM (1988) Bumpy muscles. Surv Ophthalmol 33:189–199

Som PM, Norton KI, Shugar JM, Reede DL, Norton L, Biller HF, Som ML (1987) Metastatic hypernephroma to the head and neck. Am J Neuroradiol 8:1103–1106

Srinivasan S, Gray DG (2003) Images in clinical medicine. Choroidal metastasis from renal-cell carcinoma. N Engl J Med 349:e22

Stattaus J, Mertens H, Mackowski JM, Hacklander T, Cramer BM (1999) Metastases of renal cell carcinoma to the pancreas and gallbladder: possibilities and limits of MRI diagnosis. Rofo Fortschr Geb Rontgenstr Neuen Bildgeb Verfahr 170:598–600

Strijk SP (1989) Pancreatic metastases of renal cell carcinoma: report of two cases. Gastrointest Radiol 14:123–126

Studer UE, Scherz S, Scheidegger J, Kraft R, Sonntag R, Ackermann D, Zingg EJ (1990) Enlargement of regional lymph nodes in renal cell carcinoma is often not due to metastases. J Urol 144:243–245

Suzuki M, Machida T, Masuda F, Yanagisawa M, Tashiro K, Onishi T, Kishimoto K, Ishikawa E (1982) A case of renal cell carcinoma invading the spleen. Nippon Hinyokika Gakkai Zasshi 73:1333–1337

Szymanski M, Szymanska A, Morshed K, Siwiec H (2004) Renal cell carcinoma metastases to nose and paranasal sinuses presenting as recurrent epistaxis. Wiad Lek 57:94–96

Takada T, Doita M, Nishida K, Miura J, Yoshiya S, Kurosaka M (2003) Unusual metastasis to the cauda equina from renal cell carcinoma. Spine 28:E114–E117

Tapper H, Klein H, Rubenstein W, Intriere L, Choi Y, Kazam E (1997) Recurrent renal cell carcinoma after 45 years. Clin Imaging 21:273–275

Tartar VM, Heiken JP, McClennan BL (1991) Renal cell carcinoma presenting with diffuse peritoneal metastases: CT findings. J Comput Assist Tomogr 15:450–453

Tatsuta M, Shiozaki K, Masutani S, Hashimoto K, Imamura H, Ikeda M, Miya A, Ishida H, Kawasaki T, Furukawa H, Satomi T, Hoshida Y (2001) Splenic and pulmonary metastases from renal cell carcinoma: report of a case. Surg Today 31:463–465

Tharakan J, Iasacs P, Morris EA (1995) Renal carcinoma metastases presenting as duodenal obstruction. Am J Gastroenterol 90:683–684

Thoroddsen A, Gudbjartsson T, Geirsson G, Agnarsson BA, Magnusson K (2002) Spontaneous regression of pleural metastases after nephrectomy for renal cell carcinoma: a histologically verified case with nine-year follow-up. Scand J Urol Nephrol 36:396–398

Thrasher JB, Paulson DF (1993) Prognostic factors in renal cancer. Urol Clin North Am 20:247–262

Tomita T, Inouye T, Shinden S, Ogawa K, Mukai M (1998) Palliative radiotherapy for lingual metastasis of renal cell carcinoma. Auris Nasus Larynx 25:209–214

Toye R, Jones DK, Armstrong P, Richman PI (1990) Numerous pulmonary metastases from renal cell carcinoma confined to the middle lobe. Clin Radiol 42:443–444

Trufflandier N, Gille O, Palussiere J, Prie L, Pointillart V, Ravaud A (2002) Symptomatic neurological epidural metastasis with interleukin-2 therapy in metastatic renal cell carcinoma. Tumori 88:338–340

Uchino A, Hasuo K, Mizushima A, Matsumoto S, Mihara F, Jimi M, Takahashi M, Masuda K (1996) Intracranial metastasis of renal cell carcinoma: MR imaging. Radiat Med 14:71–76

Vassalli L, Ferrari VD, Simoncini E, Rangoni G, Montini E, Marpicati P, Mambrini A, Pagani M, Agazzi C, Marini G (2001) Solitary breast metastases from a renal cell carcinoma. Breast Cancer Res Treat 68:29–31

Vespasiani G, Porena M, Virgili G, Costantini E, Bonacina R, Mearini E, Rosi P, Micali F (1990) Renal cell carcinoma with synchronous adrenal metastases. Acta Urol Belg 58:197–203

Vleeming R, Dabhoiwala NF, Bosch DA (1994) Ten years survival after recurrent intracranial metastases from a renal cell carcinoma. Br J Neurosurg 8:229–231

Ware GT, Haik BG, Morris WR (1999) Renal cell carcinoma with involvement of iris and conjunctiva. Am J Ophthalmol 127:460–461

Wyczolkowski M, Klima W, Bieda W, Walas K (2001) Spontaneous regression of hepatic metastases after nephrectomy and metastasectomy of renal cell carcinoma. Urol Int 66:119–120

Yamashita K, Yamamoto M, Nishimura H, Akiyama H, Tsuchiya E, Tanaka S (2000) Hilar lymph node metastasis in renal cell carcinoma. Jpn J Thorac Cardiovasc Surg 48:194–197

Yavascaoglu I, Korun N, Oktay B, Simsek U, Ozyurt M (1999) Renal cell carcinoma with solitary synchronous pancreaticoduodenal and metachronous periprostatic metastases: report of a case. Surg Today 29:364–366

Yokoyama Y, Sato S, Kawaguchi T, Saito Y (1998) A case of concurrent uterine cervical adenocarcinoma and renal-cell carcinoma, and subsequent vaginal metastasis from the renal-cell carcinoma. J Obstet Gynaecol Res 24:37–43

Yu CC, Huang JK, Tzeng WS, Wu JD, Lee YH, Jiaan BP (1992) Simultaneous bilateral adrenal metastases from renal cell carcinoma. Surgical implications and review of the literature. Eur Urol 22:335–338

Zhao B, Kimura W, Futakawa N, Muto T, Haida K (1997) Renal cell carcinoma of the spindle cell type with metastasis to the pancreas: a case report. Jpn J Clin Oncol 27:58–61

17 Imaging of Bone Metastases

Heung Sik Kang and Jung Ah Choi

CONTENTS

17.1
Introduction

Renal cell carcinoma is the most common malignant neoplasm of the kidney. About 25,000 cases are diagnosed annually in the United States (Brodsky and Garnick 1989), of which 20–60% have distant metastases at the time of diagnosis (Bohnenkamp et al. 1980; Skinner et al. 1971; Takashi et al. 1995). These metastases account for about 10% of all pathologic bone fractures and 5% of cases with spinal cord compression (Nielsen et al. 1991).

Following the lung, the skeleton is the second most common site of metastasis, accounting for about 20–40% of metastases (Bohnenkamp et al. 1980; Henriksson et al. 1992). In many cases, the metastasis is diagnosed before the primary tumor. In fact, renal cell carcinoma is said to be the prototype of a tumor that presents as skeletal metastasis with a clinically occult primary tumor (Tongaonkar et

H. S. Kang, MD, PhD
Professor, Department of Radiology, President, Seoul National University Bundang Hospital, Seoul National University College of Medicine, 300 Gumi-dong, Bundang-gu, Seong Nam, Gyeonggi-Do 463-707, South Korea
J. A. Choi, MD, PhD
Instructor, Department of Radiology, Seoul National University Bundang Hospital, Seoul National University College of Medicine, 300 Gumi-dong, Bundang-gu, Seong Nam, Gyeonggi-Do 463-707, South Korea

al. 1992). Such cases comprise up to 48% of patients with osseous involvement (Nielsen et al. 1991) and 4% of all patients with renal cell carcinoma (Forbes et al. 1977); therefore, renal cell carcinoma must be strongly considered among differential diagnoses for any metastatic bone tumor with an unknown primary tumor (Dorfman and Czerniak 1998).

Solitary osseous metastases are relatively frequent in renal cell carcinoma, occurring in 2.5% of all renal cell carcinoma patients (Ghert et al. 2001; Saitoh 1981; Tongaonkar et al. 1992; Wilner 1982). Conversely, the most common site of solitary metastases is bone (Althausen et al. 1997; Saitoh 1981; Tongaonkar et al. 1992). Dissemination by solitary or multiple metastases will occur eventually in up to 50% of patients initially treated for localized disease (Henriksson et al. 1992; Saitoh 1981), sometimes following a long quiescent period of 10, 20, or even 30 or more years after removal of the primary tumor (Forbes et al. 1977). The reason for this long quiescent period is unknown; hypotheses include an underlying tumor-host interaction or an immune response (Hrushesky and Murphy 1973; Varkarakis et al. 1974).

Partial or complete regression of metastatic renal cell carcinoma has been reported, either spontaneously or associated with reduction of the primary tumor burden (Fidler 1992; Ibayashi et al. 1993; Kerbl and Pauer 1993); however, the reported prognoses vary widely, from dismal in some reports, with an average life expectancy of 12–24 months or even less (Dekernion et al. 1978; Jung et al. 2003; Middleton 1967; Montie et al. 1977; Skinner et al. 1971; Thompson et al. 1975), to more favorable in others, with more than a 50% survival rate after 5 years (Althausen et al. 1997).

Although the majority of skeletal metastases from renal cell carcinoma are relatively resistant to radiation and chemotherapy (Jung et al. 2003), patients with a solitary metastasis are known to have prolonged survival, especially after aggressive therapy such as radical surgical excision (Dineen et al. 1988; Huguenin et al. 1998; Middleton 1967; Montie et al. 1977; Tolia and Whitmore 1975; Tongaonkar et al. 1992). Surgical resection of solitary skeletal metastases has been reported to significantly prolong life (Kozlowski 1994; Smith et al. 1992; Takashi et al. 1995); therefore, it is important to recognize and diagnose skeletal metastases, to provide appropriate treatment, and to prolong survival.

17.2
Pathophysiology

Metastatic renal cell carcinomas typically have clear cell features, which are seen on microscopic examination of biopsy samples of skeletal metastases (Fig. 17.1) and which suggest a primary tumor of renal origin. About 10% of renal cell carcinomas undergo dedifferentiation into high-grade spindle cell or pleomorphic sarcomatoid carcinoma. When sarcomatoid elements are the only components present in the metastatic lesions, the lesion may be misdiagnosed as a primary bone lesion, such as a fibrosarcoma or malignant fibrous histiocytoma. In such cases, clinical findings together with appropriate markers may help to identify the metastatic nature of the lesion (Dorfman and Czerniak 1998).

Renal cell carcinomas are highly vascular tumors, and similar to their primary tumors, osseous metastases are reported to be hypervascular in 65–75% of cases (Barton et al. 1996). Life-threatening blood loss at surgery may be reduced by preoperative angi-

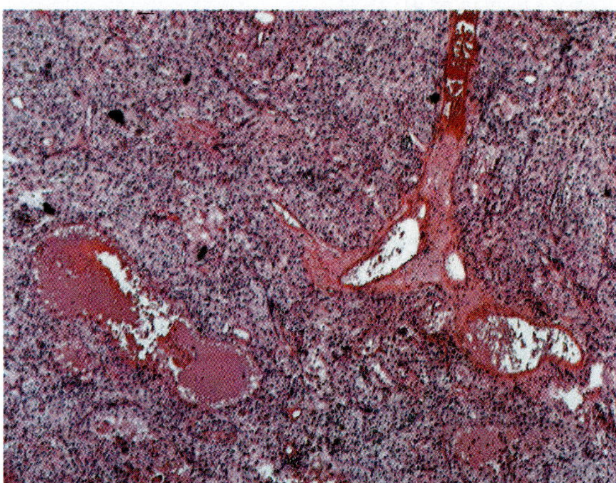

Fig. 17.1. Microscopic findings of metastatic renal cell carcinoma in the femur of a 66-year-old man. Numerous vascular structures with red blood cells surrounded by tubules and nests of cells containing small nuclei set in abundant and clear cytoplasm can be seen (Hematoxylin and eosin stain; original magnification, ×100).

ography and embolization (Layelle et al. 1998; Sun and Lang 1998).

Renal cell carcinoma spreads mainly in three ways: (a) by direct extension; (b) by involvement of lymphatic channels, including lymph nodes of the renal pedicle, that ultimately drain into the paraaortic, hilar, paratracheal, and mediastinal regions; and (c) by invasion of renal veins with subsequent extension to the inferior vena cava, right atrium, and pulmonary vessels, which results in pulmonary metastasis (Kim et al. 1983; Resnick and Niwayama 1995; Wilner 1982). Paravertebral vein plexus involvement results in metastasis to the axial skeleton (Kim et al. 1983).

17.3
Imaging Findings

17.3.1
Radiographic Findings

The most common sites of metastasis are the thoracolumbar spine, pelvic bone, ribs, and proximal humerus and femur, with solitary metastases most often found in the pelvis, spine, and long tubular bones (Resnick and Niwayama 1995; Saitoh 1981; Wilner 1982). Metastases in the small bones of the extremities are also reported (Forbes et al. 1977; Ghert et al. 2001). Most lesions develop in the metaphysis, but epiphyseal extension or diaphyseal lesions are also observed (Forbes et al. 1977).

The predominant radiographic finding is osteolysis (Resnick and Niwayama 1995). The lesions are either purely osteolytic or predominantly osteolytic in about 90% of cases (Figs. 17.2a, 17.3a; Wilner 1982). Mixed osteolytic and osteosclerotic patterns are found in only a minority of lesions (Fig. 17.4; Wilner 1982). Very occasionally, osteoblastic metastasis has been reported (Neugut et al. 1981). Lytic lesions may consist of a single large lytic lesion (Fig. 17.5) or patchy moth-eaten areas of bone destruction (Fig. 17.4; Wilner 1982).

Cortical involvement is another predominant and constant feature of the metastatic lesions. Erosion or gross destruction of the cortex may be present (Figs. 17.6, 17.7a; Forbes et al. 1977; Wilner 1982). Most lesions extend into the surrounding soft tissue after local destruction of the cortex; Less frequently, intramedullary extension with widening and endosteal scalloping of the lesions occurs (Fig. 17.8; Forbes et al. 1977). Periosteal reaction is rare, and if pres-

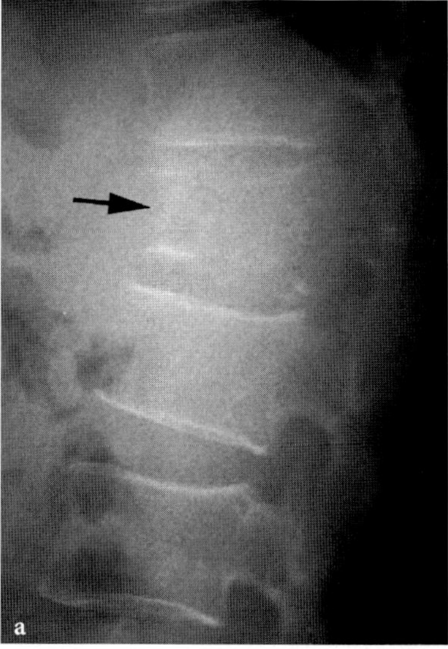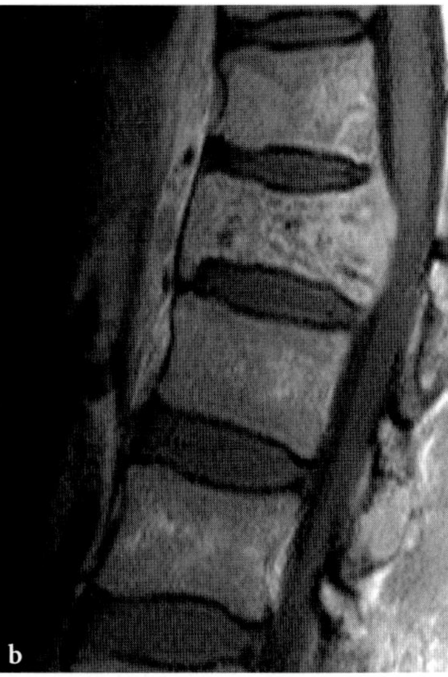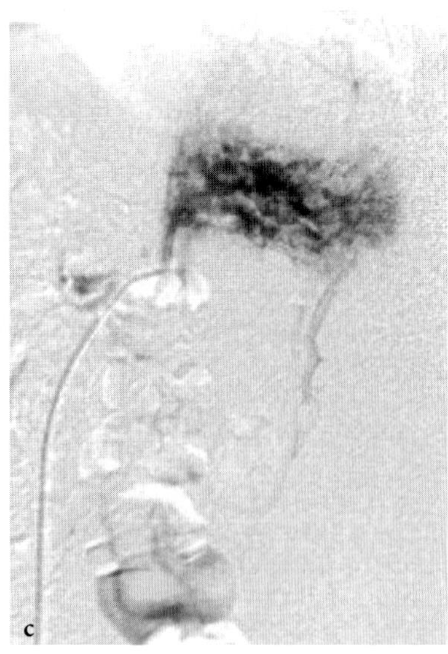

Fig. 17.2a-c. Osteolytic vertebral bone metastasis in a 54-year-old man. **a** Lateral radiograph of lumbar spine shows an osteolytic lesion at the L1 vertebral body (*arrow*), with anterior wedging, indicative of compression fracture. **b** Sagittal spin-echo T1-weighted MR image shows intermediate signal intensity masses in the T12 and L1 vertebral bodies with multiple dot-like and tubular hypointense structures within the L1 vertebral body. **c** Lateral selective angiogram shows engorged vessels with arteriovenous shunting in the L1 vertebral body. (With permission from CHOI et al. 2003)

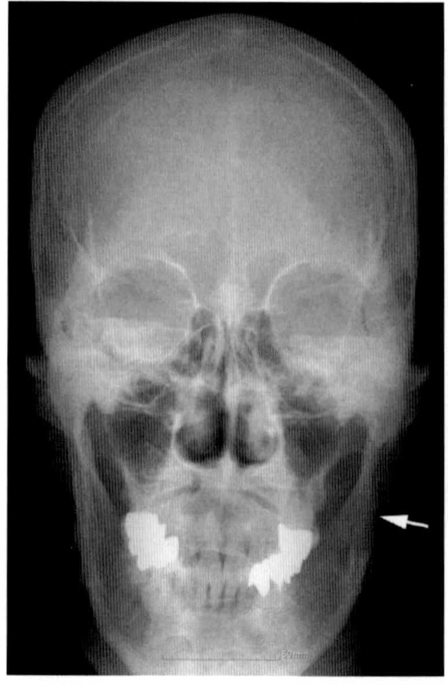

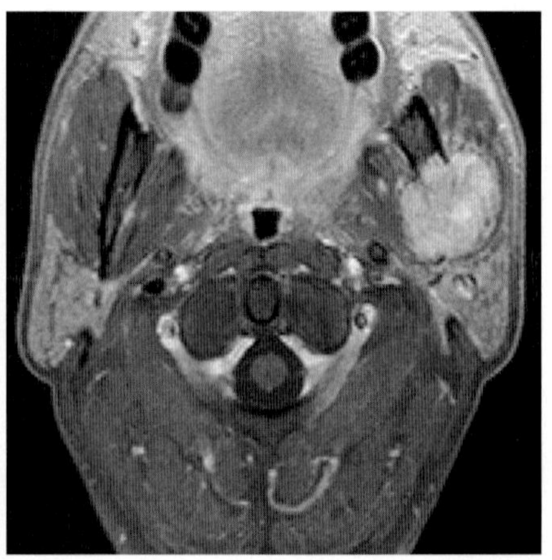

Fig. 17.3a,b. Osteolytic bone metastasis in a 64-year-old man. **a** Anteroposterior radiograph of the skull shows an osteolytic bone lesion of the left mandible ramus (*arrow*). **b** Axial contrast-enhanced fat-suppressed T1-weighted MR image shows enhancing, lobulated soft tissue mass replacing the destroyed bone in the left mandibular ramus.

ent, only faint or moderate (WILNER 1982). Margination has been described as indistinct in most cases (Fig. 17.9; FORBES et al. 1977), and more apparent than in other metastases (Figs. 17.5, 17.10a) in other reports (WILNER 1982). Margination may become more distinct after radiation therapy, but this does not have favorable implications (FORBES et al. 1977).

Another feature of the metastatic lesions is a septate appearance (Fig. 17.10a), with large, well-defined, coarse, heavy septa that traverse the area of destruction, and which is seen in about 17% of cases (WILNER 1982). Although in some studies the septate form has been deemed distinctive enough to suggest that the primary tumor is a renal cell carcinoma (WILNER 1982), the findings are neither sensitive nor specific and cannot be considered pathognomonic.

Another feature is the presence of a periosteal soft tissue mass (Figs. 17.3b, 17.11), which is related to the

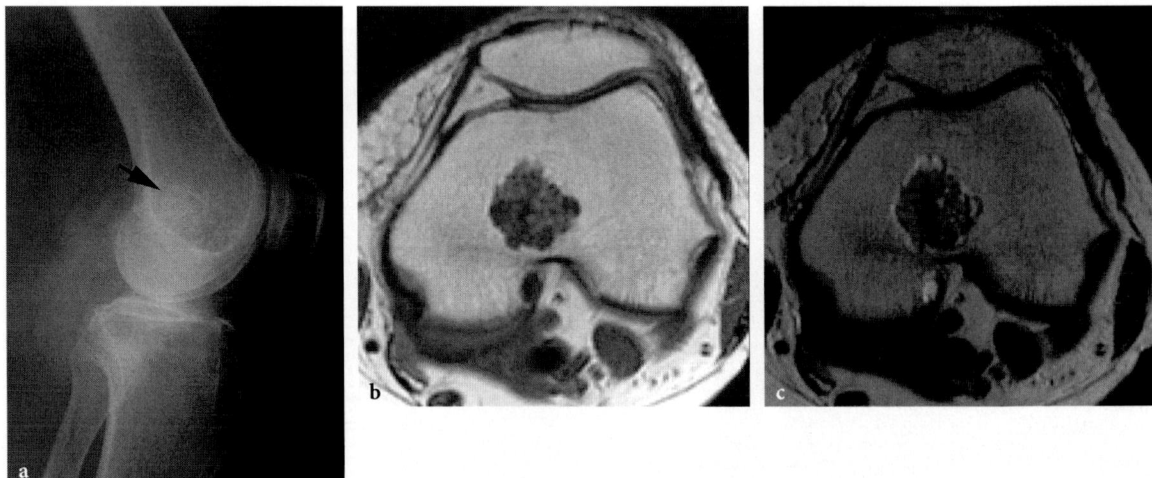

Fig. 17.4a-c. Mixed bone metastasis in an 81-year-old woman. **a** Lateral radiograph of the left knee shows an ill-defined permeative lesion with mixed osteolytic and osteoblastic foci (*arrow*) in the left distal femur. This lesion shows mixed signal intensity on axial **b** unenhanced T1- and **c** T2-weighted MR images.

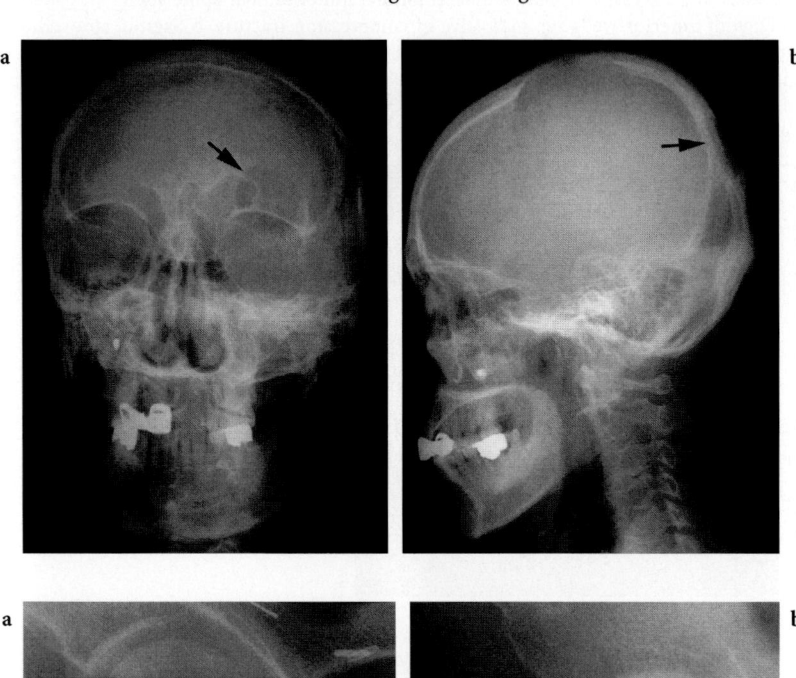

Fig. 17.5a,b. Osteolytic bone metastasis in a 67-year-old man. **a** Anteroposterior and **b** lateral radiographs of the skull show a single, large, relatively well-defined osteolytic lesion (*arrow*) with bulging soft tissue density at the left occipital bone.

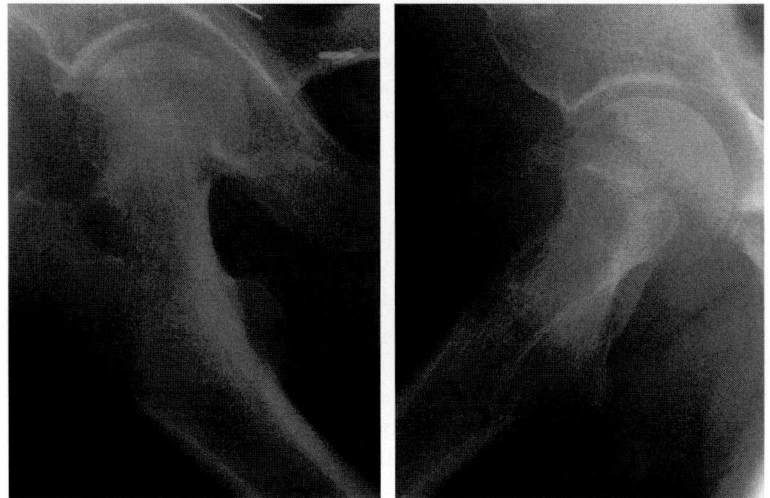

Fig. 17.6a,b. Osteolytic bone metastasis in a 66-year-old man. **a** Anteroposterior and **b** lateral radiographs of the right proximal femur show an ill-defined osteolytic lesion of slightly expansile nature accompanied by focal destruction of the cortex, mainly involving the greater trochanter area.

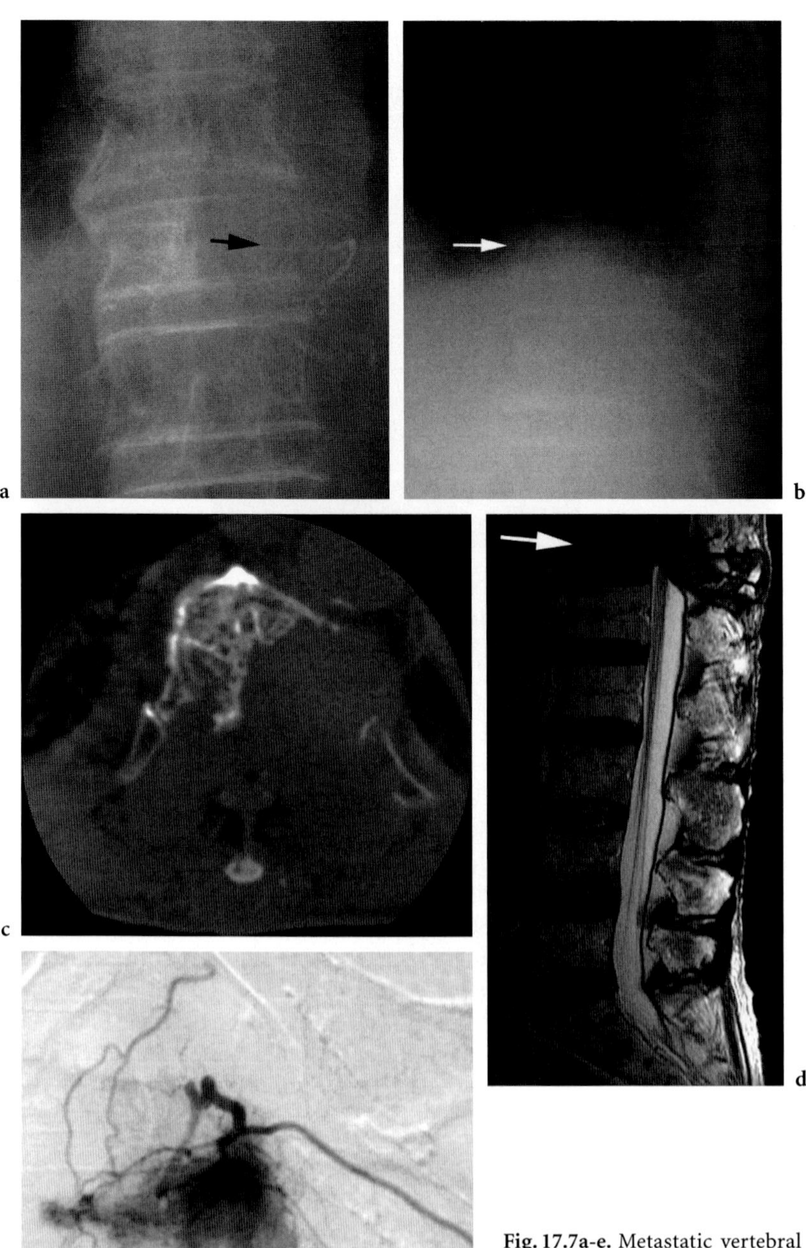

Fig. 17.7a-e. Metastatic vertebral compression fracture in an 87-year-old man. **a** Anteroposterior radiograph of the thoraco-lumbar spine junction shows cortex destruction at the left side of the T12 vertebral body with obliteration of the left pedicle (*arrow*). **b** Lateral radiograph of the thoraco-lumbar spine shows decreased vertebral body height of the T12 vertebral body (*arrow*). **c** Axial CT scan at the level of the T12 shows bone destruction with soft tissue mass formation. **d** Sagittal T2-weighted MR image demonstrates compression fracture with fracture line (*arrow*). **e** Selective angiogram shows hypervascular mass with supply from the T11 intercostal artery.

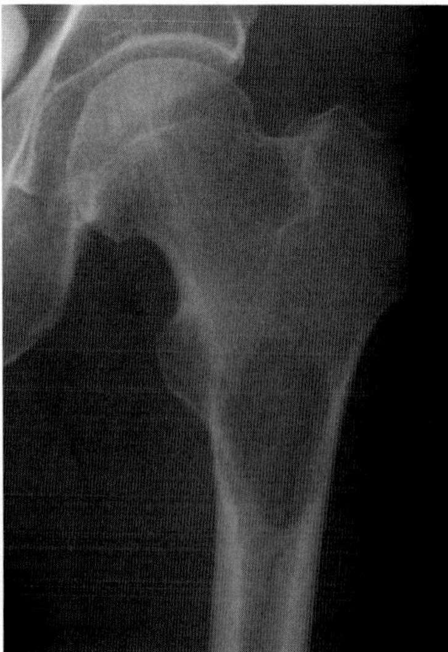

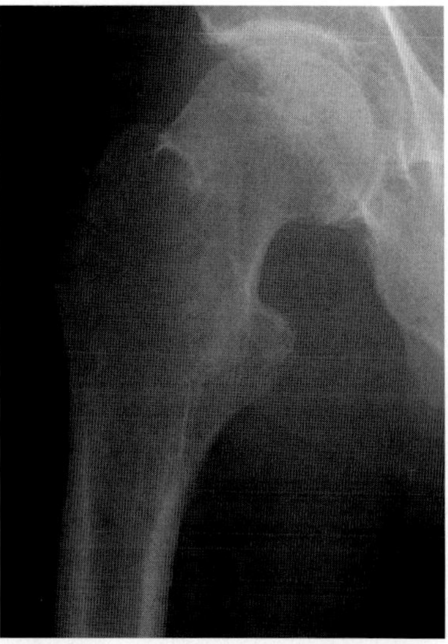

Fig. 17.8. Osteolytic bone metastasis in a 65-year-old man. Anteroposterior radiograph of the left proximal femur shows an ovoid, somewhat ill-defined osteolytic metadiaphyseal lesion with intramedullary extension and slight endosteal scalloping.

Fig. 17.9. Osteolytic bone metastasis in a 67-year-old man. Anteroposterior radiograph of the right proximal femur shows an ill-defined osteolytic metaphyseal lesion.

size of the osseous component of the tumor (FORBES et al. 1977; WILNER 1982). Pathologic fracture may occur, most frequently in the spine (Figs. 17.2a, 17.7b) and long tubular bones, and may be accompanied by marked bone destruction (FORBES et al. 1977; WILNER 1982).

Calcifications are only rarely seen (Fig. 17.11d) before radiation therapy but are seen more frequently in either the adjacent soft tissue or within the bone itself after radiation therapy (FORBES et al. 1977).

Joint destruction or involvement of a synovial-lined joint is unusual, although lesions in the pelvis or sacrum with extension across the sacroiliac joint

are seen occasionally (Fig. 17.12a; FORBES et al. 1977).

When a septate, osteolytic solitary lesion is seen, differential diagnoses may include giant cell tumor, angiomatous lesions, solitary myeloma, and metastatic tumors of nonrenal primary origin (WILNER 1982). When an osteolytic lesion is located in the cortex, further differential diagnoses may include subperiosteal osteosarcoma, chondrosarcoma, or a primary soft tissue sarcoma with bone invasion (COERKAMP and KROON 1988). When a solitary cortical lesion with distinct margin is observed, diagnostic considerations may include fibrous cortical

a

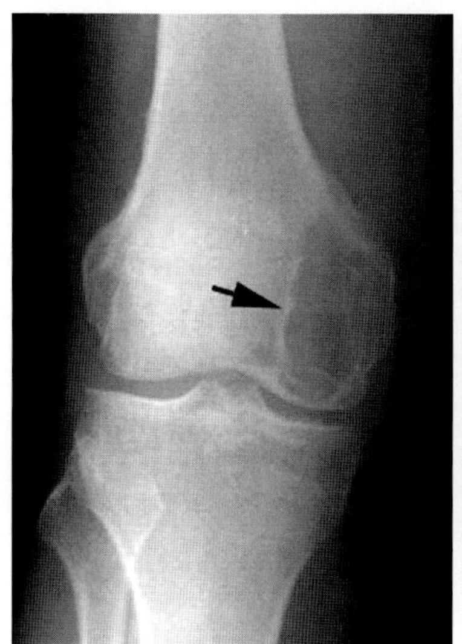

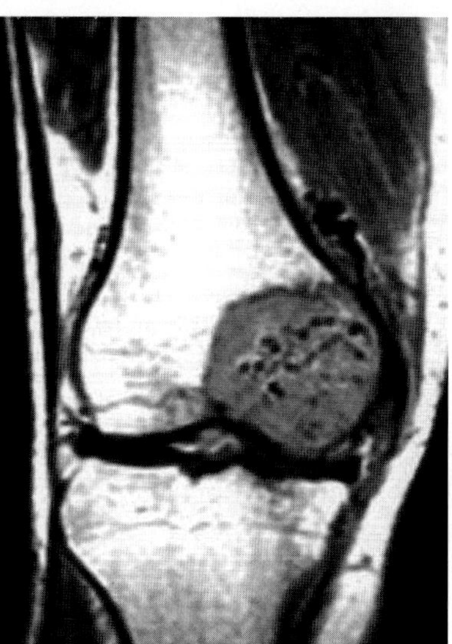

b

Fig. 17.10a,b. Osteolytic bone metastasis in a 61-year-old man. **a** Anteroposterior radiograph of the right knee shows a partially well-defined osteolytic lesion with suspicious internal septa (*arrow*) in the medial femoral condyle epiphysis. **b** Coronal spin-echo T1-weighted MR image shows hypointense mass with multiple, very hypointense dot-like or tubular structures inside and adjacent to the mass. (With permission from CHOI et al. 2003)

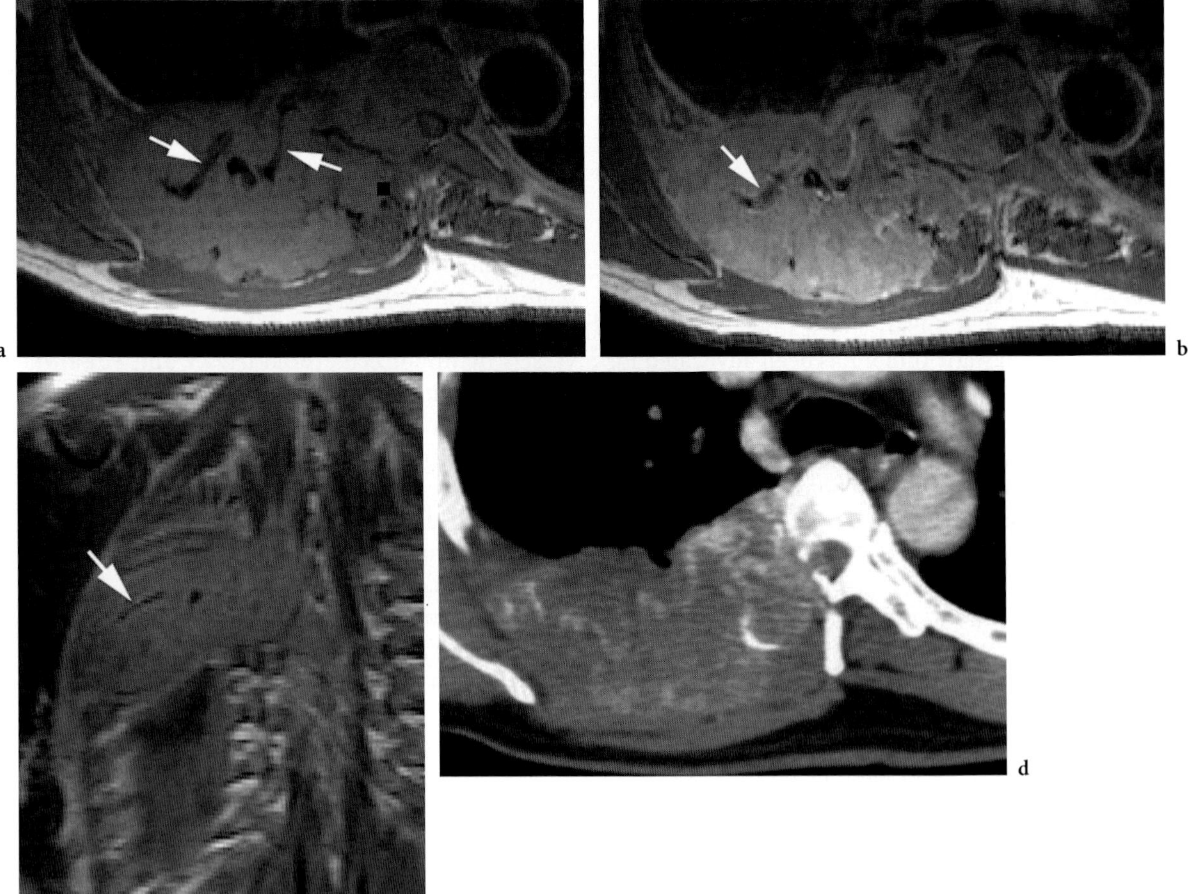

Fig. 17.11a-d. Rib metastasis in a 54-year-old man. **a** Axial unenhanced T1-weighted MR image shows a large hyperintense soft tissue mass lesion with signal intensity higher than muscle. The lesion demonstrates enhancement on **b** axial and **c** coronal contrast-enhanced T1-weighted MR images. On all MR images, multiple tubular and dot-like dark signal intensity structures (*arrows*) are noted within the mass, suggestive of "flow void". **d** Axial CT scan shows hyperdense foci within the lesions, which are partly due to enhancing vessels as well as to calcifications probably from bone destruction. (With permission from CHOI et al. 2003)

defect, brown tumor in hyperparathyroidism, osteoid osteoma, fibrous dysplasia, Brodie abscess, plasmacytoma, adamantinoma, lipoma, or hemangioma (WILLINSKY et al. 1982).

17.3.2
CT and MR Imaging Findings

Little has been reported about the CT and MR imaging findings of metastatic lesions from renal cell carcinoma, probably due to the lack of specificity of the findings. Magnetic resonance imaging has become a common technique for evaluation of bone and soft tissue tumors and yet it lacks specificity. A case report on the tissue characterization of renal cell carcinoma and its osseous metastasis on MR imaging reported similar signal intensities from the renal cell carcinoma and the metastatic lesion (PETTERSSON et al. 1985); however, signal intensity of the lesions varies (CHOI et al. 2003). Most lesions show enhancement well (CHOI et al. 2003). There is a report on the significance of the "flow-void" sign seen in osseous metastases of renal cell carcinoma on MR imaging, which are numerous dot-like or tubular structures of low signal intensity and represent dilated vessels supplying or draining the tumor (Figs. 17.2b, 17.10b, 17.11). Although the sensitivity and specificity of this sign have not been determined, awareness of the sign may help in suggesting the diagnosis and planning treatment of an occult or forgotten primary renal tumor (CHOI et al. 2003).

Both CT and MR imaging may help in visualization of the bone destruction and defining the extent of the tumor (Figs. 17.12a, 17.13). In addition, Computed tomography may help to detect the presence and amount of calcification (Fig. 17.11d) or new bone formation.

17.3.3
Angiography

Angiography reveals the hypervascular nature of the metastatic lesions in renal cell carcinoma (Figs. 17.2c, 17.7e; BOWERS et al. 1982). Transcatheter embolization of the metastatic tumor has been advocated for preoperative arterial embolization to reduce bleeding at surgery, to reduce the viable tumor burden in patients with unresectable metastases, and to relieve pain in intractable cases with bone pain (BARTON et al. 1996; BOWERS et al. 1982).

17.3.4
Radionuclide Imaging

Bone scanning has been deemed superior to radiography, although a normal bone scan result does not mean the absence of bone metastases (COLE et al. 1975; KIM et al. 1983).

Different tracers have been used in skeletal bone scintigraphy for screening of metastases, including Tc-99m methylene diphosphate (MDP), Tc-99m sodium medronate, Tc-99m pyrophosphate, and Tc-99m 2,3 dimercaptosuccinic acid (BORZUTZKY and TURBINER 1985). Scanning of photopenic metastases, i.e., metastases with an absence of uptake on bone scans, may be affected by the following factors: size of the lytic area; relative lack of reactive new bone formation; lack of significant hyperemia; and infarction of area due to obstruction of its supply vessels by tumor cells (BORZUTZKY and TURBINER 1985). The sensitivity of bone scanning is reported to vary, from 33 to 94%, and specificity is reported to be 86% (KOGA et al. 2001; WILNER 1982).

In a relatively recent report, the authors advocated omitting bone scans in patients with stage T1-3aN0M0 tumors and no pain (KOGA et al. 2001); however, bone scans still remain useful in early detection of metastasis and localizing the site of metastasis (Fig. 17.12b; KOGA et al. 2001).

The role of positron emission tomography (PET) in oncology is expanding rapidly (HAIN and MAISEY 2003). In renal cancer, PET can define the primary tumor, provide better staging of local recurrence than CT, and can define metastatic disease (HAIN

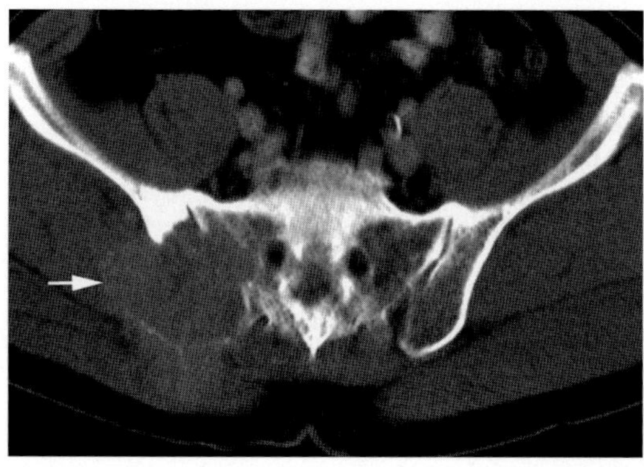

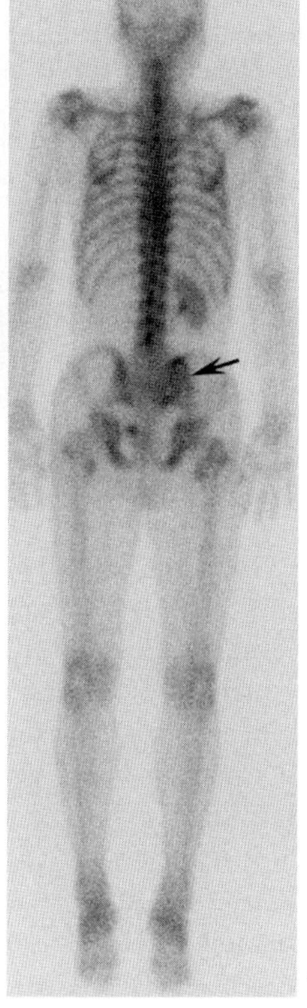

Fig. 17.12a,b. Osteolytic bone metastasis in a 62-year-old man. **a** Axial contrast-enhanced CT scan of the pelvis shows an osteolytic lesion with soft tissue mass formation and extension into the right sacral ala well (*arrow*). **b** Posterior view of whole-body Tc-99m MDP bone scan shows increased uptake around the right sacroiliac joint area (*arrow*).

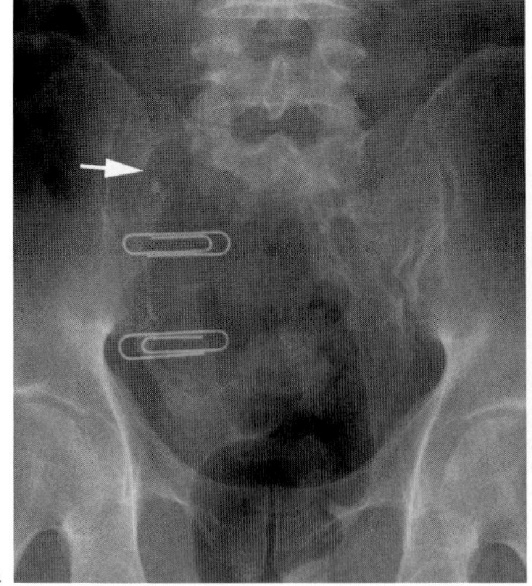
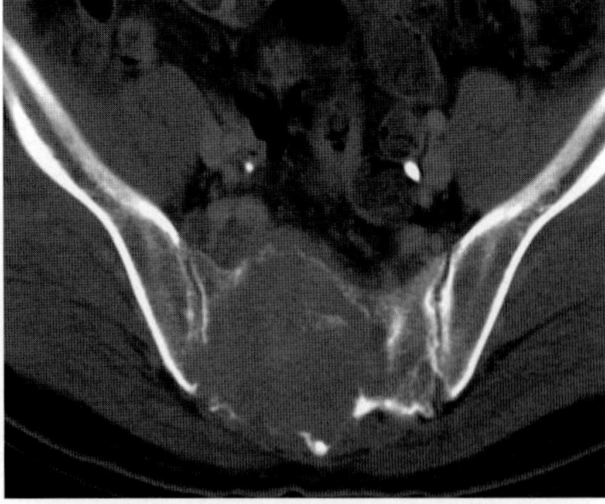
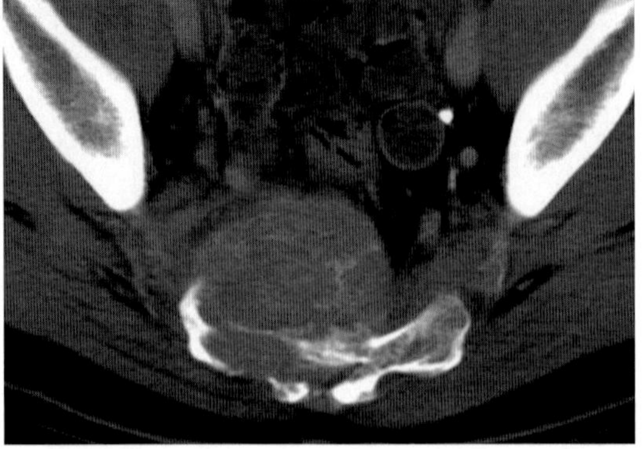

Fig. 17.13a-c. Sacral bone metastasis in a 60-year-old man. **a** Anteroposterior radiograph of the pelvis shows ill-defined osteolytic lesion in right sacral ala (*arrow*). The extent of the lesion is not well visualized due to overlapping large bowel gas. The extent of the bone destruction and soft tissue mass are better defined on axial CT scans (**b, c**) of the pelvis, which show slight extension of the soft tissue mass across the right sacroiliac joint into the right ileum.

and MAISEY 2003). Although PET has been deemed not as good as bone scans for defining bone metastases, there have been case reports in which PET detected bone metastases not identified on bone scanning as well as intramedullary spinal cord metastases (POGGI et al. 2001; SETO et al. 2000). The role of PET in imaging of bone metastases in renal cell carcinoma remains to be clarified.

17.4
Skeletal Metastases in Pediatric Renal Tumors

Many pediatric tumors metastasize to the skeleton. The best-known metastasizing tumor of renal origin in children is Wilms tumor. The reported incidence of skeletal metastases from Wilms tumor varies, ranging from 0.5 to 13% (LAMEGO and ZERBINI 1983; MARSDEN and LAWLER 1978). Skeletal metastases, when present, are associated with widespread tumor (BOND and MARTIN 1975). The metastatic lesions of Wilms tumor have been described as predominantly lytic with either permeative, or more

commonly, geographic patterns of bone destruction and poorly defined margins (MASSELOT et al. 1972; RUDHE 1969).

However, results of several studies analyzing bone-metastasizing renal tumors of children indicate that in many of the cases the bone metastases were actually from primary renal tumors other than Wilms tumor (LAMEGO and ZERBINI 1983; MARSDEN and LAWLER 1978). This distinct type of tumor became known as "bone metastasizing renal tumor of childhood" as described by MARSDEN et al. (1978) after its first identification by KIDD (1970). Then the tumor was renamed with the descriptive term "clear cell" proposed by Beckwith and Palmar to distinguish it from malignant rhabdoid tumor of the kidney (PARIKH et al. 1998); hence, it became known as clear cell sarcoma of the kidney. It is an uncommon tumor and accounts for about 4% of all pediatric renal tumors, primarily affecting young children with a mean age of 3 years (DORFMAN and CZERNIAK 1998; PARIKH et al. 1998). It is an entity distinct from Wilms tumor, with an aggressive clinical behavior and poorer prognosis than Wilms tumor and a very high rate of skeletal metastases, ranging from 42 to 69% (PARIKH et al. 1998; GREEN

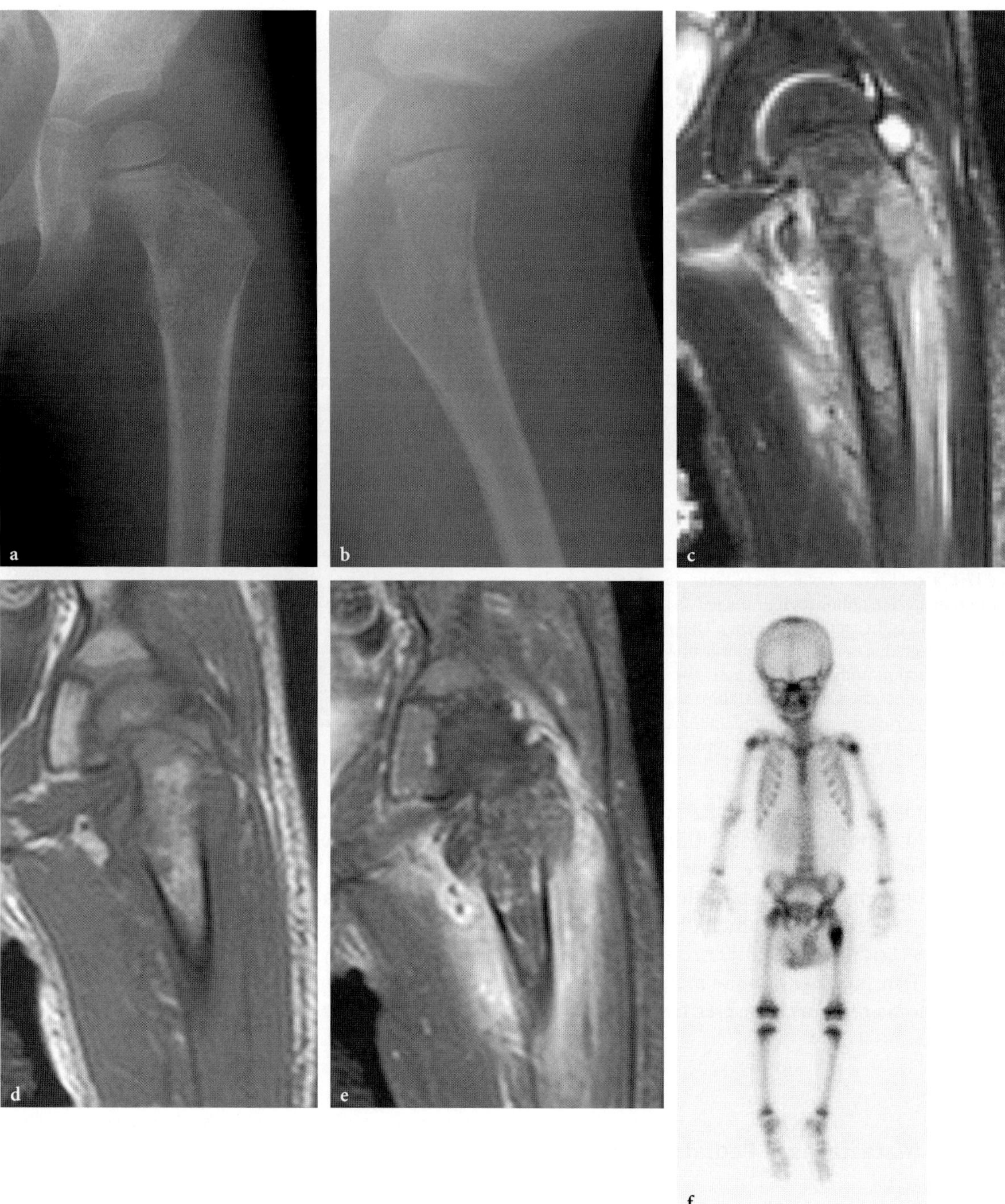

Fig. 17.14a-f. Osteolytic bone metastasis in a 3-year-old girl with clear cell sarcoma of the kidney diagnosed 6 months previously. **a** Anteroposterior and **b** lateral radiographs of the left femur reveal an ill-defined osteolytic lesion at the left proximal femoral metadiaphysis. **c** Coronal fat-suppressed T2-weighted MR image shows cortex destruction and extension of hyperintensity into surrounding muscles. **d** Coronal unenhanced T1-weighted MR image shows an infiltrative hypointense lesion at the left proximal femur. **e** Coronal contrast-enhanced fat-suppressed T1-weighted MR image shows diffuse and heterogeneous enhancement within the lesion and in the surrounding muscles. **f** Anteroposterior whole-body Tc-99m MDP bone scan shows intense focal uptake in the left proximal femur.

et al. 1997). In one series, the radiological aspects of the metastases were variable, with some lytic lesions (Fig. 17.14) as well as violently permeative lesions (LAMEGO and ZERBINI 1983). In other studies, the osseous metastases consisted mainly of multiple lytic lesions (MARSDEN et al. 1978; MARSDEN and LAWLER 1980). Not much is known about the CT and MR imaging findings of clear cell sarcoma metastasis (Fig. 17.14).

Similar to renal cell carcinoma in adults, skeletal metastases are frequently manifestations of an occult primary tumor (DORFMAN and CZERNIAK 1998). Microscopically, they are described as having a somewhat variable pattern of undifferentiated round-cell and clear-cell features that are negative for epithelial cell markers and that stain with vimentin (DORFMAN and CZERNIAK 1998).

17.5
Conclusion

In conclusion, osseous metastases from renal cell carcinoma are characterized by mainly osteolytic lesions in the metaphysis of, most commonly, the spine, pelvic bone, ribs, and proximal long bones with cortical involvement. Solitary lesions with septa are not uncommon. Both CT and MR imaging may help in defining the extent of the lesion and presence of a periosteal soft tissue mass. The presence of "flow-void" sign on MR imaging may suggest the primary origin of a metastatic bone lesion and also suggest its hypervascular nature, which may also be confirmed by angiography. Bone scanning is still used in detection of metastasis and may help in localization.

Although a rare entity, clear cell sarcoma of the kidney in children metastasizes to the bone readily and is characterized by osteolytic lesions, which may be the first manifestation of a clinically occult tumor.

Acknowledgements
We thank K.R. Son and K.H. Lee for their help in preparing the chapter.

References

Althausen P, Althausen A, Jennings LC, Mankin HJ (1997) Prognostic factors and surgical treatment of osseous metastases secondary to renal cell carcinoma. Cancer 80:1103–1109

Barton PP, Waneck RE, Karnel FJ, Ritschl P, Kramer J, Lechner GL (1996) Embolization of bone metastases. J Vasc Interv Radiol 7:81–88

Bohnenkamp B, Rhomberg W, Sonnentag W, Feldmann U (1980) Prognosis of metastatic renal cell carcinoma related to the pattern of metastasis. J Cancer Res Clin Oncol 96:105–114

Bond JV, Martin EC (1975) Bone metastases in Wilms' tumour. Clin Radiol 26:103–106

Borzutzky CA, Turbiner EH (1985) Renal cell carcinoma presenting as a "hot" lesion in kidney, with "cold" metastasis in the skeleton. Clin Nucl Med 10:710–712

Bowers TA, Murray JA, Charnsangavej C, Soo CS, Chuang VP, Wallace S (1982) Bone metastasis from renal carcinoma. The preoperative use of transcatheter arterial occlusion. J Bone Joint Surg Am 64:749–754

Brodsky G, Garnick MG (1989) Renal tumors in the adult patient. In: Tishder CC, Brenner BM (eds) Renal pathology. Lippincott, Philadelphia, pp 1540–1567

Choi JA, Lee KH, Jun WS, Yi MG, Lee S, Kang HS (2003) Osseous metastasis from renal cell carcinoma: "flow-void" sign at MR imaging. Radiology 228:629–634

Coerkamp EG, Kroon HM (1988) Cortical bone metastases. Radiology 269:525–528

Cole AT, Mandell J, Fried FA, Stabb EV (1975) The place of bone scan in the diagnosis of renal cell carcinoma. J Urol 114:364–365

Dekernion JB, Ramming KP, Smith RB (1978) The natural history of metastatic renal cell carcinoma: a computer analysis. J Urol 120:148–152

Dineen MK, Pastore RD, Emrich LJ, Huben RP (1988) Results of surgical treatment of renal cell carcinoma with solitary metastasis. J Urol 140:277–279

Dorfman HD, Czerniak B (1998) Bone tumors. Mosby, St. Louis

Fidler IJ (1992) The biology of renal cancer metastasis. Semin Urol 10:3–11

Forbes GS, McLeod RA, Hattery RR (1977) Radiographic manifestations of bone metastases from renal carcinoma. Am J Roentgenol 129:61–66

Ghert MA, Harrelson JM, Scully SP (2001) Solitary renal cell carcinoma metastasis to the hand: the need for wide excision or amputation. J Hand Surg [Am] 26:156–160

Green DM, Coppes MJ, Breslow NE et al. (1997) Wilms tumor. In: Pizzo PA, Poplack DG (eds) Principles and practice of pediatric oncology. Lippincott-Raven, Philadelphia, pp 737–738

Hain SF, Maisey MN (2003) Positron emission tomography for urological tumours. BJU Int 92:159–164

Henriksson C, Haraldsson A, Aldenborg F, Lindberg S, Pettersson S (1992) Skeletal metastases in 102 patients evaluated before surgery for renal cell carcinoma. Scand J Urol Nephrol 26:363–366

Hrushesky WJ, Murphy GP (1973) Investigation of a new renal tumor model. J Surg Res 15:327–336

Huguenin PU, Kieser S, Glanzmann C, Capaul R, Lutolf UM (1998) Radiotherapy for metastatic carcinomas of the kidney or melanomas: an analysis using palliative end points. Int J Radiat Oncol Biol Phys 41:401–405

Ibayashi K, Ando M, Gotoh E (1993) Regression of pulmonary and multiple skeletal metastases from renal cell carcinoma by nephrectomy and alpha-interferon therapy: a case report. Jpn J Clin Oncol 23:378–383

Jung ST, Ghert MA, Harrelson JM, Scully SP (2003) Treatment of osseous metastases in patients with renal cell carcinoma. Clin Orthop 409:223–231

Kerbl K, Pauer W (1993) Spontaneous regression of osseous metastasis in renal cell carcinoma. Aust N Z J Surg 63:901–903

Kidd JM (1970) Exclusion of certain renal neoplasm from the category of Wilms tumor. Am J Pathol 59:16a (Abstract)

Kim EE, Bledin AG, Gutierrez C, Haynie TP (1983) Comparison of radionuclide images and radiographs for skeletal metastases from renal cell carcinoma. Oncology 40:284–286

Koga S, Tsuda S, Nishikido M, Ogawa Y, Hayashi K, Hayashi T, Kanetake H (2001) The diagnostic value of bone scan in patients with renal cell carcinoma. J Urol 166:2126–2128

Kozlowski JM (1994) Management of distant solitary recurrence in the patient with renal cancer: contralateral kidney and other sites. Urol Clin North Am 21:601–624

Lamego CM, Zerbini MC (1983) Bone-metastasizing primary renal tumors in children. Radiology 147:449–454

Layelle I, Flandroy P, Trotteur G, Dondelinger RF (1998) Arterial embolization of bone metastases: Is it worthwhile? J Belge Radiol 81:223–225

Marsden HB, Lawler W (1978) Bone-metastasizing renal tumour of childhood. Br J Cancer 38:437–441

Marsden HB, Lawler W (1980) Bone metastasizing renal tumour of childhood: histopathological and clinical review of 38 cases. Virchows Arch A Pathol Anat Histol 387:341–351

Marsden HB, Lawler W, Kumar PM (1978) Bone metastasizing renal tumor of childhood: morphologic and clinical features, and differences from Wilms' tumor. Cancer 42:1922–1928

Masselot J, Bergiron C, Tchernia G, Tournade MF, Markovits P (1972) Radio-clinical study of bone metastases in nephroblastoma. Apropos of 19 cases. Ann Radiol (Paris) 15:1–12

Middleton RG (1967) Surgery for metastatic renal cell carcinoma. J Urol 97:973–977

Montie JE, Stewart BH, Straffon RA, Banowsky LH, Hewitt CB, Montague DK (1977) The role of adjunctive nephrectomy in patients with metastatic renal cell carcinoma. J Urol 117:272–275

Neugut AI, Casper ES, Godwin TA, Smith J (1981) Osteoblastic metastases in renal cell carcinoma. Br J Radiol 54:1002–1004

Nielsen OS, Munro AJ, Tannock IF (1991) Bone metastases: pathophysiology and management policy. J Clin Oncol 9:509–524

Parikh SH, Chintagumpala M, Hicks MJ, Trautwein LM, Blaney S, Minifee P, Woo SY (1998) Clear cell sarcoma of the kidney: an unusual presentation with review of the literature. J Pediatr Hematol Oncol 20:165–168

Pettersson H, Springfield D, Hamlin D, Scott K (1985) Magnetic resonance imaging and tissue characterization of renal cell carcinoma and its osseous metastasis. Report of a case. Acta Radiol Diagn (Stockh) 26:193–195

Poggi MM, Patronas N, Buttman JA, Hewitt SM, Fuller B (2001) Intramedullary spinal cord metastases from renal cell carcinoma: detection by positron emission tomography. Clin Nucl Med 26:837–839

Resnick D, Niwayama G (1995) Tumors and tumor-like diseases. In: Resnick D, Niwayama G (eds) Diagnosis of bone and joint disorders. Saunders, Philadelphia, pp 4019–4021

Rudhe V (1969) Skeletal metastases in Wilms' tumour: a roentgenologic study. Ann Radiol (Paris) 12:337–342

Saitoh H (1981) Distant metastasis of renal adenocarcinoma. Cancer 48:1487–1491

Seto E, Segall GM, Terris MK (2000) Positron emission tomography detection of osseous metastases of renal cell carcinoma not identified on bone scan. Urology 55:286

Skinner DG, Colvin RB, Vermillion CD, Pfister RC, Leadbetter WF (1971) Diagnosis and management of renal cell carcinoma: a clinical and pathologic study of 309 cases. Cancer 28:1165–1177

Smith EM, Kursh ED, Makley J, Resnick MI (1992) Treatment of osseous metastases secondary to renal cell carcinoma. J Urol 148:784–787

Sun S, Lang EV (1998) Bone metastases from renal cell carcinoma: preoperative embolization. J Vasc Interv Radiol 9:263–269

Takashi M, Takagi Y, Sakata T, Shimoji T, Miyake K (1995) Surgical treatment of renal cell carcinoma metastases: prognostic significance. Int Urol Nephrol 27:1–8

Thompson IM, Shannon H, Ross J, Montie J (1975) An analysis of factors affecting survival in 150 patients with renal cell carcinoma. J Urol 114:694–696

Tolia BM, Whitmore WF (1975) Solitary metastasis from renal cell carcinoma. J Urol 114:836–838

Tongaonkar HB, Kulkarni JN, Kamat MR (1992) Solitary metastases from renal cell carcinoma: a review. J Surg Oncol 49:45–48

Varkarakis MJ, Bhanalaph T, Moore RH, Murphy GP (1974) Prognostic criteria of renal cell carcinoma. J Surg Oncol 6:97–107

Willinsky RA, Rubenstein JD, Cruickshank B (1982) Case report 216. Skeletal Radiol 9:137–139

Wilner D (1982) Radiology of bone tumors and allied disorders. Saunders, Philadelphia

18 Renal Lymphoma

SHEILA SHETH and ELLIOT K. FISHMAN

CONTENTS

18.1
Introduction

Malignant lymphomas, broadly categorized into Hodgkin and non-Hodgkin lymphomas, constitute a heterogeneous group of cancers arising from the lymphoreticular system. The incidence of these tumors has been growing (approximately 50,000 new cases are diagnosed in the United States each year) and effective treatments prolong the survival of many

S. SHETH, MD
Associate Professor of Radiology and Pathology, Johns Hopkins University School of Medicine, Director, Biopsy Service, Department of Radiology, Johns Hopkins Hospital, 600 North Wolfe Street, HAL B176D, Baltimore, MD 21287, USA
E. K. FISHMAN, MD, FACR
Professor of Radiology and Oncology, Johns Hopkins University School of Medicine, Director, Diagnostic Radiology and Body CT, Department of Radiology, Johns Hopkins Outpatient Center, 601 North Caroline Street, Room 3254, Baltimore, MD 21287, USA

affected patients. Thus, imaging studies are routinely requested for diagnosis and management. While the most common manifestation of malignant lymphomas is lymphadenopathy, visceral involvement is diagnosed with increasing frequency. Excluding the hematopoietic and reticuloendothelial organs, the genitourinary tract is the most commonly affected system (RICHMOND et al. 1962).

18.2
Secondary vs Primary Renal Lymphoma

Renal lymphoma usually occurs in the setting of widespread non-Hodgkin lymphoma (NHL), typically B-cell type intermediate or high-grade tumors or Burkitt lymphoma (Figs. 18.1, 18.2). Involvement with Hodgkin disease is much less common, found in less than 1% of patients at presentation (CHEPURI et al. 2003; GUERMAZI et al. 2001).

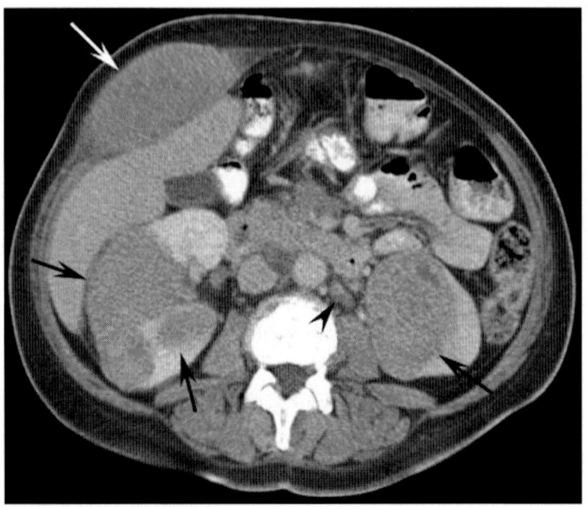

Fig. 18.1. Widespread B-cell non-Hodgkin lymphoma in a 65-year-old woman. Axial contrast-enhanced CT scan of the mid-abdomen shows soft tissue masses in both kidneys (*black arrows*). The tumor infiltrates around the left renal pelvis without causing obstruction. Note the retroperitoneal adenopathy (*arrowhead*) as well as the large mass in the abdominal wall (*white arrow*).

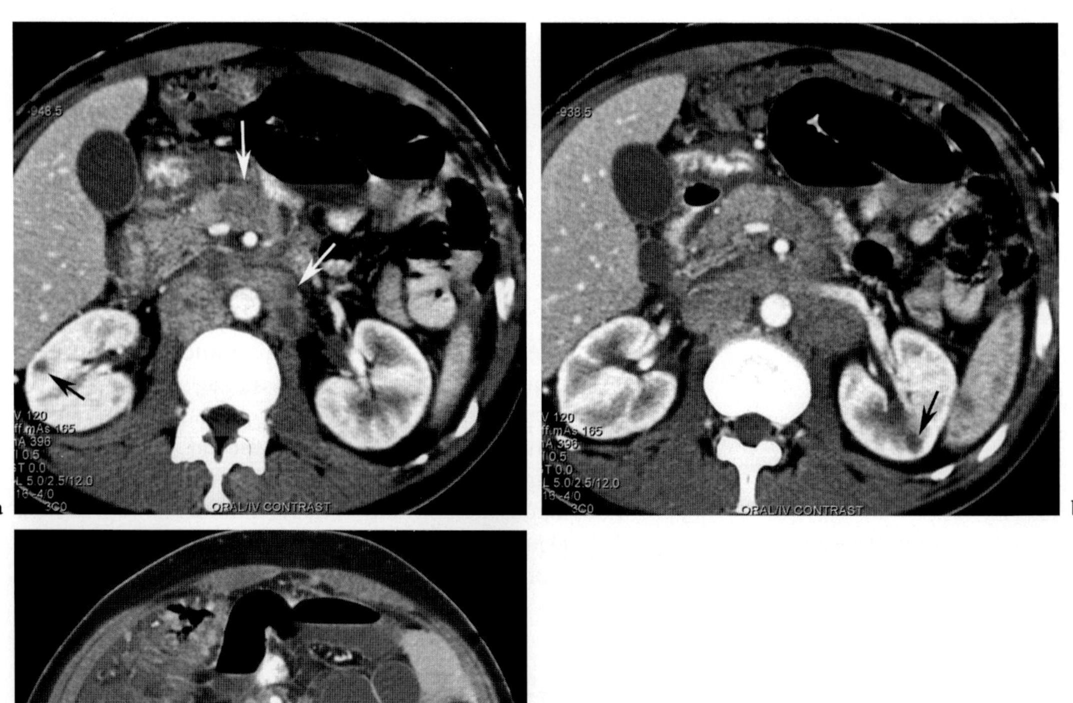

Fig. 18.2a-c. Subtle renal masses in a 40-year-old HIV-positive man with widespread large B-cell lymphoma. **a** Axial contrast-enhanced CT scan shows extensive retroperitoneal adenopathy (*white arrows*). There is a subtle hypodense lesion in the right kidney (*black arrow*). **b** A similar lesion is seen in the left kidney (*arrow*). **c** Axial contrast-enhanced CT scan also shows extensive infiltration of the cecum (*arrow*). (With Permission from URBAN and FISHMAN 2000)

Foci of lymphoma are found in the kidneys of 37 to nearly 50% of patients in autopsy series (RICHMOND et al. 1962; EISENBERG et al. 1994). Surprisingly, the diagnosis of renal lymphoma by cross-sectional imaging has been reported to reach only 3–8% of cases (CHEPURI et al. 2003; COHAN et al. 1990; REZNEK et al. 1990; URBAN and FISHMAN 2000). This apparent discrepancy between the pathological and radiological literature can be explained by several factors: renal lymphoma is often poorly documented as renal biopsy or nephrectomy are rarely indicated to confirm the diagnosis in the context of systemic disease; these numbers were gathered before the widespread use of helical single and multidetector computed tomography (CT) when older-generation scanners underestimated the frequency of renal lesions. It is anticipated that superior evaluation of the renal parenchyma afforded by modern imaging techniques will allow detection of renal lymphoma in many more patients (URBAN and FISHMAN 2000).

In the majority of cases, renal lymphoma is clinically asymptomatic. Its detection on imaging studies may, however, influence staging and type and length of treatment. Follow-up data in patients with renal lymphoma suggest that while involvement of the kidneys at the time of presentation does not necessarily indicate a poor prognosis, renal recurrence is associated with increased mortality (CHEPURI et al. 2003; RICHARDS et al. 1990).

Primary renal lymphoma, arising in the renal parenchyma and not associated with systemic manifestation, is uncommon, accounting for less than 1% of cases of extranodal disease. Its origin is somewhat speculative. As the renal parenchyma normally does not contain lymphoid tissue, several mechanisms have been postulated to account for the development of lymphoma in the kidney: the tumor may originate in the lymphatic-rich renal capsule or the perinephric fat and invade the parenchyma, or can arise from lymphocytes present in areas of chronic inflammation (STALLONE et al. 2000). It is usually a B-cell NHL and affects middle-age to older patients. Patients present with flank pain, hematuria, or non-specific symptoms of fever and night sweats (YASUNAGA et al. 1997). Renal insufficiency from extensive lymphomatous infiltration of both kidneys is rare (MALBRAIN et al. 1994; MILLS et al. 1992). The prognosis is generally poor.

18.3
Imaging Techniques for Renal Lymphoma

Several radiographic techniques are available to evaluate the kidneys. Cross-sectional imaging modalities, such as CT, ultrasound (US), or magnetic resonance (MR) imaging, are progressively replacing the traditional intravenous urography, although the latter remains the most sensitive method for detecting subtle lesions of the collecting system and diagnosing delay in renal excretion caused by hydronephrosis.

18.3.1
Computed Tomography

Helical (single or multidetector) CT is the imaging modality of choice in evaluating patients with suspected or known renal lymphoma. It not only depicts the renal lesions but also most accurately identifies extension to adjacent anatomic structures such as the perirenal space and the retroperitoneum and defines the systemic spread of the disease. Administration of intravenous contrast is essential to allow the depiction of subtle renal parenchymal abnormalities. Image acquisition in the corticomedullary and nephrographic phases of renal enhancement is generally sufficient. Small masses and subtle infiltration can be missed without the nephrographic phase, whereas the corticomedullary phase allows optimal demonstration of vascular encasement. If the tumor is predominantly central and affects the hilar region, or when the collecting system appears to be involved, excretory phase acquisition is necessary. This latter phase also best demonstrates obstruction of the collecting system by retroperitoneal masses. Images obtained prior to contrast injection are seldom required but may better demonstrate calcifications or areas of recent hemorrhage. In patients who are unable to receive intravenous contrast material, renal lymphoma can often be suspected in the presence of asymmetric size of the kidneys, focal bulge, and large retroperitoneal adenopathy.

18.3.2
Ultrasound

Ultrasound is less sensitive than CT both in detecting the presence of disease as well as the number of lesions (HEIKEN et al. 1983; WEINBERGER et al. 1990); however, it may be the first test requested for the rare patient who presents with renal insufficiency. Ultrasound is also helpful in patients who are unable to receive intravenous iodinated contrast and is the ideal guidance modality during percutaneous biopsy.

18.3.3
Magnetic Resonance Imaging

The role of MR imaging in renal lymphoma is not clearly established. It may be useful in patients with iodinated contrast allergy or renal insufficiency. In addition, MR imaging has been proven superior to CT in depicting involvement of the bone marrow.

18.3.4
Positron Emission Tomography

Positron emission tomography (PET) is a very useful technique for staging of lymphomas and detection of recurrences. Because it detects increased metabolic activity within lymphomatous deposits, fluorodeoxyglucose PET is more sensitive and specific than conventional anatomic imaging studies in detecting small additional tumor deposits (MOOG et al. 1998). The combination of PET and CT data acquisition at the same time (PET/CT) is emerging as a powerful tool for observing the metabolic activity of tumors with anatomic detail, allowing precise location and potentially earlier detection (Fig. 18.3; METSER et al. 2004).

18.4
Imaging Characteristics of Renal Lymphoma

18.4.1
Radiologic–Pathologic Correlation

Renal lymphomas display a variety of imaging appearances depending on their histological pattern of proliferation (HARTMAN et al. 1982).

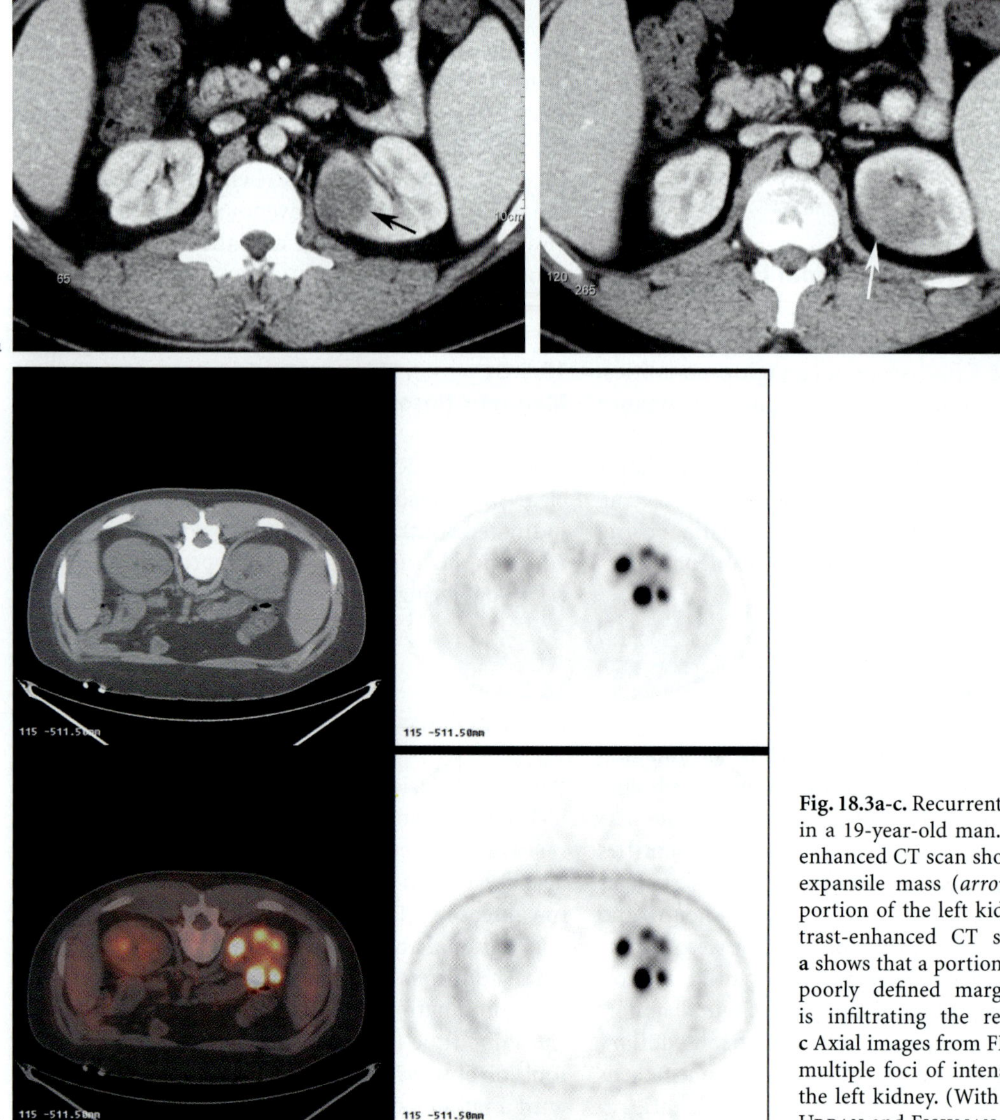

Fig. 18.3a-c. Recurrent B-cell lymphoma in a 19-year-old man. **a** Axial contrast-enhanced CT scan shows a well-defined expansile mass (*arrow*) in the medial portion of the left kidney. **b** Axial contrast-enhanced CT scan cephalad to **a** shows that a portion of the tumor has poorly defined margins (*arrow*) and is infiltrating the renal parenchyma. **c** Axial images from FDG-PET/CT show multiple foci of intense activity within the left kidney. (With Permission from URBAN and FISHMAN 2000)

Malignant lymphocytes reach the renal parenchyma via hematogenous spread and proliferate within the interstitium, using the nephrons, collecting tubules, and blood vessels as a scaffolding for further growth. Alternatively, some tumors spread by contiguous extension from the retroperitoneum penetrating through the renal capsule. Once the tumor reaches the kidneys, its radiological appearance is determined by its predominant proliferation mechanism. If the tumor follows an infiltrative growth pattern, and malignant cells proliferate along the scaffolding of the normal interstitial tissue, the kidneys enlarge but their reniform shape is pre-served. The lesions have ill-defined borders and may be quite subtle (PICKHARDT et al. 2000). In many cases, however, malignant lymphocytes proliferate focally, destroying the adjacent renal parenchyma and forming single, or more commonly, bilateral expansile lesions with well-defined margins. Small masses may coalesce, grow, and distort the renal contour (HARTMAN et al. 1982). In practice. a combination of the two types is not unusual.

Most cases of renal lymphoma occur in patients with systemic disease and do not generally pose a diagnostic dilemma (SHEERAN and SUSSMAN 1998). If, however, renal involvement is isolated or the appearance of the renal lesions is atypical, further investigations, including percutaneous biopsy, may be indicated.

Radiological appearances associated with renal lymphoma include multiple masses, solitary lesion, direct extension from retroperitoneal adenopathy, predominant involvement of the perinephric space, and diffuse infiltration of one or both kidneys. Lymphoma less commonly affects the renal sinus and collecting system. In a large autopsy series of 696 patients with lymphoma, RICHMOND et al. (1962) observed multiple renal masses in 61% of cases. Solitary renal nodule or mass or direct invasion from retroperitoneal adenopathy were equally common.

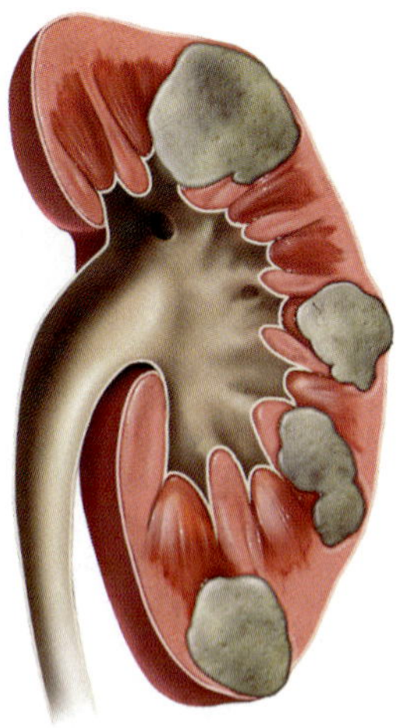

Fig. 18.4. The characteristic appearance of multiple masses in renal lymphoma. (With permission from URBAN and FISHMAN 2000)

18.4.2
Multiple Renal Masses

The most common appearance of renal lymphoma on imaging is multiple masses of variable size, typically 1–3 cm in diameter (Fig. 18.4). This pattern is seen in 50–60% of cases. The lesions are most often bilateral but can be unilateral (CHEPURI et al. 2003; COHAN et al. 1990; HEIKEN et al. 1983; REZNEK et al. 1990; URBAN and FISHMAN 2000).

On unenhanced CT, these masses appear as soft tissue lesions slightly more hyperdense than the surrounding parenchyma. Calcifications are rare. Administration of intravenous contrast is essential for detection if the lesions are small and do not distort the renal outline (Fig. 18.5). Small tumors are best demonstrated in the nephrographic phase of renal enhancement (SZOLAR et al. 1997). Lymphomatous deposits enhance less than the normal renal tissue and appear as relatively homogeneous masses that are hypodense compared with the surrounding cortex (Figs. 18.1, 18.5, 18.6). Large lesions tend to be more heterogeneous and may contain hypodense areas suggesting necrosis, particularly after chemotherapy. The presence of retroperitoneal adenopathy is an additional clue to the diagnosis.

Few reports have described the MR imaging appearance of renal lymphomas (SEMELKA et al. 1996). Tumors are hypointense compared with normal cortex on T1-weighted images and iso- or hypointense on T2-weighted images. They enhance less than the renal parenchyma following gadolinium administration.

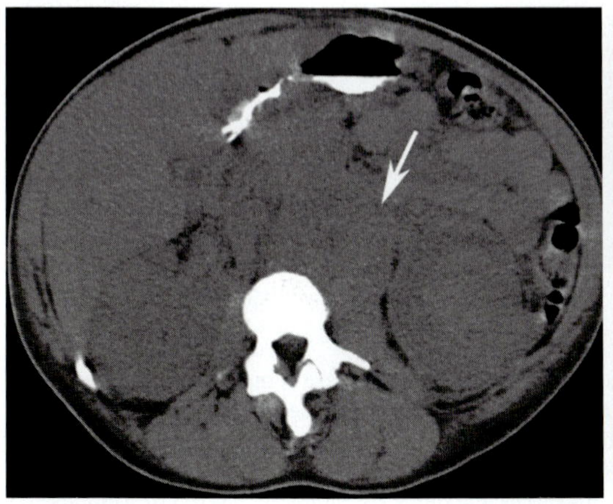
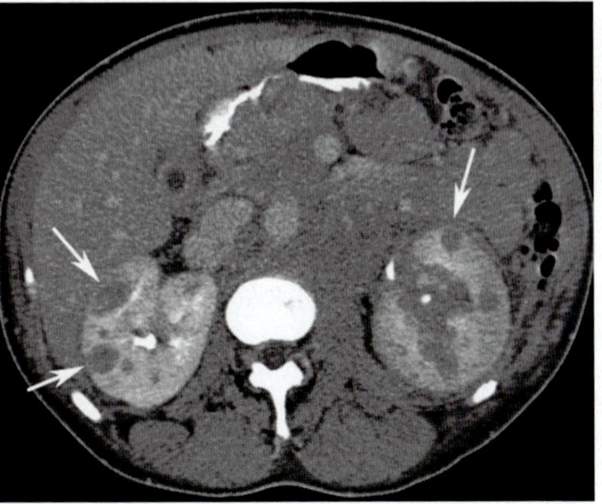

Fig. 18.5a,b. Large B-cell non-Hodgkin lymphoma in a 41-year-old HIV-positive man. **a** Axial unenhanced CT scan of the mid-abdomen shows a soft mass in the region of the great vessels suspicious for retroperitoneal adenopathy (*arrow*). The kidneys do not demonstrate any abnormality in contour. **b** Axial contrast-enhanced CT scan of the mid-abdomen shows bilateral soft tissue masses in both kidneys (*arrows*). Note that these masses do not deform the contour of the kidneys. The para-aortic retroperitoneal adenopathy is seen much better. (With Permission from URBAN and FISHMAN 2000)

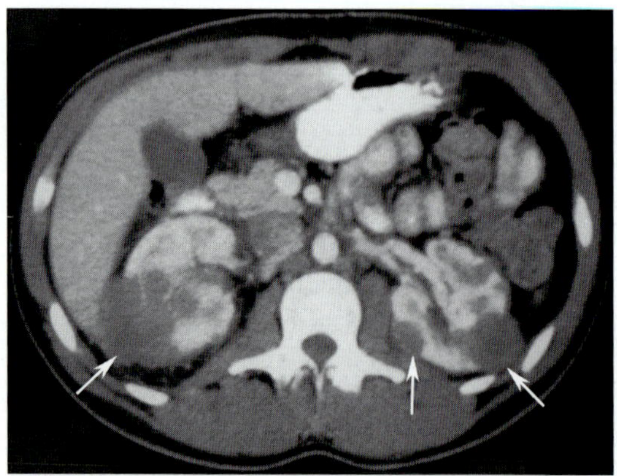

Fig. 18.6. Renal non-Hodgkin lymphoma in a 46-year-old woman. Axial contrast-enhanced CT scan of the kidneys shows multiple soft tissue masses in both kidneys (*arrows*).

On US, lymphomatous masses are typically hypoechoic and homogeneous (Fig. 18.7). The US appearance reflects the underlying homogeneity of lymphoma deposits which offer very few tissue interfaces to the insonating beam. Color or power Doppler US shows displacement of normal renal vessels with little vascularity within the lesions.

Radiologically, multifocal renal lymphoma must be differentiated from metastatic disease to the kidneys. Primary tumors that frequently spread to the kidneys include lung and breast cancer as well as melanoma (Fig. 18.8). In the absence of relevant clinical history, image-guided biopsy is indicated. Unlike lymphoma, multiple synchronous renal cell carcinomas are generally hypervascular (Fig. 18.9).

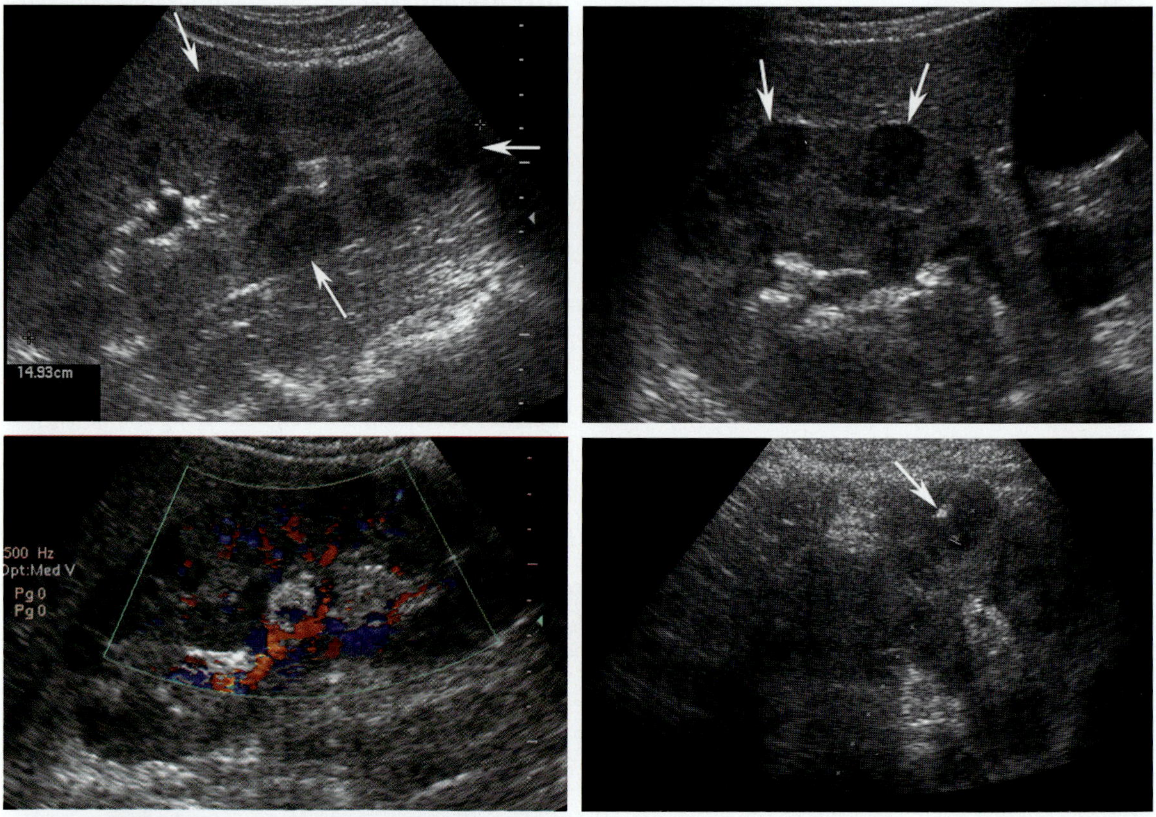

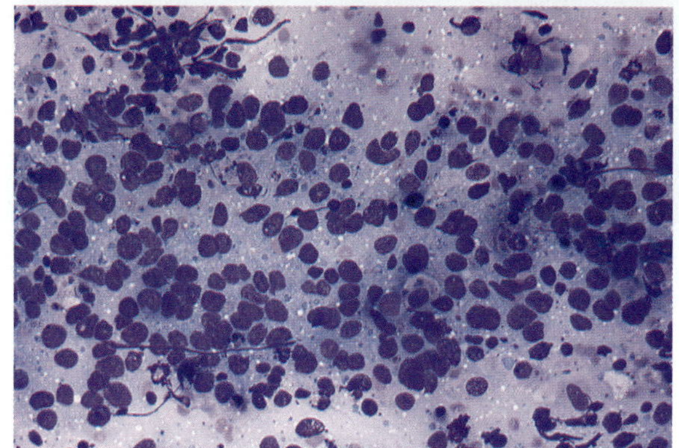

Fig. 18.7a-e. Renal non-Hodgkin lymphoma in a 33-year-old man. **a** Sagittal and **b** transverse ultrasound images of the right kidney show multiple hypoechoic soft tissue masses in the parenchyma (*arrows*). Note that the kidney is enlarged but preserves its reniform shape. **c** The color Doppler US image shows displacement of the renal vessels by the masses. **d** Transverse ultrasound image of the right kidney during the ultrasound-guided biopsy procedure shows that the echogenic needle tip (*arrow*) is clearly seen within the hypoechoic mass. **e** Analysis of the fine-needle-aspiration sample shows malignant lymphocytes (Diff-Quik stain on site). (With Permission from Urban and Fishman 2000)

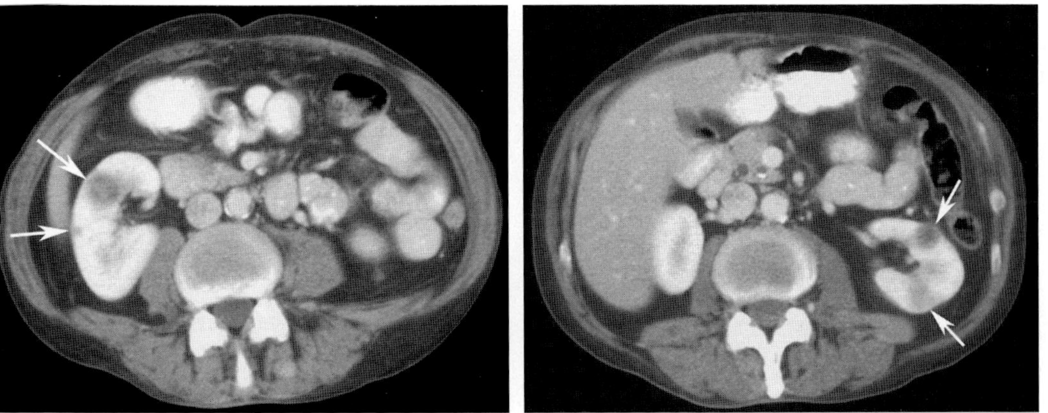

Fig. 18.8a,b. Metastatic melanoma in a 65-year-old man. **a** Axial contrast-enhanced CT scan at the nephrographic phase shows at least two soft tissue masses in the right kidney (*arrows*). **b** Axial contrast-enhanced CT scan in the nephrographic phase shows similar findings in the left kidney (*arrows*).

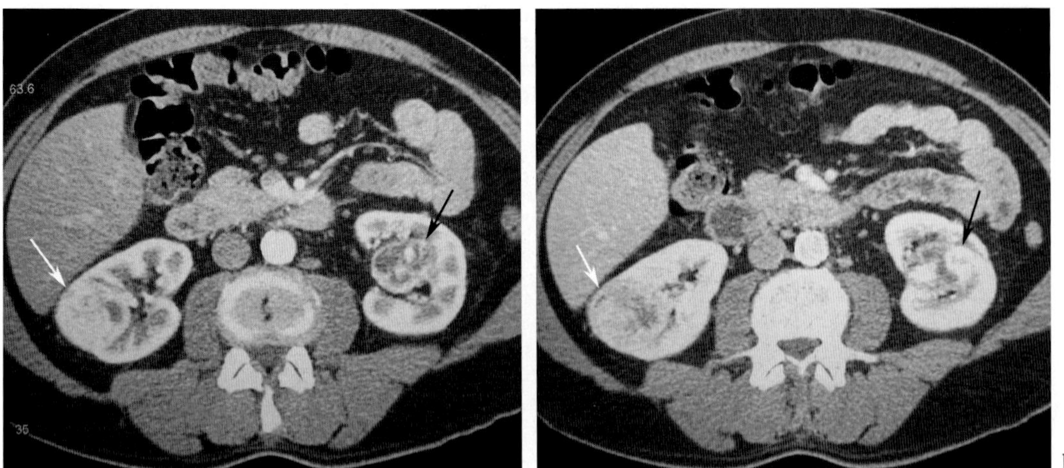

Fig. 18.9a,b. Multifocal renal cell carcinoma in a 68-year-old man with right upper quadrant pain. Axial CT scan of the kidneys at the **a** arterial phase and **b** venous enhancement show bilateral hypervascular heterogeneous masses (*arrows*). This enhancement pattern is seen more commonly in renal cell carcinoma. The diagnosis was confirmed on percutaneous ultrasound-guided biopsy and the patient was treated with partial right nephrectomy and total left nephrectomy. (With Permission from URBAN and FISHMAN 2000)

18.4.3
Solitary Mass

A solitary renal mass is reported in 10–20% of patients with renal lymphoma (Fig. 18.10). The mass characteristically demonstrates little enhancement following intravenous contrast administration (Figs. 18.11, 18.12). This feature is helpful in differentiating lymphoma from conventional renal cell carcinoma which usually enhances in the arterial phase (Fig. 18.13); however, some primary renal tumors, such as the papillary variant of renal cell carcinoma, may not exhibit this classic enhancement (Fig. 18.14). Percutaneous biopsy is required for definitive diagnosis to exclude an atypical renal cell carcinoma or a solitary metastasis.

18.4.4
Cystic Mass

Cystic appearance is distinctly unusual in renal lymphoma: Of 28 cystic Bosniak III lesions reviewed by HARSINGHANI et al. (2003), only one turned out to be a lymphoma at biopsy; however, focal lesions can appear markedly hypoechoic on US and even exhibit some degree of enhancement through transmission mimicking a cystic mass.

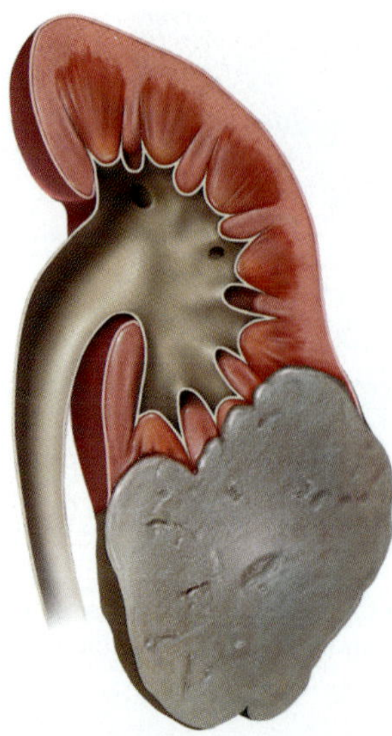

Fig. 18.10. The characteristic appearance of a dominant solitary lymphomatous renal mass. (With Permission from URBAN and FISHMAN 2000)

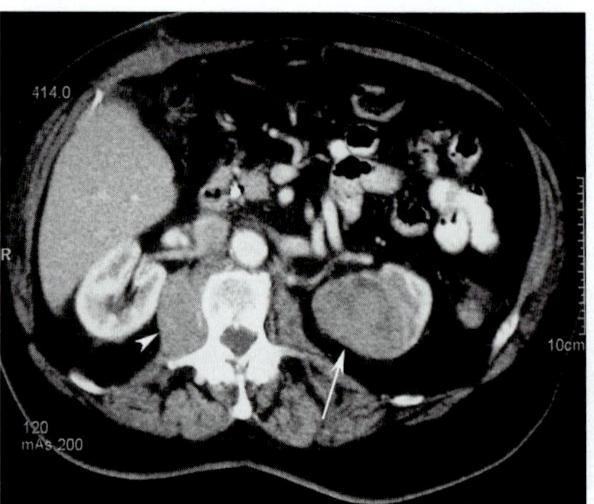

Fig. 18.11. Carlson large B-cell non-Hodgkin lymphoma in a 72-year-old man with a history of prostate cancer. Axial contrast-enhanced CT scan of the kidneys shows an expansile well-defined mass (*arrow*) in the left kidney. No other renal solid masses were present, but the right psoas muscle is enlarged (*arrowhead*). The diagnosis was established by ultrasound-guided percutaneous biopsy of the left renal mass. (With Permission from URBAN and FISHMAN 2000)

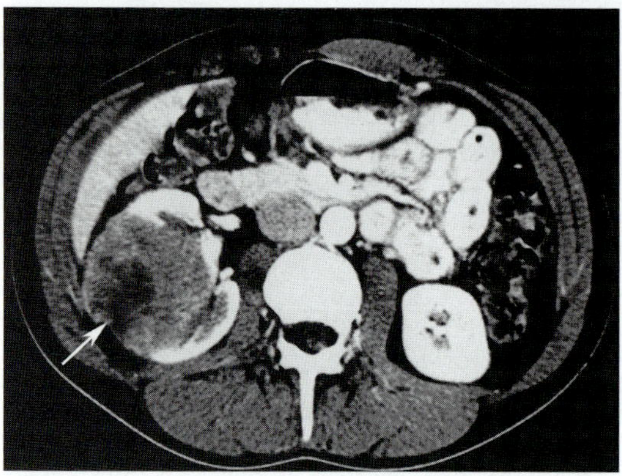

Fig. 18.12. Recurrent non-Hodgkin lymphoma in the right kidney mimicking a renal cell carcinoma in 41-year-old woman with a history of lymphoma. Axial contrast-enhanced CT scan of the kidneys shows a solitary heterogeneous mass (*arrow*) in the right kidney. The diagnosis was established by percutaneous biopsy.

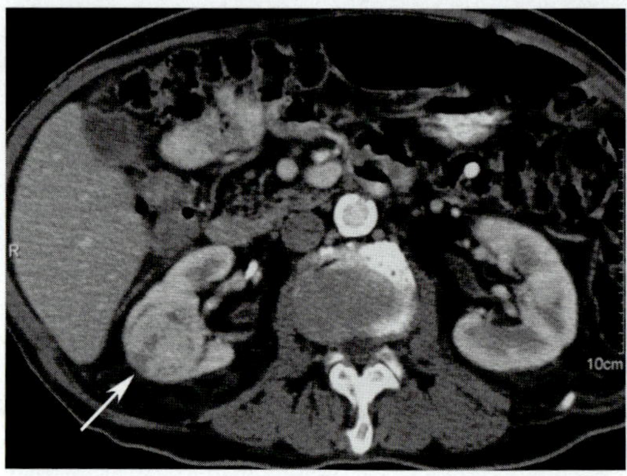

Fig. 18.13. Renal cell carcinoma in an 80-year-old man. Axial contrast-enhanced CT scan in the corticomedullary phase shows a single hypervascular mass (*arrow*) in the right kidney. This is the classic appearance of renal cell carcinoma and nephrectomy was recommended. (With Permission from URBAN and FISHMAN 2000)

18.4.5
Direct Extension from Retroperitoneal Lymphoma

Contiguous extension from large retroperitoneal masses is the second most common pattern, present in 25–30% of cases (Fig. 18.15; COHAN et al. 1990). These patients usually have widespread disease with bulky tumors and many are immunocompromised. The CT appearance is that of large retroperitoneal masses invading or displacing the adjacent kidney (Fig. 18.16). Hydronephrosis caused by entrapment of

the ureters is common; however, occlusion or thrombosis of major renal arteries and veins is rare despite extensive tumor encasement (Figs. 18.17, 18.18).

18.4.6
Perinephric Disease

Although perirenal spread from retroperitoneal lymphoma is not uncommon, isolated perinephric lymphoma is unusual, present in less than 10% of cases (Fig. 18.19; COHAN et al. 1990; REZNEK et al.

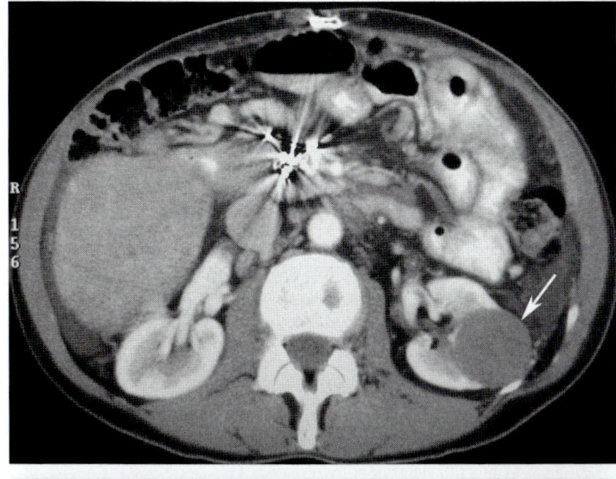

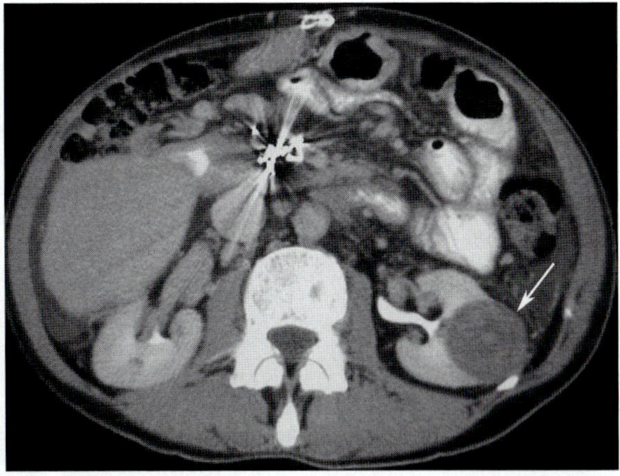

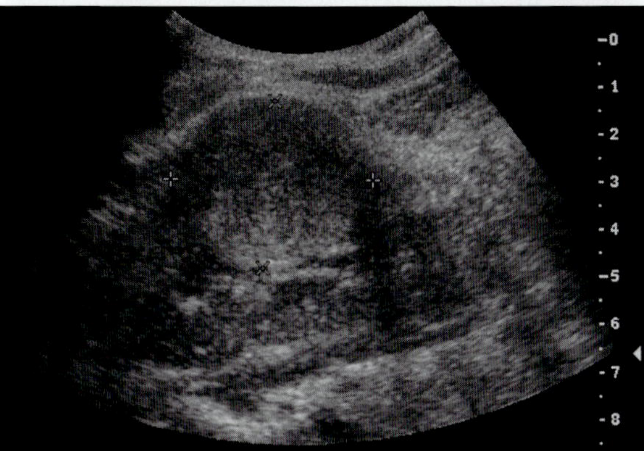

Fig. 18.14a-c. Papillary renal cell carcinoma mimicking lymphoma in a 57-year-old woman with history of liver transplant and a new renal mass. a Axial contrast-enhanced CT scan at the corticomedullary phase shows a hypovascular solitary mass (*arrow*) in the left kidney. This pattern is atypical for renal cell carcinoma. b Axial contrast-enhanced CT scan at the early excretory phase shows that the mass remains hypodense to the normal renal parenchyma in this phase (*arrow*). c Sagittal US image of the left kidney obtained at the time of biopsy shows a mildly echogenic mass (*calipers*). Note that lymphomas are generally hypoechoic. The pathological diagnosis based on the percutaneous biopsy was papillary renal cell carcinoma and the patient underwent a left nephrectomy. (With Permission from URBAN and FISHMAN 2000)

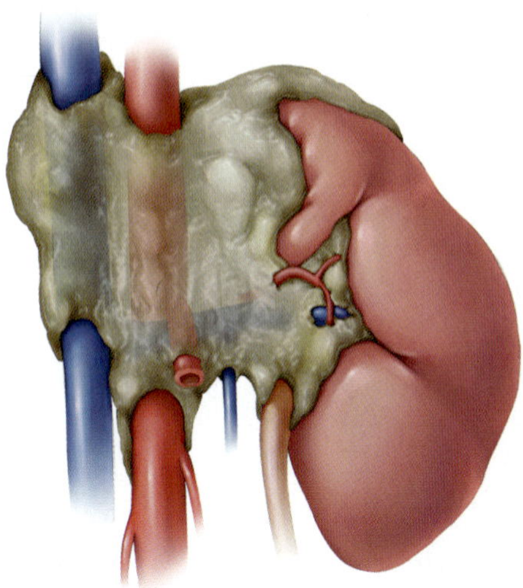

Fig. 18.15. The characteristic appearance of a bulky retroperitoneal mass invading the renal hilum and enveloping the renal vessels. (With Permission from URBAN and FISHMAN 2000)

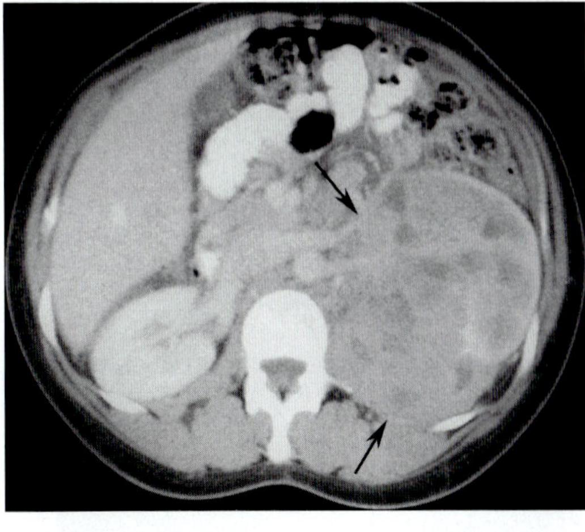

Fig. 18.16. Large B-cell non-Hodgkin's lymphoma in a 36-year-old HIV-positive woman. Axial contrast-enhanced CT scan of the abdomen shows a large heterogeneous left retroperitoneal mass extending into and infiltrating the left kidney (*arrows*). Note that the mass is encasing the left renal artery and vein.

1990). The CT images acquired after administration of intravenous contrast are invaluable to demonstrate a ring of homogeneous perinephric soft tissue compressing the normal parenchyma without causing significant impairment in renal function (Fig. 18.20). In less dramatic cases, findings include thickening of Gerota's fascia, or plaques and nodules in the perirenal space (Fig. 18.21; SHEERAN

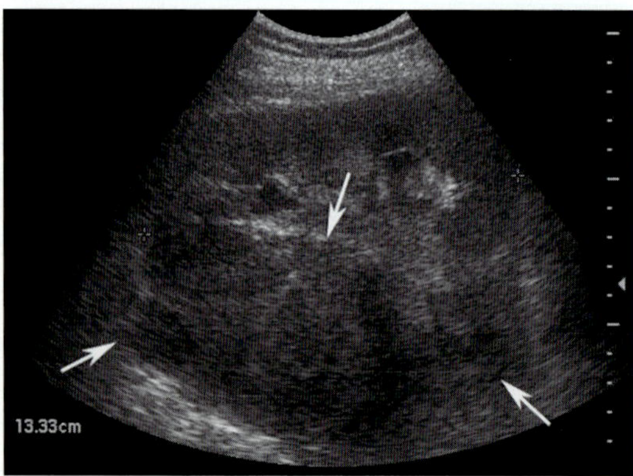

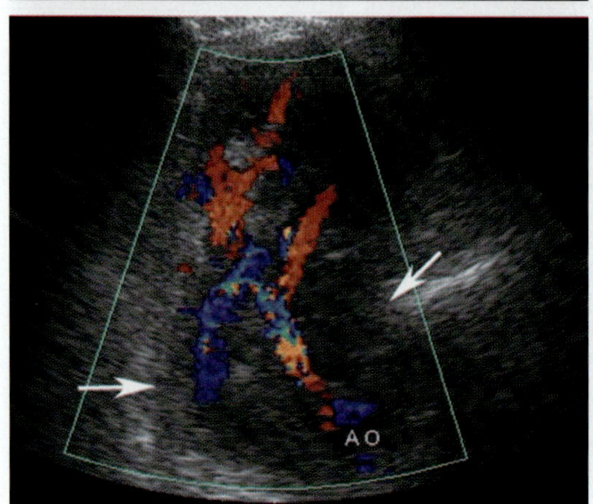

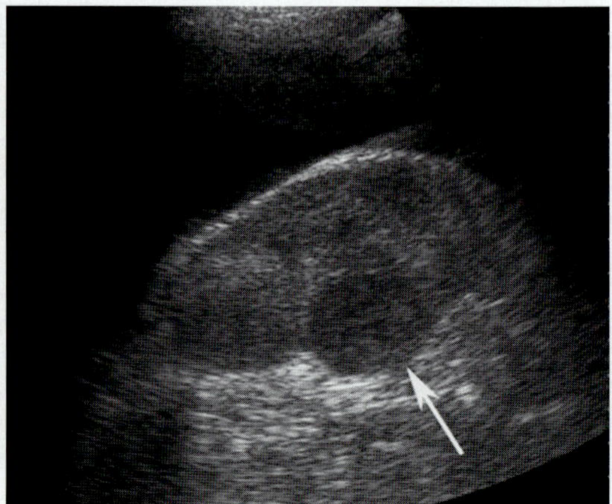

Fig. 18.17a-c. Burkitt lymphoma affecting the retroperitoneal nodes, adrenal glands, and both kidneys in a 46-year-old man. **a** Sagittal ultrasound image of the left kidney shows a large hypoechoic mass (*arrows*) displacing and infiltrating the left kidney. Note the mild left hydronephrosis. **b** Transverse color Doppler ultrasound image shows encasement of the left renal artery and vein by the mass (*arrows*). **c** Sagittal ultrasound image of the right kidney shows a hypoechoic renal mass (*arrow*). The right adrenal was also enlarged (not shown). (With Permission from URBAN and 2000)

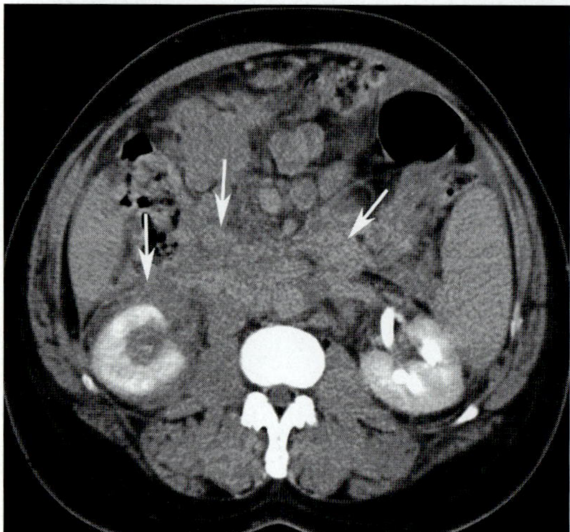

Fig. 18.18. Large B-cell lymphoma in a 52-year-old man with history of chronic lymphocytic leukemia. Axial contrast-enhanced CT scan shows tumor extension from the retroperitoneum into the right renal sinus fat and the perinephric space (*arrows*). Note delayed enhancement of the right kidney.

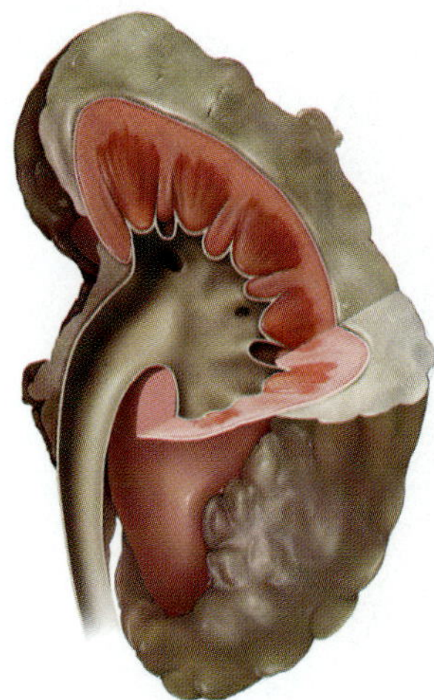

Fig. 18.19. The characteristic appearance of isolated perirenal lymphoma, which surrounds but does not destroy the underlying kidney. (With Permission from URBAN and FISHMAN 2000)

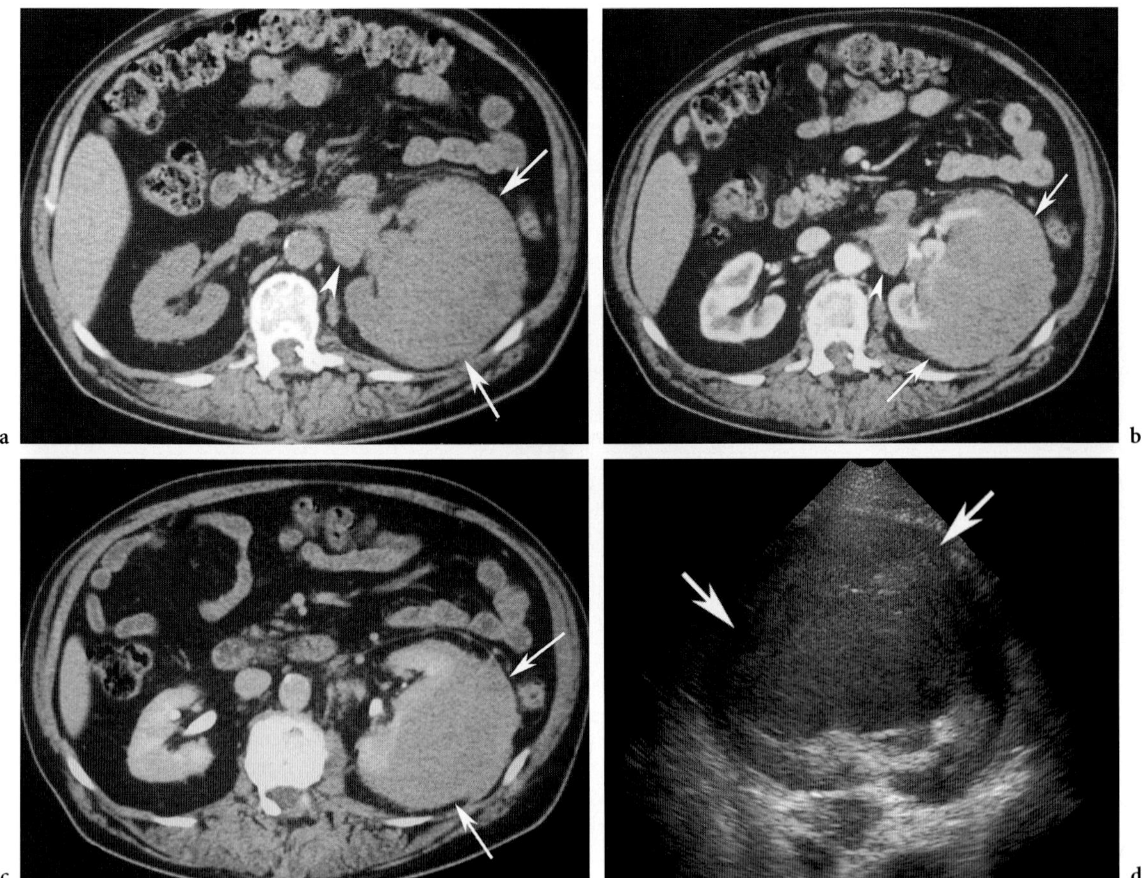

Fig. 18.20a-d. Incidental finding of left renal mass in a 66-year-old man. **a** Axial unenhanced CT scan shows marked enlargement of the left kidney (*arrows*). A left para-aortic lymph node is also present (*arrowhead*). **b** Axial contrast-enhanced CT scan in the corticomedullary phase shows a large hypovascular mass which is primarily in the perinephric space (*arrows*). The mass appears to invade the left renal parenchyma. Note that there is no significant delay in enhancement of the left renal parenchyma compared with the right kidney. **c** Axial contrast-enhanced CT scan in the excretory phase shows compression and invasion of the renal parenchyma by the mass (*arrows*). **d** Sagittal ultrasound image of the left kidney at the time of the biopsy shows a hypoechoic mass surrounding and partially invading the left kidney (*arrows*). Percutaneous biopsy yielded B-cell non-Hodgkin lymphoma. (With Permission from URBAN and FISHMAN 2000)

and SUSSMAN 1998). On US, hypoechoic tissue of variable thickness surrounds the kidney (Fig. 18.20; CADMAN et al. 1988). Differential diagnoses to consider include sarcoma arising from the renal capsule and metastases to the perinephric space as well as benign conditions such as perinephric hematoma, retroperitoneal fibrosis, amyloidosis, and extramedullary hematopoiesis (BECHTOLD et al. 1996; SHEERAN and SUSSMAN 1998).

18.4.7
Nephromegaly

Nephromegaly without distortion of the normal reniform shape of the kidneys results from diffuse infiltration of the renal interstitium by malignant lymphocytes (Figs. 18.22, 18.23). This appearance is more common in Burkitt lymphoma, either the disseminated form or limited to the kidneys (primary renal lymphoma; STALLONE et al. 2000). Acute renal failure caused by destruction of the normal renal architecture may bring the patient to seek medical attention. In such cases, both kidneys are usually affected.

Although the diagnosis can be suspected in the presence of global renal enlargement, administration of intravenous contrast is critical to demonstrate heterogeneous enhancement of the kidneys and loss of the normal differential enhancement between the cortex and the medulla in the corticomedullary phase. Alternatively, the renal parenchyma is replaced by poorly

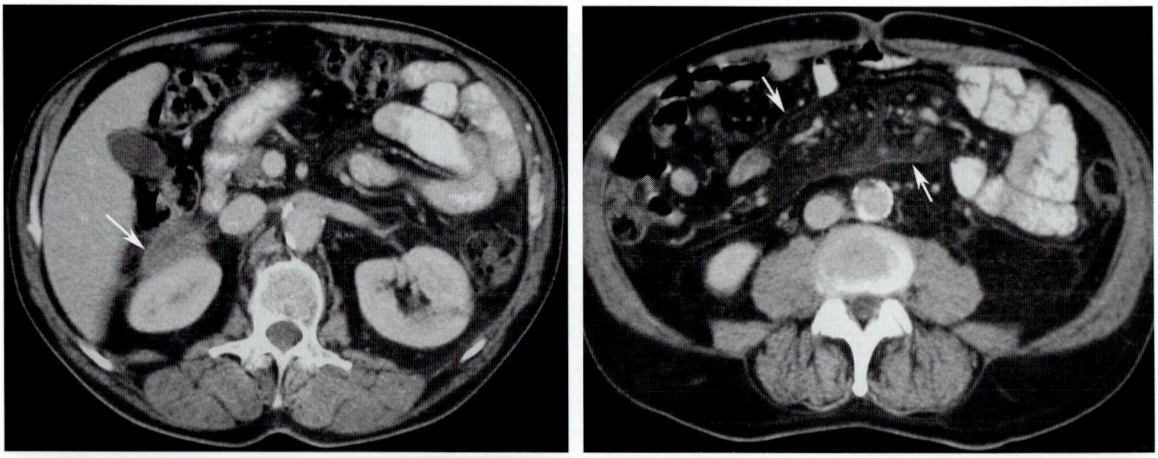

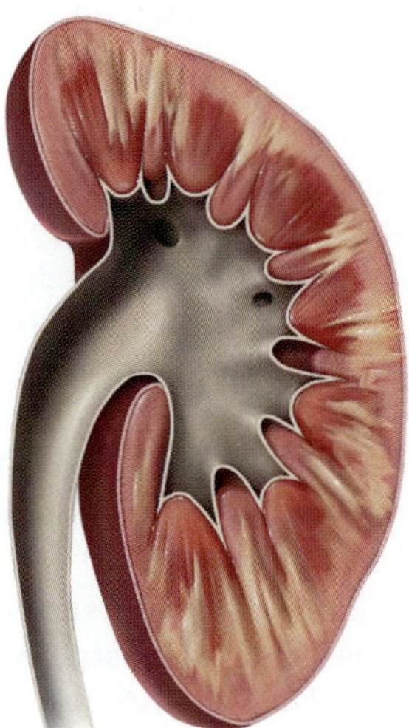

Fig. 18.21a-c. Routine follow-up CT in a 62-year-old man with a history of follicular non-Hodgkin lymphoma. **a** Axial contrast-enhanced CT scan in the portal venous phase shows a mildly enhancing mass in the right anterior pararenal space (*arrow*). This was a new finding for this patient. **b** Axial contrast-enhanced CT scan in the portal venous phase shows stranding in the mesenteric fat (*arrows*), suggestive of a "misty mesentery." This finding was also new. An ultrasound-guided biopsy of the perirenal mass yielded aggressive B-cell non-Hodgkin lymphoma. **c** Analysis of the fine-needle-aspiration sample shows malignant lymphocytes (Diff-Quik stain on site). (With Permission from URBAN and FISHMAN 2000)

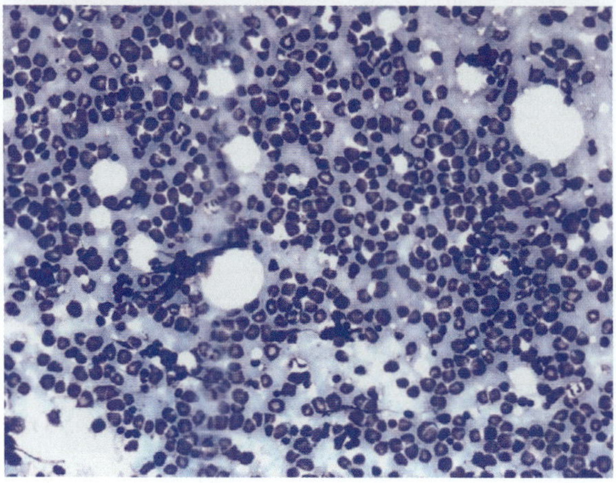

Fig. 18.22. The characteristic appearance of infiltrative lymphoma within the interstitium of the renal parenchyma. (With Permission from URBAN and FISHMAN 2000)

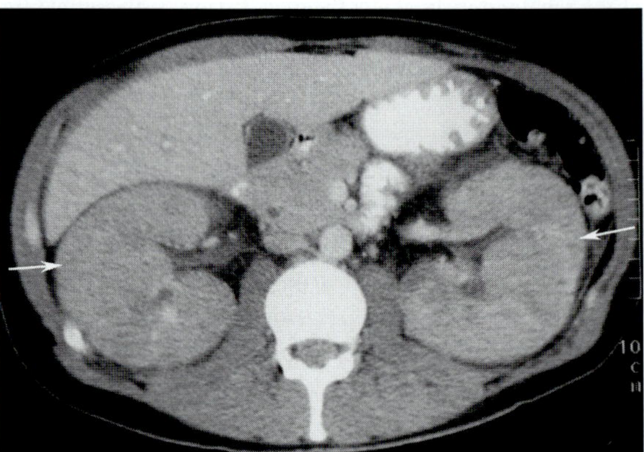

Fig. 18.23. Primary renal non-Hodgkin lymphoma involving both kidneys in a 41-year-old HIV-positive man who presented with renal failure. Axial contrast-enhanced CT scan of the kidneys in the nephrographic phase shows bilateral renal enlargement (*arrows*). There is heterogeneously decreased enhancement of the renal parenchyma. The diagnosis was established by renal biopsy. (With Permission from URBAN and FISHMAN 2000)

defined hypodense lesions. The collecting system is often encased, stretched, or attenuated rather than displaced. Occasionally, lymphoma infiltrates and destroys the renal parenchyma extensively and presents as a large non-functioning kidney (AMBOS et al. 1977; HARTMAN et al. 1988).

The US manifestations of infiltrative renal lymphoma are often subtle: they include globular enlargement of the kidneys with heterogeneous echotexture of the parenchyma and loss of the normal echogenic renal sinus (HARTMAN et al. 1988).

In some cases, the infiltrative process is unilateral or asymmetric. Diffuse infiltration of the kidney can also be caused by transitional cell carcinoma, collecting duct or medullary carcinoma of the kidneys, or severe pyelonephritis (Fig. 18.24).

18.4.8
Renal Sinus Involvement

Lymphoma can affect the renal sinus, although this is uncommon. On CT, the normal renal sinus is replaced by a homogeneous soft tissue mass (CHANG et al. 2002). The degree of enhancement within the mass is less than the normal parenchyma. Vascular encasement is common but, because of the pliable nature of the tumor, resulting hydronephrosis is often mild (Fig. 18.25). Transitional cell carcinoma is usually associated with a greater degree of obstruction to the collecting system. Castleman disease occurs occasionally in the renal hilum but cannot be differentiated without histological sampling (NISHIE et al. 2003).

On US, this type of lymphoma appears as a hypoechoic mass infiltrating the renal sinus. This should be differentiated from heterogeneous sinus fat which is usually bilateral (Figs. 18.25, 18.26). If the mass is markedly hypoechoic, it can mimic hydronephrosis.

18.5
Role of Image-Guided Renal Biopsy in the Diagnosis of Renal Lymphoma

Image-guided percutaneous biopsy is a minimally invasive method to diagnose a variety of renal masses (CAOILI et al. 2002). It is particularly helpful in avoiding unnecessary nephrectomy if the diagnosis of renal lymphoma is suspected on imaging (STALLONE et al. 2000). Core biopsy as well as flow

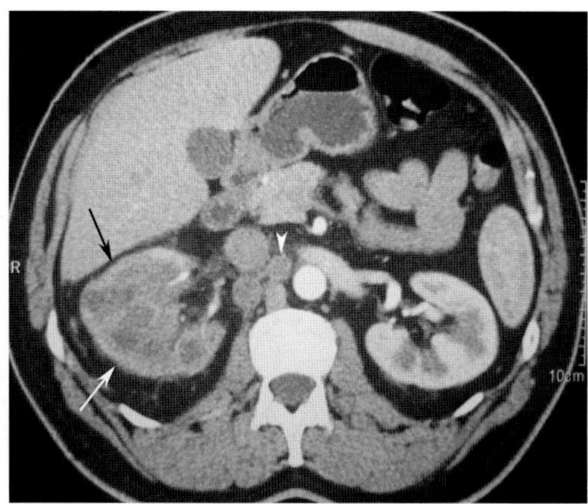

Fig. 18.24. Transitional cell carcinoma infiltrating the right kidney in a 44-year-old man with right flank pain. Contrast-enhanced CT in the corticomedullary phase shows a mass infiltrating the right kidney (*arrows*). Note that there is delayed enhancement in the right kidney and paracaval adenopathy (*arrowhead*). The diagnosis was established by percutaneous biopsy. (With Permission from URBAN and FISHMAN 2000)

cytometric studies are useful to confirm the diagnosis and classify the lymphoma prior to therapy (TRUONG et al. 2001).

At our institution, US is the preferred guidance modality for percutaneous biopsy. Its real-time capability allows the needle to be guided into suspicious lesions under direct visualization, allowing for quick adjustment if necessary (Fig. 18.7). This results in faster procedure time compared with CT, as well as more accurate diagnosis even when the target is small or deep (MEMEL et al. 1996; MIDDLETON et al. 1997). Lack of ionizing radiation, easy availability, and reduced cost are added benefits of US.

18.6
Conclusion

The urinary tract is a common site for extranodal spread of lymphoma, particularly non-Hodgkin lymphoma. Contrast-enhanced CT remains the preferred imaging modality for the detection of renal lymphoma. Magnetic resonance imaging is useful in special circumstances, particularly when the patient cannot tolerate intravenous contrast. Ultrasound has only a limited role except as a guidance modality for percutaneous biopsy.

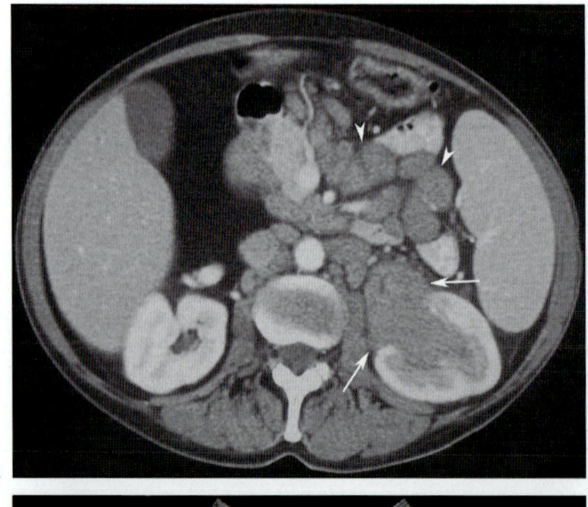

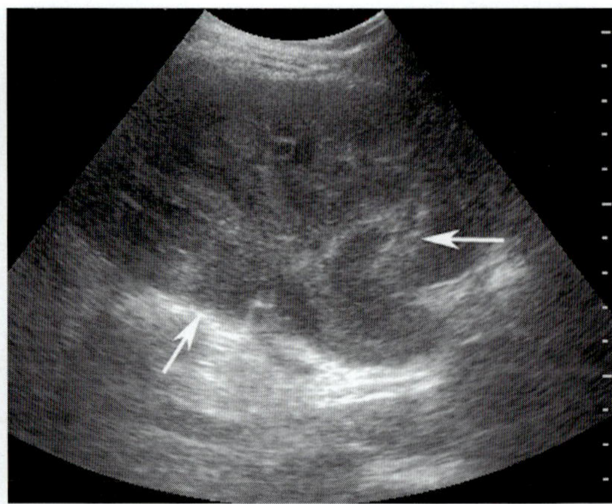

a

b

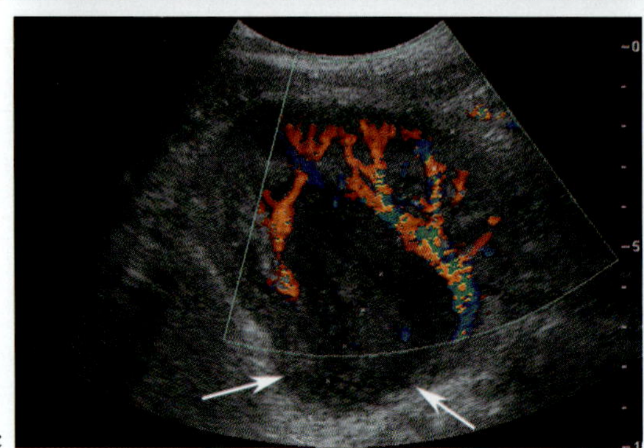

c

Fig. 18.25a-c. B-cell non-Hodgkin lymphoma in a 70-year-old woman. **a** Axial contrast-enhanced CT scan of the mid-abdomen shows a homogeneous soft tissue mass (*arrows*) in the left renal sinus. Note the lack of significant hydronephrosis and the presence of mesenteric (*arrowheads*) and retroperitoneal adenopathies. **b** Sagittal ultrasound image of the left kidney shows an infiltrating poorly defined mass (*arrows*) in the region of the renal pelvis and confirms the absence of hydronephrosis. **c** On color Doppler ultrasound image, the kidney is well vascularized and the mass is hypovascular (*arrows*). (With Permission from URBAN and FISHMAN 2000)

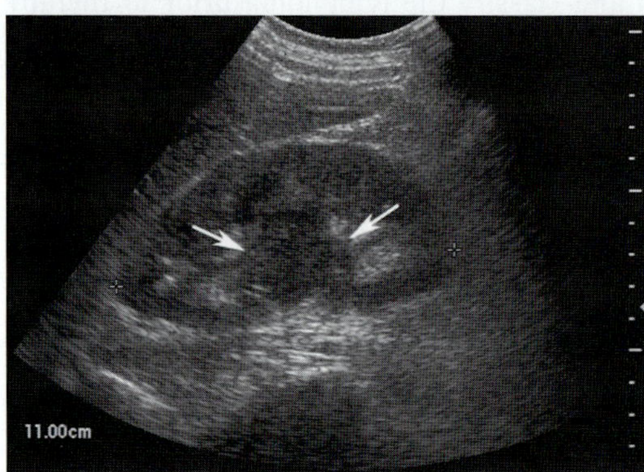

Fig. 18.26. Recurrent Hodgkin disease in a 29-year-old man presenting as a right renal hilar mass. Sagittal ultrasound image of the right kidney shows an ill-defined hypoechoic mass (*arrows*) infiltrating the renal sinus fat. The diagnosis was confirmed by percutaneous fine-needle aspiration and core biopsy performed under ultrasound guidance. (With Permission from URBAN and FISHMAN 2000)

References

Ambos MA, Bosniak MA, Madayag MA, Lefleur RS (1977) Infiltrating neoplasms of the kidney. Am J Roentgenol 129:859–864

Bechtold RE, Dyer RB, Zagoria RJ, Chen MY (1996) The perirenal space: relationship of pathologic processes to normal retroperitoneal anatomy. Radiographics 16:841–854

Cadman PJ, Lindsell DR, Golding SJ (1988) An unusual appearance of renal lymphoma. Clin Radiol 39:452–453

Caoili EM, Bude RO, Higgins EJ, Hoff DL, Nghiem HV (2002) Evaluation of sonographically guided percutaneous core biopsy of renal masses. Am J Roentgenol 179:373–378

Chang SS, Nayak R, Cookson MS (2002) Lymphoma presenting as a solitary renal hilar mass. Urology 59:134–135

Chepuri NB, Strouse PJ, Yanik GA (2003) CT of renal lymphoma in children. Am J Roentgenol 180:429–431

Cohan RH, Dunnick NR, Leder RA, Baker ME (1990) Computed tomography of renal lymphoma. J Comput Assist Tomogr 14:933–938

Eisenberg PJ, Papanicolaou N, Lee MJ, Yoder IC (1994) Diagnostic imaging in the evaluation of renal lymphoma. Leuk Lymphoma 16:37–50

Guermazi A, Brice P, de Kerviler E, Ferme C, Hennequin C, Meignin V, Frija J (2001) Extranodal Hodgkin disease: spectrum of disease. Radiographics 21:161–179

Harisinghani MG, Maher MM, Gervais DA, McGovern F, Hahn P, Jhaveri K, Varghese J, Mueller PR (2003) Incidence of malignancy in complex cystic renal masses (Bosniak category III): Should imaging-guided biopsy precede surgery? Am J Roentgenol 180:755–758

Hartman DS, David CJ Jr, Goldman SM, Friedman AC, Fritzsche P (1982) Renal lymphoma: radiologic–pathologic correlation of 21 cases. Radiology 144:759–766

Hartman DS, Davidson AJ, Davis CJ Jr, Goldman SM (1988) Infiltrative renal lesions: CT–sonographic–pathologic correlation. Am J Roentgenol 150:1061–1064

Heiken JP, Gold RP, Schnur MJ, King DL, Bashist B, Glazer HS (1983) Computed tomography of renal lymphoma with ultrasound correlation. J Comput Assist Tomogr 7:245–250

Malbrain ML, Lambrecht GL, Daelemans R, Lins RL, Hermans P, Zachee P (1994) Acute renal failure due to bilateral lymphomatous infiltrates. Primary extranodal non-Hodgkin's lymphoma (p-EN-NHL) of the kidneys: does it really exist? Clin Nephrol 42:163–169

Memel DS, Dodd GD III, Esola CC (1996) Efficacy of sonography as a guidance technique for biopsy of abdominal, pelvic, and retroperitoneal lymph nodes. Am J Roentgenol 167:957–962

Metser U, Goor O, Lerman H, Naparstek E, Even-Sapir E (2004) PET-CT of extranodal lymphoma. Am J Roentgenol 182:1579–1586

Middleton WD, Hiskes SK, Teefey SA, Boucher LD (1997) Small (1.5 cm or less) liver metastases: US-guided biopsy. Radiology 205:729–732

Mills NE, Goldenberg AS, Liu D, Feiner HD, Gallo G, Gray C, Lustbader I (1992) B-cell lymphoma presenting as infiltrative renal disease. Am J Kidney Dis 19:181–184

Moog F, Bangerter M, Diederichs CG, Guhlmann A, Merkle E, Frickhofen N, Reske SN (1998) Extranodal malignant lymphoma: detection with FDG PET versus CT. Radiology 206:475–481

Nishie A, Yoshimitsu K, Irie H, Aibe H, Tajima T, Shinozaki K, Nakayama T, Kakihara D, Naito S, Ono M, Muranaka T, Honda H (2003) Radiologic features of Castleman's disease occupying the renal sinus. Am J Roentgenol 181:1037–1040

Pickhardt PJ, Lonergan GJ, Davis CJ Jr, Kashitani N, Wagner BJ (2000) From the archives of the AFIP. Infiltrative renal lesions: radiologic–pathologic correlation. Armed Forces Institute of Pathology. Radiographics 20:215–243

Reznek RH, Mootoosamy I, Webb JA, Richards MA (1990) CT in renal and perirenal lymphoma: a further look. Clin Radiol 42:233–238

Richards MA, Mootoosamy I, Reznek RH, Webb JA, Lister TA (1990) Renal involvement in patients with non-Hodgkin's lymphoma: clinical and pathological features in 23 cases. Hematol Oncol 8:105–110

Richmond J, Sherman RS, Diamond HD, Craver LF (1962) Renal lesions associated with malignant lymphomas. Am J Med 32:184–207

Semelka RC, Kelekis NL, Burdeny DA, Mitchell DG, Brown JJ, Siegelman ES (1996) Renal lymphoma: demonstration by MR imaging. Am J Roentgenol 166:823–827

Sheeran SR, Sussman SK (1998) Renal lymphoma: spectrum of CT findings and potential mimics. Am J Roentgenol 171:1067–1072

Stallone G, Infante B, Manno C, Campobasso N, Pannarale G, Schena FP (2000) Primary renal lymphoma does exist: case report and review of the literature. J Nephrol 13:367–372

Szolar DH, Kammerhuber F, Altziebler S, Tillich M, Breinl E, Fotter R, Schreyer HH (1997) Multiphasic helical CT of the kidney: increased conspicuity for detection and characterization of small (<3 cm) renal masses. Radiology 202:211–217

Truong LD, Caraway N, Ngo T, Laucirica R, Katz R, Ramzy I (2001) Renal lymphoma. The diagnostic and therapeutic roles of fine-needle aspiration. Am J Clin Pathol 115:18–31

Urban BA, Fishman EK (2000) Renal lymphoma: CT patterns with emphasis on helical CT. Radiographics 20:197–212

Weinberger E, Rosenbaum DM, Pendergrass TW (1990) Renal involvement in children with lymphoma: comparison of CT with sonography. Am J Roentgenol 155:347–349

Yasunaga Y, Hoshida Y, Hashimoto M, Miki T, Okuyama A, Aozasa K (1997) Malignant lymphoma of the kidney. J Surg Oncol 64:207–211

19 Lymphoproliferative Neoplasms

CLARA G. C. OOI and ALI GUERMAZI

CONTENTS

19.1 Introduction

The kidney is the fifth most commonly affected organ in myeloproliferative and lymphoproliferative disorders at autopsy (BARCOS et al. 1987; XIAO et al. 1997). There is, however, a discrepancy between the incidence found at autopsy and that found clinically or on imaging (EISENBERG et al. 1994; GEOFFAY et al. 1984; RICHMOND et al. 1962; ROSENBERG et al. 1961). This discrepancy has been explained by the supposition that renal involvement represents a late manifestation of the disease, and one which is frequently clinically asymptomatic unless infection or obstruction supervenes (EISENBERG et al. 1994). However, with improved technology in cross-sectional imaging, such as computed tomography (CT) and magnetic resonance (MR) imaging, and their increased utilization in the routine staging of hematological malignancies, the detection rate of renal involvement by these conditions will invari-

ably rise (EISENBERG et al. 1994; ROSENBERG et al. 1961; REZNEK et al. 1990).

The prevalence of renal involvement at autopsy varies with the different hematological malignancies in question. It is reported in up to 45% of acute myeloid leukemia (AML), 38% of chronic myeloid leukemia (AML), 53% of acute lymphoblastic leukemia (ALL), and 60–90% of chronic lymphoblastic leukemia (CLL; BARCOS et al. 1987; SCHWARTZ and SHAMSUDDIN 1981; XIAO et al. 1997). The incidence of lymphomatous infiltration of the kidney ranges from 33.5 to 62% at autopsy (KIELY et al. 1969; MARTINEZ-MALDONADO and RAMIREZ DE ARELLANO 1966; RICHMOND et al. 1962; XIAO et al. 1997). Using radiographic techniques prior to the advent of CT (FERRY et al. 1995; ROSENBERG et al. 1961), the incidence was reported to be less than 1%, but with CT it has increased to 8% (CHEPURI et al. 2003; COHAN et al. 1990; ELLERT and KREEL 1980; GEOFFAY et al. 1984; HURII et al. 1983).

Extramedullary plasmacytoma of the kidney occurs either as a primary event without bone marrow involvement or as a manifestation of disseminated multiple myeloma and is extremely rare (SOESAN et al. 1992). In an autopsy series of 120 cases of lymphoproliferative and myeloproliferative disorders, myelomatous involvement of the kidney was found in only 12% (XIAO et al. 1997).

Although renal involvement, such as urinary obstruction, uric acid, light-chain and drug-related nephropathies, glomerulopathies secondary to amyloidosis, cryoglobulinemia, and glomerulonephritis, is a common association in hematological malignancies, particularly the leukemias and myeloma, this chapter deals only with imaging of direct tumor infiltration or involvement of the kidney.

C. G. C. OOI, MD
Associate Professor and Honorary Consultant, Department of Diagnostic Radiology, Queen Mary Hospital, University of Hong Kong, Room 405, Block K, Pokfulam Road, Hong Kong SAR, China
A. GUERMAZI, MD
Senior Radiologist, Scientific Director, Oncology Services, Department of Radiology Services, Synarc Inc., 575 Market Street, 17th Floor, San Francisco, CA 94105, USA

19.2 Leukemia

Although the kidney is one of the most common sites of involvement at autopsies in the leukemias, particularly lymphoblastic leukemia, radiological evidence in the living patient is rarely encountered. The reason is most likely that up to 67% of renal involvement in leukemia is microscopic (BASKER et al. 2002; TANAKA et al. 2004). When it occurs, renal involvement is more common at relapse than at initial presentation, as the kidneys, like the central nervous system and testes, are "sanctuary sites" where relapse may occur even in bone marrow remission (TANAKA et al. 2004). However, despite its prevalence in CLL, leukemic infiltration is rarely associated with renal failure and may therefore be clinically asymptomatic.

Interstitial infiltration by leukemic cells crowds out normal structures, and although both the renal medulla and cortex are usually involved simultaneously, XIAO et al. (1997) reported a predilection for the renal cortex in CLL with bilateral involvement more common than unilateral (Fig. 19.1).

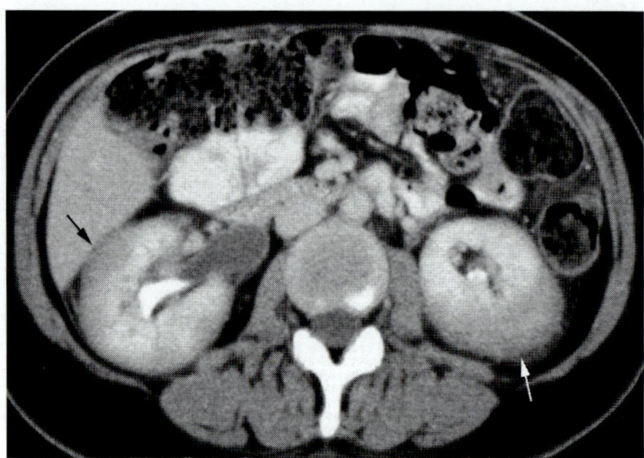

Fig. 19.1. Chronic lymphoblastic leukemia in a 51-year-old woman. Axial contrast-enhanced CT scan shows ill-defined hypodense lesions on both kidneys (*arrows*). (Image courtesy of P. PICKHARDT)

There are four patterns of infiltration: bilateral diffuse renal infiltration; unilateral renal infiltration; focal masses; and perirenal/renal hilar infiltration.

Bilateral and diffuse renal enlargement with preservation of the reniform shape is the most common presentation (BOUDVILLE et al. 2001; COMERMA-COMA et al. 1998; GUPTA and KEANE 1985; PARKER 1997), although a lobulated appearance may be encountered (BASKER et al. 2002). The bilateral diffuse renal enlargement can be observed on intravenous urography (IVU) with marked stretching of the calyces and infundibula (GUPTA and KEANE 1985) simulating polycystic kidneys; however, absence of cysts on cross-sectional imaging should exclude polycystic kidneys. On ultrasound (US), the infiltrated kidneys may be normal (BOUDVILLE et al. 2001; PARKER 1997) or hypoechogenic (GATES 1978; TEELE 1977), although cases of hyperechogenicity have been reported (Fig. 19.2) (PARKER 1997). On CT, the bilateral diffuse infiltration is depicted as thickened renal parenchyma, which may be isodense or hypodense with compression of the pelvicalyceal system (Fig. 19.3; ARAKI 1982). The masses are minimally enhancing and remain hypodense relative to normal renal tissue after contrast administration (Fig. 19.4). These imaging features, however, are not specific and are also found with glycogen storage diseases and amyloidosis.

Unilateral diffuse renal enlargement can be confused with compensatory renal hypertrophy when renal function is unimpaired and with renal vein thrombosis when renal dysfunction is present (ARAKI 1982). In cases where there is bilateral but asymmetrical involvement, the smaller kidney may be erroneously diagnosed as normal on imaging.

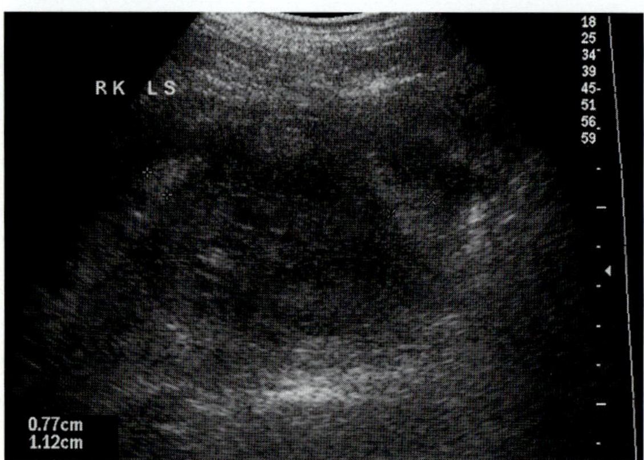
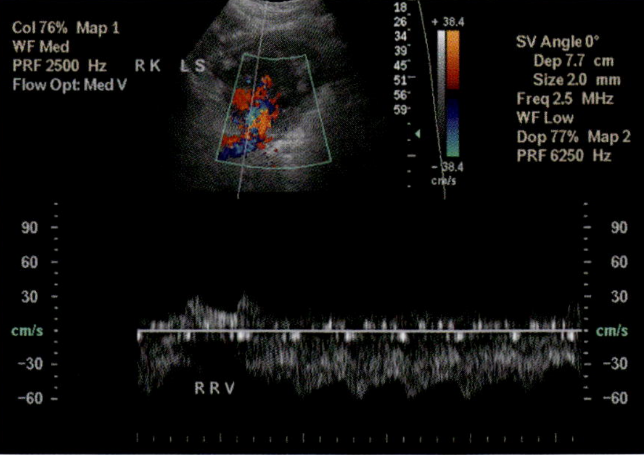

Fig. 19.2a,b. Acute myeloblastic leukemia in a 59-year-old man. **a** Longitudinal ultrasound image of the right kidney shows echogenic tissue (*calipers*) surrounding the kidney in the perinephric space. **b** On Doppler ultrasound image, the renal hilar vessels are noted to be patent.

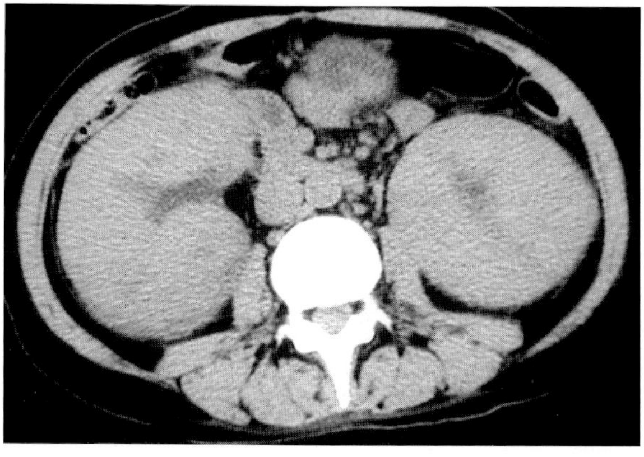

Fig. 19.3. Acute lymphoblastic leukemia in a 48-year-old woman who relapsed after bone marrow transplantation. Axial unenhanced CT scan of the abdomen shows bilateral diffuse renal enlargement by tissue isodense to muscle attenuation. Note para-aortic lymphadenopathy.

A third pattern of leukemic infiltration is the focal mass, which can be multiple, unilateral, or bilateral (COMERMA-COMA et al. 1998; TEELE 1977). The masses may appear hypoechoic on US (GOH et al. 1978) and hypodense on CT (COMERMA-COMA et al. 1998; TEELE 1977). This form of infiltration is rare in leukemia, although it is more common in lymphoma. The fourth pattern of leukemic renal infiltration manifests as enlarged peri-hilar or peri-renal masses (Fig. 19.5), which may cause hydrone-phrosis and renal distortion (TEELE 1977). These masses share the same US and CT characteristics as the other forms of renal leukemic infiltration.

19.3
Myeloid Sarcoma

Myeloid sarcoma, previously known as chloroma or granulocytic sarcoma, is an extremely rare extramed-ullary manifestation of myeloid leukemia (VARDIMAN et al. 2002). Myeloid sarcoma is defined as an extra-medullary localized tumor composed of immature granulocytic precursors. Although usually associ-ated with systemic disease in acute myeloid leukemia, granulocytic sarcoma may herald leukemic trans-formation in myelodysplastic disorders or diseases including chronic myeloid leukemia, polycythemia rubra vera, myelofibrosis, and chronic eosinophilic leukemia (LIU et al. 1973; NEIMAN et al. 1981). The overall incidence of myeloid sarcoma is 2.5–8%, and it is more common in children than in adults (13 vs 5%) with acute myeloid leukemia (LIU et al. 1973; PUI et al. 1994). There is a predilection for bone and peri-neural tissue (NEIMAN et al. 1981). Renal involvement is extremely rare and is usually reported at autopsy rather than in living patients (BREATNACH 1985; LIU et al. 1973; PARK et al. 2003). Renal myeloid sarcoma may manifest as diffuse enlargement of the affected kidney, which may be isodense or hypodense on CT, long-segment ureteral involvement, and enlarged retroperitoneal lymph node (BAGG et al. 1994; BREATNACH 1985; PARK et al. 2003).

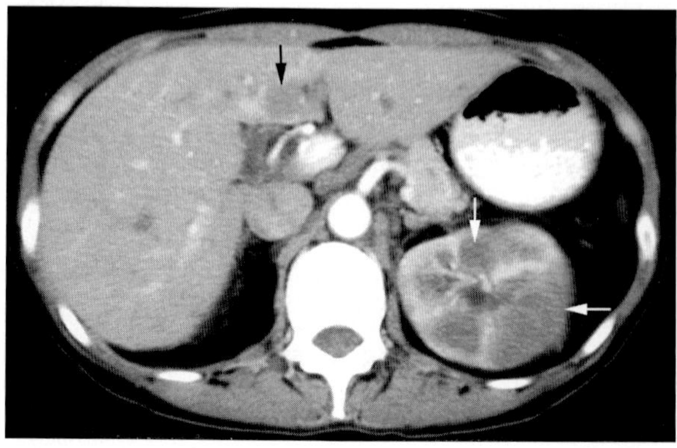
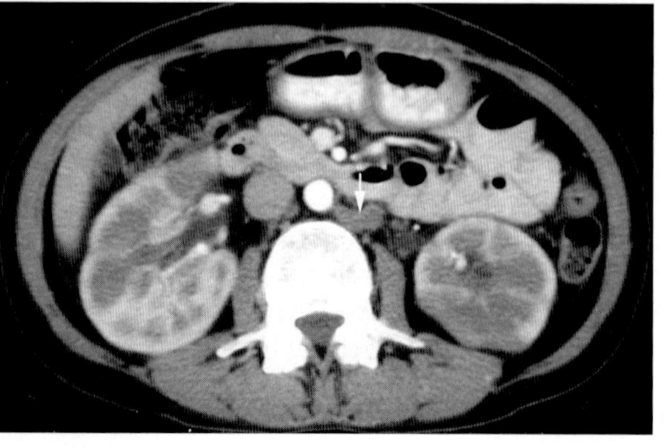

Fig. 19.4a,b. Acute lymphoblastic leukemia in a 52-year-old man. a Axial contrast-enhanced CT scan through the abdomen shows diffuse hypodense leukemic infiltration (*white arrows*) of the left kidney and a hypodense nodule (*black arrow*) in the segment IV of the liver. b Axial contrast-enhanced CT scan obtained caudad to a shows bilateral diffuse renal involvement and retroperitoneal lymphadenopathy (*arrow*).

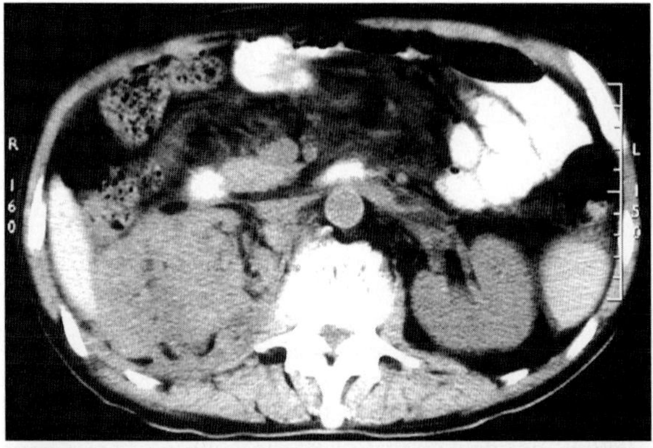
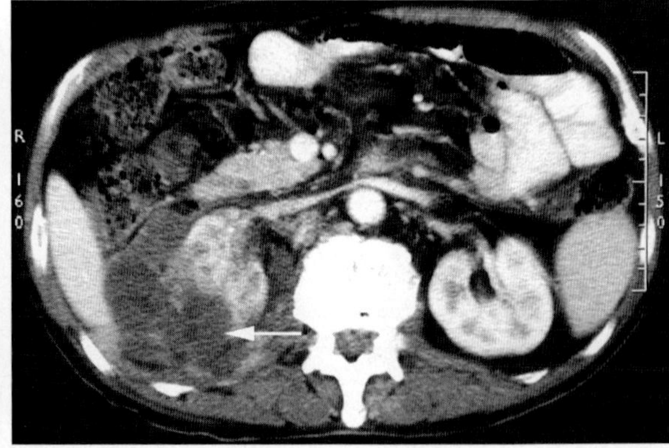
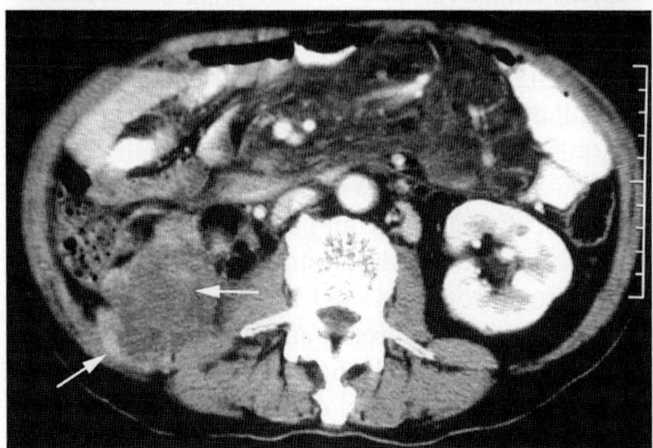

Fig. 19.5a-c. Acute myeloblastic leukemia in a 59-year-old man who relapsed after chemotherapy and bone marrow transplantation. **a** Axial unenhanced CT scan through the kidneys show irregular and heterogeneous enlargement of the right kidney with abnormal infiltration of the peri-renal space. **b** Axial contrast-enhanced CT scan demonstrates a peri-renal mass, isodense relative to normally enhancing renal tissue, which has infiltrated through the capsule of the right kidney to involve the parenchyma (*arrow*). The left kidney is normal. **c** Axial contrast-enhanced CT scan obtained caudad to **b** shows inferior extension of the heterogeneously hypodense peri-renal mass (*arrows*) within the peri-renal fat.

19.4
Hodgkin Disease

Renal involvement by non-Hodgkin lymphoma is common in disseminated disease, with an incidence of up to 62% at autopsy (KIELY et al. 1969; MARTINEZ-MALDONADO and RAMIREZ DE ARELLANO 1966; RICHMOND et al. 1962; XIAO et al. 1997). It is, however, extremely rare and seldom encountered clinically in Hodgkin disease, being documented in less than 1% of patients at diagnosis (COHAN et al. 1990; FERRY et al. 1995; PILATRINO et al. 2003; REZNEK et al. 1990). In general, lymphomatous infiltration is nearly always secondary to hematogenous spread or contiguous involvement from retroperitoneal lymphoma. Renal lymphoma arising de novo in the renal parenchyma as a primary tumor, and not from invasion of adjacent retroperitoneal lymphoma or as extranodal manifestation of disseminated lymphoma, is extremely rare. Due to the lack of specific symptoms, renal involvement in lymphoma is rarely diagnosed pre-operatively (KANDEL et al. 1987) and is often diagnosed late in the disease. Symptoms cover the whole gamut of renal disease, but the most common are flank pain, hematuria, anemia, and weight loss. Imaging features are similar in Hodgkin and non-Hodgkin lymphoma of the kidneys.

The imaging features of renal lymphoma depend on the mechanism of spread to the kidney (hematogenous vs direct invasion), pattern of intrarenal growth (interstitial or expansile), and degree of extension beyond the kidney. Hematogenous seeding results in multiple nodular lesions in the renal parenchyma, which are localized to the cortex initially. Retroperitoneal lymphomatous masses involve the kidneys in two ways: via perinephric tissue with transcapsular spread through the renal capsule into the renal cortex or via the renal pelvis into the renal medulla (trans-sinus growth; HARTMAN et al. 1982). Once in the renal parenchyma, tumor infiltration is interstitial, growing in between the nephrons, blood vessels, and collecting ducts, using them as scaffolding. The kidneys maintain their reniform configuration and renal function during this phase, and on imaging, particularly on IVU, no or very subtle abnormalities are found (COHAN et al. 1990). Expansile growth follows with destruction of the "scaffolding" resulting in enlarged kidneys with compressed and deformed calyces. Uneven growth results in a lobulated outline with masses extending outside the renal contour. More commonly even growth results in multiple nodules in both kidneys. With continued growth there the entire renal parenchyma would be replaced.

In general, IVU is not a sensitive modality for evaluating renal lymphoma (EISENBERG et al. 1994). Computed tomography is the preferred modality for evaluating the kidney, its adjacent retroperitoneal space, and the rest of the abdomen. Five patterns of

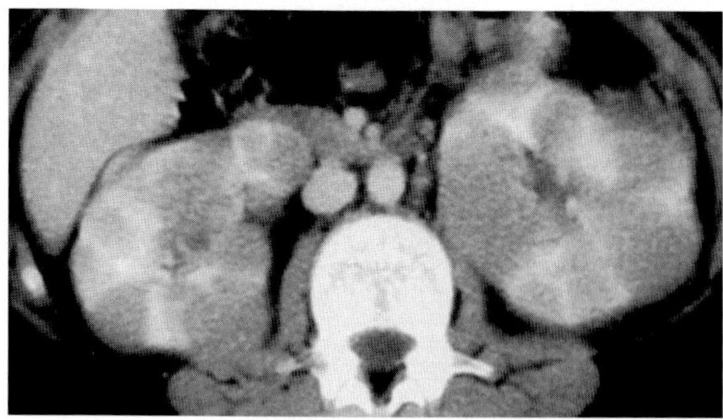

Fig. 19.6. Renal involvement by recurrent Hodgkin disease in a post-gestational 24-year-old woman. Axial contrast-enhanced CT scan shows bilateral involvement of the kidneys by several rounded hypodense lesions. This is a typical appearance of systemic involvement. Kidneys returned to normal after four chemotherapy courses of BEACOPP. (Image courtesy of L. DOBROVOLSKIENE)

renal lymphoma have been described on CT: multiple renal masses (Fig. 19.6); direct invasion from contiguous retroperitoneal lymphoma; solitary focal masses (Fig. 19.7); diffuse infiltration (Fig. 19.8); and perirenal/perihilar disease. Multiple renal masses ranging from 1 to 3 cm, which can affect one or both kidneys, is most commonly followed by direct invasion of the kidney from contiguous retroperitoneal lymphomatous masses (COHAN et al. 1990; HEIKEN et al. 1983; PILATRINO et al. 2003; REZNEK 1990). In general, renal lymphoma lesions are usually hypo- or isodense before contrast, and remain hypodense relative to normal-enhancing renal parenchyma after contrast administration (CHEPURI et al. 2003; COHAN et al. 1990; HARTMAN et al. 1982; PILATRINO et al. 2003; REZNEK 1990). On US, the lesions are hypoechoic with well-defined borders. Trans-sinus growth obliterates normally echogenic renal sinus fat, whereas perirenal lymphoma is depicted as a hypoechoic "halo" around the kidney (CRUZ et al. 1995). Perirenal lymphoma results from trans-capsular spread from within the kidney or from infiltration by retroperitoneal disease (CRUZ et al. 1995).

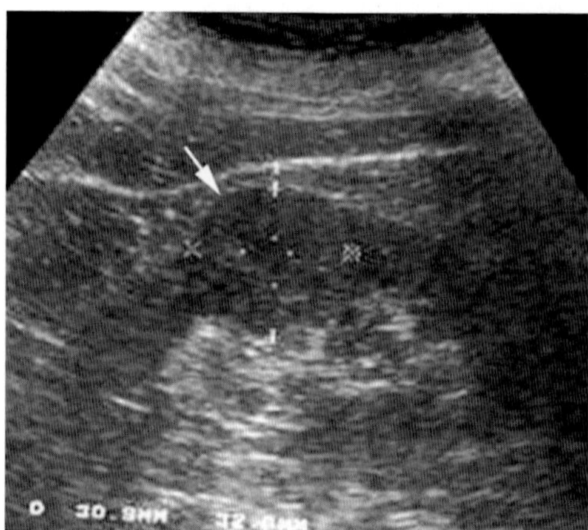

a

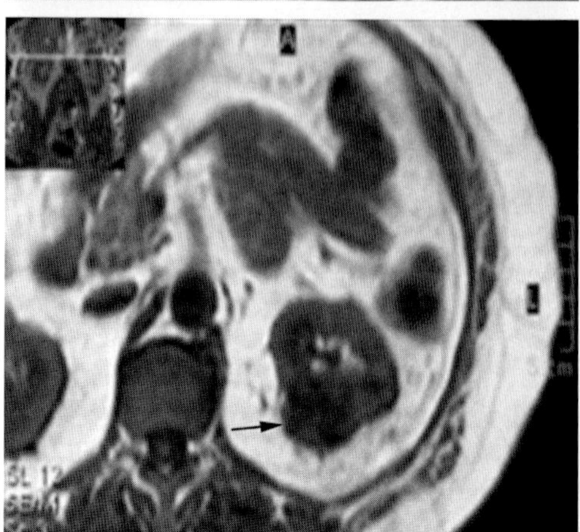

b

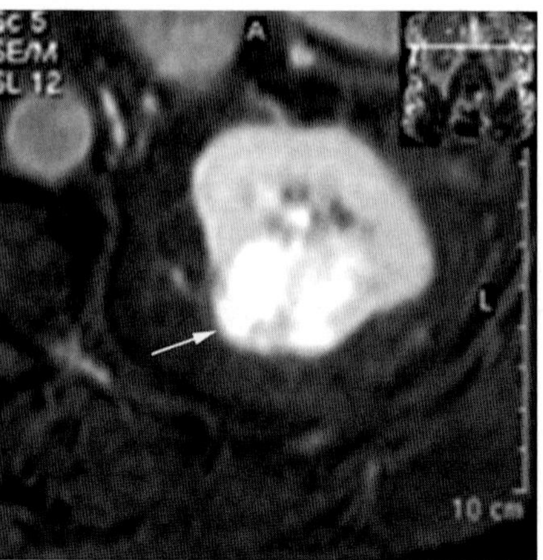

c

Fig. 19.7a-c. Stage IV Hodgkin disease of the kidney in a 62-year-old man with hematuria and enlarged mediastinal lymph nodes. **a** Longitudinal US image shows an isoechoic mass (*arrow*) of the left kidney deforming the renal contours. **b** Axial unenhanced T1-weighted MR image shows the mass (*arrow*) to be isointense to the renal parenchyma with **c** strong enhancement after contrast administration and fat suppression. Radiological imaging features were of renal cell carcinoma. Nephrectomy showed that the kidney was involved by Hodgkin disease.

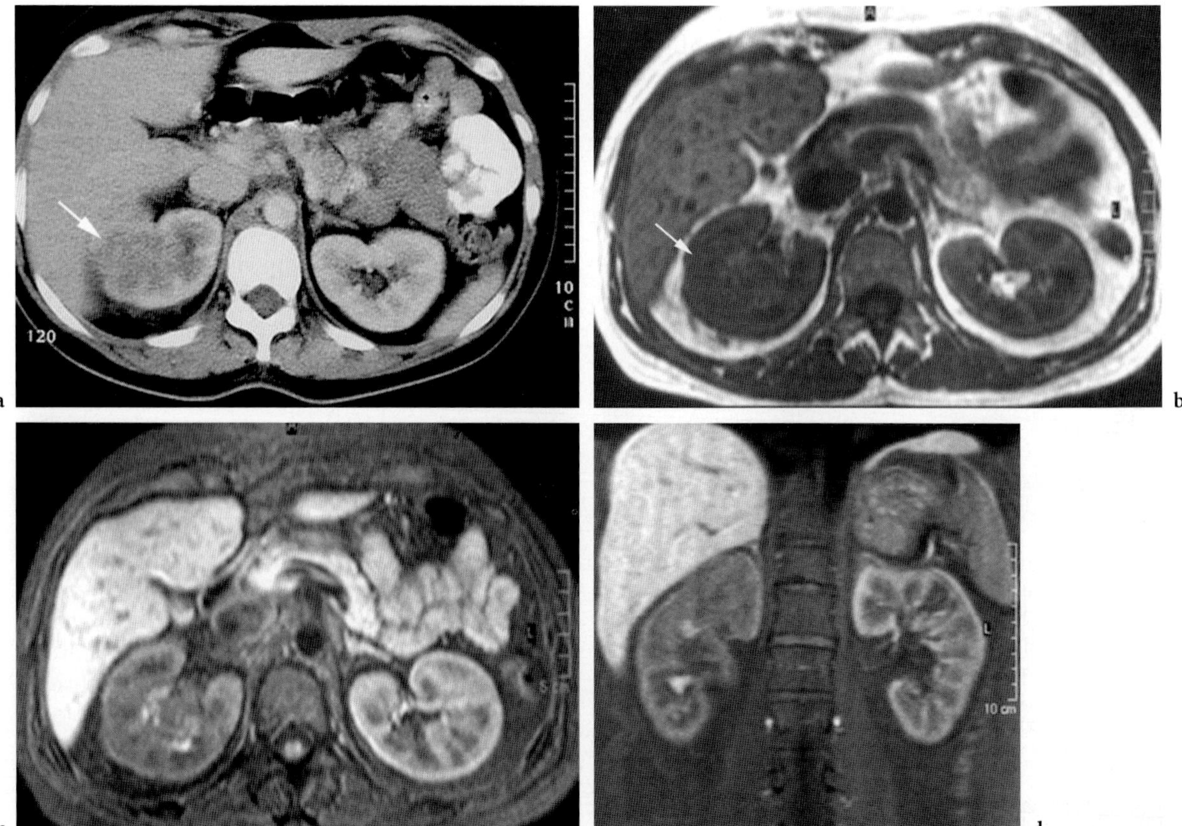

Fig. 19.8a-d. Infiltrative renal Hodgkin disease in a 32-year-old woman. **a** Axial contrast-enhanced CT scan shows hypodense infiltration (*arrow*) of the right kidney. The kidney is very slightly enlarged in comparison with the left kidney. **b** Axial unenhanced T1-weighted MR image shows the infiltration (*arrow*) to be slightly hypointense relative to the renal cortex. This infiltration obliterates the normally hyperintense renal sinus fat. **c** Axial and **d** coronal fat-suppressed contrast-enhanced T1-weighted MR images show minimal enhancement of the cortex of the right kidney due to diffuse infiltration. The reniform shape of the right kidney is maintained. (Image courtesy of L. Dobrovolskiene)

Gallium-67 citrate scanning has been used in the detection of lymphoma, with variable sensitivities depending on the site of involvement and cell type. It has the highest sensitivity (over 70%) in Hodgkin disease and diffuse large-cell malignant lymphoma, but poor sensitivity (<50%) in other cell types such as diffuse malignant lymphoma (Eisenberg et al. 1994; Hartman et al. 1982). The combination of single photon emission computed tomography (SPECT) with gallium scanning has been shown to be useful in differentiating lymphoma from benign tissue. Positron emission tomography (PET) has a better resolution than gallium scanning with increased sensitivity and shorter procedural time (Mavromatis and Cheson 2002). Its lack of specificity does not lend itself as an initial diagnostic tool in lymphoma, but it is useful in monitoring response (Romer and Schwaiger 1998).

19.5
Post-Transplantation Renal Allograft Lymphoproliferative Disorder

Post-transplantation lymphoproliferative disorders (PTLD) are a direct consequence of chronic immunosuppression, and their pathogenesis is strongly related to the Epstein-Barr virus (EBV). Most post-transplant malignancies are non-melanotic squamous cell carcinoma of the skin and lips (37%) followed by lymphomas (16%; Penn 1996). The incidence of PTLD varies with the organ transplanted. Due to aggressive immunosuppression, heart–lung transplantation has the highest incidence (4.6–25%) followed by liver (2.2–6.7%) and heart transplantations (1.8–5.1%; Penn 1996). The overall incidence of PTLD in renal transplants is 1–2%, which represents 21% of all malignancies in graft recipients

(COCKFIELD et al. 1993; DODD et al. 1992; LUTZ and HEEMANN 2003). The renal allograft is the most common site of PTLD (47%) after renal transplantation (MILLER et al. 1997; VOSE et al. 1996), although secondary involvement of the kidney from an extrarenal primary is also frequent (FRICK et al. 1984). Non-Hodgkin lymphoma is the most common type of lymphoma to arise in renal allografts.

Although the imaging features of transplant lymphoma have been described as resembling those in non-transplant patients (FRICK et al. 1984), a certain predilection for the allograft pedicle (Fig. 19.9) alludes to a predisposition for PTLD to occur at the anastomotic site (ALI et al. 1999; LOPEZ-BEN et al. 2000). Allograft pedicle involvement was described in 4 of 5 (80%), and 12 of 16, (75%) patients with renal allograft lymphoproliferative disorders (ALI et al. 1999; LOPEZ-BEN et al. 2000). Vascular encasement is a common feature. The PTLD masses are generally hypoechoic, although they may be heterogeneous at the renal hilum. On CT, they are hypodense masses (Fig. 19.9a) which can be non-enhancing, mildly enhancing, or peripherally enhancing (LOPEZ-BEN et al. 2000; VRACHLIOTIS et al. 2000). Tumoral extension around the ureter from the renal pedicle can also be present (Fig. 19.9d). The MR findings include iso- to hypointensity on T1-weighted images and hypointensity on T2-weighted images, with mild and/or peripheral enhancement (ALI et al. 1999; LOPEZ-BEN et al. 2000). In the context of post-transplantation evaluation of a renal allograft, US is usually the initial modality. Presence of a complex mass, particularly at the hila, requires exclusion of non-neoplastic conditions such as resolving hematoma, seroma, abscesses, and complicated lymphocele, using other imaging techniques (LOPEZ-BEN et al. 2000). Doppler US is useful in delineating the relationship between renal hilar vessels and the mass. Both MR imaging and CT can further characterize renal masses and evaluate tumor extension, retroperitoneal lymphadenopathy, and involvement of other extranodal sites.

Differential diagnosis of masses located within and around the graft pedicle includes other compli-

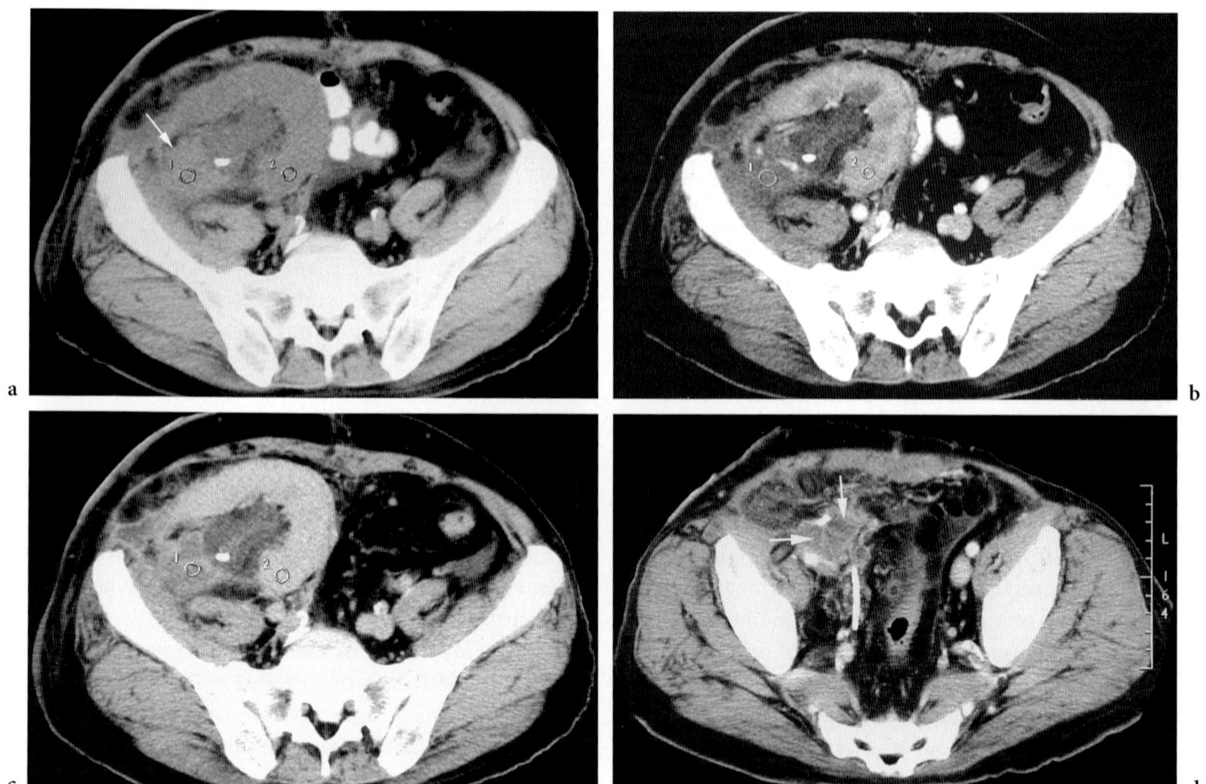

Fig. 19.9a-d. Post-transplantation lymphoproliferative disorder arising from the renal allograft in a 49-year-old woman. **a** Axial unenhanced CT scan through the pelvis shows a soft tissue thickening (*arrow*) at the renal pedicle. Note a JJ drainage stent at the pelviureteric junction. **b** Axial CT scan at the arterial phase of contrast administration show minimal contrast enhancement of the renal pedicle mass, which is hypodense relative to normally enhancing renal tissue and remains hypodense on **c** the venous phase of contrast administration. **d** The mass has extended inferiorly along and surrounding the ureter (*arrows*).

cations that occur after renal transplantation such as hematomas, perirenal lymphoceles, or abscesses (CLAUDON et al. 1998). Urinomas should be considered particularly in the presence of hydronephrosis.

19.6
AIDS-Related Lymphoma

Renal manifestations of acquired immunodeficiency syndrome (AIDS) include intrarenal infections, neoplastic disorders, acute tubular necrosis, glomerulonephritis, interstitial nephritis, and drug toxicity, among others (MILLER et al. 1993). Compared with lymphoma in immunocompetent patients, AIDS-related lymphoma is much more aggressive and is associated with higher histological grades, wider extent of disease, greater incidence of extranodal disease, and poorer prognosis (JEFFREY et al. 1986; SISKIN et al. 1995; TOWNSEND et al. 1989). The liver and spleen are the two most common intraabdominal extranodal sites (up to 90%) of AIDS-related lymphoma on imaging, whereas renal involvement is reported in up to 12% of adults who are imaged (CLIFTON and BAILY 1991; MOORE et al. 1995; NYBERG et al. 1986; SISKIN et al. 1995). AIDS-related lymphoma manifests as solitary or multiple discrete nodules that are hypoechoic on US and hypodense on CT (NYBERG et al. 1986; SISKIN et al. 1995).

19.7
Waldenström Macroglobulinemia

Waldenström macroglobulinemia is a low-grade lymphoma characterized by malignant proliferation of mature plasmacytoid lymphocytes, which produce its hallmark monoclonal immunoglobulin M (IgM). The clinical presentation is a direct reflection of the effects of malignant infiltration of tissues, circulating IgM and tissue deposition of IgM. The bone marrow is the most common site of involvement followed by the reticuloendothelial system. Renal involvement is unusual and is reported in 6% of patients with this condition (MOORE et al. 1995). Primary involvement is even rare (2.7%). Small nodular lesions and perinephric masses with imaging characteristics similar to other lymphomas have been reported (Fig. 19.10; CLIFTON and BAILY 1991; MOORE et al. 1995).

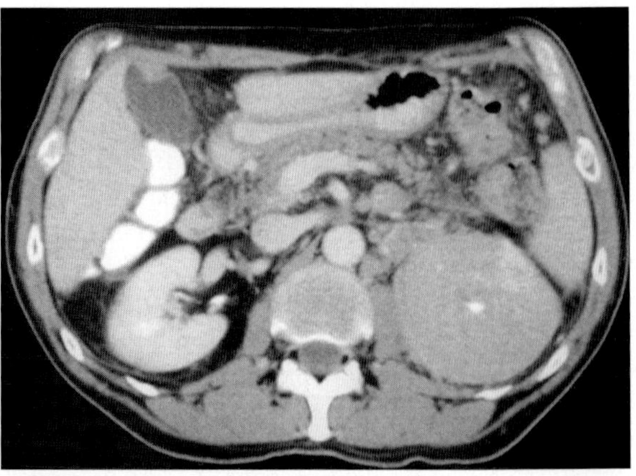

Fig. 19.10. Waldenström macroglobulinemia in a 70-year-old man with renal involvement. Axial contrast-enhanced CT scan of the abdomen shows hypodense left renal mass, which conforms to the contour of the kidney.

19.8
Multiple Myeloma and Plasmacytoma

Plasmacytoma is a malignant monoclonal proliferation of the B-cell line and a form of plasma cell tumor that can occur in any organ outside the bone marrow (ALEXIOU et al. 1999). Plasmacytoma may arise either from osseous (medullary) or non-osseous (extramedullary) sites (ALEXIOU et al. 1999; BOLEK et al. 1996; GALIENI et al. 1995; THE INTERNATIONAL MYELOMA WORKING GROUP 2003). Primary extramedullary plasmacytoma (EMP) is rare, accounting for 4% of all plasma cell tumors, and is defined as monoclonal plasma cell proliferation that develops in the absence of multiple myeloma elsewhere. Secondary EMP arises as an extramedullary manifestation of disseminated multiple myeloma. The EMP lesions classically arise in the upper aero-digestive tract (80%) with a predilection for the head and neck, followed by skin and gastrointestinal tract (BOLEK et al. 1996; IGEL et al. 1991; THE INTERNATIONAL MYELOMA WORKING GROUP 2003). Renal plasmacytoma is extremely rare (ALEXIOU et al. 1999).

Renal EMPs are vascular renal masses (Fig. 19.11; IGEL et al. 1991; KANDEL et al. 1984). In eight cases of renal plasmacytoma reviewed by KANDEL et al. (1984), neovascularity was demonstrated in all five cases in which angiography was performed. Clinical presentations were also similar to those of renal cell carcinoma, the most common being palpable abdominal mass (50%) followed by gross hematuria (25%). Renal plasmacytomas can be large, associated with enlarged retroperitoneal lymph nodes (Fig. 19.12;

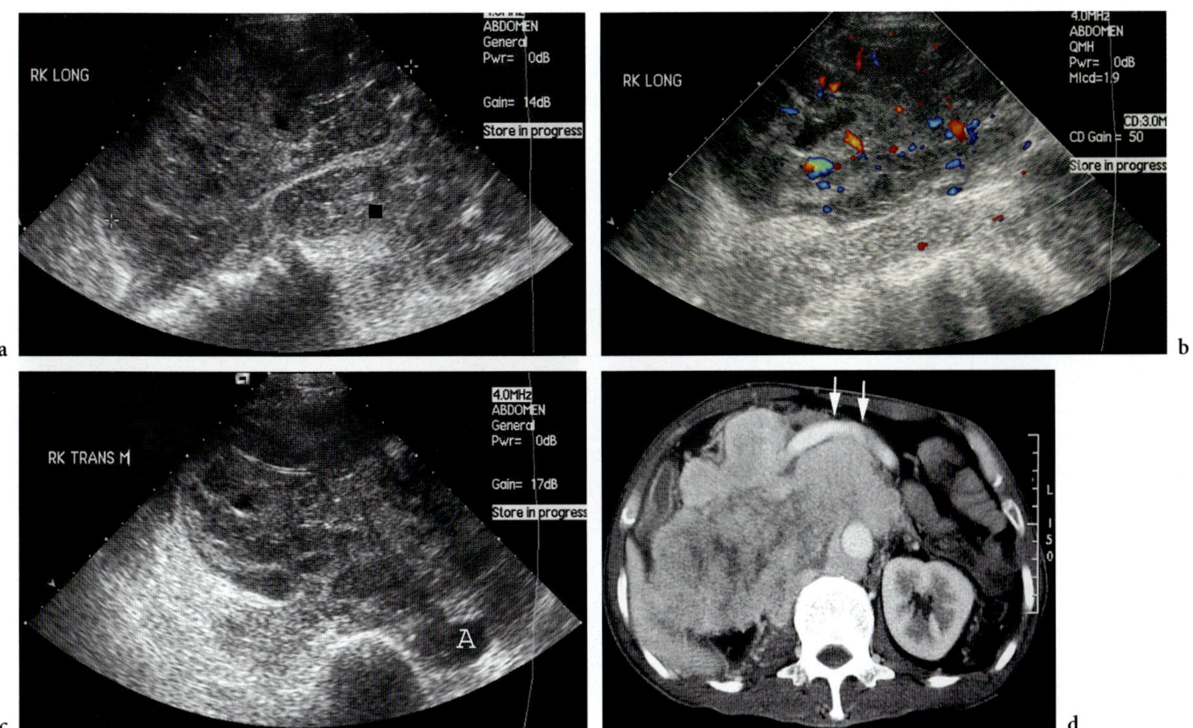

Fig. 19.11a-d. Extramedullary plasmacytoma arising from the right kidney in a 55-year-old woman. **a** Longitudinal US image of the right kidney shows diffuse replacement of normal renal tissue by a heterogeneous mass. **b** Color Doppler US image confirms vascularity of the mass. **c** Transverse US image of the right kidney illustrates the extent of the mass, which has displaced the aorta (*A*) to the left. **d** On axial contrast-enhanced CT scan, the mass is heterogeneously enhancing, and vascular encasement of the aorta and displacement of the portal vein (*arrows*) are better represented.

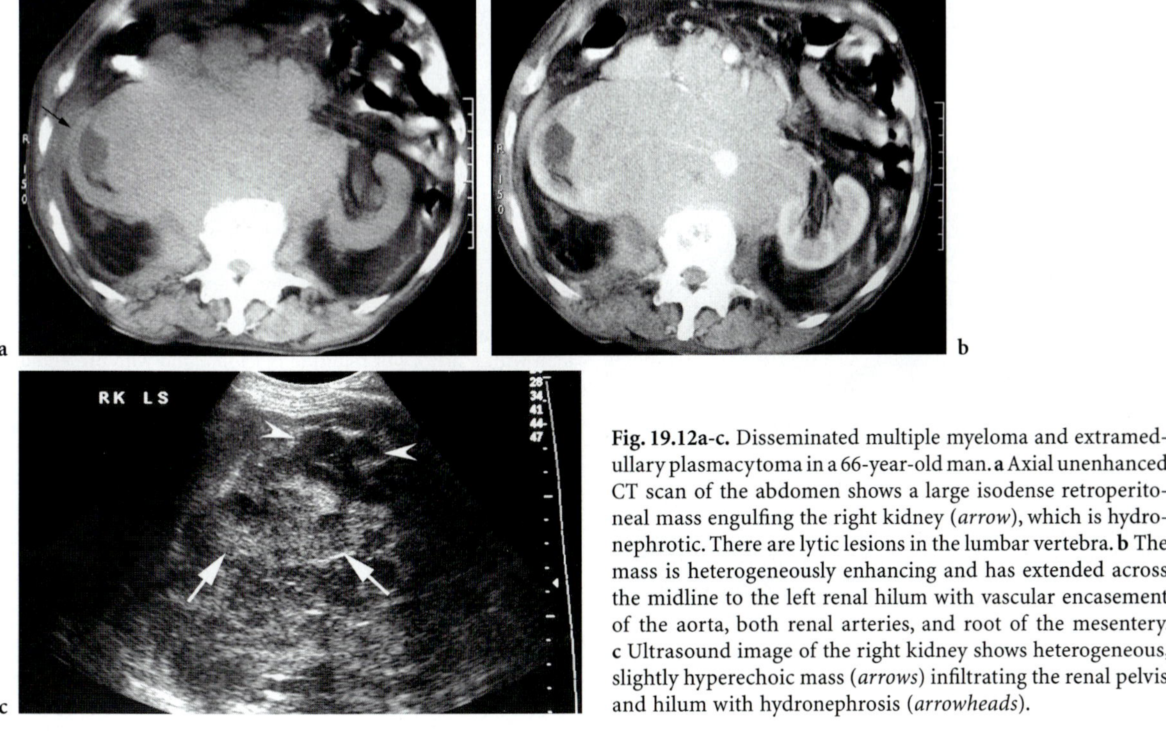

Fig. 19.12a-c. Disseminated multiple myeloma and extramedullary plasmacytoma in a 66-year-old man. **a** Axial unenhanced CT scan of the abdomen shows a large isodense retroperitoneal mass engulfing the right kidney (*arrow*), which is hydronephrotic. There are lytic lesions in the lumbar vertebra. **b** The mass is heterogeneously enhancing and has extended across the midline to the left renal hilum with vascular encasement of the aorta, both renal arteries, and root of the mesentery. **c** Ultrasound image of the right kidney shows heterogeneous, slightly hyperechoic mass (*arrows*) infiltrating the renal pelvis and hilum with hydronephrosis (*arrowheads*).

Kanoh et al. 1993), vascular encasement (Figs. 19.11, 19.12), and involvement of the renal vein (Jaspan and Gregson 1984; Sered and Nikolaidis 2003). Other manifestations include masses arising from the perinephric area (Figs. 19.13, 19.14; Sered and Nikolaidis 2003) similar to lymphoma or metastases, and the renal pelvis simulating transitional cell carcinoma (Igel et al. 1991; Kandel et al. 1984). Renal plasmacytomas have heterogeneous echogenicity on US (Figs. 19.11, 19.12), are isodense on unenhanced CT, and demonstrate heterogeneous enhancement, which can simulate renal cell carcinoma (Figs. 19.11, 19.15, 19.16). Ultrasound, CT, IVU, and angiography have thus far been unable to differentiate renal plasmacytomas from other malignant renal masses, particularly renal or transitional cell carcinoma (Igel et al. 1991; Kandel et al. 1984; Solomito and Grise 1972); however, in the presence of Bence-Jones proteinuria,

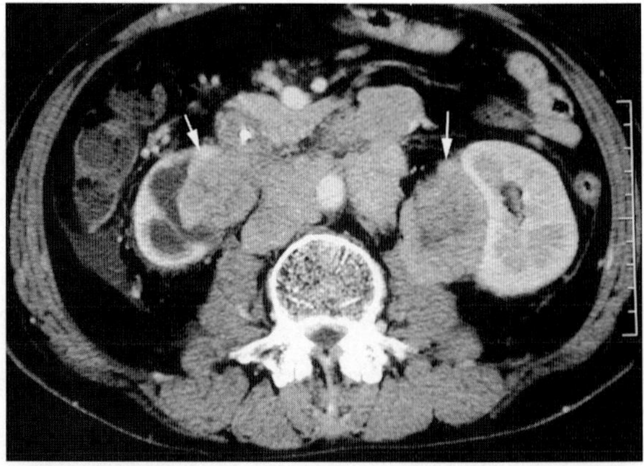

Fig. 19.13. Multiple myeloma complicated by extramedullary plasmacytoma in a 46-year-old man. Axial contrast-enhanced CT scan shows enhancing perinephric masses (*arrows*) at the medial aspects of the kidneys, with retroperitoneal lymphadenopathy. There is hydronephrosis of the right kidney.

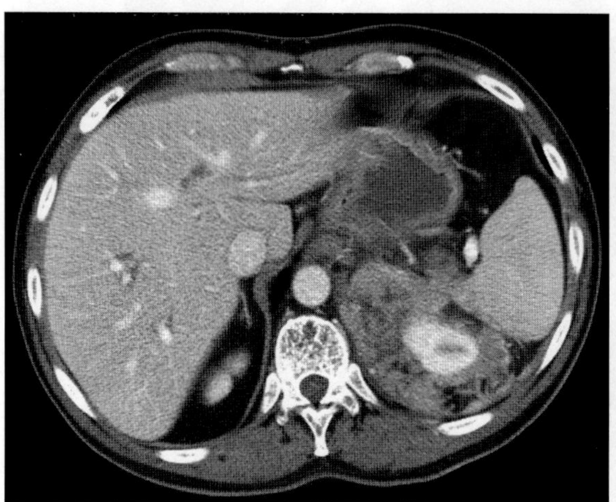

a

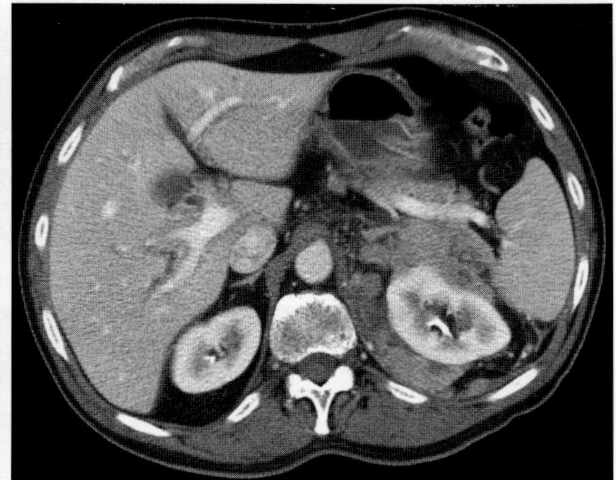

b

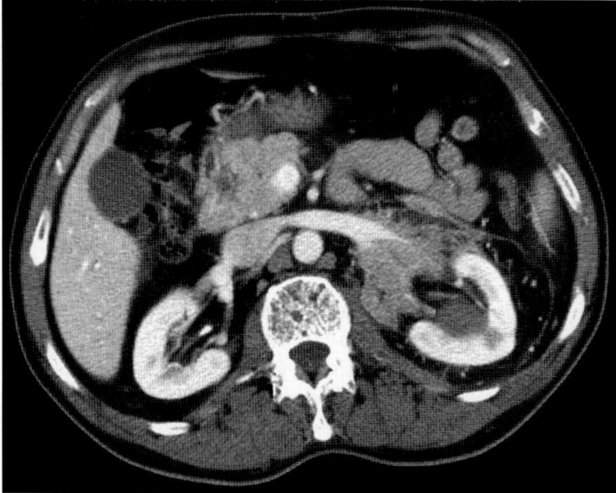

c

Fig. 19.14a-c. Extramedullary plasmacytoma in a 53-year-old man with a history of multiple myeloma and who presented with severe left flank pain. Axial contrast-enhanced CT scans show left perirenal soft-tissue-density mass encapsulating the **a** upper pole and **b** mid-portion of the left kidney. **c** The left renal artery and vein are also encased and narrowed by the mass. The kidneys enhance symmetrically without evidence of hydronephrosis. Axial contrast-enhanced CT scan obtained 2 weeks after the completion of chemotherapy showed near complete resolution of the left perirenal mass (not shown). (Image courtesy of P. Nikolaidis).

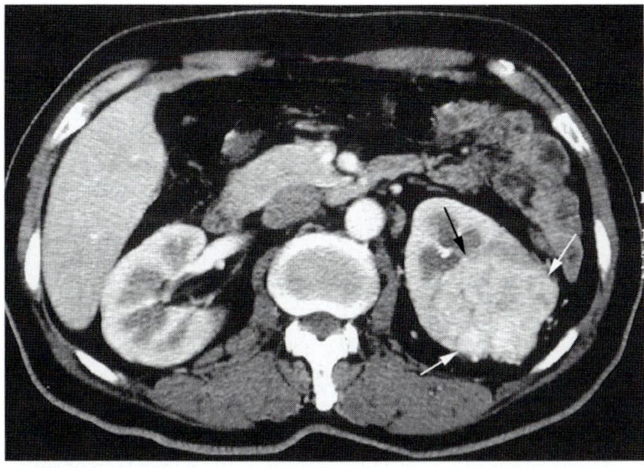

Fig. 19.15. Renal plasmacytoma in a 58-year-old man without bone marrow evidence of multiple myeloma. Axial contrast-enhanced CT scan shows a heterogeneously enhancing mass (*arrows*) arising from the left kidney.

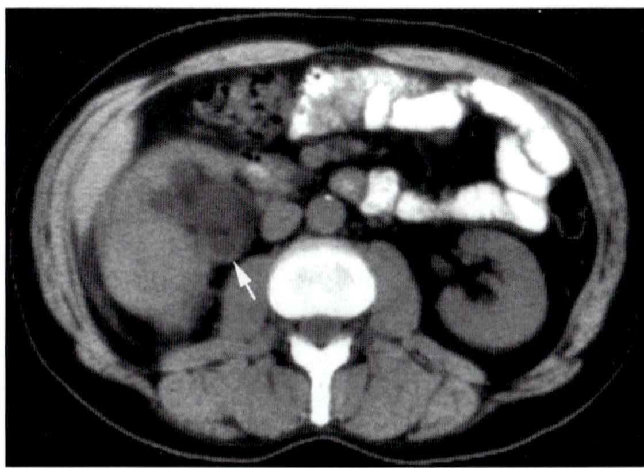

a

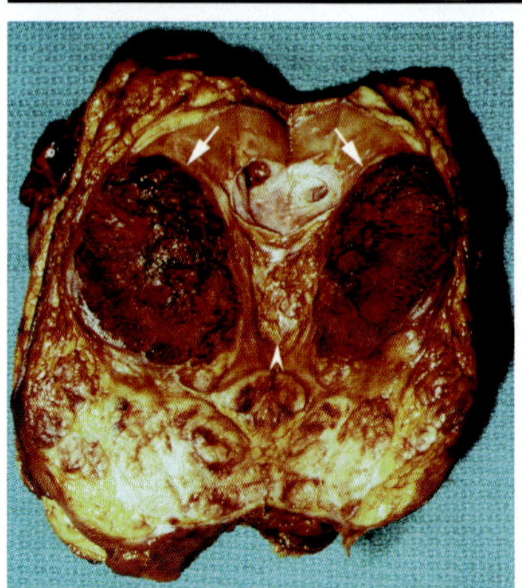

b

Fig. 19.16a,b. Renal plasmacytoma in a 59-year-old man with a recent significant weight loss. a Axial unenhanced CT scan shows an enlarged and irregular right kidney with a hypodense and lobulated mass (*arrow*) in the region of the renal hilum. b Photograph of the bivalved specimen shows the mass (*arrows*) in the mid-portion of the kidney, with extension into the renal pelvis (*arrowhead*). (Image courtesy of G. LONERGAN)

and/or history of previous plasmacytoma or multiple myeloma, the presence of a documented renal mass should raise the suspicion of a renal plasmacytoma.

19.9 Conclusion

Renal involvement in myeloproliferative and lymphoproliferative disorders is generally not routinely imaged, as in most instances they are asymptomatic owing to preserved renal function. Symptoms arise as a result of compression, renal obstruction, infection, or hemorrhage. Ultrasound and CT remain the imaging modalities of choice due to their availability, relatively short scan times, and reduced costs compared with MR imaging. Computed tomography in particular is extremely good at depicting renal, perirenal, and intra-abdominal pathology. However, nuclear medicine imaging, particularly PET, is proving useful in post-treatment monitoring of disease activity. Although there are no specific imaging features that differentiate these entities from other disease processes that can affect the kidney, in general, leukemia and lymphoma are iso- or hypoechoic on US, and iso- or hypodense on CT. Lymphomas are hypovascular, showing minimal or no enhancement after contrast administration on CT. Extramedullary plasmacytomas are heterogeneous on US, isodense on CT, and demonstrate heterogeneous enhancement.

Acknowledgements
We extend sincere thanks to L. Dobrovolskiene, G. Lonergan, P. Nikolaidis, and P. Pickhardt for providing us with their excellent images.

References

Alexiou C, Kau RJ, Dietzfelbinger H, Kremer M, Spiess JC, Schratzenstaller B, Arnold W (1999) Extramedullary plasmacytoma: tumor occurrence and therapeutic concepts. Cancer 85:2305–2314

Ali MG, Coakley FV, Hricak H, Bretan PN (1999) Complex posttransplantation abnormalities of renal allografts: evaluation with MR imaging. Radiology 211:95–100

Araki T (1982) Leukemic ivolvement of the kidney in children: CT features. J Comput Assist Tomogr 6:781–784

Bagg MD, Wettlaufer JN, Willadsen DS, Ho V, Lane D, Thrasher JB (1994) Granulocytic sarcoma presenting as a diffuse renal mass before hematological manifestations of acute myelogenous leukemia. J Urol 152:2092–2093

Barcos M, Lane W, Gomez GA, Han T, Freeman A, Preisler H, Henderson E (1987) An autopsy study of 1206 acute and chronic leukemias (1958 to 1982). Cancer 60:827–837

Basker M, Scott JX, Ross B, Kirubakaran C (2002) Renal enlargement as primary presentation of acute lymphoblastic leukaemia. Indian J Cancer 39:154–156

Bolek TW, Marcus RD, Mendenhall NP (1996) Solitary plasmacytoma of bone and soft tissue. Int J Radiat Oncol Biol Phys 36:329–333

Boudville N, Latham B, Cordingly F, Warr K (2001) Renal failure in a patient with leukaemic infiltration of the kidney and polyomavirus infection. Nephrol Dial Transplant 16:1059–1061

Breatnach E, Stanley RJ, Carpenter JT Jr (1985) Intrarenal chloroma causing obstructive nephropathy: CT characteristics. J Comput Assist Tomogr 9:822–824

Chepuri NB, Strouse PJ, Yanik GA (2003) CT of renal lymphoma in children. Am J Roentgenol 180:429–431

Claudon M, Kessler M, Champigneulle J, Lefevre F, Hestin D, Renoult E (1998) Lymphoproliferative disorders after renal transplantation: role of medical imaging. Eur Radiol 8:1686–1693

Clifton AG, Baily GG (1991) Case report: renal lymphoma in a patient with Waldenstrom's macroglobulinemia. Clin Radiol 43:285–286

Cockfield SM, Preiksaitis JK, Jewell LD, Parfrey NA (1993) Posttransplant lymphoproliferative disorder in renal allograft recipients. Clinical experience and risk factor analysis in a single center. Transplantation 56:88–96

Cohan RH, Dunnick NR, Leder RA, Baker ME (1990) Computed tomography of renal lymphoma. J Comput Assist Tomogr 14:933–938

Comerma-Coma MI, Sans-Boix A, Tuset-Andujar E, Andreu-Navarro J, Perez-Ruiz A, Naval-Marcos I (1998) Reversible renal failure due to specific infiltration of the kidney in chronic lymphatic leukaemia. Nephrol Dial Transplant 13:1550–1552

Cruz Villalon F, Escribano Fernandez J, Ramirez Garcia T (1995) The hypoechoic halo: a finding in renal lymphoma. J Clin Ultrasound 23:379–381

Dodd GD III, Greenler DP, Confer SR (1992) Thoracic and abdominal manifestations of lymphoma occurring in the immunocompromised patient. Radiol Clin North Am 30:597–610

Eisenberg PJ, Papanicolaou N, Lee MJ, Yoder IC (1994) Diagnostic imaging in the evaluation of renal lymphoma. Leuk Lymphoma 16:37–50

Ellert J, Kreel L (1980) The role of computed tomography in the initial staging and subsequent management of the lymphomas. J Comput Assist Tomogr 4:368–391

Ferry JA, Harris NL, Papanicolau N, Young RH (1995) Lymphoma of the kidney. A report of 11 cases. Am J Surg Pathol 19:134–144

Frick MP, Salomonowitz E, Hanto DW, Gedgaudas-McClees K (1984) CT of abdominal lymphoma after renal transplantation. Am J Roentgenol 142:97–99

Galieni P, Cavo M, Avvisati G, Pulsoni A, Falbo R, Bonelli MA, Russo D, Petrucci MT, Bucalossi A, Tura S (1995) Solitary plasmacytoma of bone and extramedullary plasmacytoma: Two different entities? Ann Oncol 6:687–691

Gates GF (1978) Atlas of abdominal ultrasonography in children. Churchill Livingston, New York

Geoffay A, Shirkhoda A, Wallace S (1984) Abdominal and pelvic computed tomography in leukemic patients. J Comput Assist Tomogr 8:857–860

Goh TS, LeQuesne GW, Wong KY (1978) Severe infiltration of the kidneys with ultrasonic abnormalities in acute lymphoblastic leukemia. Am J Dis Child 132:1024–1025

Gupta S, Keane S (1985) Renal enlargement as a primary presentation of acute lymphoblastic leukaemia. Br J Radiol 58:893–895

Hartman DS, Davis CJ Jr, Goldman SM, Friedman AC, Fritzsche P (1982) Renal lymphoma: radiologic–pathologic correlation of 21 cases. Radiology 144:759–766

Heiken JP, Gold RP, Schnur MJ, King DL, Bashist B, Glazer HS (1983) Computed tomography of renal lymphoma with ultrasound correlation. J Comput Assist Tomogr 7:425–450

Hurii SC, Bosniak MA, Megibow AJ, Raghavendra BN (1983) Correlation of CT and ultrasound in the evaluation of renal lymphoma. Urol Radiol 5:69–76

Igel TC, Engen DE, Banks PM, Keeney GL (1991) Renal plasmacytoma: Mayo Clinic experience and review of the literature. Urology 37:385–389

Jaspan T, Gregson R (1984) Extramedullary plasmacytoma of the kidney. Br J Radiol 57:95–97

Jeffrey RB Jr, Nyberg DA, Bottles K, Abrams DI, Federle MP, Wall SD, Wing VW, Laing FC (1986) Abdominal CT in acquired immunodeficiency syndrome. Am J Roentgenol 146:7–13

Kandel LB, Harrison LH, Woodruff RF, Williams CD, Ahl ET Jr (1984) Renal plasmacytoma: a case report and summary of reported cases. J Urol 132:1167–1169

Kandel LB, McCullough DL, Harrison LH, Woodruff RD, Ahl ET Jr, Munitz HA (1987) Primary renal lymphoma. Does it exist? Cancer 60:386–391

Kanoh T, Katoh H, Izumi T, Tsuji M, Okuma M (1993) Renal plasmacytoma. Rinsho Ketsueki 34:1470–1473

Kiely JM, Wagoner RD, Holley KE (1969) Renal complications of lymphoma. Ann Intern Med 71:1159–1175

Liu PI, Ishimaru T, McGregor DH, Okada H, Steer A (1973) Autopsy study of granulocytic sarcoma (chloroma) in patients with myelogenous leukemia, Hiroshima–Nagasaki 1949–1969. Cancer 31:948–955

Lopez-Ben R, Smith JK, Kew CE II, Kenney PJ, Julian BA, Robbin ML (2000) Focal posttransplantation lymphoproliferative disorder at the renal allograft hilum. Am J Roentgenol 175:1417–1422

Lutz J, Heemann U (2003) Tumours after kidney transplantation. Curr Opin Urol 13:105–109

Martinez-Maldonado M, Ramirez de Arellano GA (1966) Renal involvement in malignant lymphoma: a survey of 49 cases. J Urol 95:485–488

Mavromatis BH, Cheson BD (2002) Pre- and post-treatment evaluation of non-Hodgkin's lymphoma. Best Pract Res Clin Haematol 15:429–447

Miller FH, Parikh S, Gore RM, Nemcek AA Jr, Fitzgerald SW, Vogelzang RL (1993) Renal manifestations of AIDS. Radiographics 13:587–596

Miller WT Jr, Siegel SG, Montone KT (1997) Post transplantation lymphoproliferative disorder: changing manifestation of disease in a renal transplant population. Crit Rev Diagn Imaging 36:569–585

Moore DF, Moulopoulos LA, Dimopoulos MA (1995) Waldenstrom's macroglobulinemia presenting as a renal or perirenal mass: clinical and radiographic features. Leuk Lymphoma 17:331–334

Neiman RS, Barcos M, Berard C, Bonner H, Mann R, Rydell RE, Bennett JM (1981) Granulocytic sarcoma: a clinico-pathologic study of 61 biopsied cases. Cancer 48:1426–1437

Nyberg DA, Jeffrey RB Jr, Federle MP, Bottles K, Abrams DI (1986) AIDS-related lymphomas: evaluation by abdominal CT. Radiology 159:59–63

Park HJ, Jeong DH, Song HG, Lee GK, Han GS, Cha SH, Ha TS (2003) Myeloid sarcoma of both kidneys, the brain and multiple bones in a non-leukemic child. Yonsei Med J 44:740–743

Parker BR (1997) Leukemia and lymphoma in childhood. Radiol Clin North Am 35:1495–1516

Penn I (1996) Cancers in cyclosporin-treated vs azathioprine-treated patients. Transplant Proc 28:876–878

Pilatrino C, Cataldi A, Guerrasio A, Saglio G (2003) Images in haematology. Renal Hodgkin's disease. Br J Haematol 116:732

Pui MH, Fletcher BD, Langston JW (1994) Granulocytic sarcoma in childhood leukemia: imaging features. Radiology 190:698–702

Reznek RH, Mootoosamy I, Webb JA, Richards MA (1990) CT in renal and perirenal lymphoma: a further look. Clin Radiol 42:233–238

Richmond J, Sherman RS, Diamond HD, Craver LF (1962) Renal lesions associated with malignant lymphomas. Am J Med 32:184–207

Romer W, Schwaiger M (1998) Positron emission tomography in diagnosis and therapy monitoring of patients with lymphoma. Clin Positron Imaging 1:101–110

Rosenberg SA, Diamond HD, Jaslowitz B, Craver LF (1961) Lymphosarcoma: a review of 1269 cases. Medicine (Baltimore) 40:31–84

Schwartz JB, Shamsuddin AM (1981) The effects of leukemic infiltrates in various organs in chronic lymphocytic leukemia. Hum Pathol 12:432–440

Sered S, Nikolaidis P (2003) CT findings of perirenal plasmacytoma. Am J Roentgenol 181:888

Siskin GP, Haller JO, Miller S, Sundaram R (1995) AIDS-related lymphoma: radiologic features in pediatric patients. Radiology 196:63–66

Soesan M, Paccagnella A, Chiarion-Sileni V, Salvagno L, Fornasiero A, Sotti G, Zorat PL, Favaretto A, Fiorentino M (1992) Extramedullary plasmacytoma: clinical behaviour and response to treatment. Ann Oncol 3:51–57

Solomito VL, Grise J (1972) Angiographic findings in renal (extramedullary) plasmacytoma: case report. Radiology 102:559–560

Tanaka N, Matsumoto T, Furukawa M, Tokuda O (2004) Leukemia. In: Guermazi A (ed) Radiological imaging in hematological malignancies. Springer, Berlin Heidelberg New York, pp 351–366

Teele RL (1977) Ultrasonography of the genitourinary tract in children. Radiol Clin North Am 15:109–128

The International Myeloma Working Group (2003) Criteria for the classification of monoclonal gammopathies, multiple myeloma and related disorders: a report of the International Myeloma Working Group. Br J Haematol 121:749–757

Townsend RR, Laing FC, Jeffrey RB Jr, Bottles K (1989) Abdominal lymphoma in AIDS: evaluation with US. Radiology 171:719–724

Vardiman JW, Harris NL, Brunning RD (2002) The World Health Organization (WHO) classification of the myeloid neoplasms. Blood 100:2292–2302

Vose JM, Bierman PJ, Anderson JR, Harrison KA, Dalrymple GV, Byar K, Kessinger A, Armitage JO (1996) Single-photon emission computed tomography gallium imaging versus computed tomography: predictive value in patients undergoing high-dose chemotherapy and autologous stem-cell transplantation for non-Hodgkin's lymphoma. J Clin Oncol 14:2473–2479

Vrachliotis TG, Vaswani KK, Davies EA, Elkhammas EA, Bennett WF, Bova JG (2000) CT findings in posttransplantation lymphoproliferative disorder of renal transplants. Am J Roentgenol 175:183–188

Xiao JC, Walz-Mattmuller R, Ruck P, Horny HP, Kaiserling E (1997) Renal involvement in myeloproliferative and lymphoproliferative disorders. A study of autopsy cases. Gen Diagn Pathol 142:147–153

20 Pediatric Kidney Cancer

Lisa H. Lowe and Eugenio M. Taboada

CONTENTS

20.1
Introduction

Wilms tumor is the most common solid pediatric renal neoplasm. In recent years, several less common renal malignancies that were previously considered subtypes of Wilms tumor have been recognized as separate pathological entities. Although the vast majority of pediatric renal masses are Wilms tumor, various other newly described lesions may have a particular clinical history or distinctive imaging features that differentiate them from Wilms tumor (Table 20.1); however, despite the use of modern imaging techniques, renal neoplasms cannot always be diagnosed with pre-operative imaging.

L. H. Lowe, MD, FAAP
Associate Professor of Pediatric Radiology, Children's Mercy Hospital and Clinics, University of Missouri, Kansas City, 2401 Gillham Road, Kansas City, Missouri 64108, USA
E. M. Taboada, MD, FACP
Assistant Professor of Pathology, Director of Surgical Pathology, Children's Mercy Hospital and Clinics, University of Missouri, Kansas City, 2401 Gillham Road, Kansas City, Missouri 64108, USA

This chapter reviews various renal masses in children, placing emphasis on imaging findings and clinical features that are especially useful in differentiating among renal masses. Malignant lesions are discussed first, including Wilms tumor, nephrogenic rests/nephroblastomatosis, clear cell sarcoma, rhabdoid tumor, renal cell carcinoma, renal medullary carcinoma, lymphoma, leukemia, and neuroblastoma. Benign lesions follow, with mesoblastic nephroma, ossifying renal tumor of infancy, multilocular cystic renal tumor, angiomyolipoma, and metanephric adenoma.

20.2
Wilms Tumor

Eighty-seven percent of pediatric renal masses are Wilms tumors. They occur in approximately 1:10,000 patients (Julian et al. 1995; Ritchey et al. 1995) with a peak age of presentation between 3 and 4 years (Charles et al. 1998). Eighty percent of lesions are discovered before the age of 5 years (Lonergan et al. 1998). Wilms tumors are rare in neonates, with fewer than 0.16% under 1 month of age (Charles et al. 1998; Glick et al. 2004). Bilateral masses are found in 4–13% of children (Lonergan et al. 1998), and may be associated with various congenital anomalies including cryptorchidism (2.8%), hypospadias (1.8%), hemihypertrophy (2.5%), and sporadic aniridia (White and Grossman 1991).

Genetic factors related to Wilms tumors are well documented and continue to be described and better understood (Shamberger 1999). Chromosome 11 is thought to have two loci that are implicated in the genesis of a small subset of Wilms tumors. Locus 11p13 and locus 11p15 are referred to as WT1 and WT2 genes (Lowe et al. 2000). In patients with WAGR (Wilms tumor, aniridia, genitourinary abnormalities, and mental retardation) and Drash (male pseudohermaphroditism and progressive glomeru-

Table 20.1. Age range, peak age at presentation, and distinct features of solid renal masses. *VHL* von Hippel-Lindau syndrome, *TS* tuberous sclerosis, *NF* neurofibromatosis

Renal neoplasia	Age range	Peak age	Distinct clinical and imaging features
Wilms tumor			
Unilateral	1–11 years	3.5 years	Most common solid renal mass of childhood. Most often large solid mass, often vascular invasion
Bilateral	2 months to 2 years	15 months	Associated with nephroblastomatosis and various syndromes
Nephroblastomatosis	Any age	6–18 months	Bilateral, multiple subcapsular focal masses, often with associated bilateral solid Wilms tumors
Clear cell sarcoma	1 to 4 years	2 years	Frequent skeletal metastases
Rhabdoid tumor	6 months to 9 years	6–12 months	Associated with posterior fossa cranial neoplasms
Renal cell carcinoma	6 months to 60 years	10–20 years (VHL)	Non-specific appearing mass, association with VHL
Renal medullary carcinoma	10–39 years	20 years	Exclusively seen in sickle cell trait or hemoglobin SC disease
Lymphoma			
Hodgkin disease	>10 years	Late teens	Frequently associated adenopathy but variable appearance
Non-Hodgkin lymphoma	Any age	<10 years	Bilateral renal enlargement with loss of architecture
Leukemia	Any age	Any age	Reniform, bilateral nephromegaly
Neuroblastoma	Any age	<5 years	Vascular encasement, calcification, neural extension
Mesoblastic nephroma	<1 year	1–3 months	Most common solid renal mass in infants and newborns
Ossifying renal tumor of infancy	6 days to 14 years	1–3 months	Calcified mass in an infant
Multilocular cystic renal tumor			
Cystic nephroma	3 months to 4 years	1–2 years	Large, multicystic mass in young children
Cystic partially differentiated	Adult women	Adult women	Large, multicystic mass in young women
Angiomyolipoma	6–41 years	10 years (VHL, TS, NF)	Fat and soft tissue mass associated with VHL, TS, NF
Metanephric adenoma	15 months to 83 years	None	Non-specific clinical or imaging features

lonephritis) syndromes, an abnormal WT1 gene is present, whereas patients with Beckwith-Wiedemann and hemihypertrophy have an abnormal WT2 gene. Abnormalities at other sites, including chromosomes 1, 12, and 8, have been recognized, leading to the belief that the genetics of Wilms tumor is multifactorial. Approximately 1% of Wilms tumors are familial, in which cases there is no associated anomaly of chromosome 11 (Charles et al. 1998). Children with increased risk for developing Wilms tumor should be screened starting at 6 months of age with an initial CT, followed by serial ultrasound (US) every 3–6 months until 7 years of age. Screening can be discontinued after age 7 years, since there is a significantly lower risk of developing Wilms tumor (Beckwith 1998; Lonergan et al. 1998).

Wilms tumor most commonly presents with a firm, palpable mass, but may be discovered incidentally after trauma in up to 10% of cases. Hematuria and pain are infrequent clinical findings, and constitutional symptoms are usually absent. Renin production by the tumor may cause hypertension in up to 25% of cases (Lonergan et al. 1998).

Wilms tumor originates from the metanephros (mesodermal precursors of renal parenchyma) or occasionally from mesonephric remnants within the extrarenal retroperitoneum (Shamberger 1999). Grossly, the tumor is usually a soft gray or tan mass that is sharply defined by a pseudocapsule. Varying amounts of blastema, stroma, and epithelium (triphasic) compose Wilms tumors on histological exam (Fig. 20.1). If there is differentiation along non-renal tissue lines, such as cartilage, bone, or muscle, then the mass is described histologically as "teratoid Wilms" (Fig. 20.2). Anaplasia (defined as nuclei with diameters at least three times those of adjacent cells with increased chromatin content; and multipolar or otherwise recognizable polyploid mitotic figures) is directly associated with poor response to chemotherapy and a poor prognosis (Charles et al. 1998).

Radiologically, most Wilms tumors are solid masses that distort the renal parenchyma, often with a visible pseudocapsule (Fig. 20.3). Tumor spread is usually by direct extension with displacement of adjacent structures, rather than encasement of ves-

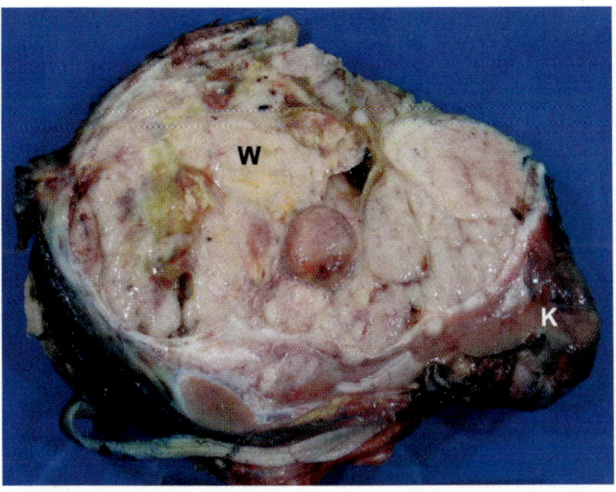

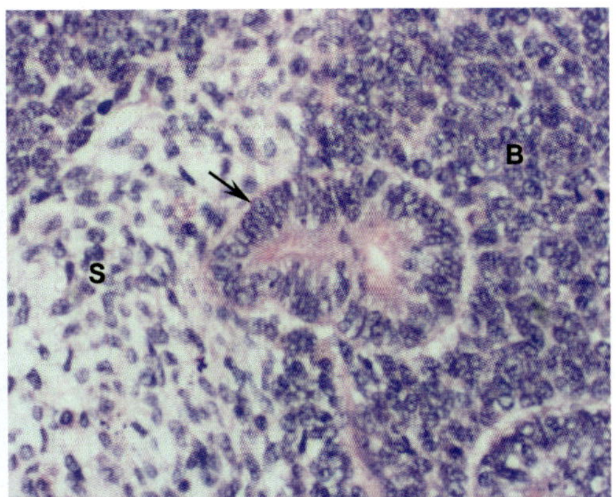

a   b

Fig. 20.1a,b. Wilms tumor in a 4-year-old-boy. **a** Gross specimen reveals a pseudocapsule and septa dividing the surface of the Wilms tumor (*W*) from the kidney (*K*). **b** Histological specimen shows the "triphasic" pattern of stromal (*S*), blastemal (*B*), and tubular (*arrow*) elements.

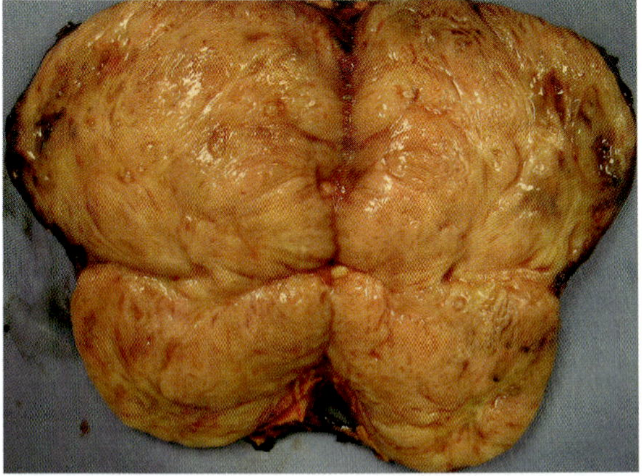

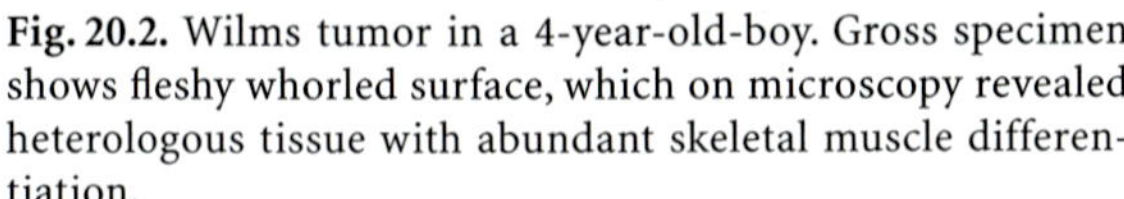

Fig. 20.2. Wilms tumor in a 4-year-old-boy. Gross specimen shows fleshy whorled surface, which on microscopy revealed heterologous tissue with abundant skeletal muscle differentiation.

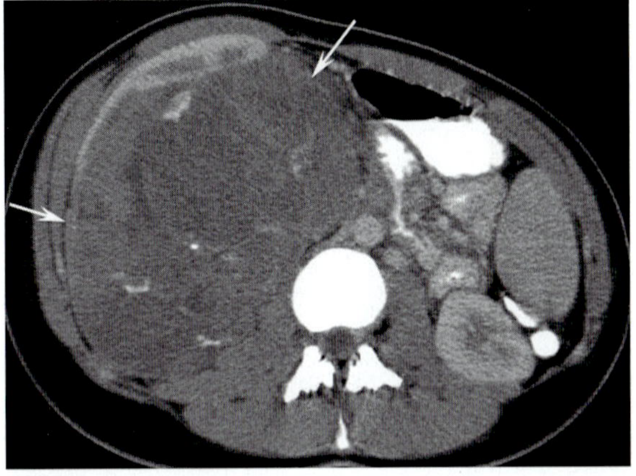

Fig. 20.3. Wilms tumor in a 5-year-old boy with an abdominal mass. Axial contrast-enhanced CT scan shows a large right renal mass (*arrows*) with heterogeneous enhancement and numerous calcifications.

sels and aortic elevation, which are characteristics that suggest neuroblastoma. Formation of a tumor thrombus in the renal vein, inferior vena cava, or right atrium is typical of Wilms tumor (Fig. 20.4). Metastases to the lungs (85%), liver, and regional lymph nodes are not uncommon (LONERGAN et al. 1998).

Areas of necrosis, hemorrhage, and/or calcification (9%), and the presence of adipose tissue within Wilms tumors, causes them to have heterogeneous echogenicity on US (LONERGAN et al. 1998; WHITE and GROSSMAN 1991). Doppler interrogation of the inferior vena cava (IVC) is useful to detect vascular invasion that may modify the surgical approach. On CT Wilms tumors are heterogeneously enhancing masses with areas of calcification, fat, or lymphadenopathy. Intravenous contrast administration is essential to detect hepatic metastases, tumor thrombus, and synchronous contralateral renal masses (LOWE et al. 2000). On MR imaging, Wilms tumor is hypointense on T1- and hyperintense on T2-weighted sequences. Although MR imaging has been reported to be the most sensitive modality for determining caval patency, patients frequently require sedation during scanning. Since Wilms tumors are often very large at presentation, severe distortion of adjacent organs, including the IVC, may prohibit a determination of venous invasion/patency. In the majority of children surgical planning is possible based on meticulous US and scrutiny of multiplanar images obtained with contrast-enhanced multidetector CT. Occasionally, Wilms tumor is mostly cystic, and it is not possible to distinguish it from multilocular cystic renal tumor (Fig. 20.5).

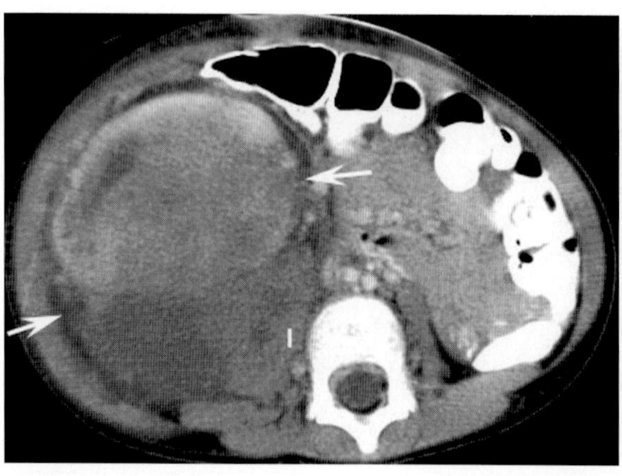 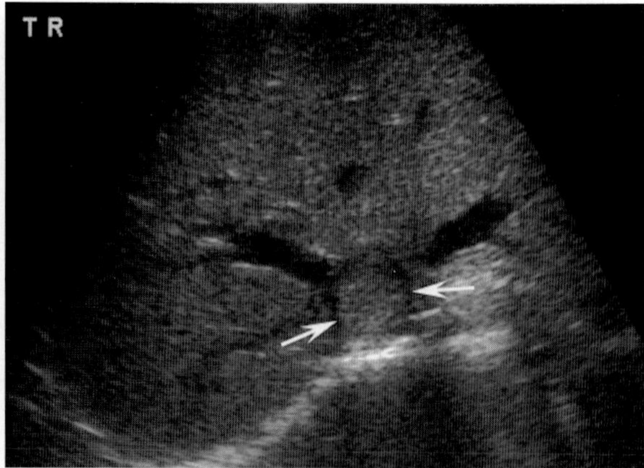

Fig. 20.4a,b. Wilms tumor in a 10-year-old girl. Axial contrast-enhanced CT scan demonstrates a large right renal mass (*arrows*) with invasion of the right iliopsoas muscle (*I*). **b** Transverse US image reveals a tumor thrombus at the confluence of the hepatic veins (*arrows*).

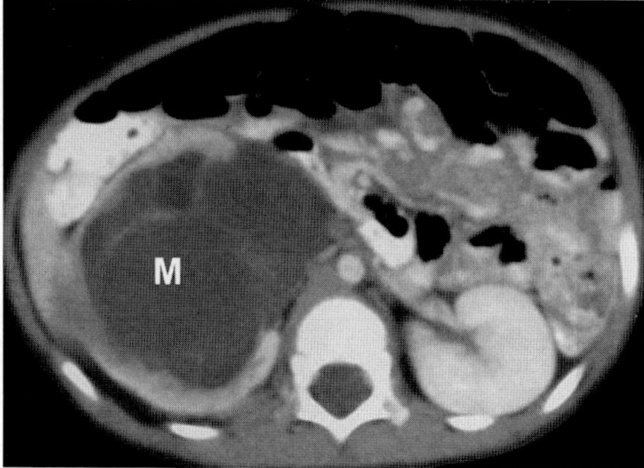

Fig. 20.5. Cystic Wilms tumor in a 3-year-old boy with an abdominal mass. Axial contrast-enhanced CT scan shows a large well-defined multiseptate cystic mass (*M*) in the right kidney. (Image courtesy of C. W. Moore)

Table 20.2. Summary of tumor prognosis

Low risk
  Wilms tumor, highly epithelial type
  Mesoblastic nephroma
  Multilocular cystic renal tumor
  Angiomyolipoma
  Ossifying renal tumor of infancy
  Metanephric adenoma

Intermediate risk
  Wilms tumor, non-anaplastic
  Neuroblastoma
  Lymphoma
  Leukemia

High risk
  Wilms tumor, anaplastic
  Renal cell carcinoma
  Renal medullary carcinoma
  Clear cell sarcoma
  Rhabdoid tumor

Treatment of unilateral Wilms tumor includes nephrectomy and chemotherapy. In very large tumors, pre-surgical chemotherapy may promote shrinkage and improve surgical outcome. Tumor bed radiation is needed in some cases, and whole abdominal irradiation is used if there is peritoneal tumor implantation or gross tumor spillage at surgery. In bilateral Wilms tumor, each kidney is staged separately and pre-operative chemotherapy is used with the goal of complete resolution of disease in one kidney (Lowe et al. 2000). If accomplished, then nephrectomy of the contralateral kidney with eventual cure may be possible. In children with bilateral Wilms tumor in whom unilateral resolution of disease is not accomplished, the current approach is tumor resection with sparing of as much normal renal parenchyma as possible. Histology and surgical stage of disease determine the

Table 20.3. Wilms tumor staging

Stage	Description
I	Can be totally resected, limited to the kidney/renal sinus, intact renal capsule
II	Can be totally resected despite local extension beyond the kidney
III	Cannot be totally resected with residual nonhematogenous disease within the abdomen (including: residual non-resected tumor, positive margins, abdominal nodes, or contamination of the peritoneum from direct extension, implants, or spillage
IV	Hematogenous spread of disease (lung, lymph nodes, liver)
V	Bilateral masses[a]

[a]Each side should also be separately staged since prognosis is dependent on the higher individual stage

rate of cure (Tables 20.2, 20.3), which has improved from 10% in the 1920s to greater than 90% presently (KALAPURAKAL et al. 2004; WHITE and GROSSMAN 1991). Fortunately, most Wilms tumors have very favorable pathology; however, long-term follow-up is important because children treated for Wilms tumor are at an increased risk of developing secondary malignancies of the kidneys and other organ systems (CHERULLO et al. 2001; PAULINO et al. 2000).

20.3
Nephrogenic Rests and Nephroblastomatosis

Foci of metanephric blastema that persist in the renal parenchyma beyond 36 weeks gestation are referred to as nephrogenic rests. When diffuse or multifocal nephrogenic rests occur, the term nephroblastomatosis is applied. Although nephrogenic rests may occur incidentally in up to 1% of infants (LONERGAN et al. 1998), it is currently believed that 30–40% of unilateral (LONERGAN et al. 1998) and up to 99% of bilateral Wilms tumors originate from these rests (WHITE and GROSSMAN 1991).

Histologically, there are four types of nephrogenic rests including dormant, sclerosing, hyperplastic, or neoplastic. While dormant and sclerosing rests are usually microscopic and do not have malignant potential, hyperplastic and neoplastic rests are grossly visible and do have malignant potential (MURPHY et al. 1994).

Grossly and on imaging, nephrogenic rests are classified according to location as perilobar and intralobar (Fig. 20.6; PERLMAN et al. 2005; LONERGAN et al. 1998). This classification system is useful to the imager because it is anatomical; however, only pathological classification is able to definitively determine the lesion type and location. The term panlobar is given when there is diffuse renal involvement (MURPHY et al. 1994). Perilobar rests, found in the peripheral cortex or columns of Bertin, are associated with Beckwith-Wiedemann syndrome, hemihypertrophy, Perlman syndrome (gigantism, cryptorchidism, visceromegaly, polyhydramnios, and characteristic facial features) and trisomy 18. Malignant degeneration into Wilms tumor occurs in up to 3% of patients with Beckwith-Wiedemann syndrome and hemihypertrophy (LONERGAN et al. 1998). Intralobar rests are much less common, and are present in 78% of patients with Drash syndrome, nearly 100% of those with sporadic aniridia, and also occur in WAGR syndrome. Malignant degeneration is much more common with intralobar than with perilobar rests.

On US, nephrogenic rests are hypoechoic and more difficult to visualize compared with MR imaging and CT. On CT they are peripheral, hypodense, poorly enhancing nodules (Figs. 20.7, 20.8). MR imaging reveals hypointensity on T1- and T2-weighted sequences. When multiple, the nephrogenic rests of nephroblastomatosis are usually bilateral, classically subcapsular in location, and often associated with larger solid masses that indicate degeneration into Wilms tumors. With US, diffuse nephroblastomatosis causes the enlarged kidneys to be hypoechoic. Diffuse nephroblastomatosis may demonstrate a thick peripheral rind of tissue causing reniform enlargement of the kidney and a striated nephrogram after contrast administration (LONERGAN et al. 1998).

The appropriate treatment for nephrogenic rests is controversial, with some authors recommending chemotherapy, whereas others maintain that close serial radiological evaluation for enlarging masses is sufficient; however, the lesions are often surgically resected since Wilms tumor must be excluded (LONERGAN et al. 1998).

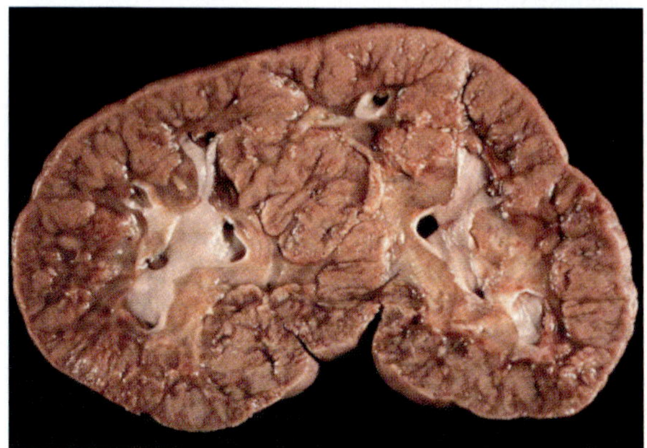

Fig. 20.6. Panlobar or universal nephroblastomatosis in a child. Gross specimen reveals complete loss of normal renal architecture within an extremely enlarged kidney. (With permission from MURPHY et al. 1994; image courtesy of M. Rodriguez)

20.4
Clear Cell Sarcoma

Clear cell sarcoma of the kidney, also known as "bone metastasizing renal tumor of childhood," was previously considered a subtype of Wilms tumor.

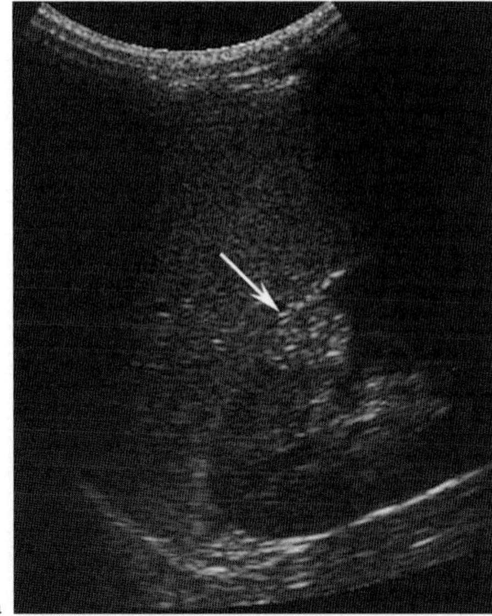

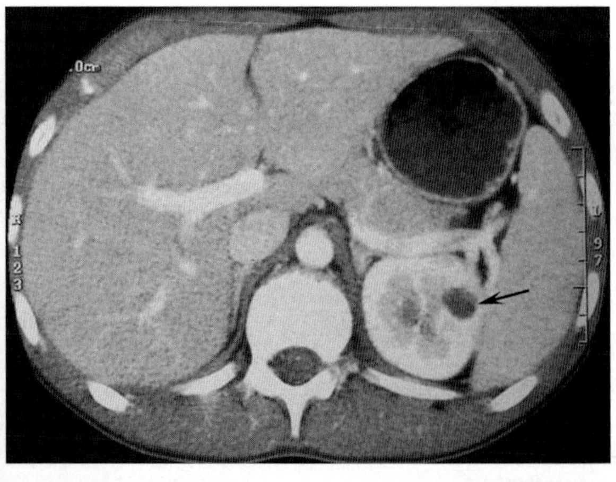

Fig. 20.7a,b. Nephrogenic rest in a 12-year-old boy with hematuria. a Longitudinal US image reveals a well-defined, hyperechoic mass (*arrow*) in the left kidney. b Axial contrast-enhanced CT scan confirms the presence of a well-defined lesion in the left kidney (*arrow*).

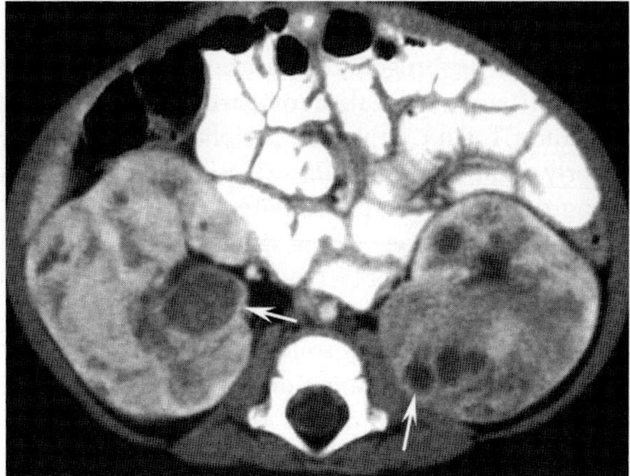

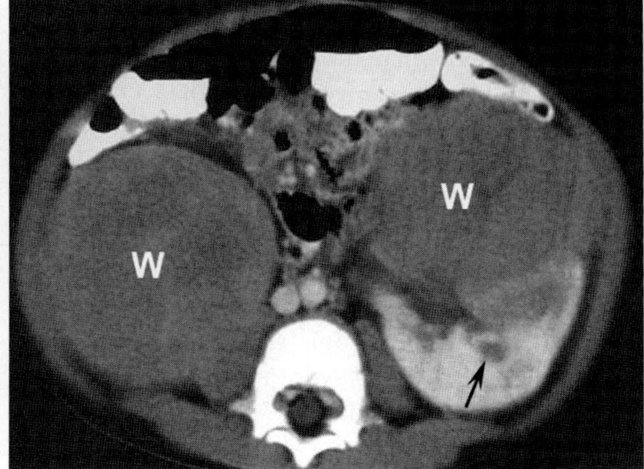

Fig. 20.8a,b. Nephroblastomatosis in a 13-month-old boy with suspected hepatosplenomegaly. a Axial contrast-enhanced CT scan demonstrates bilateral replacement of normal parenchyma with numerous nephrogenic rests (*arrows*), some of which are large and worrisome for developing Wilms tumor. b Axial contrast-enhanced CT scan of the same child 6 months later reveals progression of multiple lesions forming bilateral Wilms tumors (*W*). A focal nephrogenic rest (*arrow*) is noted.

In recent years, specific pathological features have allowed better classification of this malignancy. Clear cell sarcoma accounts for 4–5% of primary pediatric renal tumors (Charles et al. 1998; Hartman et al. 1982b) and boys are more often affected. All reported cases are unilateral and the age of peak incidence is from 1 to 4 years (Charles et al. 1998). The clinical presentation is non-specific but most often includes an abdominal mass.

Grossly, a well-circumscribed, soft mass is seen. On histological examination, small cells with inconspicuous nucleoli, ill-defined cell membranes, abundant cytoplasmic vesicles, and a prominent capillary network are characteristic (Fig. 20.9; Murphy et al. 1994); however, there is a spectrum of disease in which only 20% have clear cells.

On imaging, a well-defined, solid renal mass without intravascular extension is identified. Unfortunately, the appearance of clear cell sarcoma is non-specific and cannot be differentiated from Wilms tumor (Fig. 20.10).

Clear cell sarcoma behaves aggressively, with a much higher rate of recurrence and mortality than Wilms tumor. It may metastasize to bone, liver, brain, lymph nodes, and lungs, in some cases long after nephrectomy. Treatment consists of chemotherapy and nephrectomy, with survival rates of up to 70% (Charles et al. 1998).

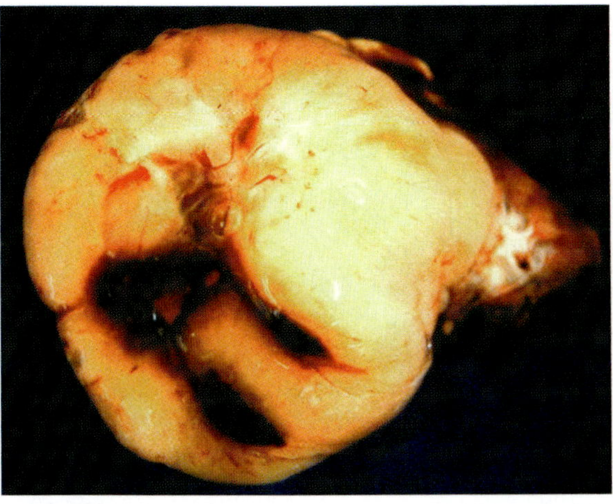
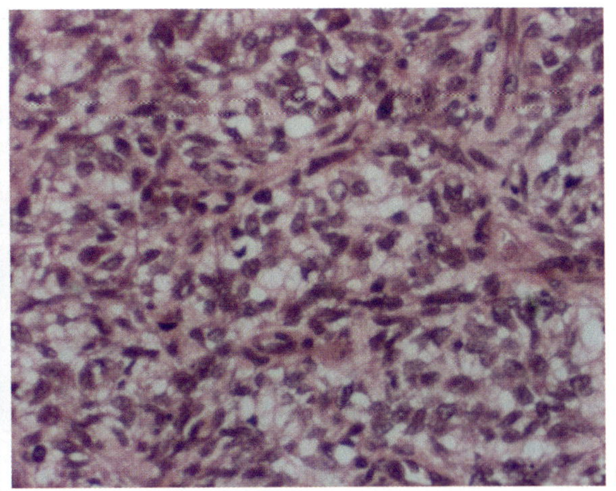

a

b

Fig. 20.9a,b. Clear cell sarcoma in a 15-month-old boy. **a** Gross specimen of a multilobulated mass. **b** Characteristic histology shows numerous cytoplasmic vesicles and delicate incomplete capillary arches. Cells contain extensive clear cytoplasm with displaced nuclei.

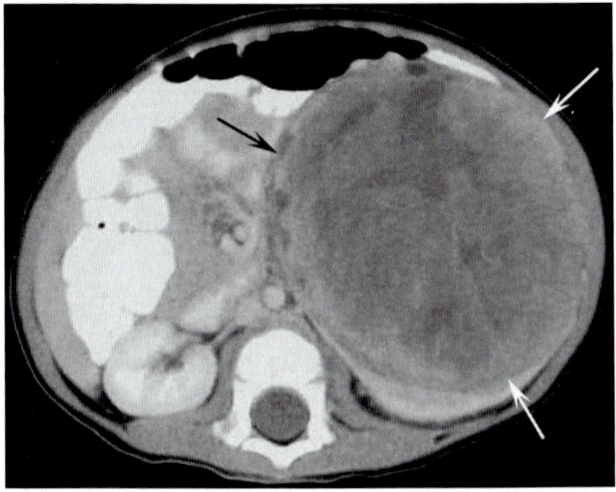

Fig. 20.10. Clear cell sarcoma in a 15-month-old boy with an abdominal mass. Axial contrast-enhanced CT scan shows a large, heterogeneously enhancing left renal mass (*arrows*).

20.5
Rhabdoid Tumor

Rhabdoid tumor, a rare, highly aggressive malignancy of early childhood, histologically resembles skeletal muscle, although a myogenic origin has not been proven. It is not related to Wilms tumor or rhabdomyosarcoma and was recently recognized as a distinct pathological entity (Lowe et al. 2000; Sacher et al. 1998). Further, recent cytogenetic studies have described a specific tumor suppressor gene on chromosome 22 in these patients. In challenging cases of rhabdoid tumor, a diagnosis is possible using cytogenetic studies, fluorescence in situ hybridiza-

tion (FISH), and molecular genetic analysis (Ogino et al. 2000).

Rhabdoid tumor includes 2% of all solid pediatric renal neoplasms. There is a male predominance of 1.5:1 (Charles et al. 1998; Hartman et al. 1982b; Sacher et al. 1998). Eighty percent of cases occur at less than 2 years of age, with a median age at diagnosis of 11 months (Charles et al. 1998). Occasionally, this renal neoplasm has been reported in children up to 9 years of age. Presenting symptoms are nonspecific, but may include hematuria, an abdominal mass, or symptoms related to metastatic disease. Elevated serum calcium due to increased parathyroid hormone levels may be found. These levels normalize following tumor resection (Hartman et al. 1982b; Sacher et al. 1998).

Synchronous or metachronous primary midline posterior fossa masses or brain metastases are a well-known, unique feature of rhabdoid tumors. Specifically, ependymoma, primitive neuroectodermal tumor (PNET), and cerebellar and brain-stem astrocytoma have all been reported (Lowe et al. 2000; Sacher et al. 1998).

Grossly, rhabdoid tumors are soft, uniform, well-defined masses without a capsule (Fig. 20.11). Microscopically, monomorphous, non-cohesive cells with prominent eosinophilic nucleoli and characteristic filamentous intracytoplasmic inclusions are characteristic (Charles et al. 1998; Murphy et al. 1994). Some tumors may have superficial areas that resemble the blastemal pattern of Wilms tumor.

The imaging appearance is often indistinguishable from Wilms tumor; however, there are several characteristics that can suggest rhabdoid tumor, including subcapsular fluid collections, tumor

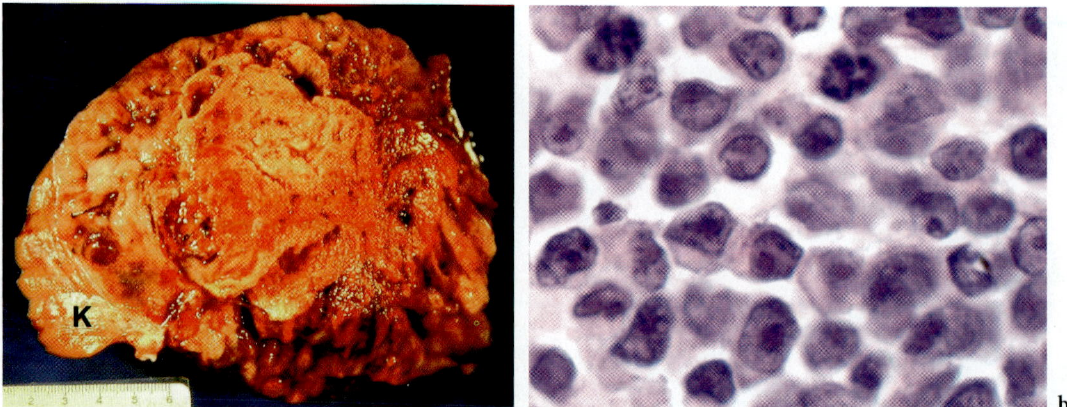

Fig. 20.11a,b. Rhabdoid tumor in a 8-month-old boy. **a** Gross specimen demonstrates a pale, well-demarcated mass without a capsule. A small amount of normal kidney (*K*) is noted on the edge of the specimen. **b** Microscopic image of Rhabdoid tumor reveals monomorphic sheets of large, loosely cohesive cells with acidophilic cytoplasm, large nucleoli and distinct cell borders.

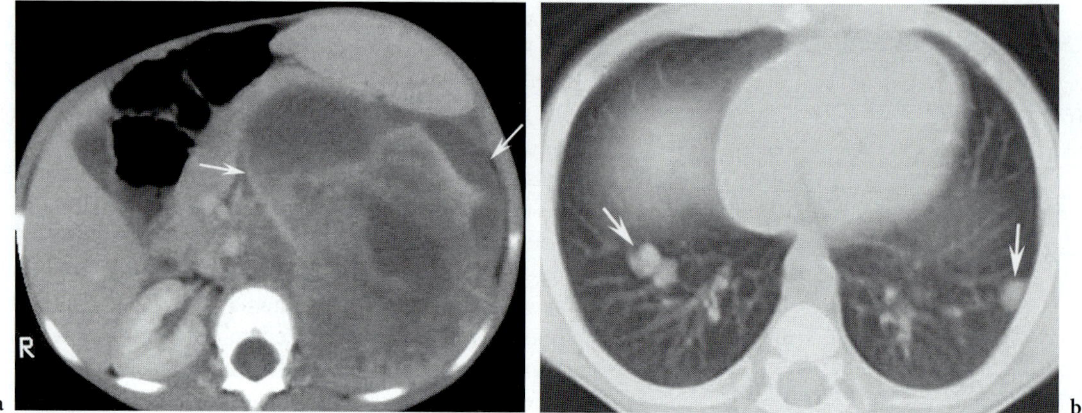

Fig. 20.12a,b. Rhabdoid tumor in an 8-month-old boy with hematuria. **a** Axial contrast-enhanced CT scan demonstrates a large left renal mass (*arrows*) with heterogeneous enhancement. Noted are subcapsular fluid collections. **b** Axial CT scan through the chest identifies multiple foci of metastatic disease (*arrows*).

lobules separated by hypodense areas of necrosis or hemorrhage, and linear calcifications outlining tumor lobules (Fig. 20.12). The mass is typically large, heterogeneous, and located near or involving the renal sinus. There may be vascular and local invasion of structures (Agrons et al. 1997; Hartman et al. 1982b; Sacher et al. 1998).

Rhabdoid tumor is extremely aggressive and has a dismal prognosis with an 18-month survival rate of only 20% (Agrons et al. 1997; Charles et al. 1998; Sacher et al. 1998). Unfortunately, most children have advanced metastatic disease at the time of presentation, most commonly to the lungs (80%), and less often the liver, abdomen, brain, lymph nodes, and skeleton.

20.6
Renal Cell Carcinoma

Renal cell carcinoma (RCC) is rare in children, including less than 7% of all primary renal masses presenting at less than 20 years of age. Although Wilms tumors are 30 times more common in children than RCC (Murphy et al. 1994), they are nearly equal in incidence in the second decade (Lack et al. 1985). The vast majority of RCC occurs in adults with fewer than 2% presenting in pediatric patients. Although RCC has been reported in infants less than 6 months of age, the peak incidence occurs in the sixth decade. Patients with von Hippel-Lindau syndrome are at an increased risk of developing RCC, in which tumors are often multiple and present at an earlier age. Because of this unique association, von Hippel-Lindau syndrome should be excluded in all children with RCC (Lack et al. 1985).

Clinically, the presentation is non-specific and the same in children as in adults. Common presenting symptoms include a palpable mass, painless gross hematuria, and flank pain. Hematuria is more common in children with RCC than those with Wilms tumor but is not useful in predicting the diagnosis or prognosis (Murphy et al. 1994).

The gross morphology of RCC is similar to that of Wilms tumor except that RCC tends to be smaller (Fig. 20.13). The normal renal architecture is usually distorted, a pseudocapsule is common, and there may be local invasion of adjacent retroperitoneal nodes. The origin of RCC remains unclear, but most authors believe that it represents an adenocarcinoma with renal tubular differentiation. Histologically, the neoplasm forms a solid infiltrative mass with variable calcification, necrosis, bleeding, and cystic degeneration (Fig. 20.14; Leuschner et al. 1991; Murphy et al. 1994). Metastases are identified at presentation in 20% of patients with the most common sites including lungs, bone, liver, and brain (Hartman et al. 1982b).

Because RCC may be somewhat small at presentation, it may be subtle on US. On CT and MR imaging, the lesion is usually easily identified as a non-specific, solid renal mass with mild contrast enhancement (Fig. 20.15). The lesion is often heterogeneous with areas of necrosis, hemorrhage, and calcification in 25% of cases (Lonergan et al. 1998). Renal cell carcinoma is treated with radical nephrectomy and regional lymphadenectomy. Unfortunately, the tumor is highly resistant to chemotherapy, making metastatic disease difficult to treat. The prognosis is mostly determined by stage at the time of presentation, with an overall survival rate of approximately 64% (Table 20.4; Geller et al. 1997).

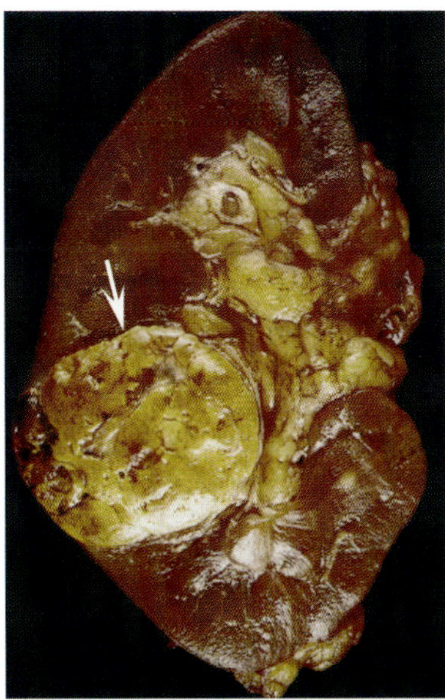

Fig. 20.13. Renal cell carcinoma in a child. Gross specimen of clear cell type of renal cell carcinoma shows a golden color (*arrow*) due to cytoplasmic lipids. (With permission from Murphy et al. 1994)

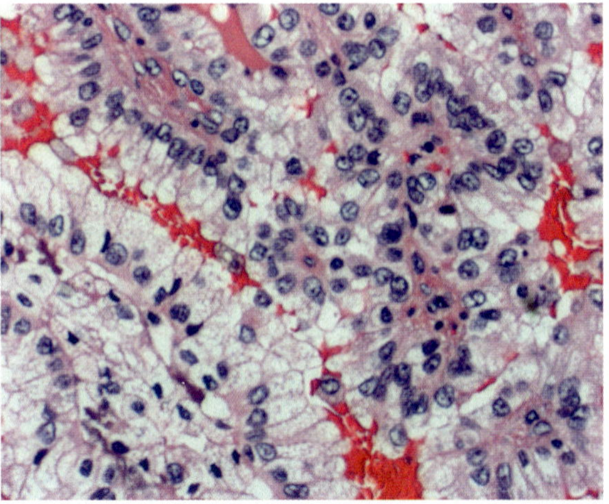

Fig. 20.14. Renal cell carcinoma in a 12-year-old boy. Histological specimen demonstrates an acinar and trabecular arrangement and clear cytoplasm.

20.7
Renal Medullary Carcinoma

Renal medullary carcinoma is a recently defined, extremely aggressive tumor occurring exclusively in teenagers and young adults with hemoglobin sickle cell (SC) disease or sickle cell trait (Davidson et al. 1995; Eble 1998). Listed as the seventh sickle cell nephropathy, the tumor does not occur in homozygous hemoglobin SS sickle cell disease (Davis et al. 1995b; Wesche et al. 1998). The mean age at presentation is 25 years (range 10–39 years). There is a male predominance (3:1) in patients under age 25 years, with an equal gender incidence over 25 years (Davis et al. 1995b). Symptoms at presentation are non-specific, including flank pain, abdominal pain, gross hematuria, weight loss, abdominal mass, and fever (Wesche et al. 1998).

Table 20.4. Renal cell carcinoma staging

Stage	Description
I	Mass <7.0 cm that is limited to the kidney
II	Mass >7.0 cm that is limited to the kidney
III	Tumor limited by Gerota's fascia (may include invasion of the ipsilateral renal vein, adrenal gland, perinephric soft tissue/fat, and/or IVC thrombus)
IV	Extension of tumor beyond Gerota's fascia

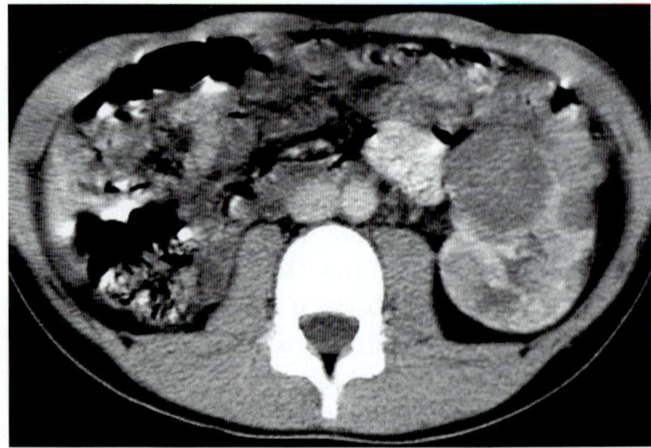

Fig. 20.15. Renal cell carcinoma in a transplanted kidney in a 12-year-old boy with suspected rejection. Axial contrast-enhanced CT scan shows multiple, well-defined foci of hypodensity within the left-lower-quadrant transplanted kidney.

The lesion arises from the epithelium at the renal pelvis–mucosa interface. Grossly, the mass fills the renal pelvis and invades adjacent vasculature and lymphatic structures (Fig. 20.16). On microscopy, drepanocytes (sickle cells), hemorrhagic foci, necrosis, stromal desmoplasia with inflammation, and a variable architectural pattern typify the lesion (WESCHE et al. 1998).

Radiographically, the infiltrative, centrally located mass causes reniform enlargement with extension into the renal sinus and collecting system. Small satellite nodules and caliectasis (hydronephrosis) are typical features (Fig. 20.17). On US and CT, the lesion shows heterogeneous echogenicity and heterogeneous enhancement. In the appropriate clinical setting the differential diagnosis is limited, including transitional cell carcinoma, which is poorly documented in children, and rhabdoid tumor, which occurs in children under 3 years old (DAVIDSON et al. 1995; LOWE et al. 2000).

The prognosis of renal medullary carcinoma is very poor, with an average survival of 15 weeks from the time of diagnosis (DAVIS et al. 1995b). The tumor usually presents with extensive metastatic disease, and there is a very poor response to radiotherapy and chemotherapy (LOWE et al. 2000).

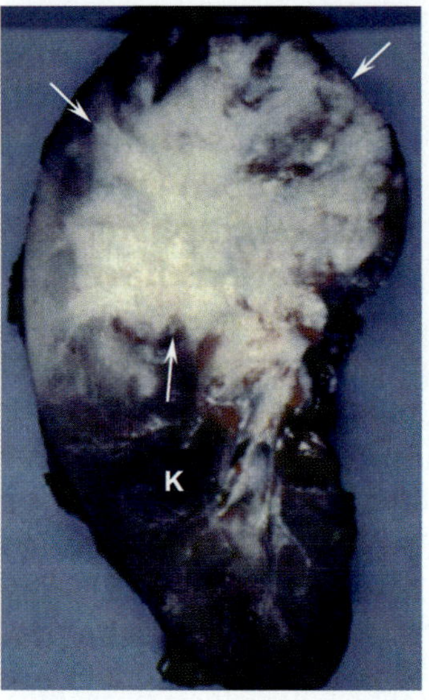

Fig. 20.16. Renal medullary carcinoma in a 16-year-old girl. Cut surface of specimen demonstrates a whorled, myomatous appearance with prominent medial extension and an ill-defined margin (*arrows*). Very little normal kidney (*K*) remains visible. (With permission from DAVIDSON et al. 1995)

20.8
Renal Lymphoma

Renal lymphoma may be the result of direct extension from the retroperitoneum or hematogenous spread. Burkitt and non-Hodgkin lymphomas are more likely to have renal involvement in children (CHEPURI et al. 2003). While less than 8% of patients with lymphoma will have their disease identified on CT, up to 62% have renal involvement on postmortem examination (REZNEK et al. 1990; SHEERAN and SUSSMAN 1998). Primary renal lymphoma is disputed as an entity by most authors due to a lack of lymphatics in the kidney (DYER et al. 1994). Primary lymphoma of the kidney has been reported only rarely and the topic remains controversial (COHAN et al. 1990). In children with lymphoma, symptoms related to the kidney usually occur late in the disease process and are non-specific, including an abdominal mass, abdominal pain, anemia, hematuria, weight loss, and occasionally hypertension (DYER et al. 1994; LACK et al. 1985).

Imaging features vary extensively, including diffuse infiltration, focal, or multiple masses, invasion from contiguous retroperitoneal lymphadenopathy, and infrequently, perinephric disease (Fig. 20.18; HARTMAN et al. 1982a). Multiple focal renal nodules that variably distort the renal capsule and collecting system are the most common presenting imaging characteristics (CHEPURI et al. 2003). On US, focal renal masses due to lymphoma are typically hypoechoic and may have increased through-transmission mimicking multiple cysts. The appearance on CT is non-specific. Diffuse infiltration may lead to

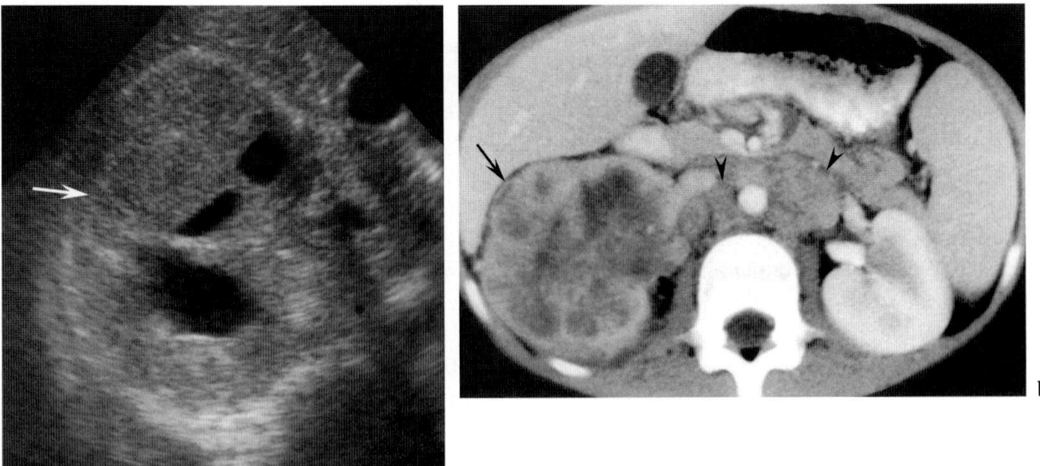

Fig. 20.17a,b. Renal medullary carcinoma in a 10-year-old boy with hematuria and sickle cell trait. **a** Transverse US image reveals loss of normal renal architecture, which is replaced by a mass (*arrow*) causing hydronephrosis. **b** Axial contrast-enhanced CT scan shows a heterogeneous mass (*arrow*) infiltrating the right kidney and adjacent retroperitoneal lymphadenopathy (*arrowheads*).

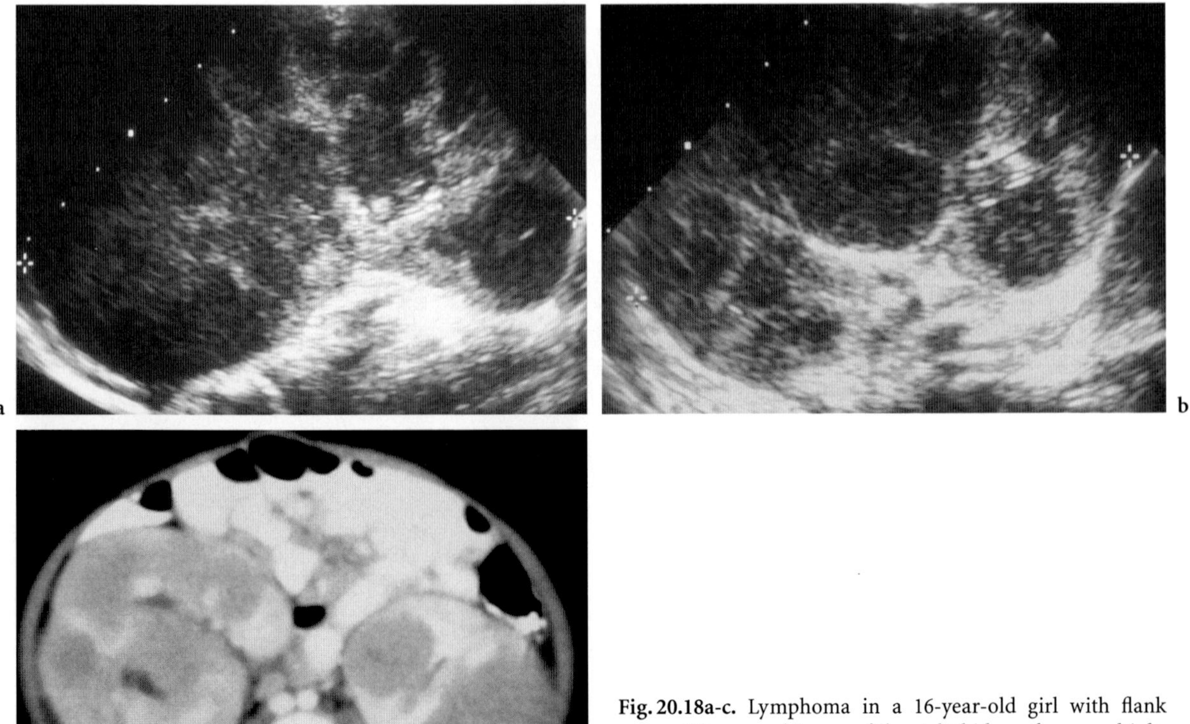

Fig. 20.18a-c. Lymphoma in a 16-year-old girl with flank pain. **a** Ultrasound image of the right kidney shows multiple, well-demarcated hypoechoic masses in the enlarged kidney. **b** Ultrasound image of the left kidney resembles the right side. **c** Axial contrast-enhanced CT scan confirms bilateral nephromegaly with multiple hypodense renal masses.

reniform enlargement, retroperitoneal disease may cause ureteral or vascular encasement, and perinephric spread may be the result of direct retroperitoneal extension or intraparenchymal invasion through the renal capsule (Chepuri et al. 2003). Focal lesions are generally homogeneous and hypodense both before and after contrast administration with some cases simulating the appearance of multiple renal cysts (Capps and Das Narla 1995). Perinephric spread may be identified as soft tissue nodules, focal curvilinear densities, thickening of the renal capsule/Gerota's fascia, or direct invasion from retroperitoneal nodes (Dyer et al. 1994). Perirenal lymphoma without renal parenchymal disease is rare, but unusual in appearance on CT (Hartman et al. 1982a) where it manifests as a hypodense soft tissue plaque encasing the kidney (Sheeran and Sussman 1998). Angiography is no longer performed but has been reported to show hypovascular foci.

Prognosis in patients with lymphoma is unrelated to the presence of renal involvement (Chepuri et al. 2003).

20.9
Leukemia

Leukemic (acute and chronic, myelogenous and lymphoblastic) involvement of the kidneys is common during the hematologically active stage of disease (Butani and Paulson 2003). The kidneys may act as a sanctuary for residual disease during remission. Clinically, symptoms related to renal leukemia are unusual but may include renal failure or hypertension. Grossly, leukemia infiltrates the kidneys causing reniform enlargement.

Imaging features are variable but may include unilateral or bilateral nephromegaly, hydronephrosis, altered architecture, abnormal echogenicity on US, and poor contrast excretion on CT (Butani and Paulson 2003).

20.10
Neuroblastoma

Neuroblastoma is the most common tumor of early childhood, occurring most often in children under age 5 years (David et al. 1989; Kushner 2004). It originates from the neural crest cells and arises most often from the adrenal medulla but may occur any-

where along the sympathetic chain from the skull base to the pelvis (Mehta et al. 2003). The presentation varies, ranging from a palpable abdominal mass, to various paraneoplastic syndromes, or symptoms related to metastatic disease (David et al. 1989; Matthay et al. 2003; Mehta et al. 2003). The diagnosis is often made by analysis of urinary catecholamines, or from bone marrow aspirates (Kushner 2004). The kidney is most often involved by invasion from an adjacent adrenal primary, or direct extension of retroperitoneal disease.

Imaging features include a solid mass with calcifications on plain radiographs and a heterogeneous mostly hyperechoic mass on US. Vascular encasement and calcification by a large, heterogeneously enhancing mass is seen on CT (Fig. 20.19). Metastatic disease is commonly detected at presentation by bone marrow aspirate, bone scan, I-131 metaiodobenzylmandelic scintigraphy (MIBG), and CT (Matthay et al. 2003; Mehta et al. 2003). In general, the prognosis is better with younger age, lower grade, lower stage, and n-myc amplification (Moore et al. 2004).

20.11
Mesoblastic Nephroma

Mesoblastic nephroma, also referred to as fetal renal hamartoma or leiomyomatous hamartoma, was originally thought to represent congenital Wilms tumor

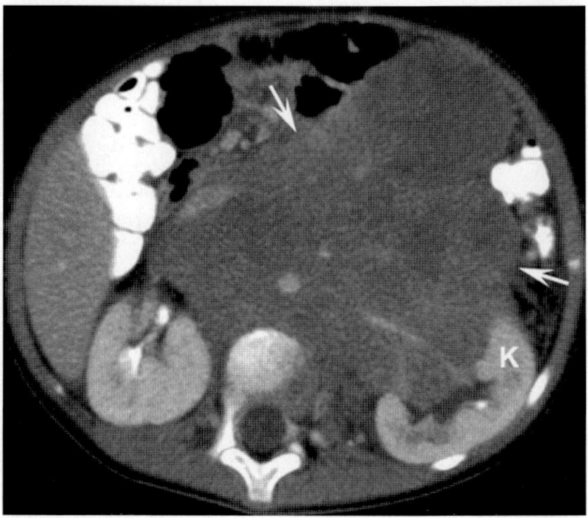

Fig. 20.19. Neuroblastoma in a 5-year-old boy with a palpable mass. Axial contrast-enhanced CT scan shows a soft tissue mass (*arrows*) centered within the retroperitoneum and extending into the left renal sinus abutting the kidney (*K*).

but is now recognized as a distinct entity. Mesoblastic nephroma is by far the most common solid renal mass in neonates (DONALDSON and SHKOLNIK 1988; GLICK et al. 2004). It is slightly more common in boys and usually presents at under 3 months of age, with 90% of lesions discovered by 12 months of age (GLICK et al. 2004; HARTMAN et al. 1982b; LOWE et al. 2000). The clinical presentation is most often a palpable abdominal mass or less frequently hematuria. Cases are increasingly detected with prenatal US. An association with hydrops, polyhydramnios, increased renin levels, and premature delivery has been described (GLICK et al. 2004).

Pathologically, mesoblastic nephroma is believed to be due to early proliferation of nephrogenic mesenchyme. On gross pathology, the tumor is usually large, rubbery, infiltrative, poorly defined, and without a capsule (Fig. 20.20). Histologically, the tumors are "monomorphic," with infiltrating finger-like projections of spindled mesenchymal cells and embryonal metaplasia of entrapped renal tissue (CHARLES et al. 1998; HARTMAN et al. 1982b).

Radiological studies demonstrate a solid intrarenal mass that often extends into the renal sinus and may have focal perinephric space infiltration. A large portion of the renal parenchyma may be replaced by the mass, which may be hemorrhagic, necrotic, or partially cystic (Fig. 20.21).

Mesoblastic nephroma is usually benign and is treated with nephrectomy (JULIAN et al. 1995). A wide surgical margin is necessary due to the infiltrative nature of the lesion which may recur locally if incompletely resected. Occasionally, metastases to lung, brain, or bones are reported. It is recommended that patients be followed closely for 1 year after surgical resection since histological characteristics cannot reliably predict biological behavior (CHARLES et al. 1998; LEUSCHNER et al. 1991). When mesoblastic nephroma is found and resected early (at <6 months of age), the prognosis is excellent (LOWE et al. 2000).

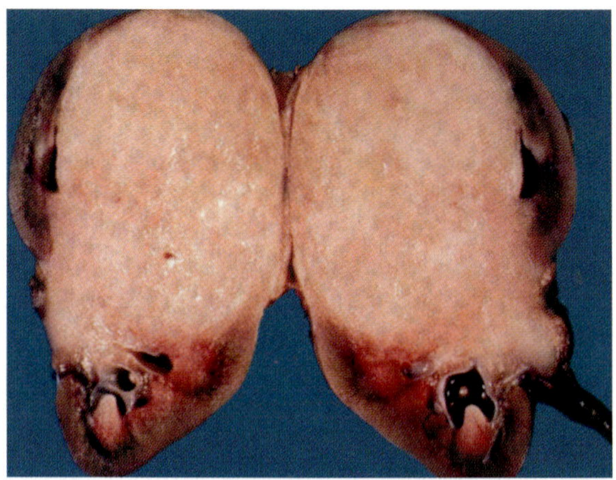

Fig. 20.20. Mesoblastic nephroma in an infant. Gross specimen shows classic whorled, myxomatous infiltrative mass with poor demarcation from the normal renal parenchyma. (With permission from MURPHY et al. 1994)

20.12
Ossifying Renal Tumor of Infancy

Ossifying renal tumor of infancy (ORTI) is a rare, benign renal mass first described in 1980

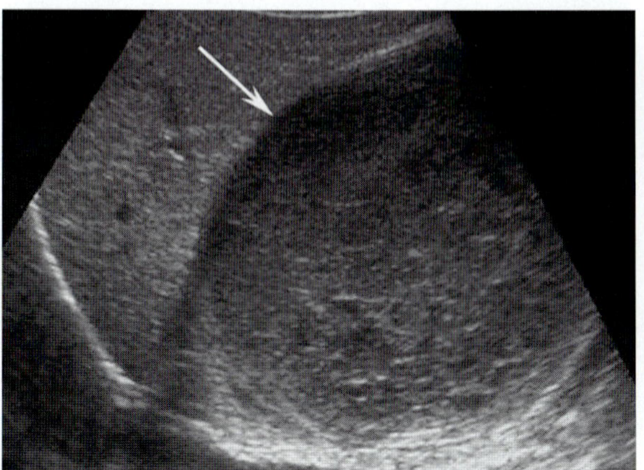

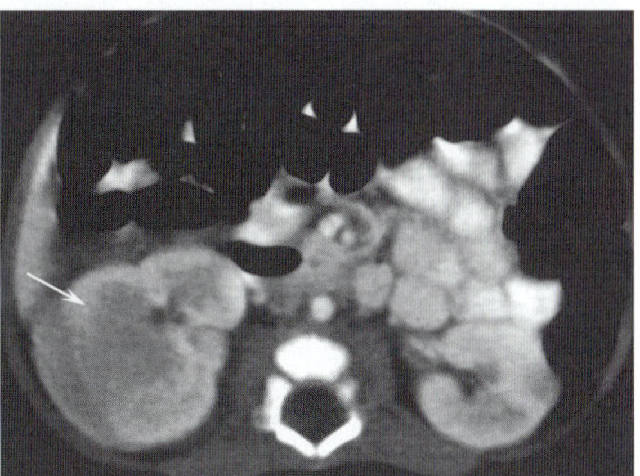

Fig. 20.21a,b. Mesoblastic nephroma in a 5-week-old infant with an in utero renal mass. a Longitudinal US image reveals a mixed echo texture mass (*arrow*) replacing most of the right kidney. b Axial contrast-enhanced CT scan reveals a hypodense, ill-defined, infiltrative, right renal mass (*arrow*).

(Chatten et al. 1980). Since then, only 11 cases have been reported in children with an age range of 6 days to 14 months (Chatten et al. 1980; Glick et al. 2004; Sotelo-Avila et al. 1995; Vazquez et al. 1998). ORTI is more common in boys (8 of 11), more common on the left side (9 of 11), and hematuria was the presenting symptom in 10 of 11 children. The upper pole calyces were involved in 7 of 11 cases (Sotelo-Avila et al. 1995).

ORTI is a urothelial lesion originating from the papillary portion of the renal pyramid. The lesion enlarges in a polypoid fashion, extending into the collecting system and usually reaching a size of no more than 2–3 cm.

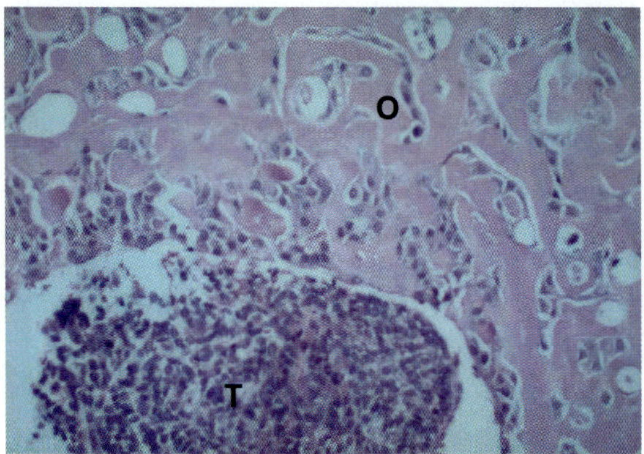

Fig. 20.22. Ossifying renal tumor of infancy in a child. Microscopic specimen reveals an osteoid core (*O*) with peripheral tubules (*T*) and mesenchyme/fibrous connective tissue. (With permission from Lowe et al. 2000)

Three basic histological components are found within the lesion: the osteoid core; osteoblasts; and spindle cells. In relatively older children, mature osteoid elements tend to be more prominent (Fig. 20.22). It is believed by some authors that the osteoid elements within the lesion are the result of urothelial cells with osteogenic potential (Chatten et al. 1980; Davis et al. 1995b). Other investigators hypothesize that spindle cells within the tumor resemble intralobular nephrogenic rests, thus indicating a mass in the pathological spectrum of Wilms tumor. Despite these two theories, Wilms tumor has never been reported in association with any of these children.

Imaging studies of ORTI typically show a calcified mass causing a filling defect and partial obstruction of the collecting system (Lowe et al. 2000). The appearance may resemble a staghorn calculus, which is not a differential consideration in a child of this age (Vazquez et al. 1998). Calcifications are present within 9 of 11 cases of ORTI with only the two youngest patients having no calcifications (Sotelo-Avila et al. 1995). Specific findings by modality include an echogenic shadowing mass with or without hydronephrosis on US, and a smoothly demarcated, poorly enhancing, calcified mass on CT (Fig. 20.23).

The prognosis of ORTI is excellent with no reports of metastatic disease or recurrence after surgical resection. Follow-up of the disease-free state has been documented from 4 months up to 23 years (Ito et al. 1998).

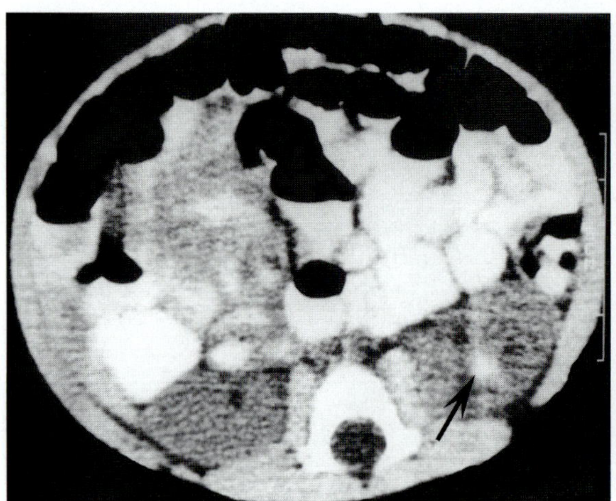
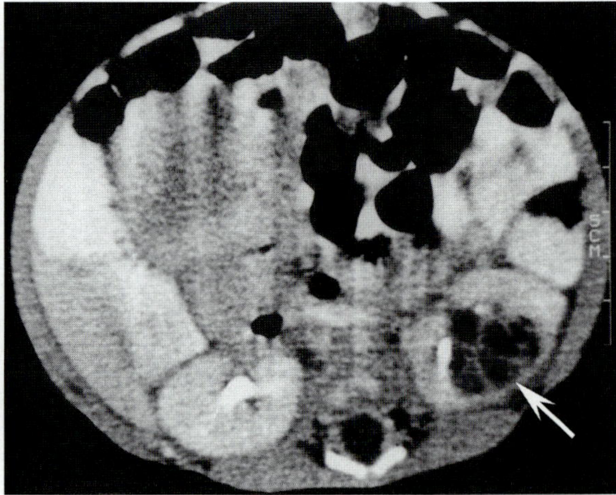

Fig. 20.23a,b. Ossifying renal tumor of infancy in a 2-month-old boy with an abdominal mass. a Axial unenhanced CT scan reveals a calcification (*arrow*) within the left kidney. b After contrast administration, axial CT scan demonstrates a hypodense mass (*arrow*) with septations. (With permission from Lowe et al. 2000)

20.13
Multilocular Cystic Renal Tumor

The term multilocular cystic renal tumor includes a group of uncommon, benign cystic renal lesions that are indistinguishable grossly and radiologically (Agrons et al. 1995; Charles et al. 1998). These masses range from purely cystic (cystic nephroma, CN), epithelial lined with fibrous septa to a mass with mature tubules and septa containing foci of blastemal cells (cystic partially differentiated nephroblastoma, CPDN; Ferrer and McKenna 1994; Shamberger 1999). Septations within the CPDN form the only solid portions of the tumor (Fig. 20.24). Cystic Wilms tumor is distinguished from CPDN by the presence of expansile solid masses of nephroblastomatous tissue.

Two distinct peak ages of incidence occur in multilocular cystic renal tumors. The first occurs in boys 3 months to 4 years, typically CN, and the second occurs in adult women, typically CPDN (Lonergan et al. 1998). The presentation is non-specific with a painless abdominal mass and occasional systemic symptoms (Sacher et al. 1998).

Cross-sectional imaging with US, CT, or MR imaging reveals a well-defined, cystic mass with enhancing septa. The cysts range in size from a few millimeters up to 4 cm, and the amount of enhancing septa determines the degree to which the lesion may appear more or less solid (Fig. 20.25). A capsule may be present and extracapsular extension may occur.

Multilocular cystic renal tumors are treated by complete surgical resection and have an excellent prognosis. Occasionally, chemotherapy or local radiation is required to treat tumor recurrence; however, there are no reports of metastatic disease (Gonzalez-Crussi et al. 1982).

20.14
Angiomyolipoma

Angiomyolipoma is a benign hamartomatous neoplasm consisting of disordered fat, smooth muscle, and vascular tissue (Chung et al. 1998; Eble 1998; Ewalt et al. 1998). It is almost always associated with tuberous sclerosis in children (Eble 1998; Lowe et al. 2000), but overall is most often sporadic (Lemaitre et al. 1995). By the age of 10 years, 80% of children with tuberous sclerosis will have angiomyolipomas (Chung et al. 1998). Other associations with angiomyolipoma include neurofibromatosis and von Hippel-Lindau syndrome. Women are affected 4:1 compared with men, and the average age at presentation for all cases is 41 years. Angiomyolipomas are typically multifocal, bilateral, and often large in size.

Lesions less than 4 cm in size are generally asymptomatic; however, larger lesions may present with symptoms such as flank pain, abdominal pain, hematuria, or severe hemorrhage (Ewalt et al. 1998; Hartman et al. 1982b). Hemorrhage within angiomyolipomas is believed secondary to bleeding aneurysms within the abundant abnormal, elastin-poor vascularity of the tumor (Eble 1998). "Wunderlich syndrome," or severe retroperitoneal hemorrhage, has been described in larger lesions and may be life-threatening (Hennigar and Beckwith 1992).

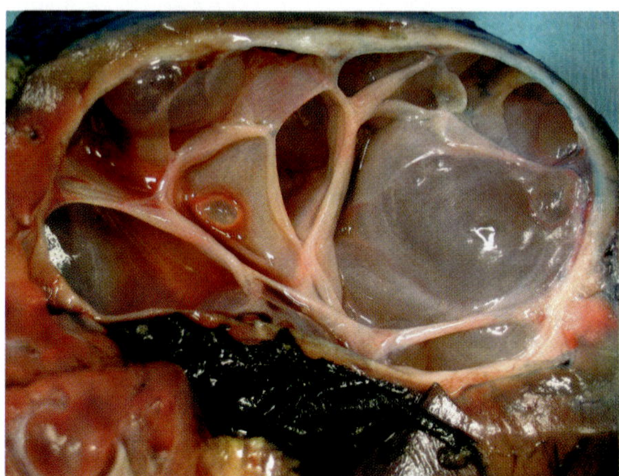
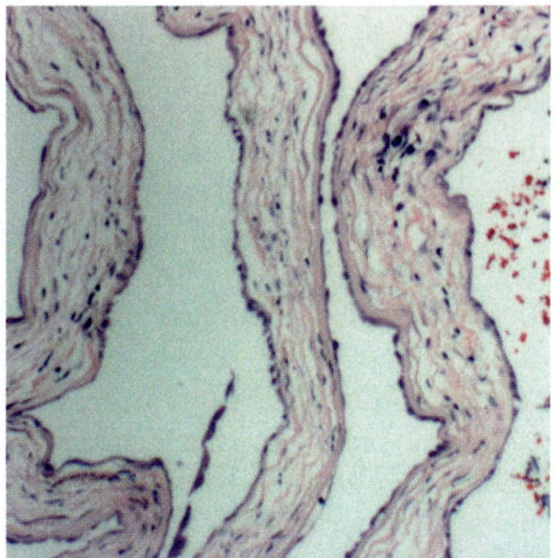

Fig. 20.24a,b. Cystic nephroma in a 2-year-old boy. **a** Gross appearance of cystic mass with well-defined, smooth margins, and multiple septations. **b** Microscopic image shows fibrous tissue in the walls of the cysts without the presence of other nephroblastic elements.

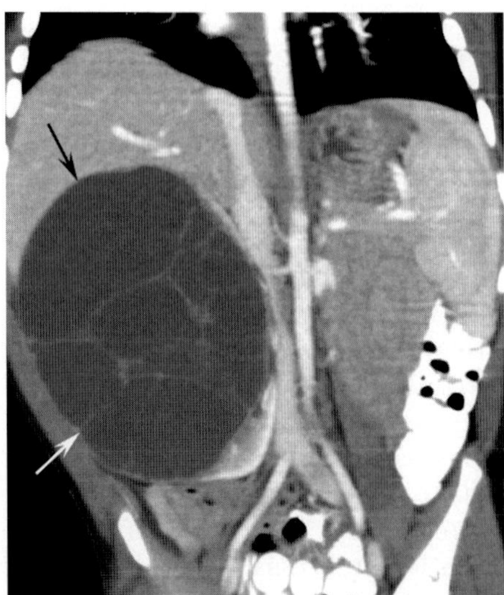

Fig. 20.25. Cystic nephroma in a 2-year-old boy with an abdominal mass on a well-child visit to the pediatrician. Coronal reconstructed contrast-enhanced CT image demonstrates a large septate right renal mass (*arrows*).

The radiological appearance of angiomyolipoma varies depending on the presence or absence of tissue components. Ultrasound reveals hyperechoic non-shadowing foci in fatty regions, iso- to hypoechoic foci in regions of soft tissue, and hypervascularity regions on color Doppler evaluation. The imaging diagnosis is often specific if fat is found in the mass on CT or MR imaging (Fig. 20.26). Catheter angiography may show characteristic dilated tortuous vessels with aneurysm formation but is not generally indicated for diagnosis. It may be necessary if intervention is required for temporization of severe bleeding. The differential diagnosis of angiomyolipoma includes Wilms tumor and renal cell carcinoma, both of which may also contain fat; however, in the appropriate clinical setting and with typical imaging features, a specific diagnosis of angiomyolipoma is usually not problematic. Although angiomyolipoma is a benign lesion, it may rarely invade neighboring structures such as lymph nodes or the inferior vena cava (Lowe et al. 2000).

Because there is a high rate of angiomyolipomas in patients with tuberous sclerosis, screening US is recommended every 2–3 years before puberty and every year thereafter to check for growing lesions (Chung et al. 1998). In children with lesions larger than 4 cm, prophylactic partial nephrectomy, or selective catheter embolization may be considered to avoid potentially life-threatening bleeding (Hartman et al. 1982b). Unfortunately, in children with tuberous sclerosis there is often replacement of a majority of normal renal parenchyma by cysts and angiomyolipomas that ultimately results in end-stage renal disease, and in these children, preservation of functional renal tissue becomes the priority.

20.15
Metanephric Adenoma

Metanephric adenoma is also known as embryonal adenoma, or nephrogenic adenofibroma (Ito et al. 1998; Navarro et al. 1999). It is a benign unilateral mass that is more common in women and has been reported from age 15 months to 83 years (Davis et al. 1995a). Presenting features include an abdominal mass, hypertension, abdominal pain, hypercalcemia, hematoma, and polycythemia. The gross appearance is non-specific, and microscopically numerous psammoma bodies can be identified among spindled mesenchymal cells that surround nodules of embryonal epithelium (Fig. 20.27; Murphy et al. 1994; Navarro et al. 1999).

Imaging features are non-specific and include a well-defined, solid lesion on US that is hypovascular with Doppler, with possible cystic change or a mural nodule (Mahoney et al. 1997). Unenhanced CT images reveal a hyper- or isodense mass that may contain small calcifications (Davis et al. 1995a; Navarro et al. 1999). After contrast administration the mass is hypodense compared with normal renal tissue (Fig. 20.28; Chefchaouni et al. 1996).

Because metanephric adenoma is a benign lesion treated with local surgical excision and normal renal parenchymal sparing, it is important to include it in

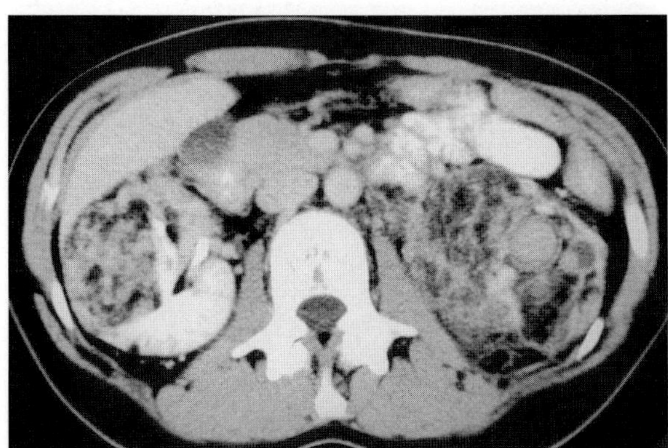

Fig. 20.26. Angiomyolipomas in a 17-year-old girl with tuberous sclerosis. Axial contrast-enhanced CT scan reveals bilateral heterogeneous enhancement of multiple renal masses containing soft tissue and fat components. Subtle, tiny peripheral renal cortical cysts are also noted.

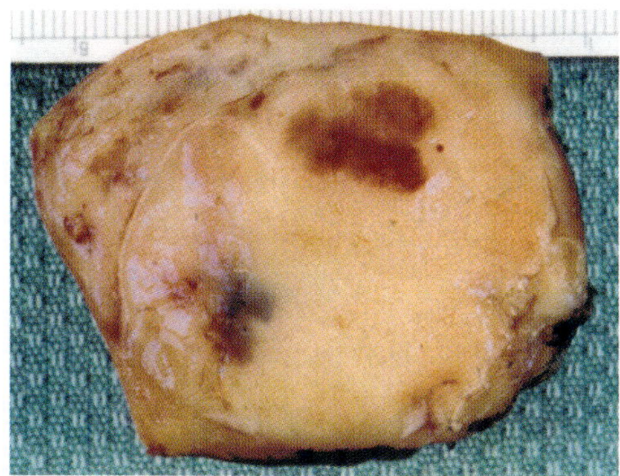
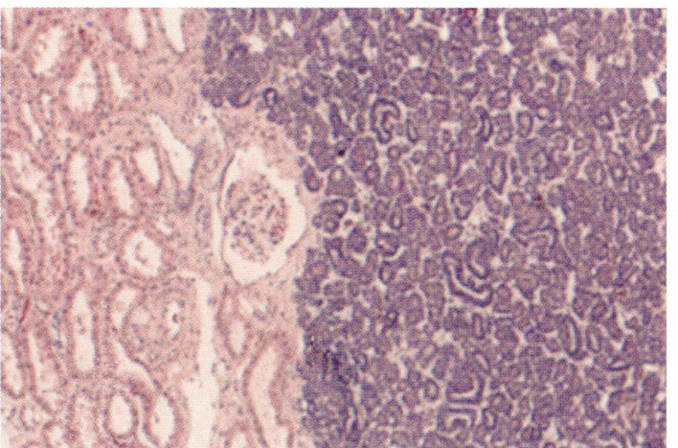

Fig. 20.27a,b. Metanephric adenoma in a 9-year-old girl. **a** Gross cut surface of mass demonstrates focus of hemorrhage without necrosis. **b** Histological specimen shows tubular and acinar structures adjacent to normal kidney on the left. Nuclei are homogenous and bland without mitotic activity (hematoxylin and eosin stain; original magnification, ×50). (With permission from Navarro et al. 1999; image courtesy of G. Taylor)

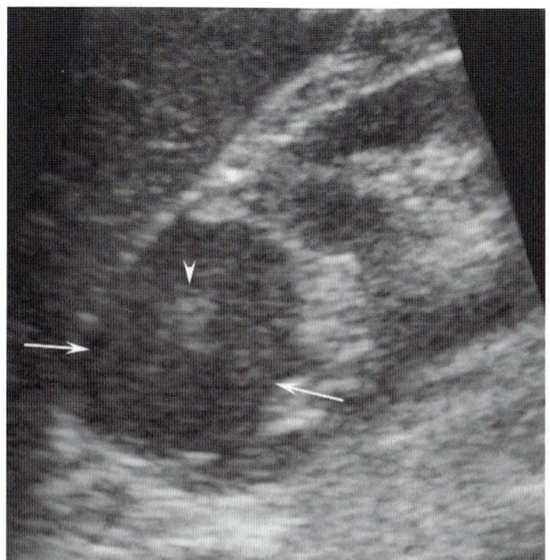
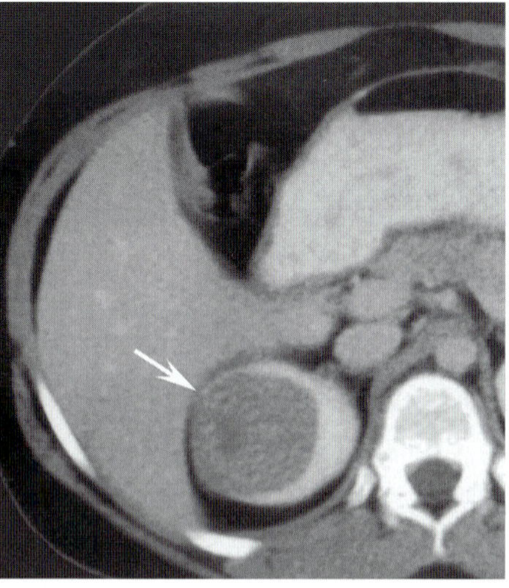

Fig. 20.28a,b. Metanephric adenoma in a 9-year-old girl with three episodes of urinary tract infection. **a** Longitudinal US image demonstrates a well-defined, hypoechoic mass (*arrows*) in the right kidney with a central focus of hyperechogenicity (*arrowhead*). **b** Axial contrast-enhanced CT scan reveals homogeneous, mildly enhancing mass (*arrow*) in the right kidney. (With permission from Navarro et al. 1999)

the differential diagnosis of pediatric renal masses (Murphy et al. 1994; Navarro et al. 1999).

20.16
Conclusion

In conclusion, Wilms tumor is characterized by displacement of structures, vascular invasion, and bilaterality in 10% of cases. Nephrogenic rests and nephroblastomatosis occur most often in neonates, and are distinguished by multiple, bilateral, subcapsular masses, and associated Wilms tumors.

Frequent skeletal metastases suggest clear cell sarcoma and a synchronous posterior fossa mass suggests rhabdoid tumor. Pediatric renal cell carcinoma occurs in the second decade and is associated with von Hippel-Lindau disease. Renal medullary carcinoma is a highly aggressive tumor seen exclusively in teenagers and young adults with sickle cell trait or SC disease. The appearance of renal lymphoma is variable, but most often includes multiple homogeneous masses with retroperitoneal lymphadenopathy. Leukemic infiltration of the kidneys causes bilateral reniform enlargement, although the diagnosis is usually not a dilemma based on the clinical history. Neuroblastoma is distinguished by direct extension of a retroperitoneal mass with vascular encasement and often has calcifications.

The primary differential diagnosis in a neonate with a solid renal mass is mesoblastic nephroma. Differentiation of ossifying renal tumor in infancy is possible by the presence of ossified elements. A large renal mass with multiple cysts and little solid tissue raises concern for multilocular cystic renal tumor. Angiomyolipomas contain fat and soft tissue, are often multiple and in children predominantly occur in association with tuberous sclerosis. Metanephric adenoma lacks specific features but is always well defined.

References

Agrons GA, Wagner BJ, Davidson AJ, Suarez ES (1995) Multilocular cystic renal tumor in children: radiologic–pathologic correlation. Radiographics 15:653–669

Agrons GA, Kingsman KD, Wagner BJ, Sotelo-Avila C (1997) Rhabdoid tumor of the kidney in children: a comparative study of 21 cases. Am J Roentgenol 168:447–451

Beckwith JB (1998) Children at increased risk for Wilms tumor: monitoring issues. J Pediatr 132:377–379

Butani L, Paulson TE (2003) Congenital acute myelogenous leukemia presenting as palpable renal masses in a neonate. J Pediatr Hematol Oncol 25:240–242

Capps GW, Das Narla L (1995) Renal lymphoma mimicking clear cell sarcoma in a pediatric patient. Pediatr Radiol 25 (Suppl 1):S87–S89

Charles AK, Vujanic GM, Berry PJ (1998) Renal tumours of childhood. Histopathology 32:293–309

Chatten J, Cromie WJ, Duckett JW (1980) Ossifying tumor of infantile kidney: report of two cases. Cancer 45:609–612

Chefchaouni MC, Zerbib M, Homsi T, Saighi D, Flam T, Thiounn N, Debre B (1996) Metanephric adenoma: an unusual tumor of the kidney. Apropos of a case. J Urol (Paris) 102:40–43

Chepuri NB, Strouse PJ, Yanik GA (2003) CT of renal lymphoma in children. Am J Roentgenol 180:429–431

Cherullo EE, Ross JH, Kay R, Novick AC (2001) Renal neoplasms in adult survivors of childhood Wilms tumor. J Urol 165:2013–2017

Chung CJ, Fordham L, Little S, Rayder S, Nimkin K, Kleinman PK, Watson C (1998) Intraperitoneal rhabdomyosarcoma in children: incidence and imaging characteristics on CT. Am J Roentgenol 170:1385–1387

Cohan RH, Dunnick NR, Leder RA, Baker ME (1990) Computed tomography of renal lymphoma. J Comput Assist Tomogr 14:933–938

David R, Lamki N, Fan S, Singleton EB, Eftekhari F, Shirkhoda A, Kumar R, Madewell JE (1989) The many faces of neuroblastoma. Radiographics 9:859–882

Davidson AJ, Choyke PL, Hartman DS, Davis CJ Jr (1995) Renal medullary carcinoma associated with sickle cell trait: radiologic findings. Radiology 195:83–85

Davis CJ Jr, Barton JH, Sesterhenn IA, Mostofi FK (1995a) Metanephric adenoma: clinicopathological study of fifty patients. Am J Surg Pathol 19:1101–1114

Davis CJ Jr, Mostofi FK, Sesterhenn IA (1995b) Renal medullary carcinoma. The seventh sickle cell nephropathy. Am J Surg Pathol 19:1–11

Donaldson JS, Shkolnik A (1988) Pediatric renal masses. Semin Roentgenol 23:194–204

Dyer RB, Lowe LH, Zagoria RJ, Amis ES Jr (1994) Mass effect in the renal sinus: an anatomic classification. Curr Probl Diagn Radiol 23:1–27

Eble JN (1998) Angiomyolipoma of kidney. Semin Diagn Pathol 15:21–40

Ewalt DH, Sheffield E, Sparagana SP, Delgado MR, Roach ES (1998) Renal lesion growth in children with tuberous sclerosis complex. J Urol 160:141–145

Ferrer FA, McKenna PH (1994) Partial nephrectomy in a metachronous multilocular cyst of the kidney (cystic nephroma). J Urol 151:1358–1360

Geller E, Smergel EM, Lowry PA (1997) Renal neoplasms of childhood. Radiol Clin North Am 35:1391–1413

Glick RD, Hicks MJ, Nuchtern JG, Wesson DE, Olutoye OO, Cass DL (2004) Renal tumors in infants less than 6 months of age. J Pediatr Surg 39:522–525

Gonzalez-Crussi F, Kidd JM, Hernandez RJ (1982) Cystic nephroma: morphologic spectrum and implications. Urology 20:88–93

Hartman DS, David CJ Jr, Goldman SM, Friedman AC, Fritzsche P (1982a) Renal lymphoma: radiologic–pathologic correlation of 21 cases. Radiology 144:759–766

Hartman DS, Davis CJ Jr, Madewell JE, Friedman AC (1982b) Primary malignant renal tumors in the second decade of life: Wilms tumor versus renal cell carcinoma. J Urol 127:888–891

Hennigar RA, Beckwith JB (1992) Nephrogenic adenofibroma. A novel kidney tumor of young people. Am J Surg Pathol 16:325–334

Ito J, Shinohara N, Koyanagi T, Hanioka K (1998) Ossifying renal tumor of infancy: the first Japanese case with long-term follow-up. Pathol Int 48:151–159

Julian JC, Merguerian PA, Shortliffe LM (1995) Pediatric genitourinary tumors. Curr Opin Oncol 7:265–274

Kalapurakal JA, Dome JS, Perlman EJ, Malogolowkin M, Haase GM, Grundy P, Coppes MJ (2005) Management of Wilms' tumour: current practice and future goals. Lancet Oncol 5:37–46

Kushner BH (2004) Neuroblastoma: a disease requiring a multitude of imaging studies. J Nucl Med 45:1172–1188

Lack EE, Cassady JR, Sallan SE (1985) Renal cell carcinoma in childhood and adolescence: a clinical and pathological study of 17 cases. J Urol 133:822–828

Lemaitre L, Robert Y, Dubrulle F, Claudon M, Duhamel A, Danjou P, Mazeman E (1995) Renal angiomyolipoma: growth followed up with CT and/or US. Radiology 197:598–602

Leuschner I, Harms D, Schmidt D (1991) Renal cell carcinoma in children: histology, immunohistochemistry, and follow-up of 10 cases. Med Pediatr Oncol 19:33–41

Lonergan GJ, Martinez-Leon MI, Agrons GA, Montemarano H, Suarez ES (1998) Nephrogenic rests, nephroblastomatosis, and associated lesions of the kidney. Radiographics 18:947–968

Lowe LH, Isuani BH, Heller RM, Stein SM, Johnson JE, Navarro OM, Hernanz-Schulman M (2000) Pediatric renal masses: Wilms tumor and beyond. Radiographics 20:1585–1603

Mahoney CP, Cassady C, Weinberger E, Winters WD, Benjamin DR (1997) Humoral hypercalcemia due to an occult renal adenoma. Pediatr Nephrol 11:339–342

Matthay KK, Brisse H, Couanet D, Couturier J, Benard J, Mosseri V, Edeline V, Lumbroso J, Valteau-Couanet D, Michon J (2003) Central nervous system metastases in neuroblastoma: radiologic, clinical, and biologic features in 23 patients. Cancer 98:155–165

Mehta K, Haller JO, Legasto AC (2003) Imaging neuroblastoma in children. Crit Rev Comput Tomogr 44:47–61

Moore SW, Satge D, Sasco AI (2004) The epidemiology of neonatal tumors. J Pediatr Surg 39:1150–1151

Murphy WM, Beckwith JB, Farrow GM (1994) Tumors of the kidney, bladder, and related urinary structures. Armed Forces Institute of Pathology, Washington, DC

Navarro O, Conolly B, Taylor G, Bagli DJ (1999) Metanephric adenoma of the kidney: a case report. Pediatr Radiol 29:100–103

Ogino S, Ro TY, Redline RW (2000) Malignant rhabdoid tumor: A phenotype? An entity?--A controversy revisited. Adv Anat Pathol 7:181-190

Paulino AC, Wen BC, Brown CK, Tannous R, Mayr NA, Zhen WK, Weidner GJ, Hussey DH (2000) Late effects in children treated with radiation therapy for Wilms' tumor. Int J Radiat Oncol Biol Phys 46:1239–1246

Perlman EJ, Faria P, Soares A, Hoffer F, Sredni S, Ritchey M, Shamberger RC, Green D, Beckwith JB (2005) Hyperplastic perilobar nephroblastomatosis: Long-term survival of 52 patients. Pediatr Blood Cancer Apr 6; [Epub ahead of print]

Reznek RH, Mootoosamy I, Webb JA, Richards MA (1990) CT in renal and perirenal lymphoma: a further look. Clin Radiol 42:233–238

Ritchey ML, Azizkhan RG, Beckwith JB, Hrabovsky EE, Haase GM (1995) Neonatal Wilms tumor. J Pediatr Surg 30:856–859

Sacher P, Willi UV, Niggli F, Stallmach T (1998) Cystic nephroma: a rare benign renal tumor. Pediatr Surg Int 13:197–199

Shamberger RC (1999) Pediatric renal tumors. Semin Surg Oncol 16:105–120

Sheeran SR, Sussman SK (1998) Renal lymphoma: spectrum of CT findings and potential mimics. Am J Roentgenol 171:1067–1072

Sotelo-Avila C, Beckwith JB, Johnson JE (1995) Ossifying renal tumor of infancy: a clinicopathologic study of nine cases. Pediatr Pathol Lab Med 15:745–762

Vazquez JL, Barnewolt CE, Shamberger RC, Chung T, Perez-Atayde AR (1998) Ossifying renal tumor of infancy presenting as a palpable abdominal mass. Pediatr Radiol 28:454–457

Wesche WA, Wilimas J, Khare V, Parham DM (1998) Renal medullary carcinoma: a potential sickle cell nephropathy of children and adolescents. Pediatr Pathol Lab Med 18:97–113

White KS, Grossman H (1991) Wilms' and associated renal tumors of childhood. Pediatr Radiol 21:81–88

21 Percutaneous Biopsy and Radiofrequency Ablation

Ajay K. Singh, Debra A. Gervais, Peter F. Hahn, and Peter R. Mueller

CONTENTS

21.1
Introduction

Traditionally solid renal masses have been managed with open surgical resection, by either complete or partial nephrectomy. This management is based on the epidemiologic and imaging data of renal cell carcinoma which accounts for the majority of solid

A. K. Singh, MD
Clinical Instructor of Radiology, Harvard Medical School, Department of Radiology, Division of Emergency Radiology, Massachusetts General Hospital, 55 Fruit Street, Boston, MA 02114, USA
D. A. Gervais, MD
Assistant Professor of Radiology, Harvard Medical School, Department of Radiology, Director of Interventional Radiology, Division of Abdominal Imaging and Interventional Radiology, Massachusetts General Hospital, 55 Fruit Street, Boston, MA 02114, USA
P. F. Hahn, MD, PhD
Associate Professor of Radiology, Harvard Medical School, Department of Radiology, Division of Abdominal Imaging and Interventional Radiology, Massachusetts General Hospital, 55 Fruit Street, Boston, MA 02114, USA
P. R. Mueller, MD
Professor of Radiology, Harvard Medical School, Department of Radiology, Division Head, Division of Abdominal Imaging and Interventional Radiology, Massachusetts General Hospital, 55 Fruit Street, Boston, MA 02114, USA

renal masses. The surgical approach is also based on the traditional belief that image-guided needle biopsy cannot adequately discriminate between renal cell carcinoma and the majority of benign masses. The management dilemma occurs when imaging alone cannot definitely classify the lesion as solid or when the lesion is small and incidentally detected on a CT performed for unrelated reasons. Similar management issues occur in patients with known primary extrarenal malignancy, when a renal mass is detected on CT. The diagnosis of these lesions with image-guided biopsy is often the basis on which the new nephron-sparing treatment procedures, including laparoscopic partial nephrectomy or image-guided radiofrequency ablation, can be performed. These less invasive procedures are associated with significantly less morbidity and shorter hospital stay, and nephron-sparing surgery, in selected cases, provides clinical outcomes similar to traditional nephrectomy. Pre-treatment investigation of some renal lesions with image-guided biopsy allows detection of benign tumors, locally advanced carcinoma, metastatic disease to the kidney, and benign lesions which are indeterminate by imaging criteria.

The characterization and treatment of renal neoplasms has gained importance with current increasing detection of incidental, localized, as well as advanced renal cell cancer (Chow et al. 1999).

In this chapter we discuss the role of image-guided biopsy and percutaneous radiofrequency ablation in the current management of focal renal lesions.

21.2
Percutaneous Biopsy

In the majority of cases the CT and MR imaging can characterize a renal lesion as solid or cystic. Most solid renal neoplasms are still treated with surgical removal, without a preceding biopsy. In the remaining lesions, the options include follow-up cross-sectional imaging, image-guided biopsy, or surgical management. With continued experience and improvements in the technique, image-guided biopsy has become a safe, accurate, and reliable method for the diagnosis of problematic cases (Caoili et al. 2002; Chow et al. 1999; Eshed et al. 2004; Mignon et al. 2001; Lee et al. 1991; Richter et al. 2000; Rybicki et al. 2003; Wood et al. 1999). The core biopsy results have been noted to modify therapeutic management in 38–41% cases and morbidity is low compared with surgery (Barriol et al. 2000; Wood et al. 1999). Metastases, lymphoma, and some cases of oncocytoma are examples of biopsy results that may preclude surgery.

21.2.1
Indications

Indications for renal biopsies include indeterminate focal lesions, which do not have all the imaging features of neoplasm; suspicion of metastases, lymphoma, angiomyolipoma (Figs. 21.1, 21.2), or oncocytoma; differentiation of transitional cell carcinoma from renal cell carcinoma; and complex cystic renal lesions (Fig. 21.3). Other indications include locally advanced renal lesion, renal transplant mass, history of tuberous sclerosis, poor surgical candidate, mass in a solitary kidney, and focal lesion in a patient with extrarenal malignancy (Hara et

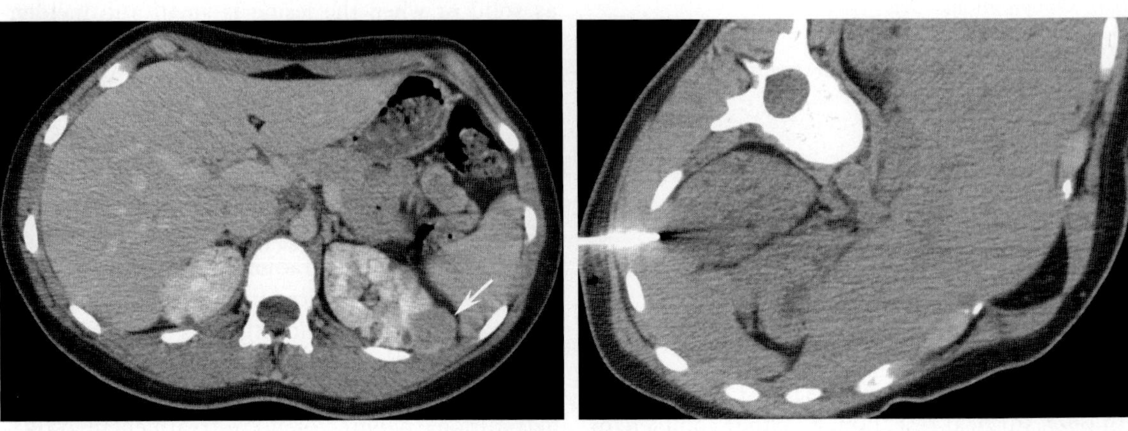

Fig. 21.1a,b. Percutaneous biopsy of multiple fat-containing tumors in a 21-year-old woman. **a** Axial contrast-enhanced CT scan shows a soft tissue density mass (*arrow*) in the left kidney. There is no fat density seen in the mass. **b** Axial unenhanced CT scan obtained in oblique prone position shows the 17-G coaxial biopsy needle tip in the renal mass. The histopathological diagnosis was angiomyolipoma.

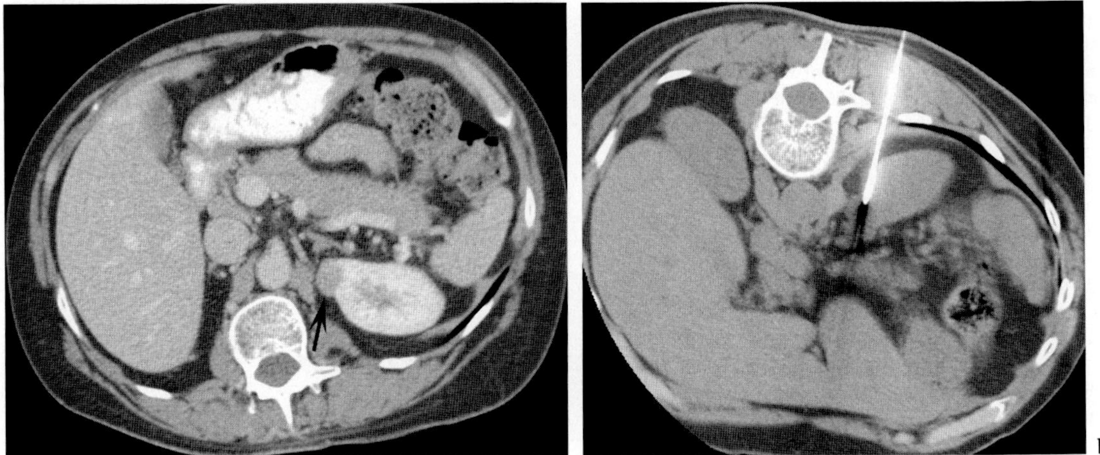

Fig. 21.2a,b. Percutaneous biopsy of soft tissue density tumor in a 61-year-old woman. **a** Axial contrast-enhanced CT scan shows a soft tissue density, exophytic mass (*arrow*) arising from the left kidney. **b** Axial unenhanced CT scan in prone position shows the 18-G needle tip in the mass. The histopathological diagnosis was angiomyolipoma.

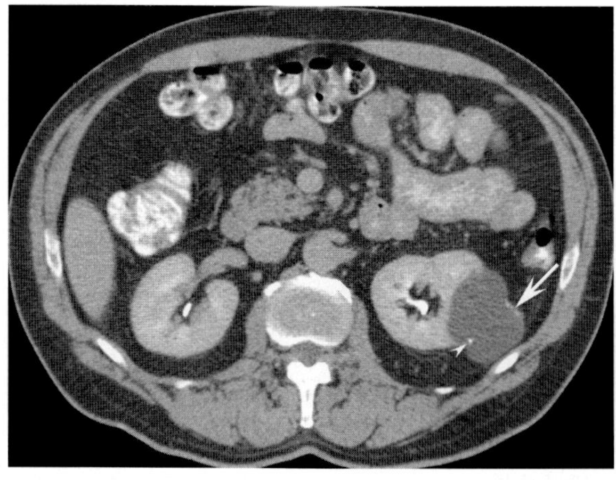
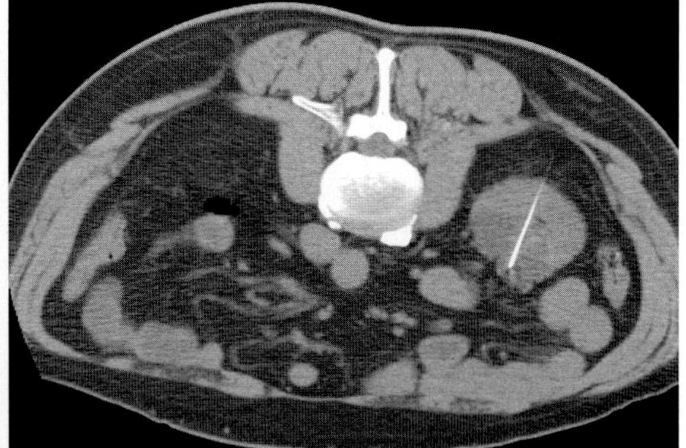
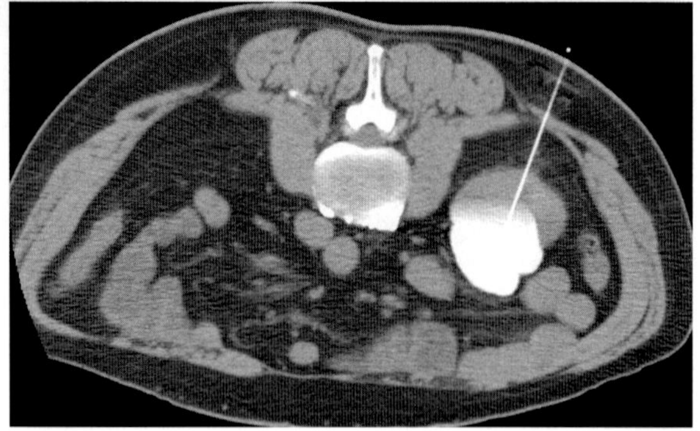

Fig. 21.3a–c. Percutaneous aspiration of cystic renal lesion in a 62-year-old man. **a** Axial contrast-enhanced CT scan shows a cystic lesion with focal thickening (*arrow*) in the lateral wall and a focus of calcification (*arrowhead*) in the medial wall. **b** Axial unenhanced CT scan in prone position shows a 20-G aspiration needle tip seen in the cystic renal lesion. **c** Contrast injection into the cyst does not demonstrate any focal intracystic solid component. The cytological analysis was negative for malignant cells.

al. 2001; LECHEVALLIER et al. 2000; MIGNON et al. 2001).

Although the traditional treatment of Bosniak category-III lesions is surgery, approximately 40% of these lesions are benign. Identification of these patients by percutaneous biopsy can obviate unnecessary surgery for patients with benign lesions (HARISINGHANI et al. 2003).

21.2.2
Technique

Image-guided renal mass biopsy procedures can be performed using CT, ultrasound (US) or, less commonly, fluoroscopic guidance. The majority of focal renal biopsy series reported in the recent literature were performed under CT guidance. In obese patients CT guidance provides better renal visibility than US (LEE et al. 1991). Ultrasound has the advantage of real-time guidance and lack of ionizing radiation and the biopsy results are comparable to those of CT guidance. Ultrasound guidance provides satisfactory results in renal biopsies for patients with and without focal renal lesion (ARENSON 1991; JUUL et al. 2004).

The biopsy needle used for renal biopsies is typically 18-G and the number of specimens obtained varies from two to five. An 18-G biopsy needle gun passed through a 17-G coaxial needle has the advantage of allowing multiple biopsies by providing a track for the core needle to be placed into the mass (Fig. 21.4). The 18-G core biopsy more often yields diagnostic results than a smaller-caliber needle (JOHNSON et al. 2001; RYBICKI et al. 2003).

In our department, the patient lies in lateral decubitus or prone position. Under image guidance the 17-G coaxial biopsy needle is placed at the edge or within the renal mass. Following this, the 18-G biopsy needle is used to obtain multiple cores. We also obtain multiple fine-needle aspiration samples using a 22-G needle, inserted through the 17-G coaxial needle. Post-procedural CT is obtained after removal of the biopsy needle to evaluate for possible complication.

Another renal biopsy technique is transjugular renal biopsy which has been used for renal biopsy in patients under evaluation for renal dysfunction (CLUZEL et al. 2000; JOUET et al. 1996; MAL et al. 1990; MAL et al. 1992; RYCHLIK et al. 2004; THOMPSON et al. 2004). This technique should be considered in patients with significantly high risk of bleeding, most often related to anticoagu-

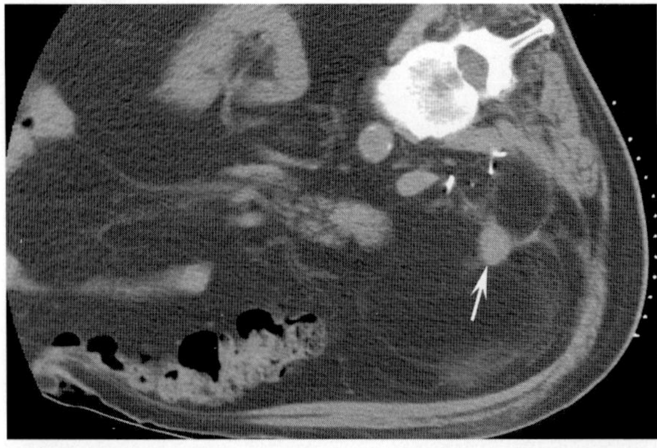
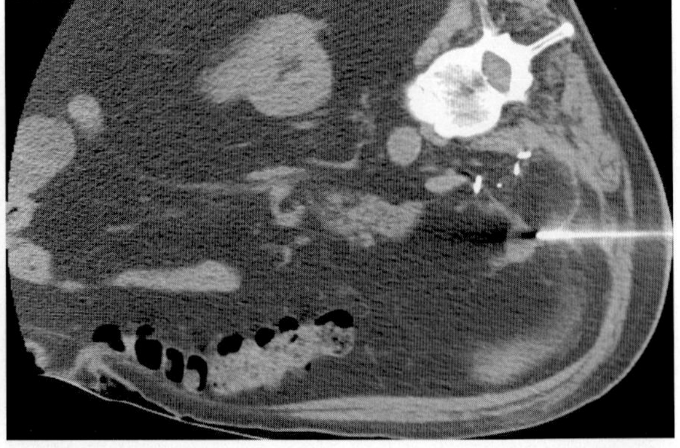

a

b

Fig. 21.4a,b. Percutaneous biopsy in a 70-year-old woman with history of renal cell carcinoma. **a** Axial postnephrectomy unenhanced CT scan in lateral position shows a soft tissue nodule (*arrow*) in the nephrectomy bed. **b** Axial unenhanced CT scan in lateral position shows the biopsy needle tip in the soft tissue nodule. The histopathological diagnosis was recurrent renal cell carcinoma.

lation use. This procedure involves placement of a 7-F jugular sheath, an inner stiffening cannula, a 5-F curved catheter, and a 19-G biopsy needle (Fig. 21.5). The biopsy is typically performed on the right kidney because of the relatively shorter length of the right renal vein and better angle for the needle fire. The adequacy rate of renal biopsy is comparable to that of percutaneous biopsy. It can be used in obese patients in whom percutaneous renal biopsy is technically more difficult due to poor visualization and longer skin to renal vein distance (FINE et al. 2004).

21.2.3
Results

Image-guided renal biopsy is a safe, sensitive, and useful procedure in the management of indeterminate renal lesions or renal lesions which are suspected to be of benign etiology. The results of 779 biopsies for focal renal lesions in 8 of the studies performed between 1999 and 2004 show that image-guided biopsies provided sufficient tissue for diagnosis in 704 (90.4%) cases (BARRIOL et al. 2000; CAOILI et al. 2002; ESHED et al. 2004; HARA et al. 2001; LECHEVALLIER et al. 2000; MIGNON et al. 2001; RICHTER et al. 2000; RYBICKI et al. 2003; WOOD et al. 1999). RICHTER et al. (2000) in a review of 393 image-guided renal mass biopsies found false diagnoses in only 7 (1.2%). The sensitivity of detection of malignancy is high and ranges from 76 to 93%. Compared with core biopsy, the limitations of fine-needle aspiration include higher false-negative rates and difficulty in diagnosis of oncocytoma

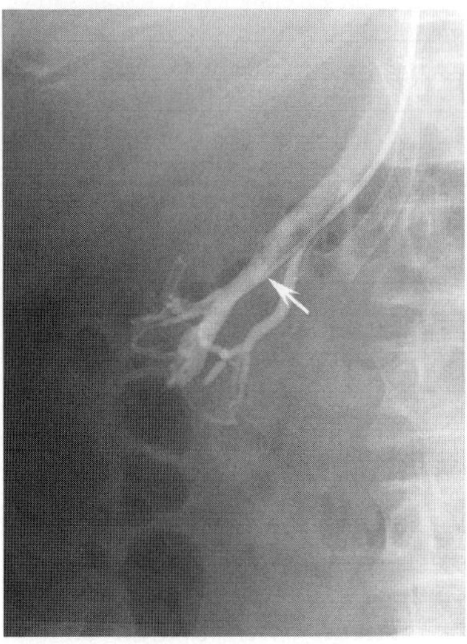

Fig. 21.5. Transjugular renal biopsy in a 75-year-old man. Right renal vein is opacified during the transjugular right renal biopsy for medical renal disease. The biopsy needle tip (*arrow*) is located in the right renal vein.

and angiomyolipoma (HARISINGHANI et al. 2003; RYBICKI et al. 2003).

Although there is a high correlation between core biopsy and histological diagnosis, insufficient tissue for diagnosis should be viewed with caution, as some of these lesions may represent neoplasm and surgical resection of localized renal cell carcinoma has a high cure rate. These lesions can be followed up on imaging or can be surgically resected (ESHED et al. 2004; RYBICKI et al. 2003).

A majority of the lesions in the study by RYBICKI et al. (2003) were biopsied with 14- to 22-G needles. In that study, all false negative results were obtained with 20- or 22-G needles, indicating a higher negative predictive value with larger needles. Some studies have found a higher incidence of insufficient material being acquired for histological evaluation when the tumor is less than 3 cm, but this result is controversial (Eshed et al. 2004; Lechevallier et al. 2000; Mignon et al. 2001; Rybicki et al. 2003). Rybicki et al. (2003) suggested caution when interpreting the results of renal masses less than 3 and more than 6 cm diameter. They showed negative predictive values of 60 and 44% for renal lesions which were less than 3 or more than 6 cm in diameter, respectively. Sampling of the necrotic area in a large mass is an important cause of sampling error. Although these results were not statistically significant, they were lower than the 89% negative predictive value for renal masses between 4 and 6 cm.

21.2.4
Complications

The complication rate from renal biopsies for focal lesions is low and most can be treated conservatively. Complications include hemorrhage (perinephric, subcapsular, and retroperitoneal) hematuria, arteriovenous fistula, pseudoaneurysm, urinoma, arterial hypertension, pneumothorax, renal abscess, and needle-track seeding (Figs. 21.6, 21.7). Hematoma in or around the kidney is a well-known post-procedural complication; however, the majority of patients do not need treatment but should be conservatively followed. Compression of the renal parenchyma by the hematoma can cause ischemia and secondary hypertension (Mackie et al. 2004; Wanic-Kossowska 1998).

Hematuria is the most common complication of percutaneous renal biopsy but usually resolves on its own. Transfusion is needed in only a minority of cases. Tumor seeding of the needle track, hemothorax, intestinal perforation, and disseminated intravascular coagulation are rare and occur only as case reports in the literature. Seeding has been reported rarely with biopsy of renal cell carcinoma, transitional cell carcinoma, Wilms' tumor, and oncocytoma (Auvert et al. 1982; Bush et al. 1977; Gibbons et al. 2004; Kiser et al. 2004; Lee et al. 1995; Shenoy et al. 1991; Slywotzky and Maya 1994). Arteriovenous fistula is most often subclinical, most commonly does not require treatment, and resolves on its own. About 30% of cases do not regress and are associated with unfavorable outcome. Uncommonly they can cause hematuria, hypertension, or

renal function impairment, and need treatment by selective coil embolization or surgical ligation (Horcicka et al. 2002; Lund-Sorensen et al. 1995; Memis et al. 1992).

Complications associated with transjugular renal biopsy include hemorrhage from capsular or pelvicalyceal system penetration. Capsular perforation is a common occurrence from the needle throw and was recorded in 73.9% of 23 patients by Thompson et al (2004). Hemorrhage can result in perinephric/retroperitoneal hematoma or hydronephrosis from clots in the pelvicalyceal system. Hypovolemic shock is an uncommon complication, but the majority of patients do not need transfusion, although they should be followed.

21.3
Radiofrequency Ablation

21.3.1
Background

With increased detection of renal masses on CT the role of the nephron-sparing procedure has become important, especially for tumors which are small or which may not be malignant. The techniques available now include laparoscopic partial nephrectomy, radiofrequency ablation (RFA), and cryoablation. Radiofrequency ablation is an alternative to nephron-sparing surgery. There is less patient morbidity

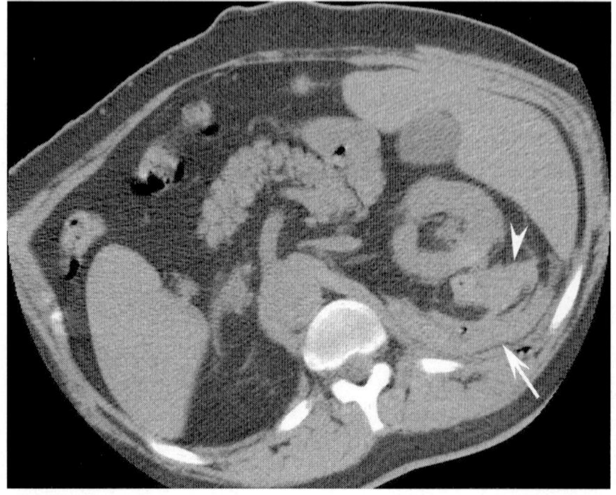

Fig. 21.6. Complication after renal biopsy in a 57-year-old man. Axial unenhanced post-procedure CT scan shows a posterior perinephric (*arrowhead*) and posterior pararenal space hematoma (*arrow*).

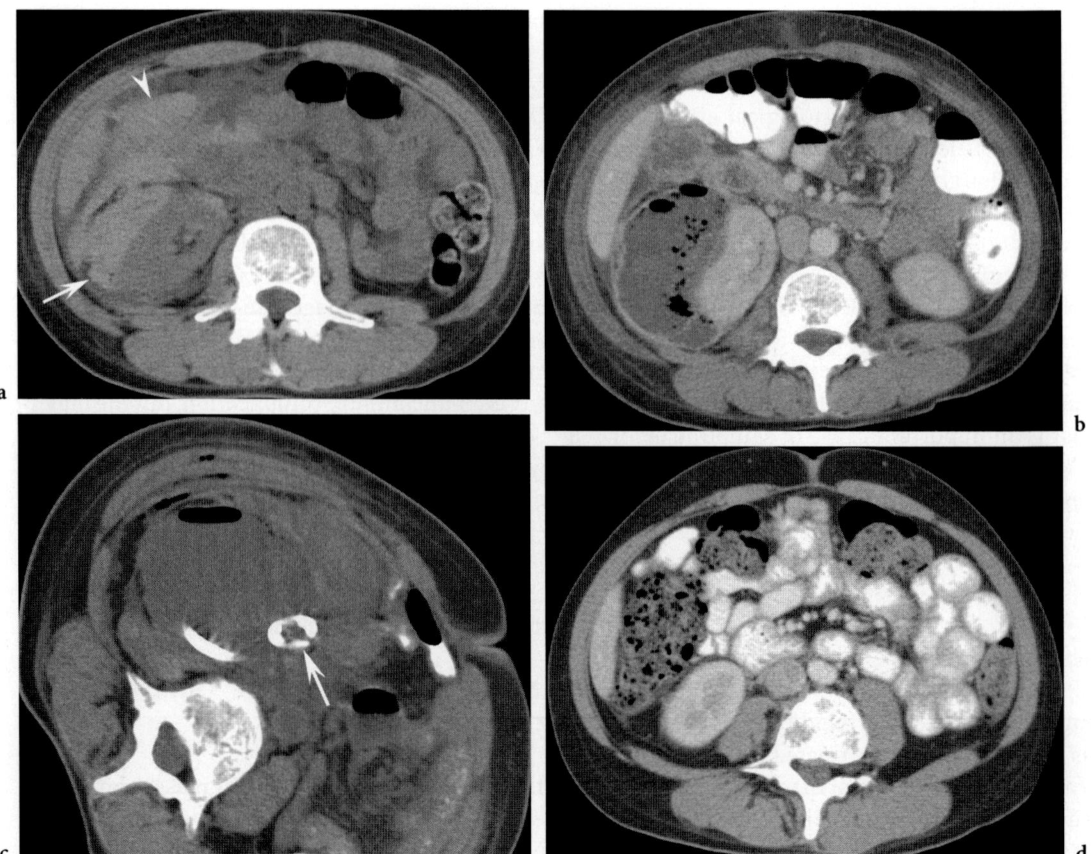

Fig. 21.7a-d. Complication after renal biopsy in a 37-year-old woman. **a** Axial unenhanced post-procedure CT scan shows a sub-capsular (*arrow*), anterior pararenal space, and Morrison's pouch (*arrowhead*) hematoma. **b** Follow-up axial contrast-enhanced CT scan shows increase in size of the collection, enhancement of wall, and development of air pockets. The findings were consistent with subcapsular abscess. **c** Post-drainage axial CT scan shows the percutaneous drainage catheter (*arrow*) in the abscess. **d** Follow-up axial CT scan shows complete resolution of the abscess.

and it can be performed under sedation in patients who are poor surgical risks.

Radiofrequency ablation has been used traditionally in the treatment of liver neoplasm but is increasingly more being used for the treatment of renal lesions in patients who are poor surgical risks or who refuse surgery (DE BAERE et al. 2002; GAZELLE et al. 2000; GOLDBERG and DUPUY 2001a; GOLDBERG and DUPUY 2001b). It is also used in patients with a solitary kidney and as an alternative to nephron-sparing surgery (FARRELL et al. 2003).

Since the description by ZLOTTA et al. (1996) of RFA of the human kidney ex vivo and in vivo, several studies have established this modality as an alternative to other nephron-sparing procedures in the treatment of renal tumors (DE BAERE et al. 2002; GAZELLE et al. 2000; GOLDBERG and DUPUY 2001a; GOLDBERG and DUPUY 2001b; ZLOTTA et al. 2004).

21.3.2
Principle

The ideal lesion for RFA is a solitary renal lesion less than 3 cm in diameter and predominantly exophytic in location. It is more difficult to treat tumors which are centrally located, due to heat dissipation by the renal vasculature. In a study by Gervais et al. (2003) only 45% (5 of 11) of central or mixed tumors were treated with technical success, which meant absence of enhancement on 1-month imaging follow-up. Peripherally located renal tumors are not found in the vicinity of large vessels and are surrounded by perinephric fat which provides insulation; therefore, the results of radiofrequency ablation are better for exophytic tumors (GERVAIS et al. 2000). Larger tumors are more difficult to treat and often need more than one overlapping treatment to cover the entire tumor volume and provide a tumor-free peripheral margin.

This is analogous to liver RFA, where smaller tumors are more likely to be completely treated than larger tumors (LIVRAGHI et al. 2000).

21.3.3
Technique

Radiofrequency ablation procedures can be performed with CT or US guidance, under sedation or general anesthesia (Figs. 21.8, 21.9). Although a number of radiofrequency generators are available, the two most commonly used are the internally cooled single or cluster electrodes with pulsed current: RITA (Radiofrequency interstitial tissue ablation) device (Rita Medical Systems, Mountain View, Calif.); and multi-timed expandable electrodes with temperature control: Radionics Device (Radionics, Burlington, Mass.). The starburst needle (Rita Medical Systems) is used to treat lesions smaller than

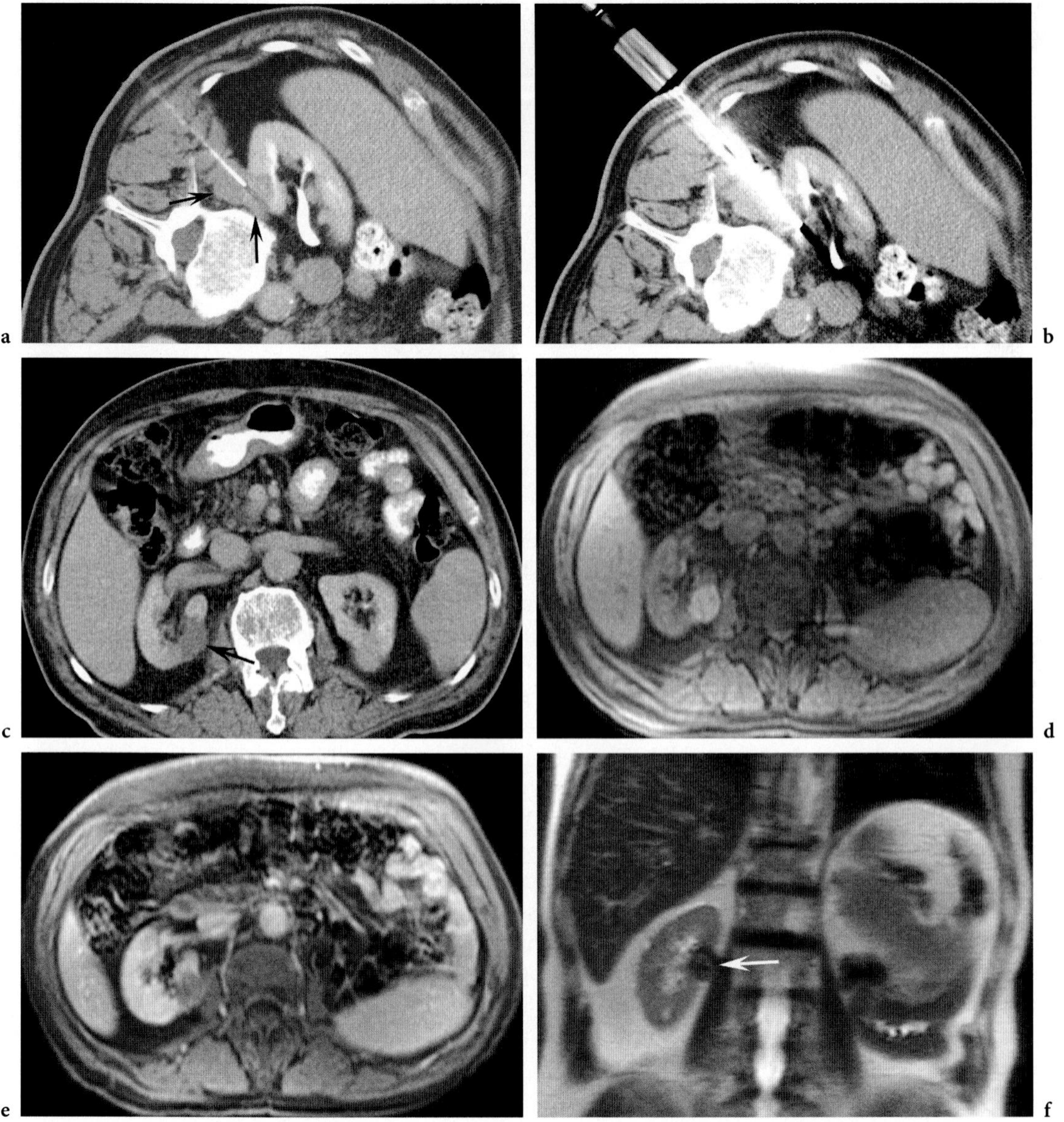

Fig. 21.8a-f. Percutaneous needle biopsy and radiofrequency ablation in a 78-year-old man with right renal mass. **a** Axial CT scan at the time of diagnosis shows the needle tip within the right renal mass (*arrows*). The histopathological diagnosis was renal cell carcinoma. **b** Axial CT scan shows that cluster probe electrodes are positioned within the right renal mass. **c** Follow-up axial CT shows a nonenhancing defect (*arrow*) in the right renal cortex, at the site of the previously seen mass. Axial **d** unenhanced T1-weighted MR image shows a focal hyperintense lesion which does not enhance on **e** contrast-enhanced T1-weighted MR image and is hypointense (*arrow*) on **f** T2-weighted MR image.

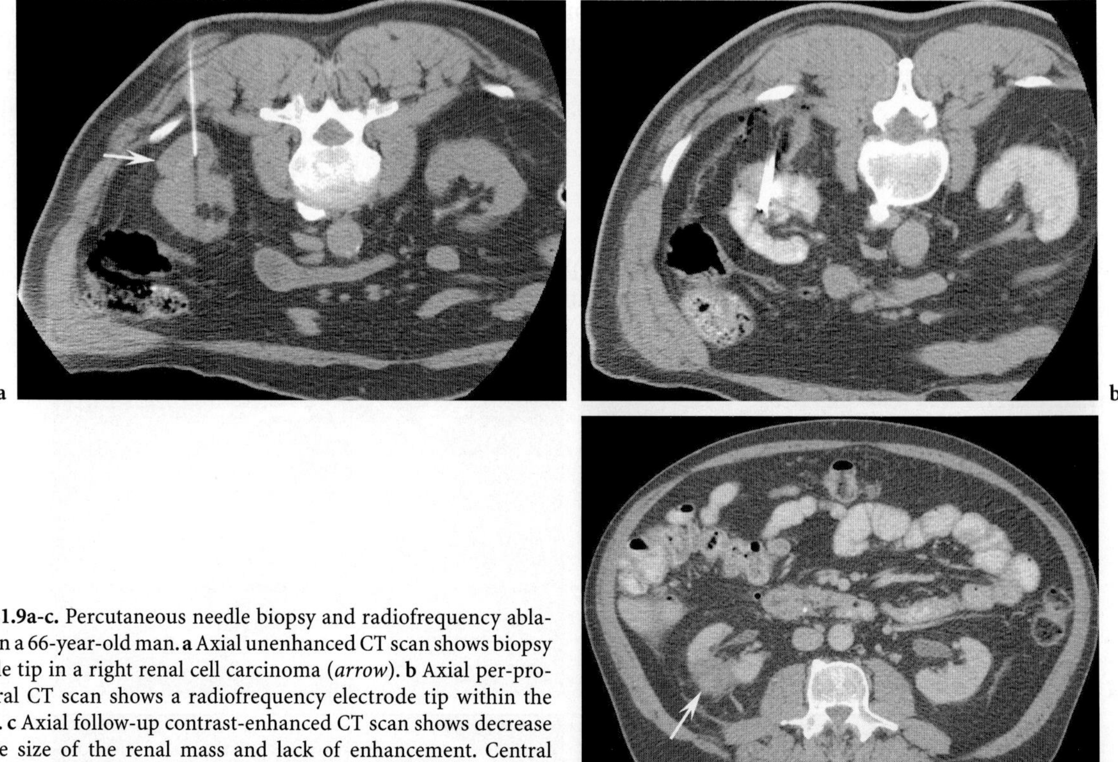

Fig. 21.9a-c. Percutaneous needle biopsy and radiofrequency ablation in a 66-year-old man. **a** Axial unenhanced CT scan shows biopsy
needle tip in a right renal cell carcinoma (*arrow*). **b** Axial per-procedural CT scan shows a radiofrequency electrode tip within the
mass. **c** Axial follow-up contrast-enhanced CT scan shows decrease
in the size of the renal mass and lack of enhancement. Central
hyperdensity (*arrow*) within the mass is due to coagulative necrosis of the neoplastic tissue.

2 cm, and the starburst XL needle (Rita Medical
Systems) is used in larger lesions.

The Radionics device includes a cool-tip single
electrode and cool-tip cluster electrode kit; the needle
length varies from 10 to 25 cm in the former and 10
to 20 cm in the latter. Each kit includes an electrode,
inflow tubing set, outflow tubing set, ground pads,
and introducer (with cluster electrode only). The
grounding pads are applied to the thighs, at an equal
distance from the treatment site. The inflow and outflow tubing are responsible for the flow of iced water
or saline to and from the electrode tip. The active tip
of the electrodes is typically 2–3 cm in length and lies
entirely inside the tumor to prevent damage to the
surrounding tissues. Care is taken to avoid damage to
important structures such as ureter or major vessels.
After positioning the electrode tip in the tumor under
image guidance, the tumor is ablated with one or
more heating cycles lasting 12 min each. The current
is pulsed in response to a rapid increase in imped-
ance, which is caused by charring of tissue and subsequent inhibition of heat diffusion. As the geometry
of the burn diameter may not cover the entire tumor,
so often more than one overlapping treatments are
required to cover the entire tumor. For example, 142

overlapping ablations were needed for the treatment
of 42 tumors in the study by GERVAIS et al. (2003).
The aim of the treatment is to produce a tumor free
margin of up to a centimeter around the tumor.

A pre-ablation biopsy at the same sitting or at
an earlier session is commonly performed and may
alter the treatment or follow-up of these patients. A
benign diagnosis on biopsy precludes an unnecessary RFA procedure.

When US guidance is used, intense echoes spreading from the electrode tip can be seen. This appearance is secondary to the microbubbles produced by
tissue ablation. This appearance is transient and the
echogenicity of the focal renal lesion becomes heterogeneous after a few minutes.

Success of RFA is indicated by lack of enhancement on follow-up CT or MR imaging. Treated tumors
are seen as a hypodense or hypointense defect in the
renal parenchyma. The exophytic tumors retain the
configuration of the original tumor with minimal
decrease in size after RFA. The findings on follow-
up CT or MR imaging also include fatty replacement at the interface with normal kidney and soft
tissue stranding in fat around the tumor (GERVAIS
et al. 2003b, MATSUMOTO et al. 2004).

21.3.4
Complications

Overall RFA is a low morbidity procedure in the treatment of renal neoplasm. Complications of RFA include hemorrhage, lumbar plexus damage, urinoma, ureteral stricture, and abscess (Figs. 21.10–21.14). Postprocedural pain along the distribution of the lumbar plexus may occur in patients treated by the posterior approach where the psoas muscle is heated. There is one report of needle-track seeding after RFA of a renal mass (MAYO-SMITH et al. 2004).

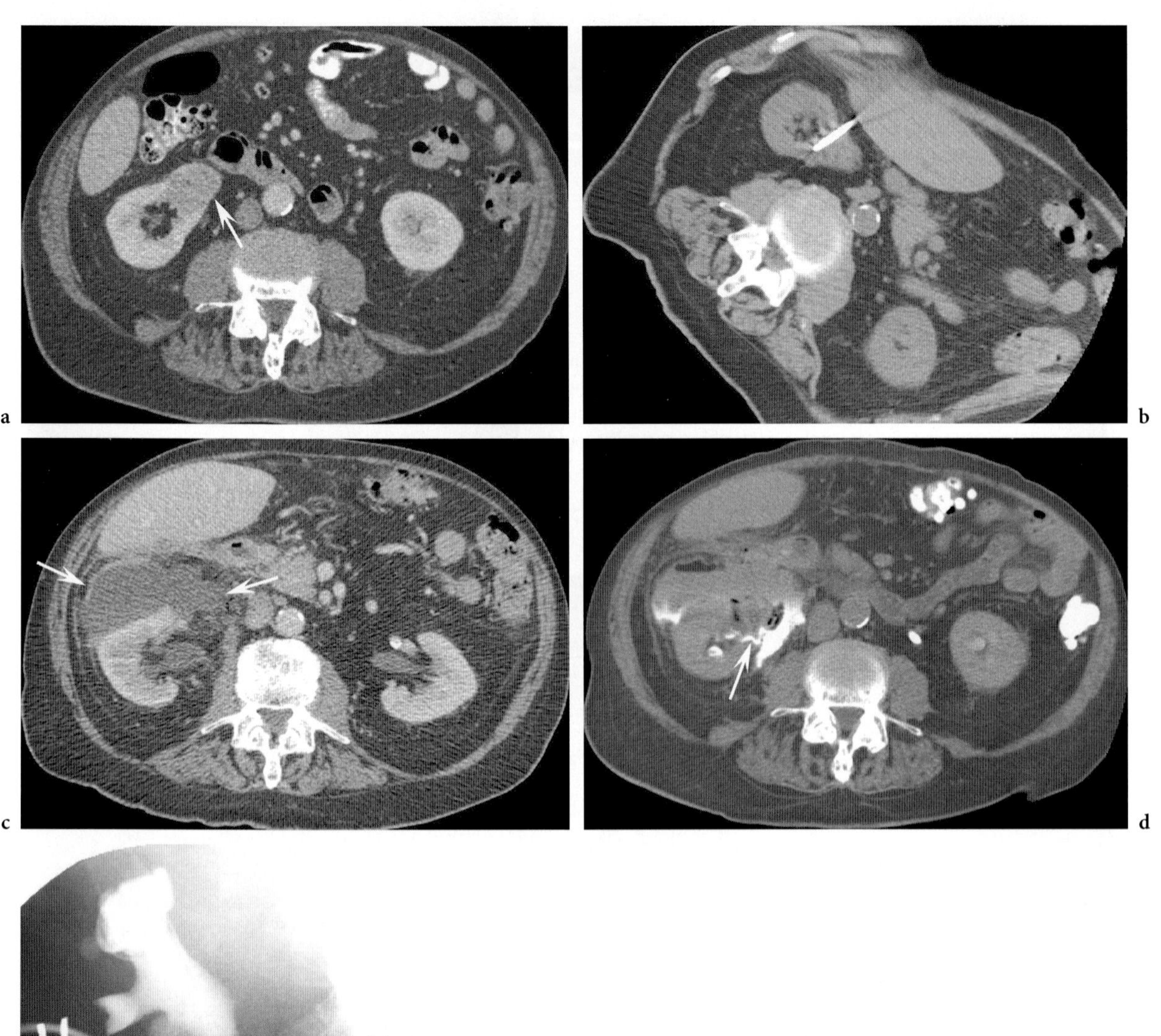

Fig. 21.10a-e. Complication after radiofrequency ablation in a 87-year-old man. **a** Axial contrast enhanced CT scan shows a right renal mass (*arrow*). **b** Axial CT scan shows Radionics electrode tip at the junction of the mass and the normal renal parenchyma. **c** Axial contrast-enhanced CT scan shows perinephric fluid collection (*arrows*). **d** Delayed axial contrast-enhanced CT scan shows communication (*arrow*) of the right pelvicalyceal system, with the anterior collection. **e** Tube injection through the percutaneous drainage catheter placed in a bilobed anterior collection (*arrow*) shows prompt opacification of the right pelvicalyceal system.

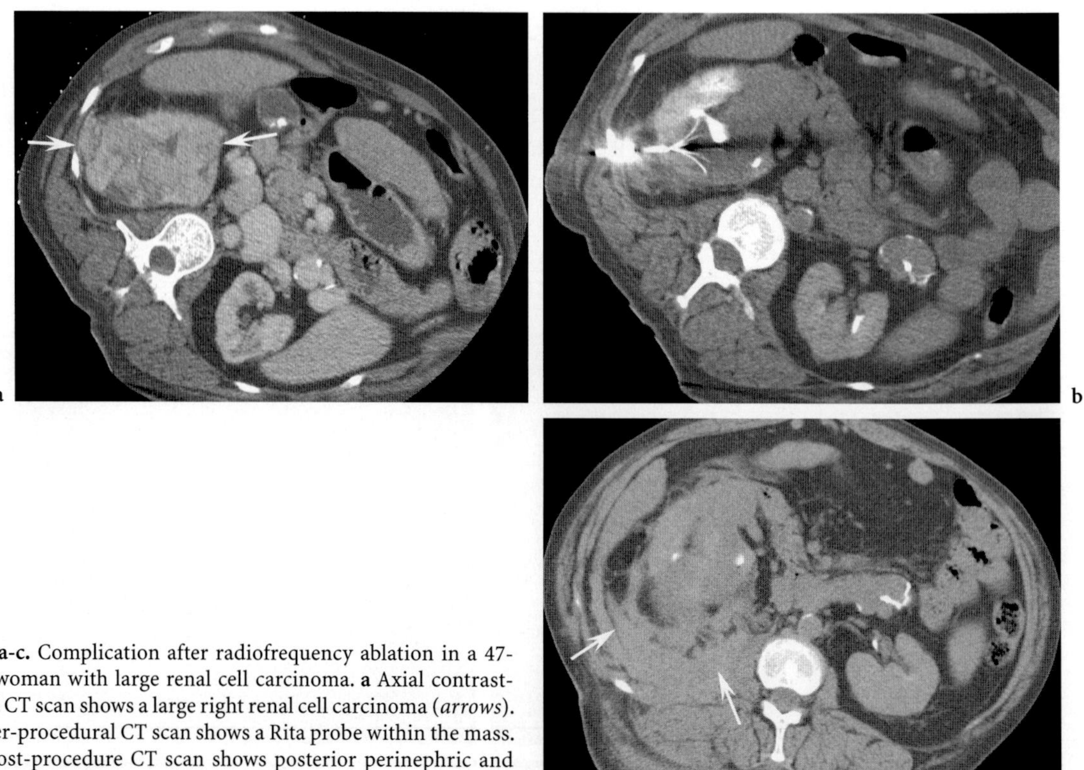

Fig. 21.11a-c. Complication after radiofrequency ablation in a 47-year-old woman with large renal cell carcinoma. **a** Axial contrast-enhanced CT scan shows a large right renal cell carcinoma (*arrows*). **b** Axial per-procedural CT scan shows a Rita probe within the mass. **c** Axial post-procedure CT scan shows posterior perinephric and posterior pararenal hematoma (*arrows*).

Fig. 21.12a-d. Complication after radiofrequency ablation in a 79-year-old man. **a** Axial contrast-enhanced CT scan shows a solid right renal mass (*arrow*). **b** Axial CT scan shows the biopsy needle tip within the renal mass. Axial post-radiofrequency ablation CT scans show clots (*arrows*) within **c** the right pelvicalyceal system and **d** urinary bladder.

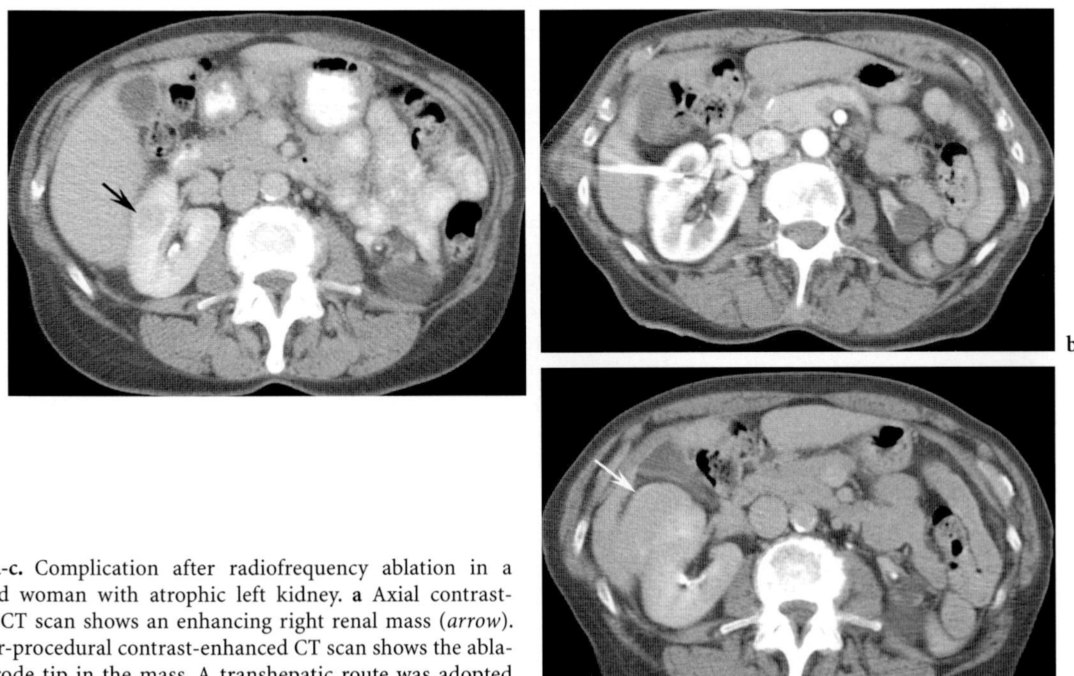

Fig. 21.13a-c. Complication after radiofrequency ablation in a 61-year-old woman with atrophic left kidney. a Axial contrast-enhanced CT scan shows an enhancing right renal mass (*arrow*). b Axial per-procedural contrast-enhanced CT scan shows the ablation electrode tip in the mass. A transhepatic route was adopted for this radiofrequency ablation. c Axial post-procedural CT scan shows an anterior perinephric hematoma (*arrow*).

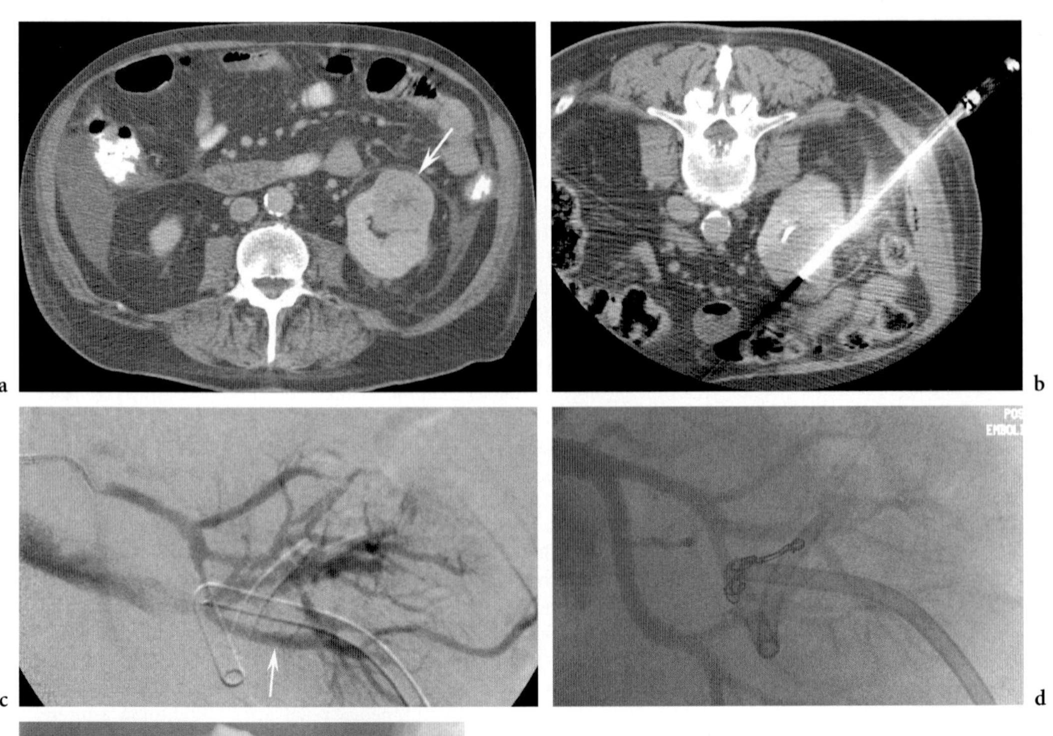

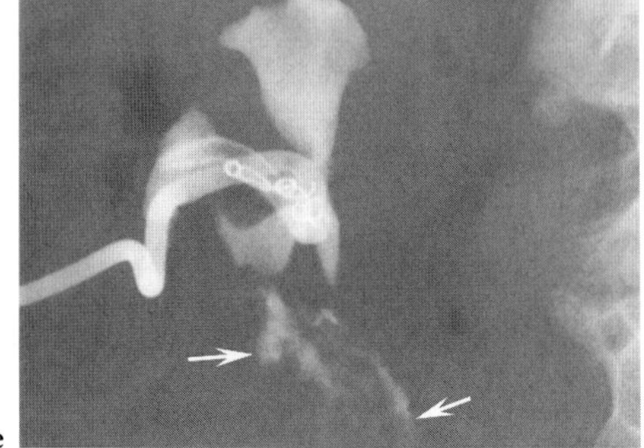

Fig. 21.14a-e. Complication after radiofrequency ablation in a 77-year-old man. a Axial contrast-enhanced CT scan shows a heterogeneously enhancing left renal mass (*arrow*). b Axial per-procedural CT scan shows that a single Radionics electrode tip is identified within the left renal mass. c Left renal angiogram after radiofrequency ablation shows an arteriovenous fistula with early opacification of renal vein (*arrow*). d Post-embolization renal angiogram shows resolution of the fistulous communication. e Tube injection through the percutaneous nephrostomy catheter shows leakage of contrast outside the pelvicalyceal system, into the urinoma (*arrows*).

21.4
Conclusion

Image-guided percutaneous renal biopsy is safe and accurate in sampling the lesion and coming to a final histopathological diagnosis. Image-guided renal mass biopsy is useful for avoiding unnecessary surgery for benign masses and in the diagnosis of renal metastases, lymphoma, differentiation of centrally located renal cell carcinoma from renal cell carcinoma, and complex cystic renal lesions. The renal biopsy can be performed with either CT or US guidance, although the majority of the current literature is based on CT-guided procedures.

Although radiofrequency ablation has been used most often for liver tumors, its use for renal masses is relatively recent and has shown promising clinical results. Long-term follow-up radiofrequency ablation results for renal masses are still being performed to define the position of this treatment in the management of renal neoplasm. The ideal lesion for radiofrequency ablation in the kidney is single, peripherally located and less than 3 cm diameter renal mass. Radiofrequency ablation of a renal mass is often useful as an alternative to nephron-sparing surgery in poor surgical risk patients and in patients with a solitary kidney.

As the frequency of detection of renal masses increases and the utility of percutaneous biopsy and radiofrequency ablation are better defined in the literature, we are likely to see these procedures become more frequent in patient management.

References

Arenson AM (1991) Ultrasound guided percutaneous renal biopsy. Australas Radiol 35:38–39

Auvert J, Abbou CC, Lavarenne V (1982) Needle tract seeding following puncture of renal oncocytoma. Prog Clin Biol Res 100:597–598

Barriol D, Lechevallier E, Andre M et al. (2000) CT-guided percutaneous fine needle biopsy of solid tumors of the kidney. Prog Urol 10:1145–1151

Bush WH Jr, Burnett LL, Gibbons RP (1977) Needle tract seeding of renal cell carcinoma. Am J Roentgenol 129:725–727

Caoili EM, Bude RO, Higgins EJ et al. (2002) Evaluation of sonographically guided percutaneous core biopsy of renal masses. Am J Roentgenol 179:373–378

Chow WH, Devesa SS, Warren JL et al. (1999) Rising incidence of renal cell cancer in the United States. J Am Med Assoc 281:1628–1631

Cluzel P, Martinez F, Bellin MF et al. (2000) Transjugular versus percutaneous renal biopsy for the diagnosis of parenchymal disease: comparison of sampling effectiveness and complications. Radiology 215:689–693

De Baere T, Kuoch V, Smayra T et al. (2002) Radiofrequency ablation of renal cell carcinoma: preliminary clinical experience. J Urol 167:1961–1964

Eshed I, Elias S, Sidi AA (2004) Diagnostic value of CT-guided biopsy of indeterminate renal masses. Clin Radiol 59:262–267

Farrell MA, Charboneau WJ, DiMarco DS et al. (2003) Imaging-guided radiofrequency ablation of solid renal tumors. Am J Roentgenol 180:1509–1513

Fine DM, Arepally A, Hofmann LV et al. (2004) Diagnostic utility and safety of transjugular kidney biopsy in the obese patient. Nephrol Dial Transplant 19:1798–1802

Gazelle GS, Goldberg SN, Solbiati L et al. (2000) Tumor ablation with radiofrequency energy. Radiology 217:633–646

Gervais DA, McGovern FJ, Wood BJ et al. (2000) Radio-frequency ablation of renal cell carcinoma: early clinical experience. Radiology 217:665–672

Gervais DA, McGovern FJ, Arellano RS et al. (2003) Renal cell carcinoma: clinical experience and technical success with radio-frequency ablation of 42 tumors. Radiology 226:417–424

Gibbons RP, Bush WH Jr, Burnett LL (2004) Needle tract seeding following aspiration of renal cell carcinoma. J Urol 118:865–867

Goldberg SN, Dupuy DE (2001a) Image-guided radiofrequency tumor ablation: challenges and opportunities – part I. J Vasc Intervent Radiol 12:1021–1032

Goldberg SN, Dupuy DE (2001b) Image-guided radiofrequency tumor ablation: challenges and opportunities, part II. J Vasc Intervent Radiol 12:1135–1148

Hara I, Miyake H, Hara S et al. (2001) Role of percutaneous image-guided biopsy in the evaluation of renal masses. Urol Int 67:199–202

Harisinghani MG, Maher MM, Gervais DA et al. (2003) Incidence of malignancy in complex cystic renal masses (Bosniak category 3): Should imaging-guided biopsy precede surgery? Am J Roentgenol 180:755–758

Horcicka V Jr, Krejci K, Zadrazil J et al. (2002) Arteriovenous fistula as a complication of renal biopsy. Vnitr Lek 48:432–437

Johnson PT, Nazarian LN, Feld RI et al. (2001) Sonographically guided renal mass biopsy: indications and efficacy. J Ultrasound Med 20:749–753

Jouet P, Meyrier A, Mal F et al. (1996) Transjugular renal biopsy in the treatment of patients with cirrhosis and renal abnormalities. Hepatology 24:1143–1147

Juul N, Torp-Pedersen S, Gronvall S et al. (2004) Ultrasonically guided fine needle aspiration biopsy of renal masses. J Urol 133:579–581

Kiser GC, Totonchy M, Barry JM (2004) Needle track seeding after percutaneous renal adenocarcinoma aspiration. J Urol 136:1292–1293

Lechevallier E, Andre M, Barriol D et al. (2000) Fine-needle percutaneous biopsy of renal masses with helical CT guidance. Radiology 216:506–510

Lee IS, Nguyen S, Shanberg AM (1995) Needle tract seeding after percutaneous biopsy of Wilms Tumor. J Urol 153:1074–1076

Lee SM, King J, Spargo BH (1991) Efficacy of percutaneous renal biopsy in obese patients under computerized tomographic guidance. Clin Nephrol 35:123–129

Livraghi T, Goldberg SN, Lazzaroni S et al. (2000) Hepatocellular carcinoma: radio-frequency ablation of medium and large lesions. Radiology 214:761–768

Lund-Sorensen N, Gudmundsen TE, Rogstad B (1995) Arteriovenous fistula as a complication of percutaneous renal biopsy. Tidsskr Nor Laegeforen 115:3625–3626

Mackie GC, Davies PF, Challis DR et al. (2004) Renal infarction secondary to subcapsular hematoma following percutaneous renal biopsy. Australas Radiol 48:207–210

Mal F, Meyrier A, Callard P et al. (1990) Transjugular renal biopsy. Lancet 335:1512–1513

Mal F, Meyrier A, Callard P et al. (1992) The diagnostic yield of transjugular renal biopsy. Experience in 200 cases. Kidney Int 41:445–449

Matsumoto ED, Watumull L, Johnson DB et al. (2004) The radiographic evolution of radio frequency ablated renal tumors. J Urol 172:45–48

Mayo-Smith WW, Dupuy DE, Parikh PM et al. (2004) Imaging-guided percutaneous radiofrequency ablation of solid renal masses: techniques and outcomes of 38 treatment sessions in 32 consecutive patients. Am J Roentgenol 180:1503–1508

Memis A, Killi R, Ozer H (1992) Renal arteriovenous fistula after kidney biopsy: color Doppler ultrasound and angiography diagnosis with embolization using same procedures. Bildgebung 59:200–202

Mignon F, Mesurolle B, Ariche-Cohen M et al. (2001) Value of CT guided renal biopsies: retrospective review of 67 cases. J Radiol 82:907–911

Richter F, Kasabian NG, Irwin RJ Jr et al. (2000) Accuracy of diagnosis by guided biopsy of renal mass lesions classified indeterminate by imaging studies. Urology 55:348–352

Rybicki FJ, Shu KM, Cibas ES et al. (2003) Percutaneous biopsy of renal masses: sensitivity and negative predictive value stratified by clinical setting and size of masses. Am J Roentgenol 180:1281–1287

Rychlik I, Petrtyl J, Tesar V et al. (2004) Transjugular renal biopsy. Our experience with 67 cases. Kidney Blood Press Res 24:207–212

Shenoy PD, Lakhkar BN, Ghosh MK et al. (1991) Cutaneous seeding of renal carcinoma by Chiba needle aspiration biopsy. Case report. Acta Radiol 32:50–52

Slywotzky C, Maya M (1994) Needle tract seeding of transitional cell carcinoma following fine needle aspiration of a renal mass. Abdom Imaging 19:174–176

Thompson BC, Kingdon E, Jhonston M et al. (2004) Transjugular kidney biopsy. Am J Kidney Dis 43:651–662

Wanic-Kossowska M (1998) Arterial hypertension due to perirenal hematoma after renal percutaneous biopsy. Pol Arch Med Wewn 100:454–457

Wood BJ, Khan MA, McGovern F et al. (1999) Imaging guided biopsy of renal masses: indications, accuracy and impact on clinical management. J Urol 161:1470–1474

Zlotta AR, Raviv G, Peny MO et al. (1996) A new method of cancer treatment: the use of radiofrequencies in urological tumors. Acta Urol Belg 64:1–5

Zlotta AR, Wildschutz T, Raviv G et al. (2004) Radiofrequency interstitial tumor ablation (RITA) is a possible new modality for treatment of renal cancer: ex vivo and in vivo experience. J Endourol 11:251–258

22 Transarterial Embolization

Jean-Pierre Pelage and Salah Dine Qanadli

CONTENTS

J.-P. Pelage, MD, PhD
Associate Professor, Department of Radiology, Ambroise Paré University Hospital, 9 avenue Charles de Gaulle, 92104 Boulogne Billancourt, France
S. D. Qanadli, MD, PhD
Associate Professor, Department of Radiology and Interventional Radiology, Centre Hospitalier Universitaire Vaudois (CHUV), 46 rue du Bugnon, 1011 Lausanne, Switzerland

22.1
Introduction

Surgical resection is the basis of treatment of localized renal cell carcinoma, as the disease is relatively resistant to both radiotherapy and chemotherapy (Giberti 1997). Recently, alternative systemic therapies, such as interleukin-2 immunotherapy and interferon, have shown promise, but objective response rates are still limited to 10–15% (Bukowski 2001; Motzer and Russo 2000). Minimally invasive therapies including transarterial embolization (TAE) and radiofrequency ablation have been recognized as new approaches to treat renal cell carcinoma and its complications. The objective of this chapter is to review the role of TAE in renal cell carcinoma management.

22.2
Technique of Transarterial Embolization

The interventional radiologist performing embolization procedures should know well the physical, chemical, and biological characteristics of embolization devices as well as the best technique for each clinical indication (Berenstein and Kricheff 1979; Segni et al. 1997). The embolic agent is selected on the basis of whether temporary or permanent occlusion is wanted, whether proximal or distal devascularization is desirable, and the individual arterial anatomy. Only if the proper choice is made for each indication will success be permanent; thus, for emergent embolization in patients with intractable hematuria or for preoperative embolization, a temporary embolic agent, such as gelatin sponge, is usually favored (Lanigan et al. 1992; Kalman and Varenhorst 1999). Conversely, a more definitive embolization using non-resorbable particles (non-spherical polyvinyl alcohol particles or calibrated microspheres) will provide targeted tumoral devascularization. Transarterial embolization can also be used in patients with bone metastases, which are usually hypervascular (CHATZIIOANNOU et al. 2000). In those patients, embolization can contribute to reduction of pain and/or control of bleeding in unresectable tumors or before surgery (CHUANG et al. 1979).

22.2.1
Transarterial Embolization Materials

22.2.1.1
Gelatin Sponge

Gelatin sponge is a foam-like material derived from gelatin that was introduced in 1945 as an aid to hemostasis in surgical procedures. Since then, gelatin sponge has been used extensively as an embolic agent for a variety of indications, including renal cell carcinoma, just before resection or gastroduodenal hemorrhage (BRACKEN et al. 1975; GOLD and GRACE 1975). It is biodegradable and considered a resorbable agent. Three forms are available from different companies: a powder containing small fragments; a sheet from which sections of different sizes can be cut; or thicker blocks or cubes for making large pledgets (Fig. 22.1). Gelatin sponge powder is associated with a high risk of ischemia and normally should not be used for arterial embolization (SEGNI et al. 1997). Pledgets or cubes measuring 1×2 to 3×3 mm are particularly suitable for preoperative embolization when temporary arterial occlusion is needed. A gelatin sponge slurry can also be obtained by mixing small pledgets with contrast. Mechanical arterial occlusion will occur followed by acute necrotizing

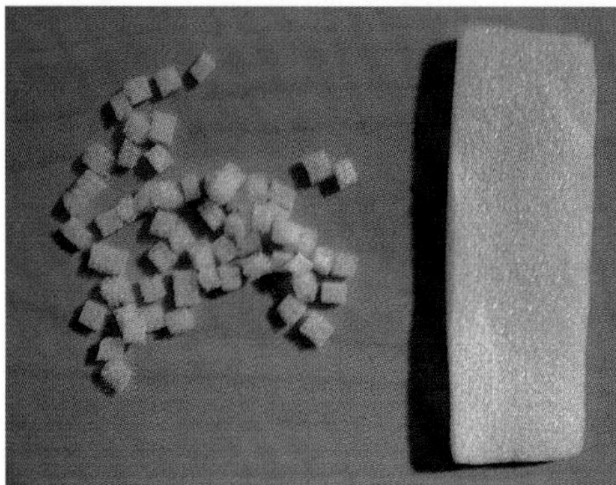

Fig. 22.1. Gelatin sponge cubes (Curaspon, Caps Recherche, Saint-Cloud, France) or pledgets obtained from sheets (Gelfoam, Kalamazoo, MI/USA) are particularly suitable for temporary embolization.

arteritis (BERENSTEIN et al. 1979). Thrombus formation is also associated with gelatin sponge. Arterial recanalization can be seen within days to weeks after embolization, although long-term occlusions have been reported occasionally.

22.2.1.2
Non-Spherical Polyvinyl Alcohol Particles

Polyvinyl alcohol particles (PVA) have been used as an embolic agent in various vascular distributions for more than 20 years (CASTANEDA-ZUNIGA et al. 1978; KERBER et al. 1978). The irregular shape of the material is associated with a larger granulometric distribution of the particles than would be expected (DERDEYN et al. 1995). In addition, there is a risk of injection of particles smaller than the theoretical size in conjunction with aggregates (REPA et al. 1989; DERDEYN et al. 1995). This potential adverse effect of PVA can lead to extensive necrosis, as has been reported several times (REPA et al. 1989). In clinical practice, clumping of PVA particles can lead to obstruction of the catheter or microcatheter or even to uncontrolled level of arterial occlusion (REPA et al. 1989; DERDEYN et al. 1995). The mechanism of arterial occlusion induced by non-spherical PVA particles is well understood: the initial incomplete lumen occlusion by the particles is associated with thrombus formation within the interstices (CASTANEDA-ZUNIGA et al. 1978). Recanalization of the embolized artery is usually observed after several months or years. Several mechanisms, such as distal migration, fragmentation, or extravascular migration of PVA particles and resorption of thrombus, may account for arterial recanalization. Non-spherical PVA particles are particularly suitable for embolization of non-resectable renal tumors or bone metastases (LANIGAN et al. 1992; CHATZIIOANNOU et al. 2000).

22.2.1.3
Calibrated Microspheres

Tris-acryl gelatin microspheres were developed in France and have been used widely in Europe since 1994 (BEAUJEUX et al. 1996; LAURENT et al. 1996). Microspheres are precisely calibrated, microporous, cross-linked acrylic beads embedded with gelatin (Fig. 22.2; LAURENT et al. 1996; DERDEYN et al. 1997). The tris-acryl polymer has been used for many years as a base material for chromatographic

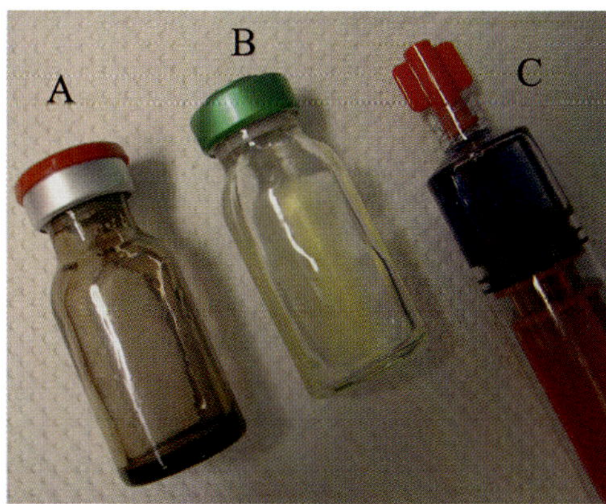

Fig. 22.2. Calibrated microspheres allow targeted devascularization of tumors. Three types of microspheres provided in prepacked syringes or vials are available for embolization: polyvinyl alcohol microspheres such as Contour SE (*A*; Boston Scientific, Natick, MA/USA), tris-acryl microspheres (*B*; Biosphere Medical, Louvres, France), or Bead Block (*C*; Biocompatibles, Farnham, UK).

filtration and is well characterized and understood. There is much experience with the use of tris-acryl microspheres in neuroradiology and for targeted devascularization of uterine fibroids in which calibration of the embolization agent is crucial to avoid complications (BEAUJEUX et al. 1996; SPIES et al. 2001). The spheres are compressible, which allows easy passage through a microcatheter with a luminal diameter smaller than that of the microspheres (DERDEYN et al. 1997). Better distribution of the tris-acryl microspheres than the non-spherical particles has been observed after injection into the renal or uterine arteries of sheep. It has been demonstrated that the degree of penetration of the particles into the vascular system is different for non-spherical PVA and tris-acryl microspheres (PELAGE et al. 2002; ANDREWS and BINKERT 2003). A significant correlation between the level of arterial occlusion and the diameter of the particles used was observed for all sizes of tris-acryl microspheres (PELAGE et al. 2002); thus, deeper penetration of embolic particles can be advantageous, leading to a more effective devascularization of many hypervascularized lesions, including renal tumors or bone metastases from renal cell carcinoma (ANDREWS and BINKERT 2003). In a renal artery embolization animal model, blood flow was more quickly and reliably reduced using tris-acryl microspheres than non-spherical PVA (ANDREWS and BINKERT 2003).

Polyvinyl alcohol particle spheres were developed in the past decade, to overcome the unpredictable behavior of non-spherical PVA particles during arterial embolization and because of the theoretical and

published advantages of tris-acryl microspheres for neurologic and gynecologic interventions (Fig. 22.2; SISKIN et al. 2003). Polyvinyl alcohol particle spheres were chosen as the core constituent based on its long track record of safety and efficacy in embolization procedures. Like tris-acryl microspheres, even large PVA spheres are easy to inject through microcatheters. Initial animal studies demonstrated that PVA microspheres are as effective for targeted renal parenchymal infarction as tris-acryl microspheres (SISKIN et al 2003).

22.2.1.4
Cyanoacrylate

N-butyl-cyanoacrylate, also called acrylic glue, is a fast-polymerization tissue adhesive of low viscosity that appears to be one of the best agents for complete occlusion of large-to-medium-sized arteries (BERENSTEIN et al. 1979; SEGNI et al. 1997). Acrylic glue polymerizes on contact with ionic solutions, such as normal saline, contrast material, and blood, and with the intima of the vessels; therefore, the delivery system must be flushed with 5% glucose to delay polymerization and avoid gluing of the vessel wall. A mechanical occlusion of the target artery is obtained followed by intense inflammatory reaction (BERENSTEIN et al. 1979; SEGNI et al. 1997). Cyanoacrylate is considered as a definitive embolic agent even if recanalization may occur in the long term. Special training is required for its use. Acrylic glue has found limited acceptance as an embolic agent (BERENSTEIN et al. 1979; SEGNI et al. 1997).

22.2.1.5
Absolute Ethanol

Ethanol administered as an intra-arterial agent induces endovascular endothelial damage and tissue protein denaturation, resulting in permanent vascular occlusion and tumor infarction. Its efficacy as an embolizing agent has been demonstrated in experimental studies and through clinical experience (EKELUND et al. 1981; ELLMAN et al. 1981). The use of balloon-assisted occlusion technique is widely accepted to reduce the risk of retrograde reflux of the agent, especially during renal procedures. For complete renal embolization, 0.2 ml/kg body weight of absolute ethanol (99% ethyl alcohol) is typically perfused in a mixture with non-ionic contrast material for appropriate control under fluoroscopy (PARK et al. 1994; Park et al. 2000). Vascular occlusion induced by the ethanol is more peripheral than most other agents (Latschaw1985). The main advantages of ethanol for embolization are its minimal cost, universal availability, high efficacy on tumor, and renal infarction, and low complication rate when used with balloon-assisted occlusion. No post-embolization recanalization of vessels embolized with ethanol has been reported in animal studies (Latschaw 1985).

22.2.1.6
Other Embolic Agents

Coils are non-resorbable non-particulate embolic agents. Initially, only stainless-steel coils were available (Segni et al. 1997), but more recently platinum coils have become available, with fibered and non-fibered variants (Fig. 22.3). Choosing the correct size is critical: too small and the coil may not occlude completely the arterial lumen; too large, and the coil may cause occlusion of proximal arterial branches or may elongate leading to recanalization. After placement of the first coil, additional coils must be positioned until arterial blood flow has ceased (Segni et al. 1997). If the number of coils is not sufficient, recanalization may also occur because of insufficient thrombosis formation (Segni et al. 1997). Therefore, coils are usually injected as a secondary embolic agent in conjunction with particles (Fig. 22.3; Lanigan et al. 1992); however, the use of coils increases the cost of the procedure and may prevent re-embolization, if necessary (Lanigan et al. 1992; Segni et al. 1997).

A new liquid embolic material obtained by partial hydrolysis of polyvinyl acetate has been used recently (Park et al. 2000).

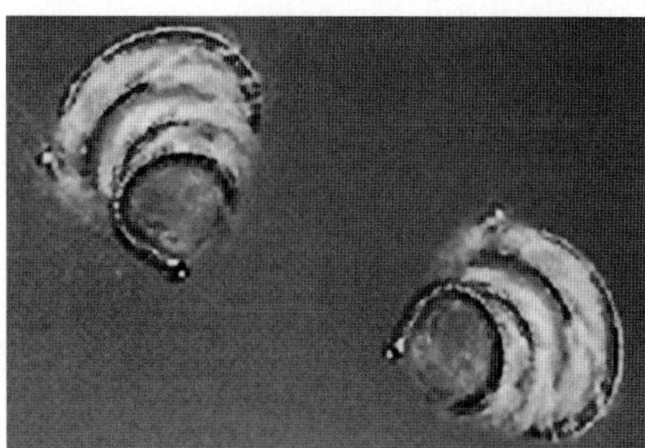

Fig. 22.3. Different types of fibered coils or microcoils allow a more permanent arterial occlusion than gelatin sponge particles.

Gelatin sponge pledgets can also be used as a secondary embolic agent in conjunction with non-spherical PVA particles or calibrated microspheres to obtain a temporary proximal arterial occlusion.

22.2.2
Transarterial Embolization Procedures

For successful renal TAE, both selection of appropriate selective or super-selective catheterization and adequate operator experience are required. To occlude the main renal artery proximally, some authors recommend balloon-assisted occlusion to exclude potential reflux, particularly when liquid embolic materials are used (Park et al. 2000). When the target vessels are distal to segmental arteries, a super-selective approach with the use of a microcatheter should be favored. Various commercially available coaxial catheters with large inner lumen can be used. Coaxial systems facilitate super-selective embolization with targeted tumoral devascularization sparing normal renal parenchyma (Beaujeux et al. 1995).

22.3
Indications for Renal Transarterial Embolization

The first description of renal TAE in humans was reported in 1973 by Almgard et al. In the early 1980s, TAE was introduced into clinical practice; however, management of renal cancer using TAE is not clearly defined and some points are still controversial. It has been suggested that TAE could be used for different situations depending on the target objective: (a) to control symptoms related to the primary tumor in patients with advanced disease; (b) to provide an alternative to radical surgery in patients; and (c) to be used as preoperative treatment.

The primary use of TAE is to control renal-cancer-related symptoms. These symptoms include hemorrhage from the tumor or after a biopsy, renal arteriovenous shunts or pseudoaneurysms (Albani and Novick 2003), pain, and compressive mass (McLean and Meranze 1985; Kuether 1996). To control hemorrhage, gelatin sponge pledgets with or without supplemental coils are the usual first recourse (Fig. 22.4).

Indications of TAE as an alternative to surgery include cancer in a solitary kidney, bilateral tumors, and end-stage renal carcinoma (Kalman and

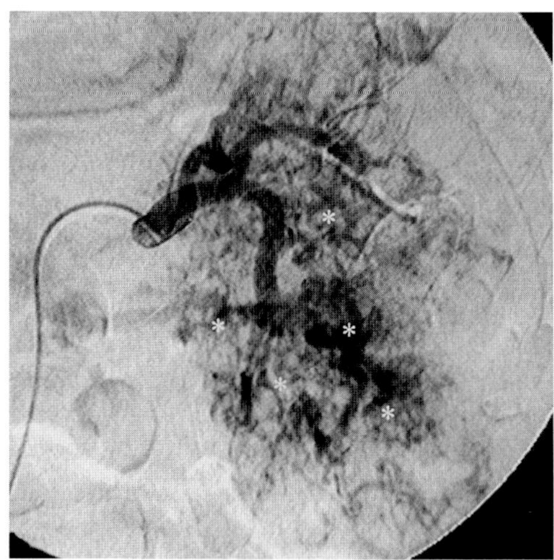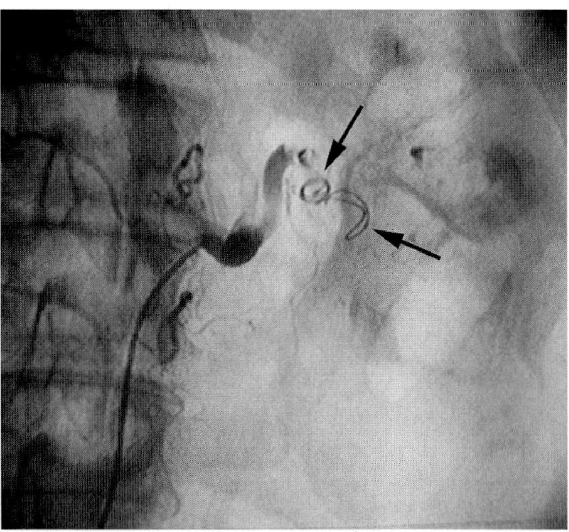

Fig. 22.4a,b. Large left renal cell carcinoma in a 67-year-old man. **a** Preoperative digital subtraction angiogram after selective injection into the left renal artery shows diffuse renal hypervascularization (*asterisks*). **b** Complete arterial occlusion is achieved after embolization using gelatin sponge pledgets and two coils (*arrows*).

VARENHORST 1999). For a more targeted devascularization of a renal cell carcinoma in these patients, non-spherical PVA particles or calibrated microspheres are usually favored (Figs. 22.5, 22.6). Combined embolization and percutaneous radiofrequency ablation of renal tumor in a solitary kidney has also been reported (HALL 2000).

Management of hemorrhage with preoperative embolization has little support in the literature. Gelatin sponge pledgets with or without coils are the usual choice (Fig. 22.7) for the immediate preoperative period (KALMAN and VARENHORST 1999).

22.4
Results of Renal Transarterial Embolization

22.4.1
Symptom Control

Many reports have indicated successful symptom control with TAE in a variety of clinical settings. NURMI et al. (1987) reported a 78% success rate for hematuria and 50% for pain. MARX et al. (1982) reported a success rate of 100% for hematuria control. In MUNRO et al. (2003), only 3 of 16 patients

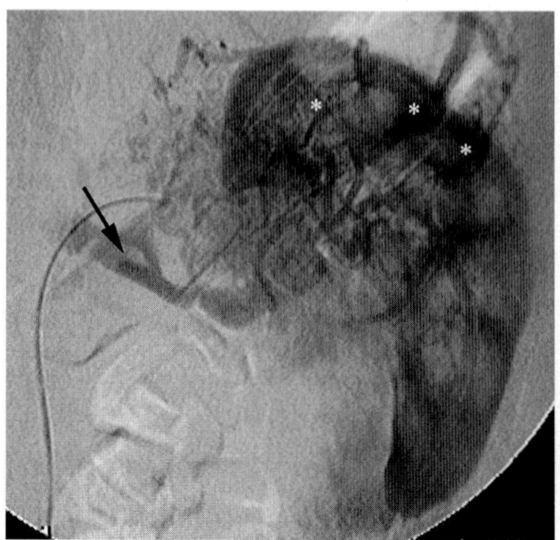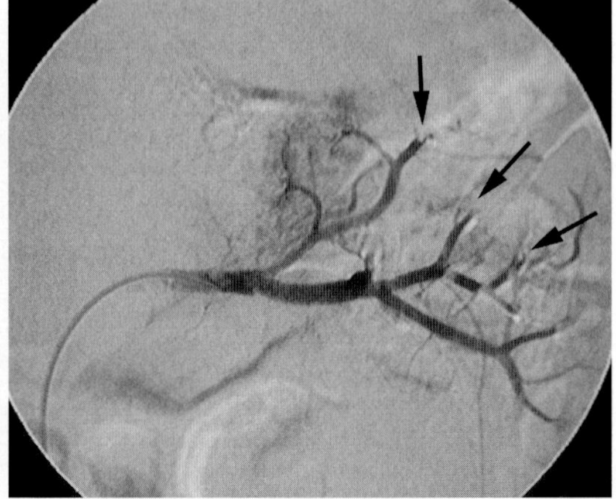

Fig. 22.5a,b. Left renal cell carcinoma of the upper pole of the kidney in a 31-year-old man with hematuria. **a** Pre-embolization digital subtraction angiogram of selective injection into the left renal artery shows diffuse tumoral hypervascularization (*asterisks*) consistent with carcinoma. Also note that a thrombus is present in the left renal vein (*arrow*). **b** Distal tumoral devascularization is seen (*arrows*) with a reduced flow in the main renal artery after arterial embolization using 300- to 500-μm tris-acryl microspheres (Embosphere) and gelatin sponge pledgets.

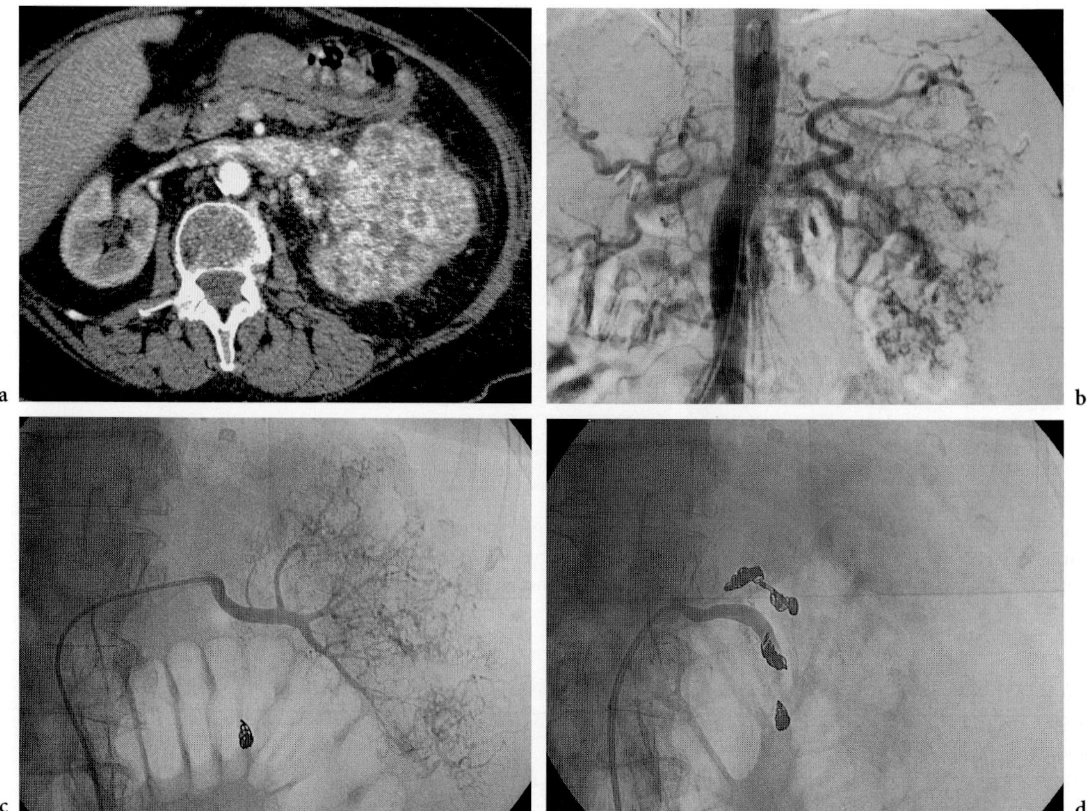

Fig. 22.6a-d. Renal cell carcinoma infiltrating whole left kidney and invading the left renal vein in a 62-year-old man. **a** Axial contrast-enhanced CT scan at the arterial phase shows a diffuse infiltration of the left kidney by a hypervascular mass. The left renal vein is filled by a hypervascular thrombus. **b** Aortogram shows the hypervascular mass in the left renal region. **c** Selective angiogram of the posterior renal branch shows the hypervascular pattern of the lesion. **d** Complete tumoral devascularization is achieved after embolization using 300- to 500-μm microspheres and supplemental coils placed in the main left renal artery.

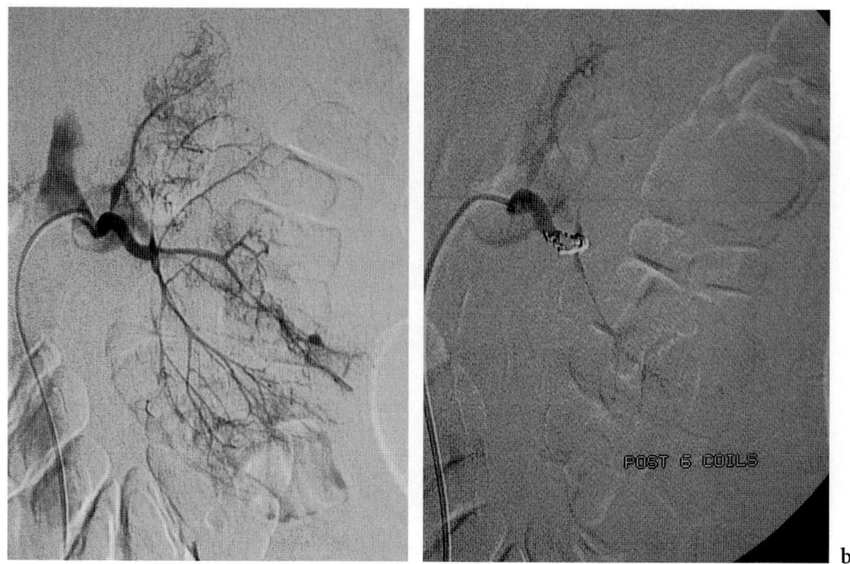

Fig. 22.7a,b. Palliative embolization of a renal urothelial tumor invading the entire left kidney in a 58-year-old woman. **a** Selective angiogram shows a moderate tumoral hypervascularization. **b** The left renal artery appears completely occluded after palliative embolization using 300- to 500-μm microspheres and coils.

treated for hematuria or pain by TAE required further treatment to control their symptoms.

22.4.2
Survival

The clinical ability of TAE to improve the prognosis in patients with disseminated disease in candidates for radical surgery is unclear.

Onishi et al. (2001) compared the outcome of 24 patients with metastatic renal cell carcinoma undergoing TAE to 30 patients without TAE. They reported that patients with unresectable disseminated renal cell carcinoma who underwent ethanol-based TAE had better prognoses (1- and 3-year survival 29 and 10%, respectively) than those who did not (1- and 3-year survival 13 and 3%, respectively), with a median survival of 229 days. These results are similar to those reported in patients with disseminated renal cell cancer treated by TAE followed by nephrectomy (1-year survival of 28% and median survival of 7 months).

Zielinski et al. (2000) reviewed a series of 474 patients with renal cell carcinoma to evaluate the value of preoperative renal embolization before radical surgery. They found that the overall 5- and 10-year survival for 118 patients who had embolization before surgery was 62 and 47%, respectively, but 35 and 23%, respectively, for a matched group of 116 patients without embolization prior to surgery; however, it is still unresolved whether the use of this technique results in increased survival.

From current reports, TAE seems to be an adequate therapeutic option; however, further studies with more data and prospective comparisons are needed to establish the prognostic value of TAE, especially regarding survival.

22.5
Renal Transarterial Embolization-Related Complications

Post-embolization syndrome occurs in most cases, as well as combined fever, back pain in the embolized site, nausea, and/or vomiting for several days. This syndrome should be considered a part of the process and is easily controlled with appropriate medication.

Overall complication rates during renal TAE reported in the literature vary from 10 to 20%. The most common cause of complications during renal TAE is unintentional embolization of non-target vessels including visceral arteries, peripheral arteries of the lower extremities, and spinal cord branches. Incidental embolism could be due to agent reflux or agent dislodgement.

Lammer et al. (1985) recorded complications of renal tumor embolization in a series of 121 procedures. They reported a mortality rate of 3.3% and major morbidity of 9.9%. The most common complications were renal failure and unintentional embolization of non-target organs including peripheral arteries, colon infarction, and spinal cord ischemia.

22.6
Transarterial Embolization for Bone Metastases

22.6.1
Indications and Technique

Metastases from renal cell carcinoma usually mimic the primary neoplasm in degree of vascularity, being hypervascular in up to 75% of cases (Fig. 22.8). After the lung, the most frequent site is the skeletal system with an incidence around 40% (Chuang et al. 1979). Several reports have addressed the issue of transarterial embolization in the management of bone metastases from renal cell carcinoma (Chuang et al. 1979; Bowers et al. 1982; Varma et al. 1984; Chatziioannou et al. 2000). Three different purposes have been promoted. Embolization can contribute to reduction of pain (Fig. 22.9; Chuang et al. 1979; Stepanek et al. 1999; Yilmaz et al. 2002). It can also be useful to control bleeding in patients with unresectable tumors (Barton et al. 1996; Chatziioannou et al. 2000); however, the most common use is preoperative embolization (Fig. 22.8; Patel et al. 1977; Bowers et al. 1982; Chatziioannou et al. 2000). Pathologic fractures associated with metastatic renal cell carcinoma usually result in significant compromise of function (Rowe et al. 1984). If feasible, operative intervention with reduction and fixation of the fracture site offers restoration of function, often for an extended time (Rowe et al. 1984). The hypervascular nature of these metastases may result in technical difficulties at surgery, and frequently heavy and intractable bleeding (Patel et al. 1977; Bowers et al. 1982; Barton et al. 1996; Chatziioannou et al. 2000). Various types of surgery may benefit from preoperative embolization including open reduction, curettage, internal fixation, bone

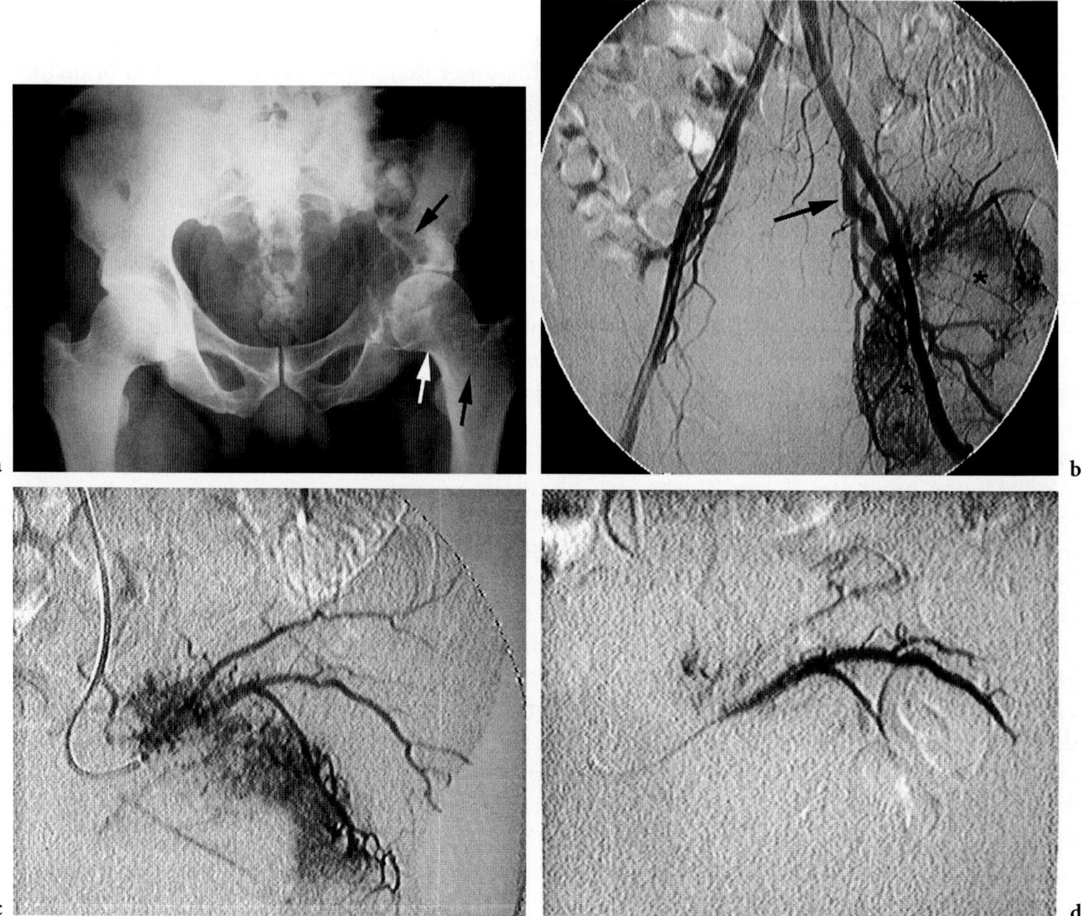

Fig. 22.8a-d. Preoperative embolization of bone metastases from renal cell carcinoma in a 59-year-old man. **a** Initial radiograph shows lytic lesions involving the left femoral neck and acetabular region (*arrows*). **b** Flush pelvic aortography demonstrates a large hypervascular metastatic lesion (*asterisks*) supplied mainly by the left hypogastric artery (*arrow*). **c** Selective injection into the left superior gluteal artery confirms the hypervascular lesion. **d** After superselective embolization using 500- to 700-μm microspheres and gelatin sponge pledgets, complete devascularization is obtained. Successful total hip replacement has been performed with minimal peri-operative blood loss.

resection, prosthetic replacement, or intramedullary nail placement (Fig. 22.8; Bowers et al. 1982; Chatziioannou et al. 2000). The most frequent locations are the femoral neck, acetabular region, pubic ramus, humerus, and scapula. Vertebral metastases may also be treated preoperatively (Fig. 22.10). In this case, special attention should be paid to the identification of the spinal artery during the initial angiographic evaluation (Fig. 22.11).

Microcatheters are frequently used access the small feeding arteries (Figs. 22.9, 22.10; Chatziioannou et al. 2000). Small non-resorbable non-spherical PVA particles or calibrated microspheres are recommended for optimal devascularization of bone metastases and to spare normal surrounding tissues (Figs. 22.9, 22.10; Chatziioannou et al. 2000; Yilmaz et al. 2002).

Fig. 22.10a-e. Preoperative embolization of vertebral metastases from renal cell carcinoma in a 54-year-old man. **a** Selective injection into the common right and left trunk (*asterisk*) of L4 demonstrates a hypervascular lesion involving the left part of the vertebral body (*arrow*). **b** Superselective catheterization of the left lumbar arterial feeder is achieved using a microcatheter (*arrow*). **c** After superselective embolization using 300- to 500-μm microspheres, complete devascularization is obtained (*arrow*). The right lumbar artery is left patent. **d** Selective injection into the common right and left trunk (*asterisk*) of L3 demonstrates a hypervascular lesion involving the left part of the vertebral body (*arrow*). **e** Superselective embolization of the left lumbar arterial feeder is achieved (*arrow*) using the same technique.

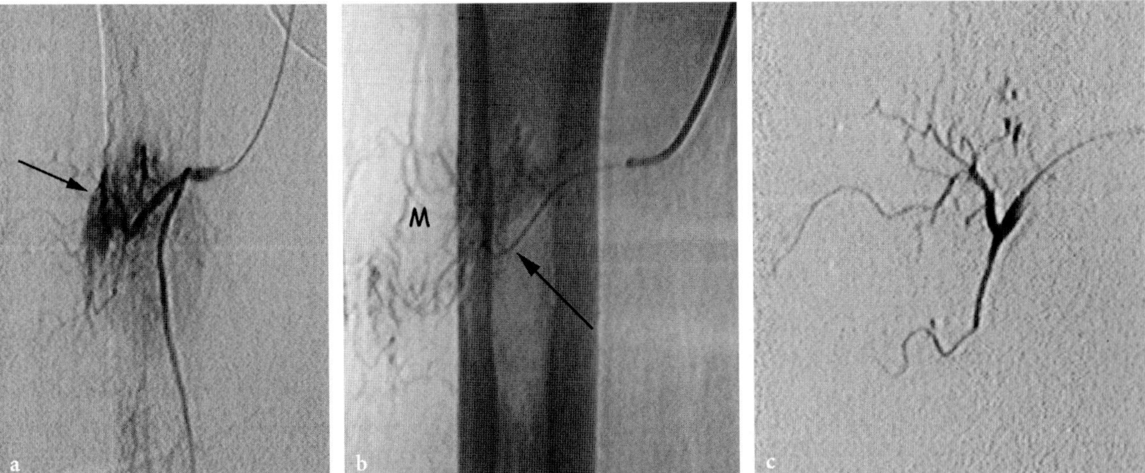

Fig. 22.9a-c. Palliative embolization of bone metastasis from renal cell carcinoma in a 71-year-old man with severe pain. **a** Pre-embolization arteriogram demonstrates a hypervascular lesion of the right femoral bone (*arrow*). **b** Superselective catheterization of the main arterial feeder is achieved using a microcatheter (*M* metastasis). **c** After superselective embolization using 300- to 500-μm microspheres, complete devascularization is obtained. Pain relief was obtained for 2 months.

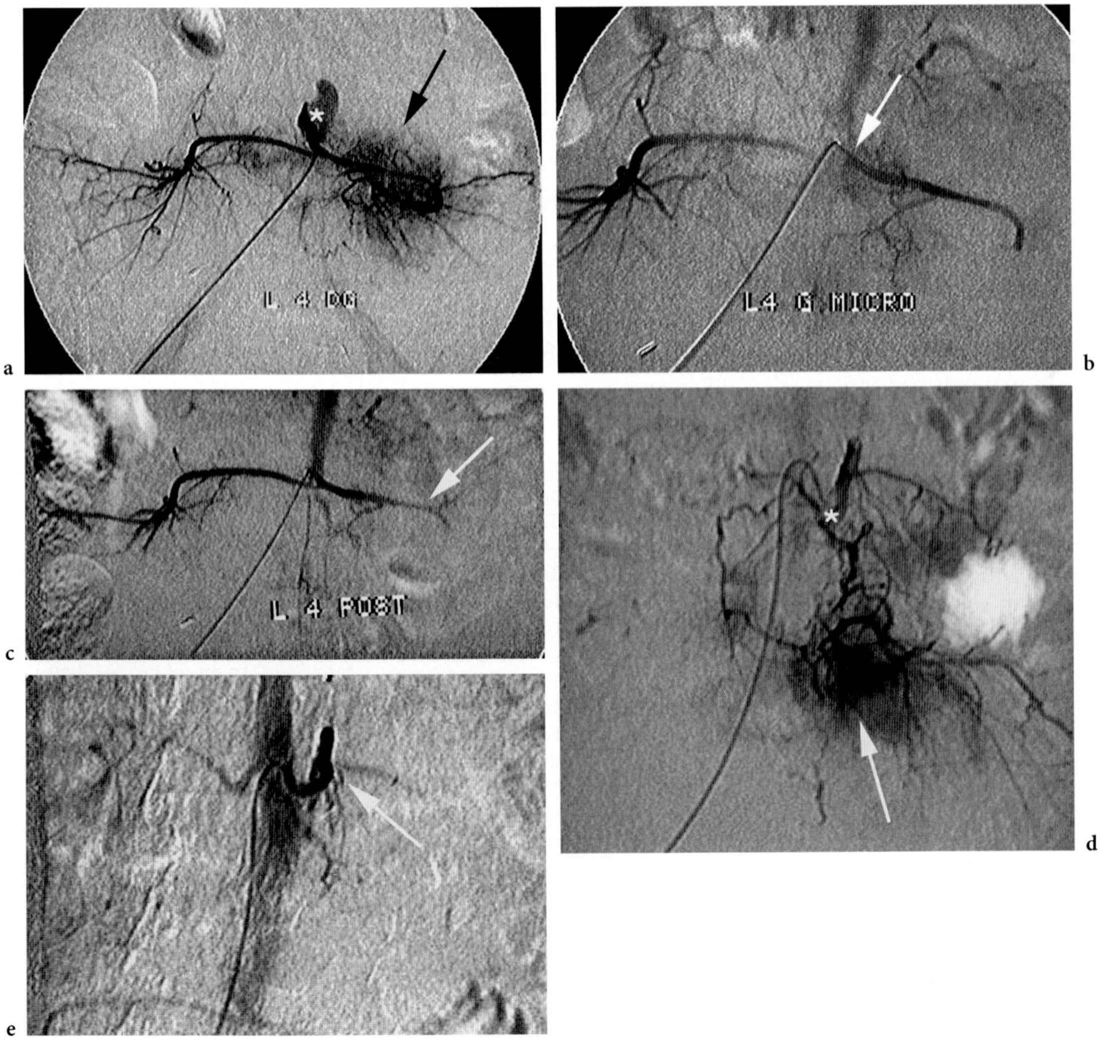

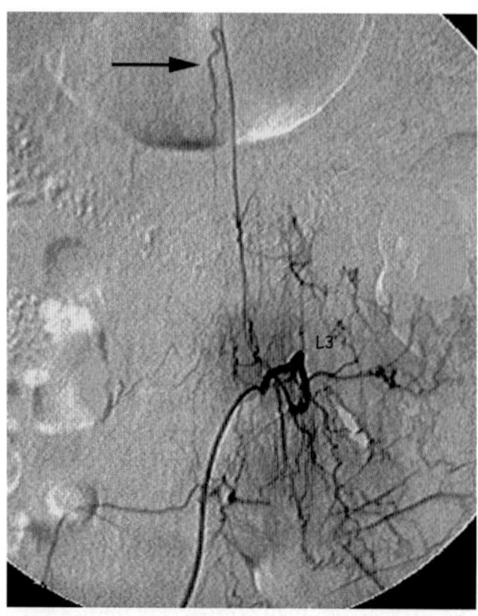

Fig. 22.11. Preoperative embolization of lumbar metastases from renal cell carcinoma in a 63-year-old woman with severe pain. Selective injection into the third left lumbar artery demonstrates a hypervascular lesion of L3. A spinal artery (*arrow*) is identified precluding further embolization.

22.6.2
Results and Complications

All published series of patients treated with preoperative embolization have reported a marked reduction in perioperative blood loss (Barton et al. 1996; Chatziioannou et al. 2000). Barton et al. (1996) reported a mean blood loss of 6800 ml in patients who underwent surgery without embolization, but only a 500- to 1500-ml blood loss after preoperative embolization. Chatziioannou et al. (2000) compared the perioperative blood loss in patients with complete tumoral devascularization and in those with incomplete embolization. They demonstrated that there was a statistically significant difference in the mean blood loss between the two groups. Patients with complete embolization had a mean blood loss of 535 vs 1247 ml in patients with incomplete embolization. Transfusion requirements were also different between the two groups. As expected, however, the degree of embolization has no effect on patient survival. No major complication has been reported in this situation (Barton et al. 1996; Chatziioannou et al. 2000). Barton et al. (1996) confirmed the reduction of blood loss at the time of surgery, and the reduction of viable tumor before radiotherapy and chemotherapy.

When embolization is performed as a palliative treatment for pain relief, elimination of pain for up to 9 months has been reported (Stepanek et al. 1999); however, most patients will require repeated embolization procedures because of recurrence (Yilmaz et al. 2002). Multiple sessions may allow patients to spend the rest of their lives almost pain free (Yilmaz et al. 2002). Complications are rarely encountered. Barton et al. (1996) reported temporary paresis in 3 of 51 patients with skeletal metastases treated with embolization.

22.7
Conclusion

Transarterial embolization is an accepted therapeutic option in palliating symptoms related to renal cancer with very high success rate and low complication rate. Proper selection of both embolic material and the catheterization approach are essential to the success of the procedure. The role of renal TAE in disease control and survival improvement seems promising. Further studies are needed to determine whether TAE improves survival in patients with disseminated disease or localized tumor. The value of TAE in patients with bone metastases has been well demonstrated to reduce pain or, if performed preoperatively, to decrease blood loss and transfusion requirements during surgery.

References

Albani JM, Novick AC (2003) Renal artery pseudoaneurysm after partial nephrectomy: three case reports and a literature review. Urology 62:227–231

Almgard LE, Fernstrom I, Haverling M, Ljungqvist A (1973) Treatment of renal adenocarcinoma by embolic occlusion of the renal circulation. Br J Urol 45:474–479

Andrews TA, Binkert CA (2003) Relative rates of blood flow reduction during transcatheter arterial embolization with tris-acryl gelatin microspheres or polyvinyl alcohol: quantitative comparison in a swine model. J Vasc Interv Radiol 14:1311–1316

Barton PP, Waneck ER, Karnel JF, Ritschl P, Kramer J, Letchner LG (1996) Embolization of bone metastases. J Vasc Interv Radiol 7:81–88

Beaujeux R, Saussine C, al-Fakir A, Boudjema K, Roy C, Jacqmin D, Bourjat P (1995) Superselective endo-vascular treatment of renal vascular lesions. J Urol 153:14–17

Beaujeux R, Laurent A, Wassef M et al. (1996) Trisacryl gelatin microspheres for therapeutic embolization, II: clinical evaluation in tumors and arteriovenous malformations. Am J Neuroradiol 17:541–548

Berenstein A, Kricheff II (1979) Catheter and material selection for transarterial embolization: technical considerations. Radiology 132:631–639

Bowers TA, Murray JA, Charnsangavej C, Soo CS, Chuang VP, Wallace S (1982) Bone metastases from renal cell cercinoma: the preoperative use of transcatheter arterial occlusion. J Bonc Joint Surg 64:749–754

Bracken RB, Johnson DF, Goldstein HM, Wallace S, Ayala AG (1975) Percutaneous transfemoral renal artery occlusion in patients with renal carcinoma. Urology 6:6–10

Bukowski RM (2001) Cytokine therapy for metastatic renal cell carcinoma. Semin Urol Oncol 19:148–154

Castaneda-Zuniga WR, Sanchez R, Amplatz K (1978) Experimental observations on short and long-term effects of arterial occlusion with Ivalon. Radiology 126:783–785

Chatziioannou AN, Johnson ME, Pneumaticos SG, Lawrence DD, Carrasco CH (2000) Preoperative embolization of bone metastases from renal cell carcinoma. Eur Radiol 10:593–596

Chuang VP, Wallace S, Swanson D et al. (1979) Arterial occlusion in the management of pain from metastatic renal carcinoma. Radiology 133:611–614

Derdeyn CP, Moran CJ, Cross DT AI et al. (1995) Polyvinyl alcohol particle size and suspension characteristics. Am J Neuroradiol 16:1031–1036

Derdeyn CP, Graves VB, Salamat MS, Rappe A (1997) Collagen-coated acrylic microspheres for embolotherapy: in vivo and in vitro characteristics. Am J Neuroradiol 18:647–653

Ekelund L, Jonsson N, Treugut H (1981) Transcatheter obliteration of the renal artery by ethanol injection: experimental results. Cardiovasc Intervent Radiol 4:1–7

Ellman BA, Parkhill BJ, Curry TS III, Marcus PB, Peters PC (1981) Ablation of renal tumors with absolute ethanol: a new technique. Radiology 141:619–626

Giberti C, Oneto F, Martorana G, Rovida S, Carmignani G (1997) Radical nephrectomy for renal cell carcinoma: long-term results and prognostic factors on a series of 328 cases. Eur Urol 31:40–48

Gold RE, Grace DM (1975) Gelfoam embolization of the left gastric artery for bleeding ulcer: experimental considerations. Radiology 116:563–567

Hall WH, McGahan JP, Link DP, deVere White RW (2000) Combined embolization and percutaneous radiofrequency ablation of a solid renal tumor. Am J Roentgenol 174:1592–1594

Kalman D, Varenhorst E (1999) The role of arterial embolization in renal cell carcinoma. Scand J Urol Nephrol 33:162–170

Kerber CW, Bank WO, Horton JA (1978) Polyvinyl alcohol foam: prepackaged emboli for therapeutic embolization. Am J Roentgenol 130:1193–1194

Kuether TA, Nesbit GM, Barnwell SL (1996) Embolization as treatment for spinal cord compression from renal cell carcinoma: case report. Neurosurgery 39:1260–1263

Lammer J, Justich E, Schreyer H, Pettek R (1985) Complications of renal tumor embolization. Cardiovasc Intervent Radiol 8:31–35

Lanigan D, Jurriaans E, Hammonds JC, Wells IP, Choa RG (1992) The current status of embolization in renal cell carcinoma. Clin Radiol 46: 176–178

Latschaw RF, Pearlman RL, Schaitkin BM, Griffith JW, Weidner WA (1985) Intraarterial ethanol as a long-term occlusive agent in renal, hepatic, and gastrosplenic arteries of pigs. Cardiovasc Intervent Radiol 8:24–30

Laurent A, Beaujeux R, Wassef M et al. (1996) Trisacryl gelatin microspheres for therapeutic embolization. I. Development and in vitro evaluation. Am J Neuroradiol 17:533–540

Marx FJ, Chaussy C, Moser E (1982) Limitations and hazards of palliative renal tumor embolization. Urologe A 21:206–210

McLean GK, Meranze SG (1985) Embolization techniques in the urinary tract. Urol Clin North Am 12:743–754

Motzer RJ, Russo P (2000) Systemic therapy for renal cell carcinoma. J Urol 163:408–417

Munro NP, Woodhams S, Nawrocki JD, Fletcher MS, Thomas PJ (2003) The role of transarterial embolization in the treatment of renal cell carcinoma. BJU Int 92:240–244

Nurmi M, Satokari K, Puntala P (1987) Renal artery embolization in the palliative treatment of renal adenocarcinoma. Scand J Urol Nephrol 21:93–96

Onishi T, Oishi Y, Suzuki Y, Asano K (2001) Prognostic evaluation of transcatheter arterial embolization for unresectable renal cell carcinoma with distant metastasis. BJU Int 87:312–315

Park JH, Kim SH, Han JK, Chung JW, Han MC (1994) Transcatheter embolization of unresectable renal cell carcinoma with a mixture of ethanol and iodized oil. Cardiovasc Intervent Radiol 17: 323–327

Park SI, Lee DY, Won JY, Park S (2000) Renal artery embolization using a new liquid embolic material obtained by partial hydrolysis of polyvinyl acetate. Korean J Radiol 1:121–126

Patel D, Crothers O, Harris WH, Waltman A, Fahmy N, Carey R (1977) Arterial embolization for radical tumor resection. Acta Orthop Scand 48:353–355

Pelage JP, Laurent A, Wassef M et al. (2002) Acute effects of uterine artery embolization in the sheep: comparison between polyvinyl alcohol particles and calibrated microspheres. Radiology 224:436–445

Repa I, Moradian GP, Dehrer LP et al. (1989) Mortalities associated with use of a commercial suspension of polyvinyl alcohol. Radiology 170:395–399

Rowe D, Becker G, Rabr F, Holden R, Richmond B, Wass J, Sequeira F (1984) Osseous metastases from renal cell carcinomas. Embolization and surgery for restoration of function. Radiology 150:673–676

Segni RD, Young AT, Qian Z, Castaneda-Zuniga WR (1997) Embolotherapy: agents, equipment and techniques. In: Castaneda-Zuniga WR, Tadavarthy SM, Qian Z, Ferral H, Maynar M (eds) Interventional radiology. Williams and Wilkins, Baltimore, pp 29–103

Siskin GP, Dowling K, Virmani R, Jones R, Todd D (2003) Pathologic evaluation of a spherical polyvinyl alcohol embolic agent in porcine renal model. J Vasc Interv Radiol 14:89–98

Spies JB, Benenati JE, Worthington-Kirsch RL, Pelage JP (2001) Initial experience with the use of trisacryl gelatin microspheres for uterine artery embolization for leiomyomata. J Vasc Interv Radiol 12:1059–1063

Stepanek E, Josph S, Campbell P, Porte M (1999) Embolization of a limb metastasis in renal cell carcinoma as a palliative treatment of bone pain. Clin Radiol 54:855–857

Varma J, Huben RP, Wajsman Z, Pontes JE (1984) Therapeutic embolization of pelvic metastases of renal cell carcinoma. J Urol 131:647–649

Yilmaz S, Sindel T, Luleci E (2002) Repeated palliative embolization of renal cell carcinoma metastases. Clin Radiol 57:319–320

Zielinski H, Szmigielski S, Petrovich Z (2000) Comparison of preoperative embolization followed by radical nephrectomy with radical nephrectomy alone for renal cell carcinoma. Am J Clin Oncol 23:6–12

23 Preoperative Navigation of Nephron-Sparing Surgery

Takuya Ueda, Hisao Ito, and Ali Guermazi

CONTENTS

T. Ueda, MD
Lecturer and Instructor, Department of Radiology, Institute of Clinical Medicine, University of Tsukuba, 1-8-1 Tennoudai, Tsukuba-city, Ibaraki 305-8575, Japan
H. Ito, MD
Professor and Chairman, Department of Radiology, Graduate School of Medicine, Chiba University, 1-8-1 Inohana, Chuoh-ku, Chiba-city, Chiba 260-8670, Japan
A. Guermazi, MD
Senior Radiologist, Scientific Director, Oncology Services, Department of Radiology Services, Synarc Inc., 575 Market Street, 17th Floor, San Francisco, CA 94105, USA

23.1 Introduction

The history of partial nephrectomy dates back to the 1880s, when Wells (1884) reported successful removal of a perirenal fibrolipoma, and Czerny (1890) performed a partial nephrectomy for a malignant renal tumor. Excessive postoperative morbidity, however, limited its widespread application. The case for partial nephrectomy was reconsidered in the 1950s, when Vermooten et al. (1950) suggested that encapsulated renal cell carcinoma (RCC) could be excised locally, leaving a margin of normal parenchyma around the tumor. Since then, nephron-sparing surgery (NSS) has largely supplanted radical nephrectomy (RN) in the treatment of RCC in patients with a compelling need for preservation of renal function, and whom RN would render anephric and requiring dialysis (Grabstald and Aviles 1968). Following the excellent results in bilateral RCC or resection of RCC in a solitary kidney (Schiff et al. 1979), indications for NSS have been expanded to localized RCC in patients with a normal contralateral kidney.

Enthusiasm for NSS has been motivated by several trends: advances in radiological imaging and expanded applications of noninvasive imaging techniques enable earlier detection of incidental RCC and detailed preoperative evaluation; improved surgical techniques minimize the risk of ischemic renal injury and hemorrhage; and better postoperative management reduces the risk of complications (Duque et al. 1998; Gacci et al. 2001).

Nephron-sparing surgery has become an established option for treatment of RCC. Although whether NSS can be recommended as standard treatment is still controversial (Schlichter et al. 2000), accumulating data have provided evidence of the long-term functional advantage gained by maximal preservation of unaffected renal parenchyma afforded by NSS, without sacrificing cancer control or patient satisfaction (Filipas et al. 2000; Fergany et al. 2000; Shinohara et al. 2001; Delakas et al. 2002).

New minimally invasive technologies are currently being applied to the field of NSS, including laparoscopic partial nephrectomy and laparoscopic cryoablation. As these modalities are very new, it is too soon to say whether their initial promise will be sustained. Early reports for these modalities have included only highly selected patients and many clinical trials are underway to assess their efficacies.

23.2
Overview of Nephron-Sparing Surgery

23.2.1
Indications

Acceptable indications for NSS can be divided into two categories: imperative and elective. Imperative indications may be subdivided into absolute and relative indications (Table 23.1).

Imperative indications apply to patients with a compelling need for the preservation of renal function. Absolute indications include RCC involving an anatomically or functionally solitary kidney due to unilateral renal agenesis, previous contralateral nephrectomy, or irreversible impairment of contralateral renal function due to a benign disorder (FERGANY et al. 2000; GACCI et al. 2001; GHAVAMIAN et al. 2002). Significant renal insufficiency is generally considered an absolute indication (SCHIFF et al. 1979). Bilateral synchronous RCC is also an absolute indication (SCHIFF et al. 1979; BALTACI et al. 2000). Relative indications are potential risk of future renal insufficiency and dialysis: when the contralateral kidney is threatened by local, systemic, or genetic conditions, that may affect future function; or when there is a likelihood of subsequent contralateral tumors in some diseases such as von Hippel-Lindau disease (UZZO and NOVICK 2001). Imperative indications compel the use of NSS even in technically difficult conditions, because the alternative would yield the patient anephric by nephrectomy (UZZO and NOVICK 2001).

Elective indications include small, localized, often incidental RCC with a normal contralateral kidney. Although patient selection for elective indication is still a matter of controversy, elective indication is generally applied to small tumors, usually 4 cm or less in diameter, and peripherally located tumors without deep invasion into renal sinus. Patient age may also influence determination of indication (HAFEZ et al. 1999; FILIPAS et al. 2000; DELAKAS et al. 2002).

23.2.2
Surgical Procedures

Nephron-sparing surgery is technically more challenging than RN. Unlike the en bloc removal of the kidney with tumor in RN, NSS requires management of the intrarenal structures including the segmental branch of the artery and vein, and the collecting system (UZZO and NOVICK 2001; GHAVAMIAN and ZINCKE 2001; NIEDER and TANEJA 2003). Radiologists should understand the procedure so that they can provide effective support to urologists.

Figure 23.1 demonstrates the general surgical procedures of NSS.

The surgical approach generally involves an extraperitoneal flank incision through the eleventh and twelfth ribs. The kidney is mobilized within Gerota's fascia while leaving the perirenal fat around the tumor intact (Fig. 23.1a, b).

The method of surgical resection is determined based on preoperative radiological evaluation and the renal function of the patient, with the aim of maximal preservation of renal parenchyma and minimizing the risk of complications while controlling the cancer without residual tumor (Fig. 23.1c, d).

Table 23.1. Indications for nephron-sparing surgery

Imperative indications		Elective indications
Absolute indications	*Relative indications*	
Anatomically or functionally solitary kidney	Future risk for dysfunction	Small, localized, often incidental RCC
Past nephrectomy by contralateral RCC	Calculus disease	with a normal contralateral kidney
Functionally solitary kidney due to	Chronic pyelonephritis	
benign renal disease	Renal artery stenosis	
Unilateral renal agenesis	Ureteral reflux	
Bilateral synchronous RCC	Systemic disease	
Severe renal insufficiency	(i.e., diabetes mellitus)	

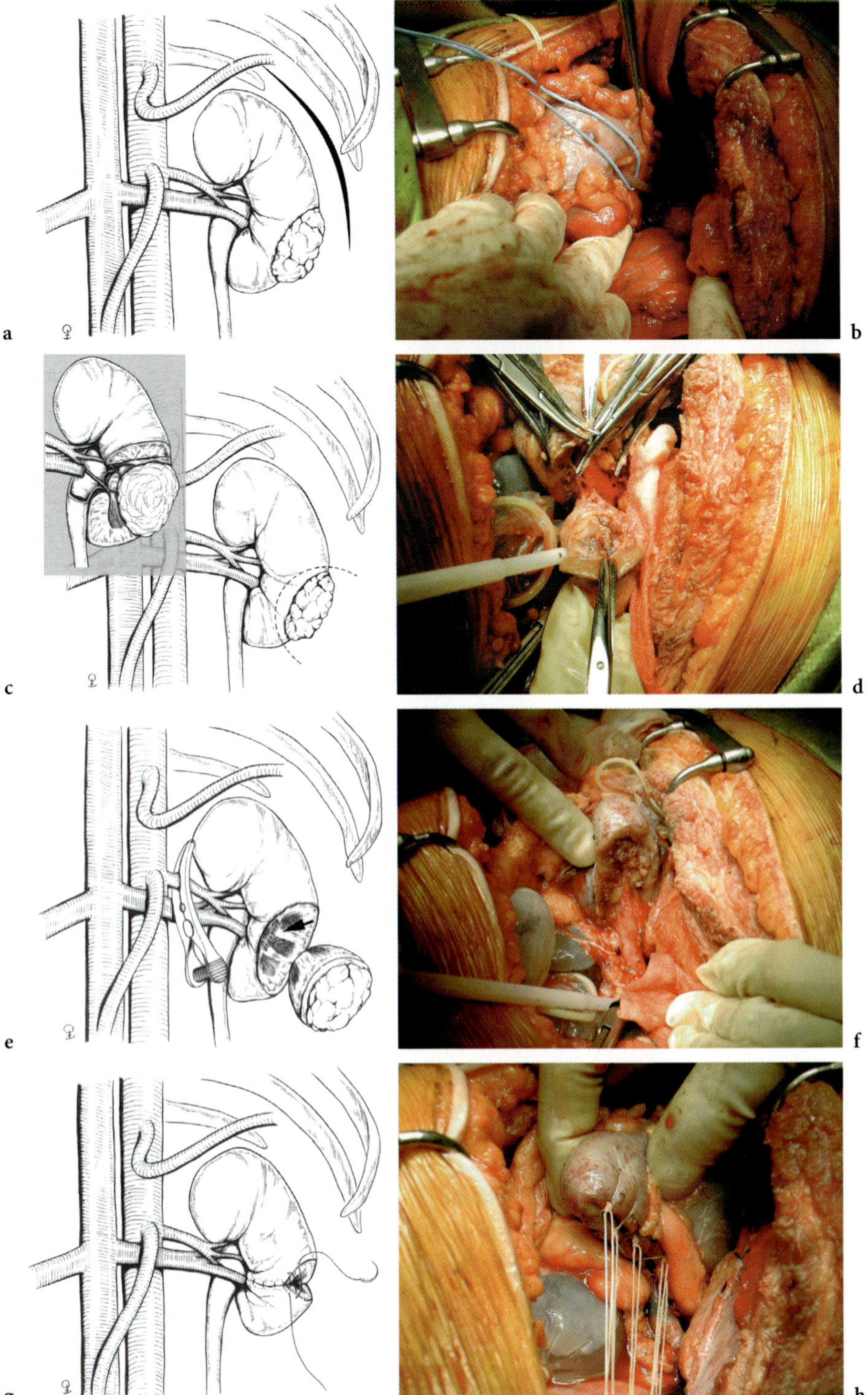

Fig. 23.1a–h. Surgical procedures during nephron-sparing surgery in a 52-year-old woman. **a** Drawing and **b** photograph show the initial surgical approach which usually starts with an extraperitoneal flank incision through the 11th and 12th ribs. **c** Drawing and **d** photograph show that the method of surgical resection is determined based on preoperative evaluation (*dotted line*). The *inset* demonstrates deep extension of the tumor into the kidney delineated by the preoperative imaging. Segmental resection was selected for this patient. **e** Drawing and **f** photograph show the tumor removed with a thin margin of adjacent normal renal parenchyma under temporary arterial occlusion. Watertight closure of the collecting system may be required to prevent urinary fistula formation (*arrow*). **g** Drawing and **h** photograph show the surgical defect closed with a figure-8 suture.

Various surgical resections are possible depending on the location and extension of the tumor (Uzzo and Novick 2001; Ghavamian and Zincke 2001). Although tumor enucleation is performed for localized and superficial tumors, indications are limited because it carries the risk of incomplete tumor resection. In the majority of patients undergoing NSS, excision is performed by wedge or segmental resection with a thin margin of adjacent normal renal parenchyma. Major transverse resection and extracorporeal NSS with autotransplantation are performed in rare cases with exceptionally large and technically challenging tumors. Preoperative planning of resection is particularly critical for patients with tumors approaching the renal sinus. The choice of surgical plane should also be reconsidered against any images just prior to resection during the surgery. In assessing the depth of resection, intraoperative ultrasound is useful for delineating the intrarenal extent of the tumor and its relationship to renal vessels and other critical adjacent structures (Campbell et al. 1996).

Temporary vascular occlusion is performed during the procedure to decrease bleeding and renal tissue turgor (Fig. 23.1e; Uzzo and Novick 2001; Ghavamian and Zincke 2001; Nieder and Taneja 2003). For centrally located tumors invading deeply into the renal parenchyma, the renal vein is also temporarily occluded (Hafez et al. 1998; Chan and Marshall 1999). Renal hypothermia, administration of intravenous mannitol before arterial clamping, and maintenance of venous patency during arterial clamping may be applied simultaneously during arterial clamping to minimize ischemic injury to the kidney (Uzzo and Novick 2001). The length of time of the vascular occlusion should be minimized. Increased duration will lead to increased risk of renal ischemic injury and the need for subsequent hemodialysis. Careful preoperative planning can reduce postoperative complications by minimizing the duration of vascular occlusion. Removal of a centrally located tumor is technically more demanding than removal of a peripheral tumor.

Watertight closure of the collecting system is required to prevent urinary fistula formation (Fig. 23.1e, f). When possible, the collecting system should be dissected and ligated before it is transected to ensure proper closure. Methylene blue is injected into the collecting system to detect urinary leakage (Uzzo et al. 2002).

Finally, the surgical defect is closed carefully after confirming that there is no bleeding or urinary leakage (Fig. 23.1g, h).

23.2.3
Complications

The complex procedures of NSS are associated with several specific complications, as summarized in Table 23.2 (Campbell et al. 1994; Polascik et al. 1995; Duque et al. 1998; Delakas et al. 2002; Ghavamian et al. 2002). Early studies of NSS described a significant risk of complications, and excessive postoperative mortality limited its widespread application. Recent studies have reported a decreased incidence of complications based on proper patient selection, progress in preoperative imaging, improved surgical techniques and postoperative management, and cumulative surgical experience. Surgical mortality is rare, 1.5% or less in most studies.

Acute renal failure is the most common complication of NSS. The risk of acute renal failure has been reported to range from 6 to 17.1%. Most cases of acute renal insufficiency are likely to be temporary and managed by conservative treatment. The need for temporary or permanent dialysis arises in 0–4% of patients. The incidence of acute renal failure may be closely related to indications and selection of patients for the procedure. Risk factors for acute renal failure with the need for dialysis include tumor size greater than 7 cm, excision of more than 50% of parenchyma, and duration of renal ischemia greater than 60 min (Uzzo and Novick 2001; Ghavamian et al. 2002). The risk of acute renal failure with the need for dialysis has significantly decreased according to recent studies, including most patients undergoing elective NSS (Delakas et al. 2002; Ghavamian et al. 2002).

Urinary fistula is another common complication after NSS, with a reported incidence ranging from 1.6 to 17.4%. Recent improvements in technical methods for watertight closure have markedly reduced the incidence of urinary fistulas (Ghavamian et al. 2002). Most urinary fistulas may be managed conservatively by observation, and with catheter insertion of a urethral stent. Percutaneous drainage may be necessary in cases developing large urinoma.

Other reported complications are postoperative hemorrhage (2.4%), infection with or without retroperitoneal abscess (3.2%), injury to adjacent viscera such as the spleen (0.6%), and perioperative medical complications. The reoperative rate after NSS remains low, 0–3% in most series (Uzzo and Novick 2001).

Detailed preoperative planning is absolutely critical for minimizing the risk of complications while maintaining excellent cancer control.

23.2.4
Patient Outcome

Initial interest in NSS for RCC was aroused when the tumor-free survival rate after NSS became comparable to that reported after RN. Many early studies of NSS were limited to high-risk cases in which NSS was the only alternative to renal replacement therapy. An early study by GRABSTALD and AVILES (1968) demonstrated a 77% tumor-free survival rate in patients with a solitary or single functioning kidney. SCHIFF et al. (1979) reported a 78% tumor-free survival rate in patients with absolute indications for NSS. These outcomes were approximately equivalent to those reported for RN (ROBSON et al. 1969). BERG et al. (1981) reviewed the role of NSS for bilateral synchronous RCC, demonstrating improved survival after NSS compared with RN.

Encouraged by these favorable results, technical improvements, and by accumulated surgical experience, the role of NSS was expanded to patients with local RCC. Further studies in a variety of clinical settings demonstrated cancer-specific survivals from 72 to 100%. In recent studies from the late 1990s, when indications for NSS were further refined, disease-specific survival rates exceeded 90% as summarized in Table 23.3.

Recently, FERGANY et al. (2000) reported the 10-year long-term outcome of patients with imperative indications of NSS. Cancer-specific survival was 88.2 and 73% at 5 and 10 years, respectively, with 26% of the patients dying of metastatic disease. Those patients with RCC less than 4 cm showed particularly satisfactory cancer-free survival rates of 98 and 92% at 5 and 10 years, respectively. Many studies have also reported excellent 10-year long-term outcomes with NSS performed in elective indications, resulting in over 95% disease-specific and cancer-free survival rates (FILIPAS et al. 2000; DELAKAS et al. 2002; ZIGEUNER et al. 2003).

Although RN has remained the standard treatment for RCC, many retrospective reviews have assessed the validity of NSS by comparing NSS and RN, controlling for differences in patient age, sex, tumor size, TNM stage, histopathological grade, and tumor location. Many reports have revealed no significant difference in outcome for patients with sporadic, localized, asymptomatic RCC less than 4 cm, and with a normal contralateral kidney (BUTLER et al. 1995; LEE et al. 2000; MARTIN et al. 2002). SHEKARRIZ et al. (2002) reviewed the costs and complications of NSS compared with RN.

Factors affecting the outcome of patients undergoing NSS may be divided into those that influence the risk of local recurrence and those that influence the risk of distant metastasis; the latter is largely due to biological characteristics of the tumor and such factors generally can not be controlled; the former is influenced considerably by the success of tumor resection (DELAKAS et al. 2002; ZIGEUNER et al. 2003). The simultaneous pursuit of complete resection of the tumor and maximal preservation of normal renal parenchyma is tied to improvement of the predictive prognosis of patients; thus, radiological preoperative evaluation for NSS should be more extensive than that for RN.

Table 23.2. Complications of nephron-sparing surgery

Reference	No. of patients	Mortality rate (%)	Acute renal failure (%)	Urinary fistula (%)
GHAVAMIAN et al. (2002)	63	0	12.7	3.2
DELAKAS et al. (2002)	118	0	17.1	1.6
DUQUE et al. (1998)	66	–	15.0	9.1
POLASCIK et al. (1995)	67	1.5	6.0	9.0
CAMPBELL et al. (1994)	259	1.5	12.7	17.4

Table 23.3. Results of nephron-sparing surgery for renal cell carcinoma

Reference	No. of patients	5-year cancer-specific survival (%)	Local recurrence (%)	Follow-up (months)
MORGAN and ZINCKE (1990)	104	89	6	56
STEINBACH et al. (1992)	106	93	2	47
LERNER et al. (2002)	185	89	5.9	44
HAFEZ et al. (1999)	485	92	3.2	47
LEE et al. (2000)	79	96	0	40
FILIPAS et al. (2000)	180	98	1.6	56
DELAKAS et al. (2002)	118	97.3	4	102

23.3
Preoperative Imaging for Nephron-Sparing Surgery

23.3.1
Overview of Preoperative Imaging

Preoperative imaging for RN is performed to assess tumor size, extent, invasion, and distant and/or lymph node metastasis according to the TNM classification, and relevant vascular anatomy.

The greater technical difficulty of NSS requires more detailed preoperative information. Urologists require this information to aid in determining the feasibility of performing NSS, to plan the surgical procedure, and to ensure complete surgical resection of the tumor while maintaining maximum preservation of normal parenchyma (SMITH et al. 1999); thus, the radiologist must provide the surgeon with the following preoperative information: position of the kidney relative to the lower rib cage as it affects the surgical approach; vascular anatomy of the renal artery and vein, especially the segmental arterial supply to the tumor; tumor location and depth of tumor extension into the kidney; and the relationship between the tumor and the collecting system. Such detailed information is essential to minimize the risk of intraoperative and postoperative complications, achieve complete tumor excision with a negative margin, and preserve maximum renal function.

Previously, arteriography and occasionally venography were performed for preoperative evaluation of vasculature, but the role of these modalities in preoperative imaging has been reduced except in special circumstances.

Multiphasic contrast-enhanced computed tomography (CT) imaging has been established as the essential imaging modality for staging and preoperative evaluation of RCC (KOPKA et al. 1997; SZOLAR 1997). The advent of multidetector-row CT (MDCT) technology and advances in the volume data processing workstation have led to frequent clinical application of high-performance three-dimensional (3D) imaging.

Currently, multiphasic contrast-enhanced CT imaging, in combination with 3D volume rendering, is the essential imaging modality for the preoperative evaluation of NSS (COLL et al. 1999).

23.3.2
Multiphasic Contrast-Enhanced CT Imaging

Helical CT is widely used for detection and staging of RCC, as it provides sufficient sensitivity and specificity, cost-effectiveness, and ready accessibility (SHETH et al. 2001). When a patient is referred for NSS, the preoperative imaging demands higher sensitivity to small tumors and more detailed visualization of anatomical structures, despite the added radiation exposure and cost. We perform dedicated multiphasic CT acquisitions in four phases together with volume data acquisition for 3D volume-rendering imaging: a combination of unenhanced CT; corticomedullary phase with 3D volume data acquisition; nephrographic phase; and excretory phase (Fig. 23.2). It is essential to review the original multiphasic CT images for all required information prior to reviewing 3D images, as they may contribute substantially to the preoperative evaluation of NSS.

Currently, MDCT has improved renal imaging, allowing rapid image acquisition covering the entire kidneys during various phases of contrast enhancement after bolus administration of contrast material. The MDCT has brought rapid and extensive changes to the CT protocols, and progress is continuing. We use a 16-channel MDCT scanner for preoperative evaluation of NSS, which can cover a 40-cm scan range in about 20 s.

It is important to understand the beneficial nature of MDCT, as well as its limitations. The superior abilities of MDCT come at the cost of significantly higher radiation exposure to the patient. Also, each examination produces a flood of images which must be reviewed by radiologists. As with any procedure, the expected benefits must be measured against the drawbacks; however, when well planned and appropriately implemented, the MDCT protocol, which varies from one hospital to another, is extremely useful, providing adequate information for NSS while minimizing CT acquisition time and exposure to radiation.

23.3.2.1
Unenhanced CT

Unenhanced CT is used to provide a baseline localization for the subsequent contrast-enhanced series (Fig. 23.2). The possible presence of renal calculus disease should be considered and excluded when reconfirming the diagnosis. Fat within the tumor should not be overlooked, as it is an important clue

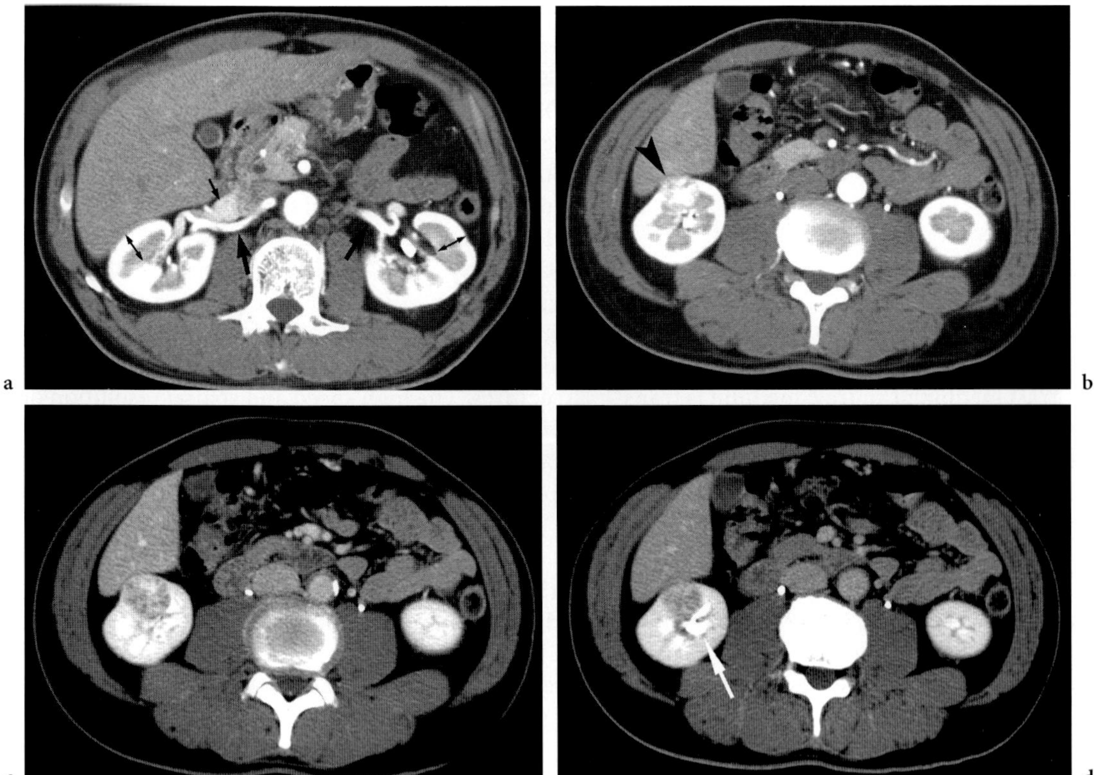

Fig. 23.2a-d. Multiphasic helical CT imaging in a 47-year-old man. **a, b** Axial contrast-enhanced CT scans during the cortico-medullary phase show maximal enhancement of the renal arteries (*large arrows*) and vein (*small arrow*). The tumor also shows strong enhancement (*arrowhead*). Note that the renal cortex and medulla demonstrate sufficient contrast (*two-headed arrows*), depicting deep extension of the tumor into the renal sinus. **c** Axial contrast-enhanced CT scan during the nephrographic phase demonstrates homogeneous enhancement of renal parenchyma. In contrast, enhancement of the tumor has been washed out, demarcating the renal parenchyma. **d** Axial contrast-enhanced CT scan during the excretory phase shows marked excretion of contrast medium into the collecting system (*arrow*), delineating the relationship of the tumor to the collecting system.

for differentiating angiomyolipoma from RCC. With unenhanced CT, a 5-mm slice is enough to localize subsequent series and to identify renal calculi and fat content within the tumor.

23.3.2.2
Corticomedullary Phase

The corticomedullary phase occurs between 25 and 70 s after starting the bolus injection of contrast medium. In this phase, the contrast medium is primarily confined to the cortical capillaries, peritubular spaces, and cortical tubular lamina, and has not yet filtered through the more distal renal tubules (SHETH et al. 2001). The CT images depict maximal enhancement of the renal arteries and veins and marked contrast between the renal cortex and medulla (Fig. 23.2a, b).

The corticomedullary phase is suitable for preoperative navigation of NSS: maximal enhancement of the renal vasculature provides the best opportunity to detect multiple renal arteries and other vascular anomalies, and the contrast between renal cortex and medulla is helpful for assessing the depth of tumor extension into the kidney.

Several pitfalls and limitations of the corticomedullary phase have been reported. A small, hypervascular tumor may occasionally be overlooked because it has enhanced to the same degree as the renal cortex (KOPKA et al. 1997; SZOLAR 1997). A centrally located tumor may be mistaken for the normal, hypoattenuating medulla (YUH and COHAN 1999). Conversely, a heterogeneously enhanced medulla may be mistaken for a renal tumor (SZOLAR 1997, YUH and COHAN 1999).

The corticomedullary phase is simultaneously used for volume data acquisition of 3D imaging.

(The details are described in section 23.2.3.) For the preoperative evaluation, the scanning range must cover from the level of the eleventh rib to the level of the common iliac arteries to prevent missing any polar or accessory renal artery.

23.3.2.3
Nephrographic Phase

The nephrographic phase occurs after at least 80 s and lasts up to 180 s after the start of bolus injection of contrast medium. Contrast medium is transferred through the glomeruli into the loops of Henle and the collecting tubules (SHETH et al. 2001). In the nephrographic phase, the renal parenchyma is enhanced homogeneously, but enhancement of the tumor has been washed out (Fig. 23.2c). The nephrographic phase is more sensitive for detecting small RCC (KOPKA et al. 1997; SZOLAR 1997). The nephrographic phase should be scanned every 3 mm, by CT if it is available, to avoid missing any undetected multicentric small RCC.

23.3.2.4
Excretory Phase

The excretory phase begins approximately 160 s after starting the injection of contrast medium. Contrast medium is excreted into the collecting system in this phase (Fig. 23.2d). The excretory phase delineates the relationship of the tumor with the collecting system, which is especially useful for centrally located tumors invading deeply into the kidney and for managing the collecting system (SHETH et al. 2001).

Recently, some reports have demonstrated the usefulness of intravenous CT urography for benign urinary tract disease (McTAVISH et al. 2002). This CT urographic technique – volume-rendering CT imaging during the excretory phase – can be applied to preoperative evaluation of NSS, allowing 3D visualization of the relationship between the collecting system and the tumor.

23.3.3
Three-Dimensional CT Imaging

Many reports have emphasized the usefulness of intravenous 3D volume-rendering CT imaging for preoperative evaluation of NSS, as it integrates essential information from angiography, venography, excretory urography, and conventional 2D CT into a single preoperative staging test (SMITH et al. 1999; COLL et al. 1999; WUNDERLICH et al. 2000; REMER et al. 2002, DERWEESH et al. 2003). The 3D imaging allows interactive stereoscopic viewing of complex anatomy from various viewpoints, delineating the tumor and its relationship to the renal surface, vascular anatomy, collecting system, and adjacent structures.

Currently, MDCT is quite useful for 3D imaging, allowing rapid image acquisition covering a wide range over the whole abdomen during optimal timing of contrast enhancement of the target structures. The high speed and spatial resolution of MDCT, and hardware advances in the volume data processing workstation, have led to frequent clinical application of 3D volume-rendering imaging.

23.3.3.1
Data Acquisition Technique

The quality of 3D volume-rendered images depends largely on the contrast of CT attenuation between the target structures and surrounding tissues. Optimizing CT volume data acquisition is necessary to acquire 3D images of excellent quality. This optimization carries implications for the hemodynamics of contrast medium administration.

The 3D imaging for preoperative evaluation of NSS is useful for assessing renal vasculatures, location and extension of tumor, and the collecting system. The protocol of contrast medium administration and the scan delay for data acquisition should be designed to provide appropriate contrast enhancement for these structures according to the contrast medium transit time.

A high level of enhancement is necessary for visualizing small accessory or polar arteries and intrarenal branches. As the degree of arterial enhancement is proportional to the iodine administration rate, a high injection flow rate is needed (FLEISCHMANN 2003). Because the duration of maximal arterial enhancement is closely tied to the duration of the administration of contrast medium, the bolus injection should continue beyond the scanning time for 3D data acquisition so that homogeneous enhancement is maintained throughout the scan. We use 120-ml bolus injection of 300 mg iodine/ml of contrast medium at a rate of 4.5 ml/s. With this protocol of contrast-enhanced administration, renal arteries and veins maintain their peak enhancement from approximately 20–40 and 25–50 s, respectively, from the beginning of the bolus injection.

To determine the depth of the tumor extension into the kidney, the renal cortex should be enhanced while maintaining proper contrast in the renal medulla. Their contrast is continued during the corticomedullary phase, occurring between 25 and 70 s. Since the contrast between artery and renal cortex and the contrast between renal cortex and medulla decreases later in the phase, CT acquisition should be completed within 50 s from the start of the injection.

Some institutions use a test bolus injection technique or automated bolus triggering technique to determine the scan delay (COLL et al. 1999). Despite their usefulness, we have not adopted these techniques. A test bolus injection technique finds the time for scan delay from sequential image acquisition, adding additional radiation exposure for the patients. Automated bolus-triggering techniques detect the arrival of contrast medium in the artery of interest, but are not entirely reliable, and sometimes fail to trigger.

Figure 23.3 illustrates our protocol of 3D volume-rendering CT imaging. For preoperative evaluation of NSS, we perform volume data acquisition for 3D volume rendering together with multiphasic CT in the corticomedullary phase using a 16-channel MDCT scanner. The scanning parameters are: 120 kVp; 250–320 mA; 16×0.625-mm with beam width of 10 mm; beam pitch of 1.375:1.0; and reconstruction thickness of 1.25 mm. With 16-channel MDCT scanners, a 40-cm scan range can be covered in about 20 s. We set 30 s for the mean scan delay from the start of bolus injection. In this phase, renal arteries and veins show superior enhancement to the renal cortex and, simultaneously, the cortex maintains proper contrast to the medulla.

Urographic imaging of the collecting system is obtained in the excretory phase. With a single bolus injection, vascular structures and the collecting system must be evaluated with separate images in the different phases. We perform a time-lapse dual-phase infusion of contrast medium: 30 ml of contrast medium is administered 5 min before the bolus injection, which results in satisfactory urographic opacification of the collecting system while maintaining high opacification of vascular structures. This integrates the preoperative information for visualizing the vascular structures and collecting system simultaneously on a 3D image. Although the technique cannot evaluate renal calculus disease, this is rarely critical in clinical applications because renal calculus diseases have already been evaluated in most patients referred for NSS.

23.3.3.2
Volume-Rendering Processing

Volume-rendering processing is the latest 3D imaging technique (CALHOUN et al. 1999, COLL et al. 1999). Two factors are essential for volume-rendering processing: the opacity curve for the volume data and the visualization method for display.

The 3D volume image is generated by summing the contributions from all the voxels along a line from any viewing angle through the volume data set of sequential CT images. Each set of data is assigned an opacity that determines its contributions to the sum, expressed as a percentage from 0 to 100%.

Volume rendering retains all the CT data during processing and requires no preliminary editing;

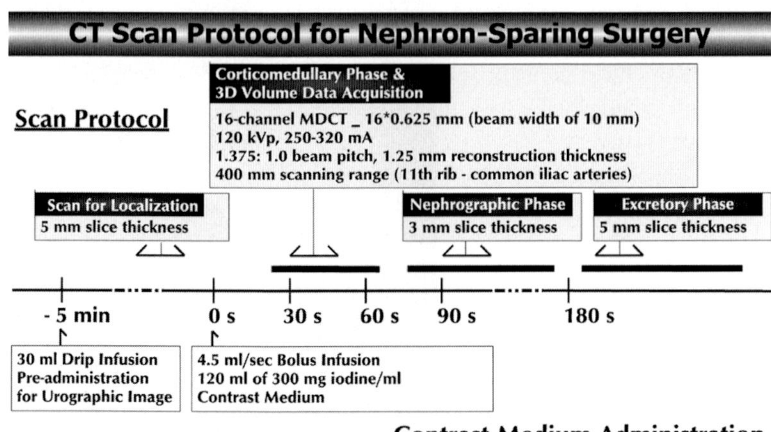

Fig. 23.3. The CT scan protocol for nephron-sparing surgery.

therefore, the resulting 3D image potentially conserves all the information from the original CT data during the processing. In contrast, other 3D processing techniques, such as shaded-surface display and maximum intensity projection (MIP), trim large parts of the voxel information and use only a small fraction of the original volume data during the process to generate and display images.

Optimization of the opacity setting is the cornerstone of volume-rendering processing, and is closely associated with that of contrast enhancement of the target structures. Adequate contrast enhancement and optimal opacity determination will produce homogeneous, high-quality generated 3D images. Rendering parameters consist of settings for opacity and color. For the opacity setting, a linear, ramp-shaped curve is used to set the upper- and lower-cutoff CT attenuation points at 0 and 100% opacity (CALHOUN 1999). Another advanced means of determining rendering parameters is the multiangular opacity curve, in which multiple segments of opacity curves with different gradients are combined (CALHOUN 1999). This method depends on the assumption that the voxel histogram of the volume data set is composed of the sum of the Gaussian distribution of intensities for given structures. Although further research is needed, this method is useful for emphasizing the target structure while decreasing the opacity of surrounding tissue. While the influence of color determination on the 3D visualization has not been fully established, color display of 3D images is widely used in routine clinical applications.

As we recognize the position information through visual perception, the volume data within the 3D vector space on the workstation has to be projected as a picture or on a computer monitor. This "virtual" display of 3D volume data on a 2D plane is called the "rendering method." Various rendering methods and tools are available depending on the clinical situation. Standard "3D imaging" is one of the rendering methods which present a view of the volume data from outside the body. The volume data can be observed from various viewpoints (Fig. 23.4). The clip plane tool can remove a segment of volume from the whole volume data (Fig. 23.5). Because many renal structures are covered with a markedly enhancing volume of renal cortex, the clip plane tool is particularly useful for renal 3D imaging as

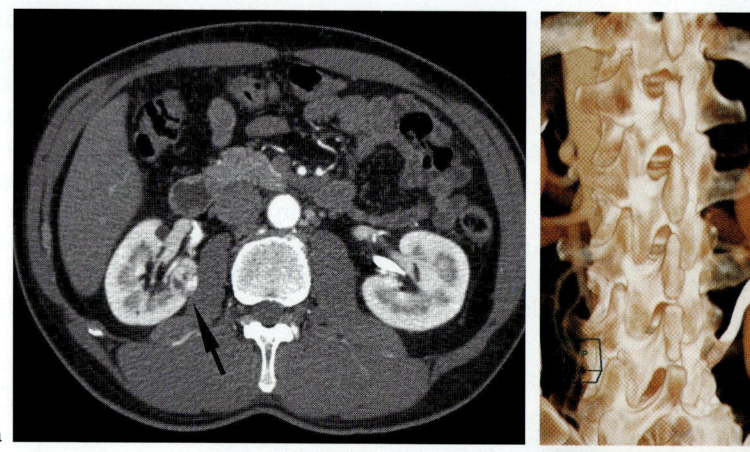

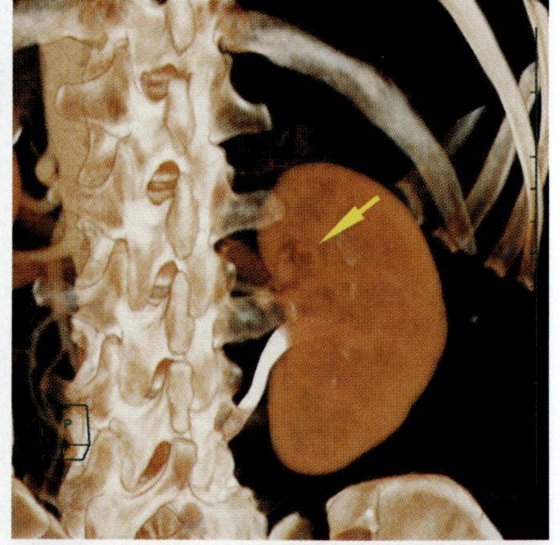

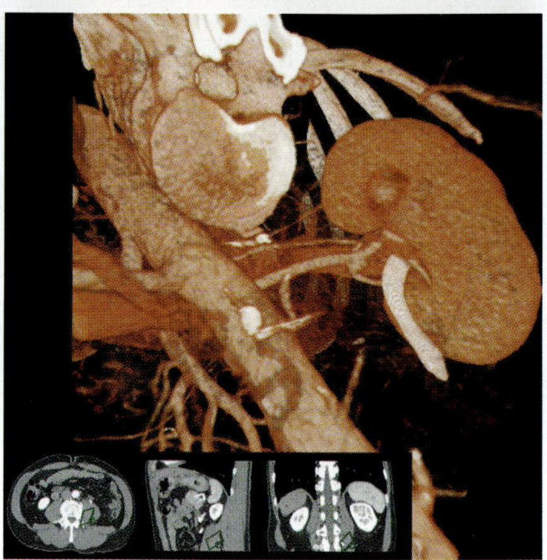

Fig. 23.4a-c. Various 3D volume-rendering displays in a 55-year-old man. **a** Axial contrast-enhanced CT scan and **b** 3D image from the posterior view demonstrate a medially located renal tumor (*arrow*) on the dorsal side of the kidney. The volume data can be projected from **c** the viewpoint inside of the volume, so-called virtual endoscopic display.

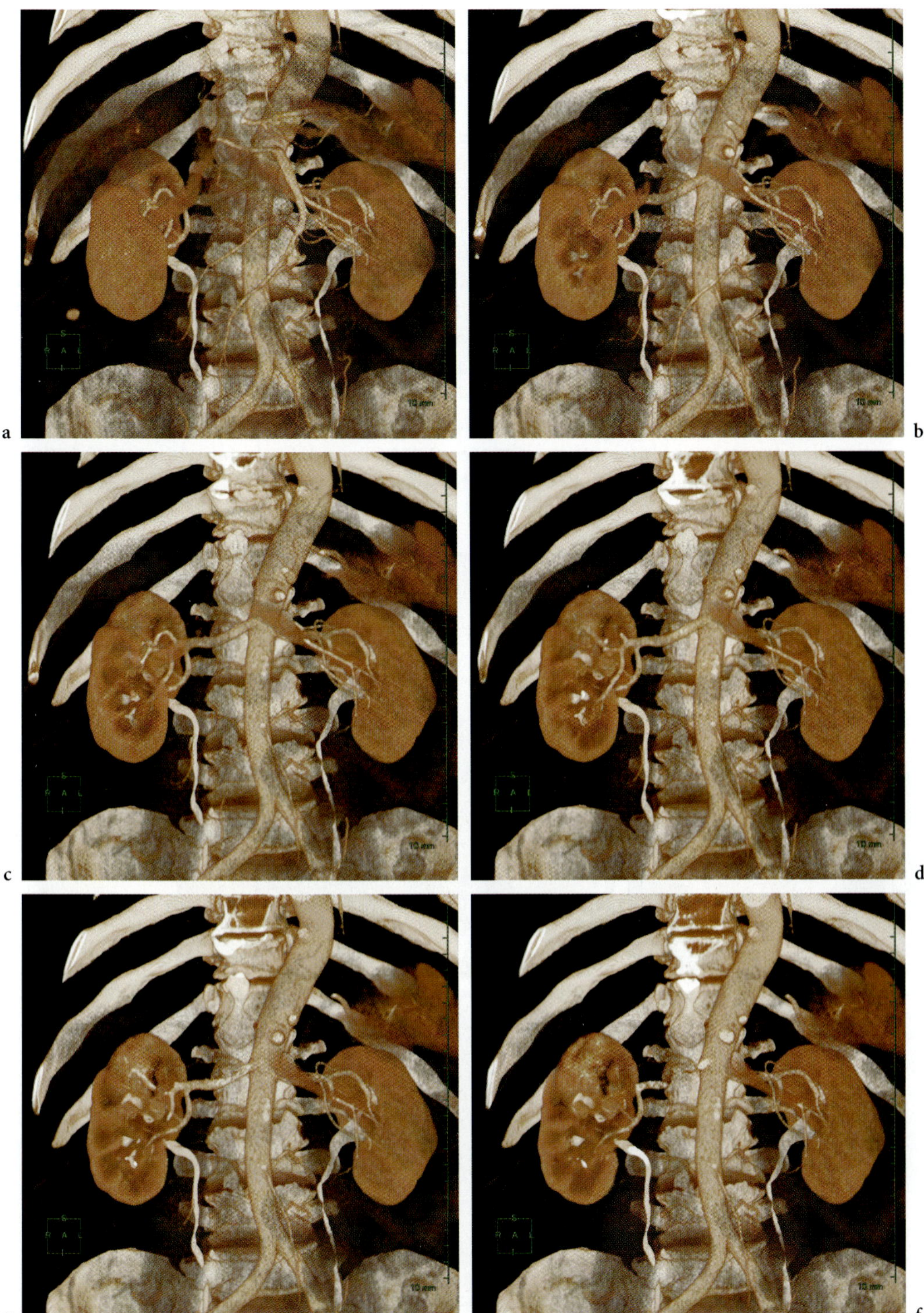

Fig. 23.5a-f. Sequential scrolling images using the clip plane tool in a 73-year-old man. **a–f** A series of 3D images visualizes the intrarenal structures, scrolling the cut planes back and forth. We generated 3D images as a video file of continuous images, as well as static print images.

it permits visualization of inner structures lying deeper within the volume. Currently, advances in 3D workstation hardware have enabled interactive settings of viewpoints and clip planes without a time lag for visualization. "Virtual endoscopic imaging" is another method of 3D volume-rendering display which presents a view of the volume data from inside the body. Virtual endoscopic imaging is helpful, especially for preoperative simulation of laparoscopic nephrectomy and laparoscopic NSS (MARUKAWA et al. 2002).

Generated 3D volume-rendered images can be formatted as a movie-like stream of continuous images, scrolling viewpoints, and cut planes (Fig. 23.5), as well as conventional static print images. This cinematic output enhances the advantages of interactive processing in 3D volume-rendering imaging.

23.3.4
Intra-arterial Three-Dimensional CT Angiography

Unlike the removal of small, peripheral tumors, which are found in a large proportion of cases, the higher risk of removing a centrally located tumor demands detailed preoperative assessment of intrarenal structures (CHAN and MARSHALL 1999; COLL et al. 1999). Nevertheless, segmental arterial branches sometimes fail to appear in patients with large and/or centrally located tumors. To solve this problem, some institutions add angiography to preoperative imaging for centrally located tumors (COLL et al. 1999).

For such centrally and/or medially located tumors, we use intra-arterial 3D volume-rendering CT angiography (Fig. 23.6). The CT volume data acquisition

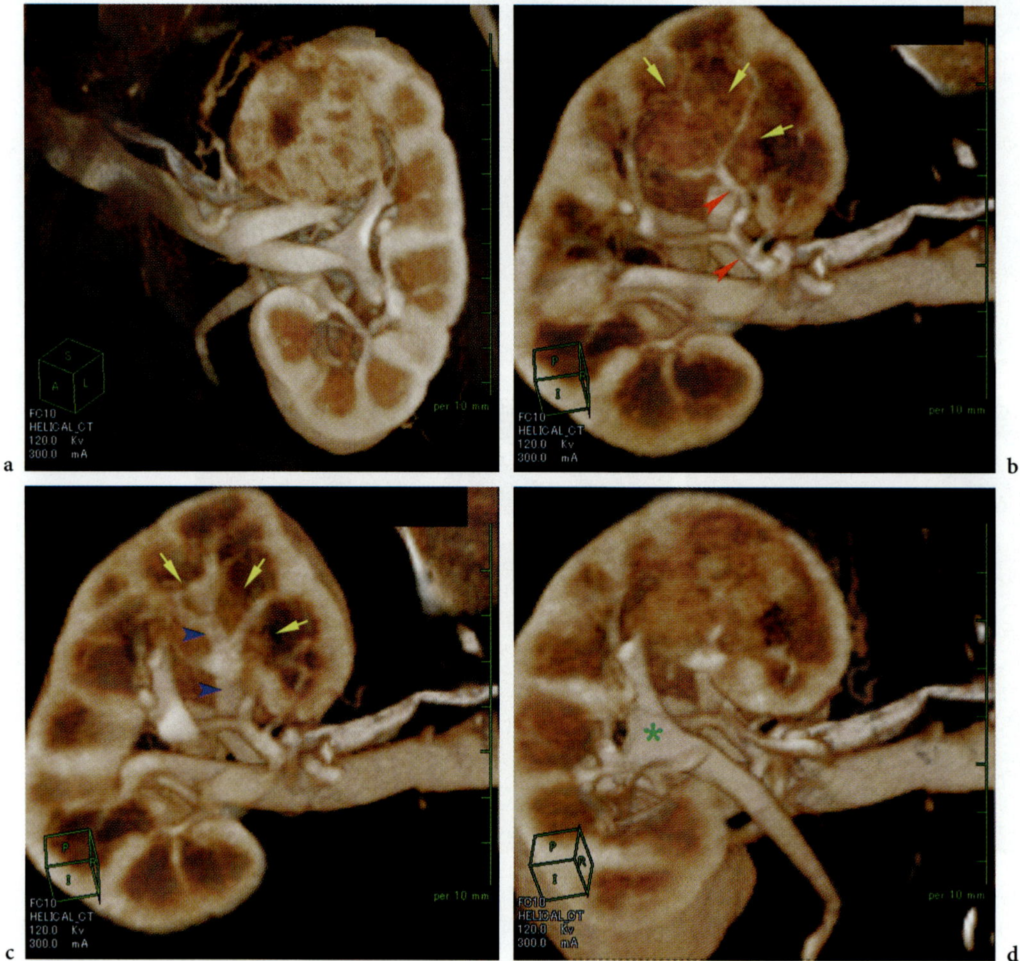

Fig. 23.6a–d. Intra-arterial 3D CT angiography in a 64-year-old man. **a** A 3D image from anterior view shows a large and centrally located renal tumor deeply extending into renal sinus. **b–d** Sequential scrolling 3D images using the cut-plane tool demonstrates the tumor (*arrows*) in relation to the intrarenal segments of the renal artery (*red arrowheads*), renal vein (*blue arrowheads*), and the collecting system (*asterisk*).

is performed with a selective renal angiographic technique using combined digital subtraction angiography and an MDCT system. For visualizing the collecting system, CT urographic technique is combined with 3D angiography under a time-lapse dual phase infusion of contrast medium. Despite some potential pitfalls and invasiveness, this intra-arterial 3D CT angiography delineates the detailed intrarenal segment of renal vasculature and tumor blood supply. For large and/or centrally located tumors, it is helpful for the guidance of tumor excision and for minimizing the complications of hemorrhage and ischemic injury (UEDA et al 2004).

23.4
Clinical Applications of Preoperative Imaging

23.4.1
Renal Position

For the initial surgical approach, urologists generally choose an extraperitoneal flank incision through the eleventh and twelfth ribs. Preoperative navigation using 3D images assists urologists to decide on the location and extent of the initial incision. The 3D imaging demonstrates the location of the kidney in relation to the lower rib cage. For this purpose, we provide two types of 3D imaging displays from the posterior view: an opaque image with visualization of the abdominal wall and a transparent image with visualization of the kidney and lower ribs (Fig. 23.7).

23.4.2
Vascular Anatomy

It is important to determine variants and identify the segmental arterial supply to the tumor before surgery. The 3D volume-rendering CT angiography allows preoperative evaluation of such anatomical information, delineating the main renal arteries with almost 100% sensitivity (PLATT et al. 1997). Arterial branches can usually be identified to the segmental level (WUNDERLICH et al. 2000; URBAN et al. 2001).

Variants of the renal artery are common, occurring in approximately 25% of all individuals (URBAN et al. 2001). Preoperative identification of arterial variants is crucial because failure to do so is directly linked to bleeding during surgery. Multiple renal arteries occur in 15% of all individuals (Fig. 23.8). Accessory arteries usually arise from the aorta or iliac arteries, from the level of the eleventh thoracic vertebra to the level of the fourth lumbar spine. The scanning range should include this area to avoid missing any aberrant accessory arteries. Accessory vessels usually course into the renal hilum to perfuse the upper or lower renal poles. Uncommonly, an aberrant artery may enter the kidney directly through an accessory renal hilum. Perihilar branching and early branching of the renal artery are other common variants (Fig. 23.8).

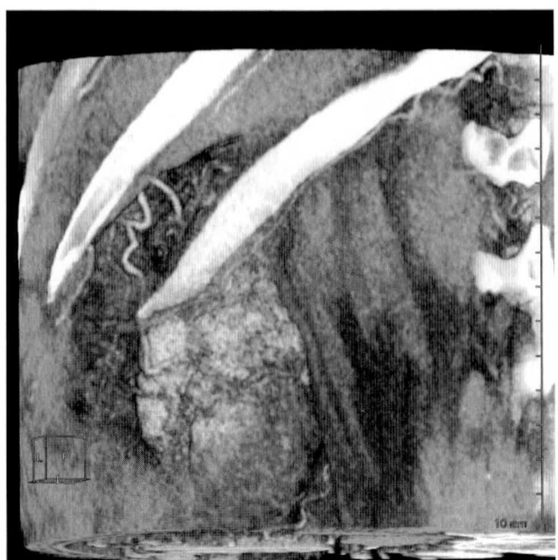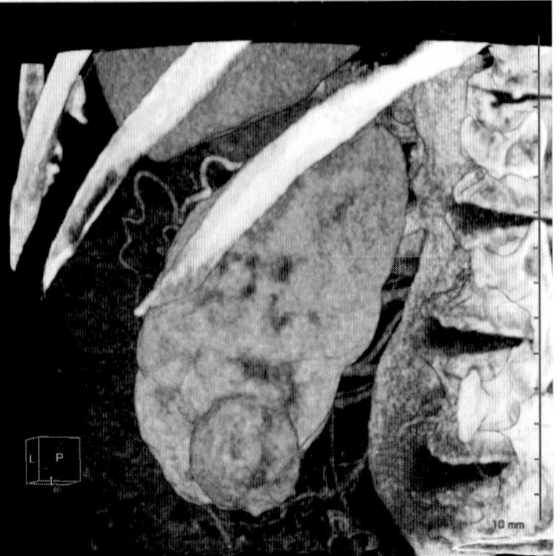

Fig. 23.7a,b. Navigation of initial excision in a 62-year-old man. **a** Opaque and **b** transparent 3D images navigate the initial surgical approach, depicting the kidney and the tumor in relation to the abdominal wall and lower ribs.

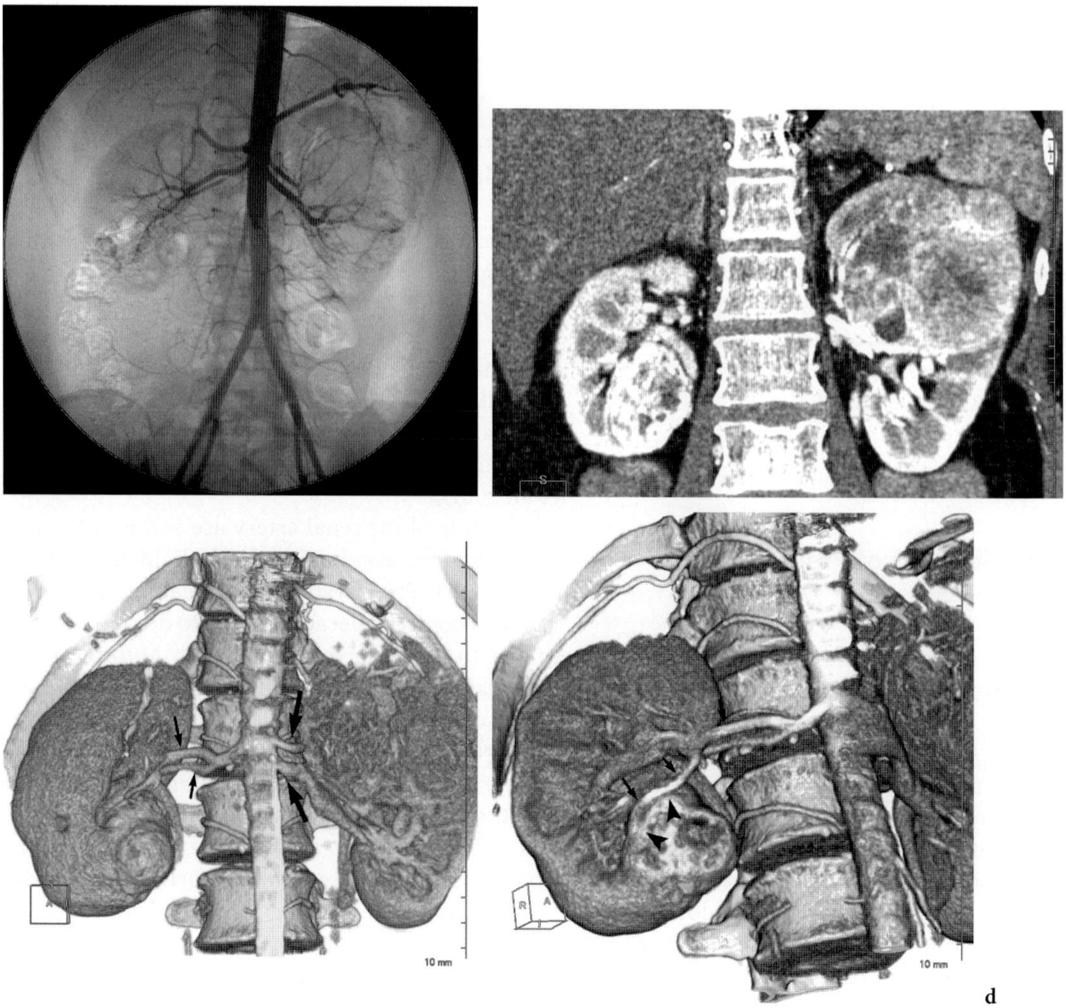

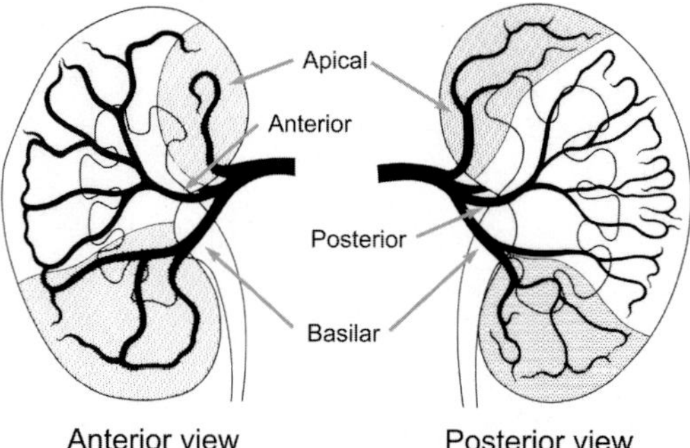

Fig. 23.8a-d. Variants of renal artery in a 52-year-old woman. **a** Anteroposterior aortography shows early branching of right renal artery and left double renal arteries. **b** Coronal contrast-enhanced CT image by multiplanar reconstruction shows bilateral synchronous renal cell carcinomas. **c** A 3D volume-rendering CT image demonstrates arterial variants of double renal arteries of the left kidney (*large arrows*) and early branching of the right renal artery (*small arrows*). **d** A 3D image using cut-plane tool demonstrates the basilar branch from the early branch (*arrows*), running adjacent to and supplying the tumor (*arrowheads*).

The kidney has four vascular regions: apical; anterior; posterior; and basilar (Fig. 23.9). One or more segmental branches are at the end of the supply of each of these regions. These segmented arteries are end arteries with little or no collateral blood flow between them (COLL et al. 1999). Knowledge of the segmental arterial supply to the tumor obviates ligation of the segmental artery supplying normal parenchyma and minimizes the risk for renal insufficiency. For centrally located tumors, detailed understanding of the segmental vascular anatomy is crucial for reducing their higher risk of vascular transection. We perform intra-arterial 3D CT angiography for centrally located tumors (Fig. 23.6).

Fig. 23.9. Drawing of the segmental arterial anatomy. Anterior (*left*) and posterior (*right*) views illustrate four segmental branches: apical; anterior; posterior; and basilar. Each shared vascular supply is expressed as the *shaded* and *white* region of the kidney.

Multiple renal veins are the most common variant, occurring in approximately 30% of all individuals (Fig. 23.10). A circumaortic renal vein is another common variant.

23.4.3
Tumor Location and Extension

The urologist must choose a method of tumor resection that balances the goals of maximal preservation of renal parenchyma, minimizing the risk of complications, and controlling the cancer without residual tumor. Careful preoperative evaluation of tumor location and extension ensures complete tumor excision and preservation of renal function. A small and peripherally located tumor (Fig. 23.11) that is localized to the renal cortex presents no serious difficulty for surgical resection and carries less risk of complications. Arterial clamping may not be required in many cases. In contrast, a large and centrally located tumor (Fig. 23.12) extending deeply into the renal sinus is technically demanding. A centrally located tumor may require ligation of segmental vessels supplying the tumor and watertight closure of the collecting system, and preoperative evaluation must rely on careful investigation of the segmental vascular anatomy and deep extension in relation to the renal calyces (Fig. 23.6). A medially located tumor (Fig. 23.13) located near the renal hilum is also technically demanding. The close proximity to the renal hilum poses a risk of transection of the major renal vasculature and the renal pelvis.

The 3D imaging readily demonstrates the orientation and depth of extension of the tumor into the kidney, and its spatial relationship to surrounding structures. A cinematic display of sequential scrolling using the clip plane tool is helpful for evaluating the deep extension of the tumor into the kidney.

23.4.4
Relationship to Collecting System

Detection of calyces adjacent to the tumor indicates the need for a watertight closure of the collecting system. This helps to minimize postoperative com-

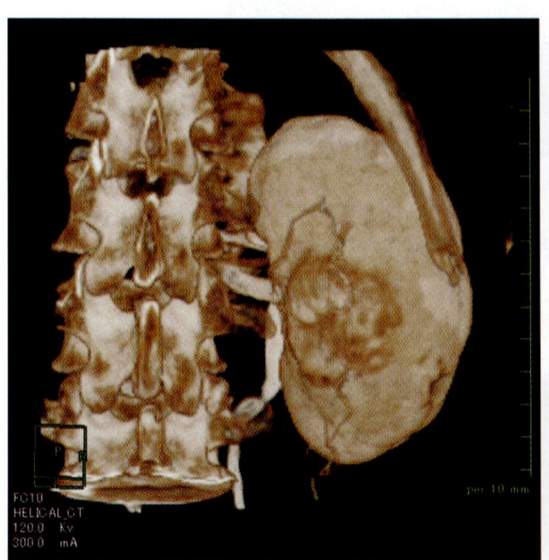

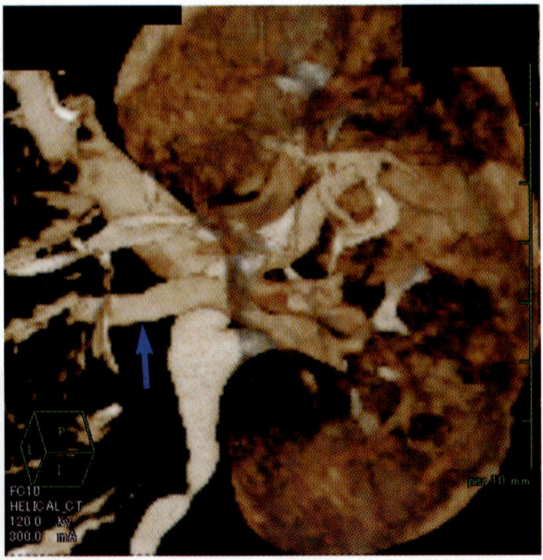

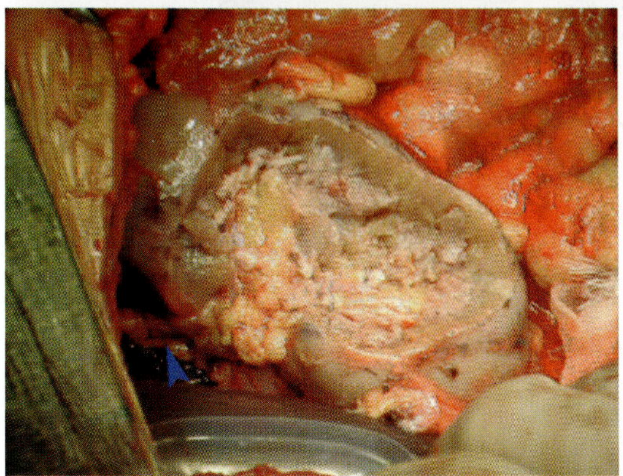

Fig. 23.10a–c. Variants of renal vein in a 69-year-old man. **a** Intra-arterial 3D CT angiography from posterior view demonstrates a large and centrally located renal tumor. **b** After volume of the tumor is removed using the cut plane tool, one branch of double renal veins is visualized immediately adjacent to the tumor (*arrow*). **c** Photograph shows this variant confirmed during the surgery (*arrowhead*).

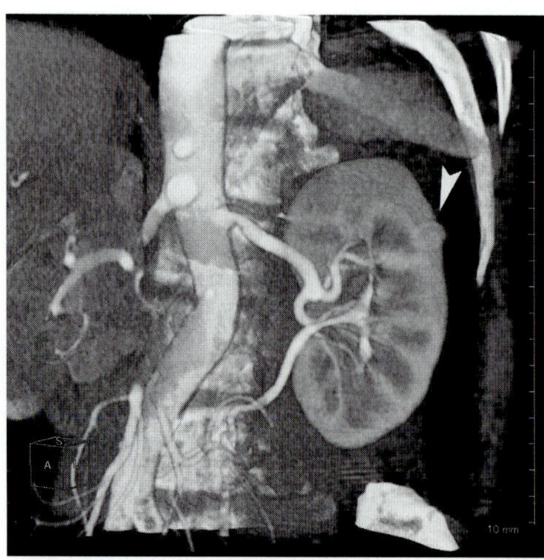

Fig. 23.11. Peripherally located renal cell carcinoma in a 60-year-old man. Coronal 3D image using cut-plane tool shows a small and peripherally located tumor (*arrowhead*) which is an ideal indication for nephron-sparing surgery.

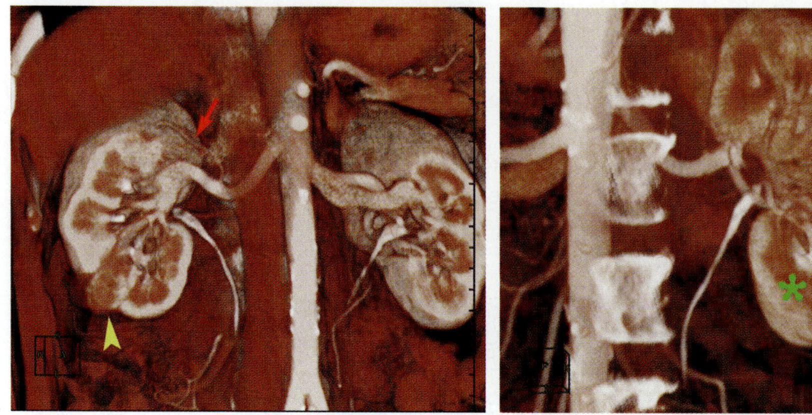

Fig. 23.12a,b. Centrally located renal cell carcinoma in a 62-year-old man. **a** Intravenous 3D volume-rendering CT from anterior view demonstrates a centrally located tumor (*arrowhead*) extending deeply into the renal sinus. An accessory upper polar branch of the right renal artery (*arrow*) is also depicted. **b** A 3D image from posterior view delineates the relationship of the tumor (*arrowheads*) with collecting system (*asterisk*).

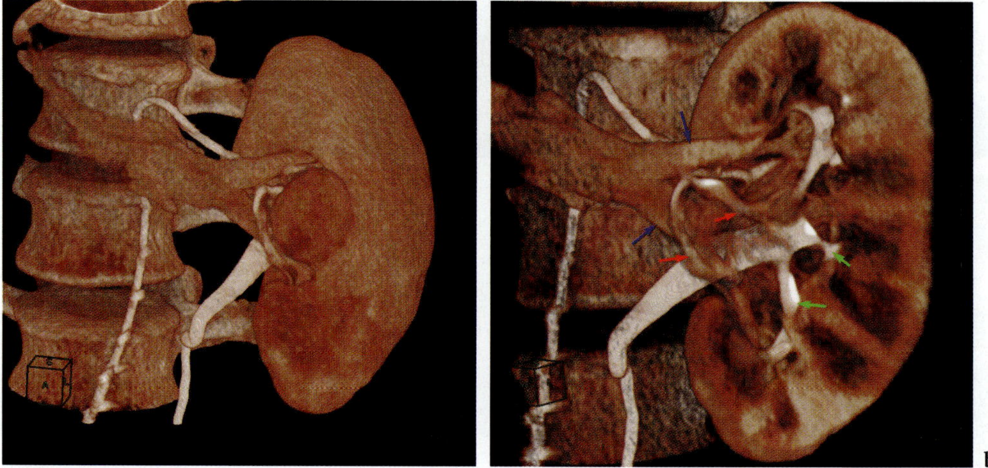

Fig. 23.13a,b. Medially located renal cell carcinoma in a 42-year-old woman. **a** Intra-arterial 3D CT angiography demonstrates a medially located renal cell carcinoma adjacent to the renal hilum. **b** The cut-plane tool delineates the segmental branches of renal artery (*red arrows*) and vein (*blue arrows*) and the collecting system (*green arrows*) behind the tumor.

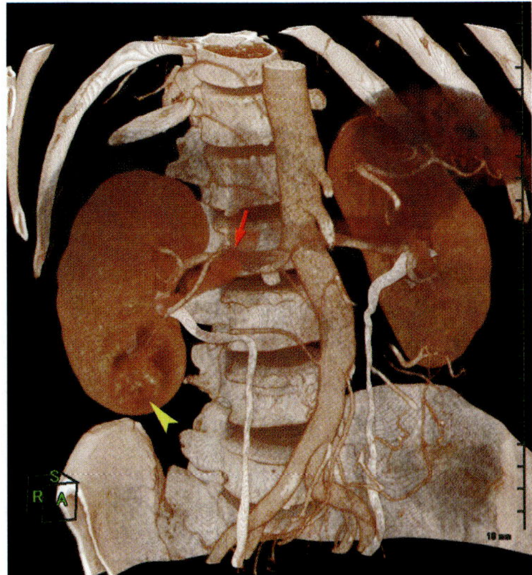
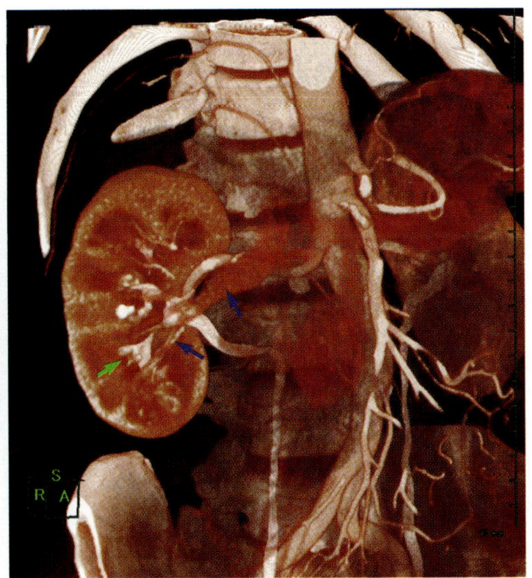

a   b

Fig. 23.14a,b. Relationship to the collecting system in a 56-year-old man. **a** Intravenous 3D volume-rendering CT images demonstrates a centrally located tumor (*arrowhead*) and early branching of the right renal artery (*arrow*). **b** A time-lapse dual-phase technique enables simultaneous visualization of the vascular anatomy of renal artery and vein (*blue arrows*), the tumor, and the collecting system (*green arrow*).

plications of urinary fistula and the time needed for reconstruction of the collecting system.

Urographic imaging of the collecting system is obtained in the excretory phase of contrast enhancement. Using the standard technique with single bolus injection, vascular structures and the collecting system are evaluated with separate images in different phases. We use a time-lapse dual phase technique for 3D imaging. This integrates the preoperative information of the vascular structures and collecting system simultaneously on a 3D image (Fig. 23.14).

23.5
Conclusion

Nephron-sparing surgery has demonstrated satisfactory cancer control and patient satisfaction. Long-term functional advantages are gained by the maximal preservation of normal renal parenchyma. Multiphasic contrast-enhanced CT in combination with 3D volume-rendering CT imaging has become established as the essential imaging modality for preoperative evaluation of NSS, providing sufficient evidence of sensitivity and specificity of RCC, cost-effectiveness, and ready accessibility. By having a better understanding of the indications, procedures, complications, and factors affecting patient outcome, radiologists can provide urologists with essential information for the preoperative planning of NSS.

Acknowledgements
We thank R. Ishimura for drawing the medical illustrations.

References

Baltaci S, Orhan D, Soyupek S et al. (2000) Influence of tumor stage, size, grade, vascular involvement, histological cell type and histological pattern on multifocality of renal cell carcinoma. J Urol 164:36–39

Butler BP, Novick AC, Miller DP et al. (1995) Management of small unilateral renal cell carcinomas: radical versus nephron-sparing surgery. Urology 45:34–31

Calhoun PS, Kuszyk BS, Heath DG et al. (1999) Three-dimensional volume rendering of spiral CT data: theory and method. Radiographics 19:745–764

Campbell SC, Novick AC, Streem SB et al. (1994) Complications of nephron sparing surgery for renal tumors. J Urol 151:1177–1180

Campbell SC, Fichtner J, Novick AC et al. (1996) Intraoperative evaluation of renal cell carcinoma: a prospective study of the role of ultrasonography and histopathological frozen sections. J Urol 155:1191–1195

Chan DY, Marshall FF (1999) Partial nephrectomy for centrally located tumors. Urology 54:1088–1082

Coll DM, Uzzo RG, Herts BR et al. (1999) 3-dimensional volume rendered computerized tomography for preoperative evaluation and intraoperative treatment of patients undergoing nephron sparing surgery. J Urol 161:1097–1102

Czerny HE (1890) Ueber Nierenextirpation. Beitr Klin Chir 6:484–486

Delakas D, Karyotis I, Daskalopoulos G et al. (2002) Nephron-sparing surgery for localized renal cell carcinoma with a normal contralateral kidney: a European three-center experience. Urology 60:998–1002

Derweesh IH, Herts B, Novick AC (2003) Three-dimensional image reconstruction for preplanning of renal surgery. Urol Clin North Am 30:515–528

Duque JL, Loughlin KR, O'Leary MP et al. (1998) Partial nephrectomy: alternative treatment for selected patients with renal cell carcinoma. Urology 52:584–590

Fergany AF, Hafez KS, Novick AC (2000) Long-term results of nephron sparing surgery for localized renal cell carcinoma: 10-year followup. J Urol 163:442–445

Filipas D, Fichtner J, Spix C et al. (2000) Nephron-sparing surgery of renal cell carcinoma with a normal opposite kidney: long-term outcome in 180 patients. Urology 56:387–392

Fleischmann D (2003) Renal vessels. In: Bonomo L, Foley DW, Imhof H, Rubin G (eds) Multidetector computed tomography: advances in imaging techniques, 1st edn. Royal Society of Medicine Press Ltd, London, pp 79–89

Gacci M, Rizzo M, Lapini A et al. (2001) Imperative indications for conservative surgery for renal cell carcinoma: 20 years' experience. Urol Int 67:203–208

Ghavamian R, Zincke H (2001) Open surgical partial nephrectomy. Semin Urol Oncol 19:103–113

Ghavamian R, Cheville JC, Lohse CM et al. (2002) Renal cell carcinoma in the solitary kidney: an analysis of complications and outcome after nephron sparing surgery. J Urol 168:454–459

Grabstald H, Aviles E (1968) Renal cancer in the solitary or sole-functioning kidney. Cancer 22:973–987

Hafez KS, Novick AC, Butler BP (1998) Management of small solitary unilateral renal cell carcinomas: impact of central versus peripheral tumor location. J Urol 159:1156–1160

Hafez KS, Fergany AF, Novick AC (1999) Nephron sparing surgery for localized renal cell carcinoma: impact of tumor size on patient survival, tumor recurrence and TNM staging. J Urol 162:1930–1933

Kopka L, Fischer U, Zoeller G et al. (1997) Dual-phase helical CT of the kidney: value of the corticomedullary and nephrographic phase for evaluation of renal lesions and preoperative staging of renal cell carcinoma. Am J Roentgenol 169:1573–1578

Lee CT, Katz J, Shi W et al. (2000) Surgical management of renal tumors 4 cm or less in a contemporary cohort. J Urol 163:730–736

Lerner SE, Hawkins CA, Blute ML et al. (2002) Disease outcome in patients with low stage renal cell carcinoma treated with nephron sparing or radical surgery. 1996. J Urol 167:884–890

Marukawa K, Horiguchi J, Shigeta M et al. (2002) Three-dimensional navigator for retroperitoneal laparoscopic nephrectomy using multidetector row computerized tomography. J Urol 168:1933–1936

Matin SF, Gill IS, Worley S et al. (2002) Outcome of laparoscopic radical and open partial nephrectomy for the sporadic 4 cm or less renal tumor with a normal contralateral kidney. J Urol 168:1356–1360

McTavish JD, Jinzaki M, Zou KH et al. (2002) Multi-detector row CT urography: comparison of strategies for depicting the normal urinary collecting system. Radiology 225:783–790

Morgan WR, Zincke H (1990) Progression and survival after renal-conserving surgery for renal cell carcinoma: experience in 104 patients and extended followup. J Urol 144:852–858

Nieder AM, Taneja SS (2003) The role of partial nephrectomy for renal cell carcinoma in contemporary practice. Urol Clin North Am 30:529–542

Platt JF, Ellis JH, Korobkin M et al. (1997) Helical CT evaluation of potential kidney donors: findings in 154 subjects. Am J Roentgenol 169:1325–1330

Polascik TJ, Pound CR, Meng MV et al. (1995) Partial nephrectomy: technique, complications and pathological findings. J Urol 154:1312–1318

Remer EM, Herts BR, Veniero JC (2002) Imaging for nephron-sparing surgery. Semin Urol Oncol 20:180–191

Robson CJ, Churchill BM, Anderson W (1969) The results of radical nephrectomy for renal cell carcinoma. J Urol 101:297–301

Schiff M, Bagley DH, Lytton B (1979) Treatment of solitary and bilateral renal carcinomas. J Urol 121:581

Schlichter A, Wunderlich H, Junker K et al. (2000) Where are the limits of elective nephron-sparing surgery in renal cell carcinoma? Eur Urol 37:517–520

Shekarriz B, Upadhyay J, Shekarriz H et al. (2002) Comparison of costs and complications of radical and partial nephrectomy for treatment of localized renal cell carcinoma. Urology 59:211–215

Sheth S, Scatarige JC, Horton KM et al. (2001) Current concepts in the diagnosis and management of renal cell carcinoma: role of multidetector CT and three-dimensional CT. Radiographics 21:237–254

Shinohara N, Harabayashi T, Sato S et al. (2001) Impact of nephron-sparing surgery on quality of life in patients with localized renal cell carcinoma. Eur Urol 39:114–119

Smith PA, Marshall FF, Corl FM et al. (1999) Planning nephron-sparing renal surgery using 3D helical CT angiography. J Comput Assist Tomogr 23:649–654

Steinbach F, Stockle M, Muller SC et al. (1992) Conservative surgery of renal cell tumors in 140 patients: 21 years of experience. J Urol 148:24–30

Szolar DH, Kammerhuber F, Altziebler S et al. (1997) Multiphasic helical CT of the kidney: increased conspicuity for detection and characterization of small (<3 cm) renal masses. Radiology 202:211–217

Ueda T, Tobe T, Yamamoto S et al. (2004) Selective intra-arterial 3-dimensional computed tomography angiography for preoperative evaluation of nephron-sparing surgery. J Comput Assist Tomogr 28:496–504

Urban BA, Ratner LE, Fishman EK (2001) Three-dimensional volume-rendered CT angiography of the renal arteries and veins: normal anatomy, variants, and clinical applications. Radiographics 21:373–355

Uzzo RG, Novick AC (2001) Nephron sparing surgery for renal tumors: indications, techniques and outcomes. J Urol 166:6–18

Uzzo RG, Cherullo EE, Myles J et al. (2002) Renal cell carcinoma invading the urinary collecting system: implications for staging. J Urol 167:2392–2396

Vermooten V (1950) Indications for concervative surgery in certain renal tumors: a study based on the growth pattern of the clear cell carcinoma. J Urol 64:200–206

Wells S (1884) Successful removal of two solid circumrenal tumours. Br Med J 1:758–767

Wunderlich H, Reichelt O, Schubert R et al. (2000) Preoperative simulation of partial nephrectomy with three-dimensional computed tomography. BJU Int 86:777–781

Yuh BI, Cohan RH (1999) Different phases of renal enhancement: role in detecting and characterizing renal masses during helical CT. Am J Roentgenol 173:747–755

Zigeuner R, Quehenberger F, Pummer K et al. (2003) Long-term results of nephron-sparing surgery for renal cell carcinoma in 114 patients: risk factors for progressive disease. BJU Int 92:567–571

24 Laparoscopic Partial Nephrectomy

RAID ABO-KAMIL and RIZK EL-GALLEY

CONTENTS

24.1
Introduction

The widespread use of imaging techniques, such as computed tomography (CT) and ultrasound (US), has resulted in an increased detection of incidental renal lesions (MEVORACH et al. 1992). The majority of these tumors are small and well localized. Radical nephrectomy is still considered the gold standard for localized renal cell carcinoma, yet nephron-sparing surgery (NSS) has gained more popularity over the past 10–15 years. Originally, NSS was reserved for patients with a solitary functioning kidney; now, it has become an option for selected patients with renal small tumors (<4 cm) and a normal contralateral kidney (FERGANY et al. 2000).

Over the past few years laparoscopic surgery has become more popular than open surgery due to the advantages of small incisions, minimal postoperative pain, and early return to normal activities. Successful laparoscopic partial nephrectomy (LPN) on a porcine was first reported in 1993 (SHALHAV et al. 1998). Later the same year, two groups reported successful clinical LPN in patients with benign disease (WINFIELD et al. 1995).

Unlike laparoscopic radical nephrectomy, the laparoscopic partial nephrectomy has proved to be a technically demanding procedure that requires an experienced laparoscopic urologist. Hemostasis during dissection of renal parenchyma presents a major challenge; however, experience with laparoscopic partial nephrectomy is growing and a number of centers have reported promising results (MCDOUGALL et al. 1998; RASSWEILER et al. 2000; SIMON et al. 2003). This chapter outlines the various LPN techniques and results with emphasis on the imaging evaluations that help to guide the surgeon for a successful outcome.

24.2
Indications and Contraindications

24.2.1
Indications

Laparoscopic partial nephrectomy has been successfully performed for benign and malignant conditions:

R. ABO-KAMIL, MD
Research fellow, Department of Surgery, Division of Urology, University of Alabama School of Medicine at Birmingham, 1530 3rd Avenue South, MEB 602, Birmingham, AL 35294-3296, USA
R. EL-GALLEY, MB BCH, FRCS
Associate Professor, Department of Surgery, Division of Urology, University of Alabama School of Medicine at Birmingham, 1530 3rd Avenue South, Birmingham, AL 35294-3296, USA

1. Benign diseases treated with laparoscopic partial nephrectomy:
   a. Poorly functioning renal moieties associated with ureteral duplication or horse shoe kidney.
   b. Hydrocalix with urolithiasis.
   c. Recurrent renal infection.
   d. Equivocal renal cyst.
   e. Indeterminate solid renal mass.
2. Malignant diseases treated with laparoscopic partial nephrectomy; renal cell cancer (RCC), for example, which meets the following criteria:
   a. Tumor size <4 cm.
   b. Unilateral tumor.
   c. Absence of multifocality.
   d. Location of the tumor should not be too close to the renal hilum to allow partial nephrectomy without injury to the major vessels or the renal pelvis.

24.2.1
Contraindications to Partial Nephrectomy

Laparoscopic partial nephrectomy is contraindicated in the following cases:
1. Lymphadenopathy.
2. Inferior vena cava involvement.
3. Extensive perinephric visceral involvement.

24.3
Preoperative Evaluation

Preoperative imaging should provide the surgeon with the following information:
1. Position of the kidney relative to the lower rib cage, spine, and iliac crest.
2. Tumor location and depth of tumor extension into the kidney.
3. Relationship of the tumor to the collecting system as well as the renal arterial and venous anatomy, especially the segmental arterial supply to the tumor.

The diagnosis of RCC is generally made by CT with intravenous injection of contrast, showing a solid mass in the parenchyma of the kidney. Fewer than 5% of all RCC have a cystic appearance with separations, irregular borders, dystrophic calcification, or other features that distinguish it from a simple renal cyst.

The differential diagnosis of the solid kidney masses include: oncocytoma (granular oncocytes on histological analysis, with a central scar in the tumor); angiomyolipoma (contains fat, seen on CT scans); xanthogranulomatous pyelonephritis (usually in patients with diabetes, with a concurrent stone in a poorly functioning kidney); fibromas; or metastasis.

Both CT and MR imaging are used to stage renal tumors. Abdominal CT is useful to show local extension of the tumor and presence of enlarged para-aortic lymph nodes. Spiral CT should be done if extensive parenchymal resection is planned to detect polar arteries and to evaluate extension of the tumor in the renal sinus and veins (COLL et al. 1999). These new imaging studies have replaced, to a large extent, venocavography and arteriography, which are more invasive. Chest radiograph or CT is routinely done to rule out pulmonary metastasis. Bone scan is required only in the presence of a large tumor or if clinical evaluation suggests skeletal metastasis.

When evaluating renal tumors, the urologist is looking for certain information to help in constructing a management plan. Here are some of the points that contribute to the surgical decision-making.

24.3.1
Is It a Tumor or a Pseudotumor?

Pseudotumors in the kidneys are rare; however, this diagnosis should be taken into consideration. A hypertrophied column of Bertin, inflammatory renal mass, or perinephric inflammation extending to the kidney may be confused with a renal tumor. A CT scan is usually very helpful in delineating the nature of the tumors. In some cases, when the nature of these masses is undetermined, a repeat CT a few weeks later shows a significant change in an inflammatory mass, whereas a tumor change is less remarkable. A hypertrophied column of Bertin has been a diagnostic problem on the intravenous pyelogram and a dimercaptosuccinic acid (DMSA) nuclear scan is required to establish the diagnosis. A column of Bertin is homogenous with the rest of the kidney tissue, whereas a tumor shows different isotope uptake. Most of these swellings, however, can be differentiated with a CT scan which obviates the need for a nuclear scan (MAZER and QUAIFE 1979; THORNBURY et al. 1980).

24.3.2
Is It a Cystic Tumor?

Cystic renal masses range from a simple cyst to cystic renal carcinoma. Characterization of cystic renal masses relies mainly on the Bosniak classification, which consists of four categories (BOSNIAK 1986; BOSNIAK 1991; BOSNIAK 1994): benign simple cysts (category I); minimally complicated cysts (category II); indeterminate cystic renal masses that include cystic renal tumors (multiloculated or not) and complex cysts (category III); and cystic renal carcinomas (category IV). Usually, category I cysts are not an indication for surgery unless they are symptomatic, category II are most likely benign and can be watched, category III are more likely to be malignant, and category IV are highly suspicious for being malignant (BOSNIAK 1997; KOGA et al. 2000).

24.3.3
Is It a Solid Tumor?

In general, a solid tumor should be considered malignant until proved otherwise, with the exception of a tumor that contains fat on the CT scan (angiomyolipoma) or tumors that do not enhance on a CT and do not grow on follow-up CT exams. Oncocytoma is another tumor that is difficult to differentiate from malignant tumors radiologically and is usually diagnosed after excision (SCHATZ and LIEBER 2003).

Surgical planning is usually dependent on radiological information. The extent of the tumor and its location in the kidney, proximity to the renal collecting system and renal vessels, and presence of fat planes between the tumor and other structures (e.g., liver, colon, posterior abdominal wall muscles) are all important information in helping the surgeon to assess the local invasiveness of the tumor.

24.3.4
Role of Intraoperative Ultrasound in Partial Nephrectomy

Ultrasound has emerged as a useful modality for intraoperative evaluation during LPN (ASSIMOS et al. 1991). In general, the kidney and associated lesions are best imaged with a 7.5-MHz probe, which is especially useful in identifying the extent of lesion depth within the parenchyma. Excellent anatomical resolution can be attained using probes of higher frequency applied to the kidney surface directly (Fig. 24.1). Since US is a dynamic study, it is equipped to identify the boundary of the surgical margin in real-time. It can also provide intraoperative detail in evaluating complicated cysts

(Figs. 24.2, 24.3). Duplex Doppler scanning is useful in assessing tumor vascularity and can help in differentiating a cyst or dilated calyx from an artery or vein. The renal vein and inferior vena cava (IVC) can easily be examined for tumor thrombus. Color Doppler can also identify deep vessels near the wall of the lesion that may be encountered during excision. The identification of these surrounding vessels a few millimeters from a hilar renal tumor may assist the surgeon planning the enucleation of a tumor in this location and can influence the decision to use cold renal ischemia.

Ultrasound has several limitations. It is unable to identify very small lesions, especially if they share a similar echo pattern with the renal parenchyma. Satellite lesions can be also missed, additionally, US

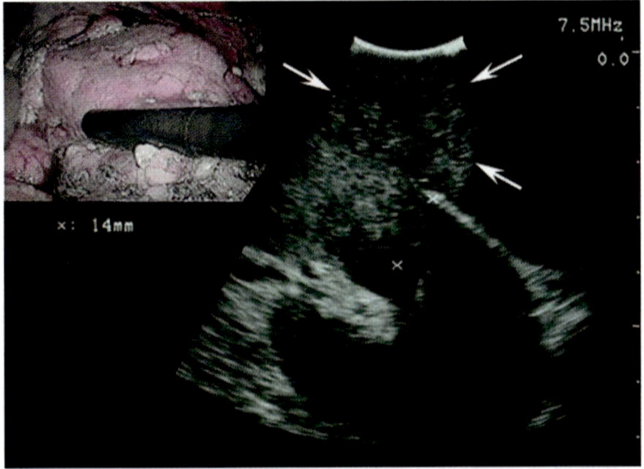

Fig. 24.1. Laparoscopic intraoperative real-time ultrasound. Intraoperative US image shows the tumor outlined by *arrows* and 14-mm distance of inner margin of tumor from caliceal system marked by two cursors (*x*). *Inset* shows picture-in-picture capability that allows visualization of location of laparoscope probe on tumorous kidney.

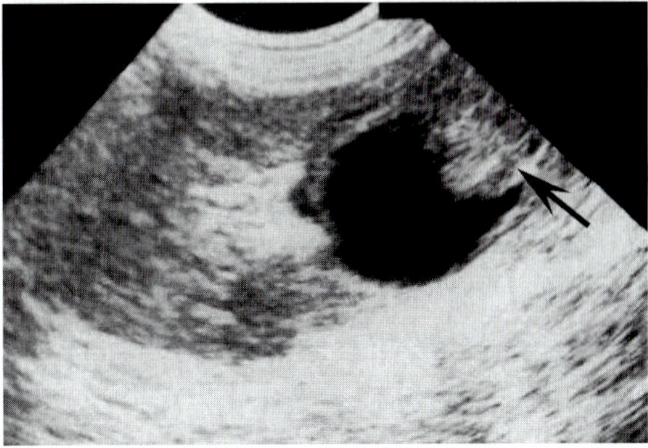

Fig. 24.2. Intraoperative real-time ultrasound. Transverse intraoperative US image shows renal tumor (*arrow*) within renal cyst.

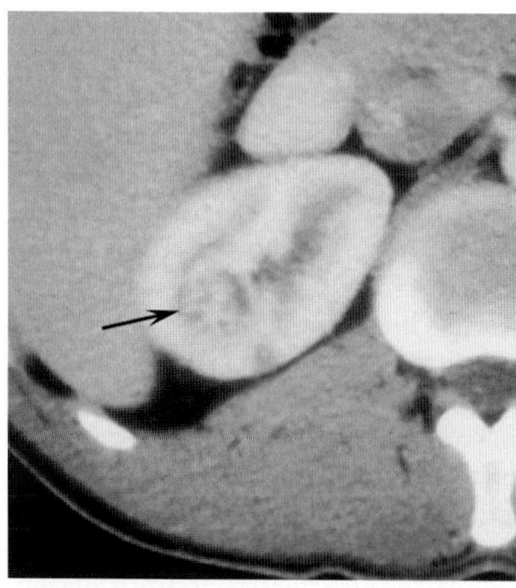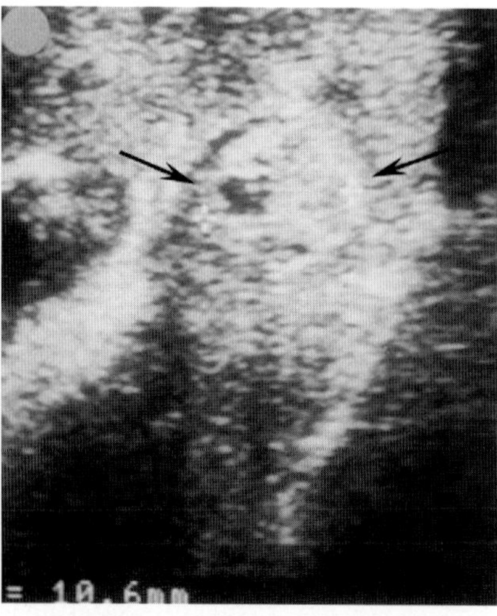

Fig. 24.3a,b. Solid renal mass. a Preoperative axial contrast-enhanced CT scan demonstrates a poorly defined mass (*arrow*) deep in surface of right kidney. b Intraoperative US image reveal 1-cm solid lesion (*arrows*) with small cystic components. Small lesion seen on CT on renal surface was fulgurated.

cannot diagnose with certainty whether a particular lesion is benign or malignant. Finally, imaging the adrenal gland is difficult, even with tumor present. The adrenal gland size, shape, anatomical position, and echo pattern are not ideal for US evaluation.

24.4
Full Laparoscopic Partial Nephrectomy Techniques

Based on the tumor location, a transperitoneal or retroperitoneal approach can be employed. Tumors on the anterior surface of the kidney are better accessed through a transperitoneal technique, whereas posterior tumors can be accessed with a retroperitoneal technique. In general, the surgeon should choose the approach with which he or she is most experienced. The transperitoneal approach has the advantage of providing a larger space which makes it easier to perform intracorporal sutures. The retroperitoneal approach provides posterior access to the kidney in addition to limiting the dissection to the retroperitoneal space. In cases where urine leaks occur, the leak is limited to the retroperitoneum avoiding peritonitis.

24.4.1
Cystoscopy Stent Placement and Positioning

The patient is given general anesthesia and positioned in a lithotomy position. A cystoscopy is per-

formed and a ureteral catheter is inserted in the corresponding ureter. Fluoroscopy is useful in confirming the position of the ureteral catheter in the ureter. Care should be taken to avoid perforating the collecting system with the guide wire or the ureteral catheter; therefore, we prefer to advance the ureteral catheter only half way in the ureter. A Foley catheter is inserted separately into the bladder and the ureteral catheter is tied or taped to it to avoid inadvertent displacement of the ureteral catheter. The ureteral catheter is then connected to a urine bag and is used to inject a diluted methylene blue solution to check for urinary leaks after excising the tumor. Exophytic tumors which are shown to be distant from the collecting system could be excised without stenting the ureter or checking for leaks, however, the authors prefer to insert the stent and check for leaks in every case. In our experience, this is the safest technique to avoid the serious complication of urine leakage.

The patient is then positioned in the lumbar position according to the side of the tumor. We prefer to put the patient in 45° lumbar position for a transperitoneal approach and 90° lumbar position for a retroperitoneal approach.

24.4.2
Transperitoneal Approach

We usually use four trocars for the transperitoneal approach; 10 mm at the umbilicus for the laparoscope, 12 mm at the ipsilateral iliac region for dissection and for admission of large instruments, 5 mm in the subcostal region for dissection, and a final 5-mm trocar in the anterior axillary line for the assistant to use for suction, retraction, or to follow the sutures.

After positioning, scrubbing the abdomen from mid-chest to upper thighs, sterile drapes are applied. The surgeon should keep the flank within the surgical field to allow conversion to open surgery in case of an emergency.

The procedure starts with insufflation. It is important to learn the insufflation technique and apply it properly because it is a blind step and can result in many complications. We use a laparoscopic insufflation needle (Veress needle) to start insufflation in the ipsilateral iliac region. In our experience this area is the most successful site for insufflation needle insertion unless the patient has a previous scar in that area. The skin is cut to about 1 cm at the site of the expected trocar, the fat is separated with a hemostat, and the insufflation needle is filled with saline and inserted. The needle should be handled with the surgeon's two hands. One hand applies pressure and the other hand holds the needle close to the skin to control the depth of insertion. The needle should pass two resistances: at external oblique aponeurosis and at the peritoneum. After insertion of the needle in the peritoneum, the valve should be opened to allow the saline in the needle to drop into the peritoneum by the intraperitoneal negative pressure. A 10-ml syringe filled with 5 ml saline is then used to aspirate from the insufflation needle looking for blood or bowel contents. If that test is negative, the saline should be injected and aspirated again to confirm that the needle is not in a blood vessel or bowel. The needle is held in place and insufflation starts with CO_2 with a low flow. The resting intraperitoneal pressure should be 4–6 mm Hg. Insufflation continues until 500 ml of CO_2 are injected in the peritoneum without a sharp rise in the abdominal pressure or uneven distention of the abdominal cavity. The flow is then increased until the peritoneal pressure reaches 15 mm Hg. The insufflation needle is then removed and the first trocar is inserted in its place. We prefer using trocars with non-cutting tips (unbladed introducers). The camera is then introduced to inspect for injures or bleeding and the insufflation is then continued through the trocar side channel.

Because insufflation is a blind step, it is more likely to result in complications; therefore, careful attention to detail is very important. The insufflation needle should be checked by the surgeon before insertion for any blockages that will give false high pressures. It should be also checked for leaks between the valve and the needle that will leak the saline and give a false saline positive test. If two resistances are not palpated by the surgeon after inserting the needle for appropriate distance, the surgeon should resist advancing the needle further. The needle should be removed, checked, and inserted again. If the pressures at the beginning of insufflation are high or rising quickly, the insufflation should be stopped and the needle removed. However, the surgeon must keep in mind that in obese patients and in very muscular patients, the intra-abdominal resting pressure can be high (10–12 mm Hg); therefore, rising pressure is more alarming than resting pressure during the initial insufflation. Most importantly, if the insufflation is not proceeding well in one area, the surgeon should try another area, e.g., periumbilical or subcostal areas.

Some surgeons prefer to avoid blind insufflation and insert the first trocar under vision through a small incision. If this is preferred, a special trocar with an inflatable cuff at the tip (Hasson trocar) should be used to avoid CO_2 from the incision. The rest of the trocars are inserted under vision using the laparoscope. It is helpful to point the laparoscope at the site of the trocar insertion and transilluminate the abdominal wall to avoid injuring the abdominal wall vessels during trocar insertion.

24.4.2.1
Dissection of the Left Kidney

The dissection of the left kidney starts with colon mobilization. An incision is made at Toldt's line from the splenic flexure to the pelvis. The colon should be completely mobilized with its mesentery to avoid colonic injury. There is a relatively avascular plane between the mesentery and Gerota's fascia covering the kidney. Excessive bleeding usually indicates that the dissection is in the wrong plane. We prefer using the laparoscopic ultrasonic shears for this purpose because they cut with mechanical friction, thus avoiding dispersing an electric current close to the colon which might cause electric burns.

The next step is usually to identify the psoas muscle below the lower pole of the kidney, then to identify the ureter and gonadal vein and follow them to the lower pole of the kidney (Fig. 24.4). There is usually a thick layer of fat between the lower pole of the kidney and the mesentery which can be divided safely as long as the ureter is protected and a con-

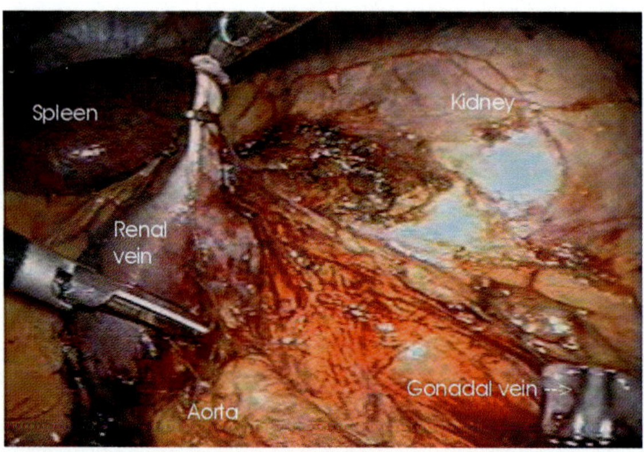

Fig. 24.4. Laparoscopic view during laparoscopic partial nephrectomy. The colon has been mobilized and the gonadal vein has been clipped and divided. The fibro-lymphatic tissue lateral to the aorta is being divided by ultrasonic laparoscopic shears.

tinuous watch is maintained for accessory arteries to the lower pole of the kidney. The gonadal vein is then followed to the renal vein which is then carefully dissected. The gonadal vein is either clipped or cauterized with a bipolar current and is divided close the renal vein. The fascia on the lateral aspect of the aortic wall is usually the easiest guide for finding the renal artery. This fascia is usually dissected with a laparoscopic J hook until the white wall of the aorta is identified. The dissection then continues behind the renal vein looking for the pulsations of the renal artery which is then dissected free from its fascia. The space between the renal artery and vein is then developed with a laparoscopic dissector.

Failure to identify the anatomical landmarks is the main reason for complications. While dissecting the colon and mesentery, the surgeon should identify the plane between these structures to avoid penetrating the mesentery or violating the Gerota's fascia. Incisions in the Gerota's fascia on top of the tumor risk contaminating the abdominal cavity with tumor cells. In addition, mobilizing the spleen gives better access to the upper pole of the kidney and helps to keep the colon and pancreas retracted from the renal hilum area.

It is important to identify the ureter after mobilization of the colon. The ureter is usually easily identifiable in front of the psoas muscle below the kidney. Identifying the ureter assists in mobilizing the lower pole and avoids ureteric injury. The surgeon should also be attentive to vasculature in the lower pole area since an accessory lower pole vessel is not unusual. While dissecting the renal pedicle the surgeon should be alert to vascular anatomy variations particularly with the venous system. Lumbar

veins should be assumed present until proven otherwise. If these veins are injured, they retract into the muscle and become hard to control. They are also close to the main renal vessels and trying to control them in the midst of bleeding can result in damaging these structures. Some patients will have a retro-aortic vein diagnosed by radiological investigations before surgery. In our experience neither retro-aortic veins nor multiple renal arteries are contraindications for laparoscopic surgery.

24.4.2.2
Dissection of the Right Kidney

The dissection of the right kidney usually starts with retracting the liver through a 5-mm trocar inserted in the midline under the xiphisternum. A laparoscopic locking grasping forceps should be passed under the falciform ligament to retract it with the liver and gallbladder and is then used to grasp the peritoneum on the lateral abdominal wall as high as possible. The right colon is then mobilized from in front of the kidney with ultrasonic scissors and the peritoneum between the kidney and the under surface of the liver is divided. The duodenum should be identified and mobilized medially. Care should be taken not to use electric cauterization close to the duodenum because it can cause thermal damage. The IVC is then identified and the gonadal vein is found. The ureter is usually easily identified lateral to the IVC below the kidney. In most patients the gonadal vein can be left intact. The renal vein is then identified and dissected carefully. The adrenal gland is also identified, but it should only be mobilized in patients with upper-pole renal tumors. The renal artery is usually found behind the renal vein on the lower side. The space between the vein and artery is dissected with a laparoscopic dissecting forceps. In some patients the artery is located on the upper side of the vein. In these circumstances it is better to mobilize the kidney completely and access the artery behind the kidney since anterior approach risks bleeding from the renal or adrenal veins that are located in that area.

The right kidney is usually easier to dissect than the left kidney. Retracting the liver at the beginning of the procedure is very important to gain access to the kidney's upper pole and avoid injuries to the liver and gallbladder. When the adrenal gland is to be dissected from the upper pole of the kidney, the surgeon should be very careful about the venous anatomy in this area. Some patients have very small veins between the adrenal gland and the renal vein that can be a source of significant bleeding. Similar to the left kidney, dissecting the right ureter early avoids its injury. The gonadal vein could be preserved in most patients; however, if it obstructs the view to the ureter or renal artery, it should be sacrificed early in the dissection to avoid its avulsion. We prefer using the bipolar coagulation to control the gonadal vein. In some patients the duodenum will look similar to the IVC at the beginning of the dissection. In other patients the duodenum is located medially and the IVC is the first structure behind the colon. Nevertheless, the structure first found behind the colon should be treated as the duodenum until the duodenum is clearly identified. Sticking to this policy helps in avoiding inadvertent duodenal injuries due to mistaking it for the IVC.

24.4.2.3
Identifying the Tumor and Planning the Excision

We prefer to locate the tumor with laparoscopic US in every case. This technique allows mapping of the excision margins. The fat on top of the tumor should be excised and sent for permanent histological study for cancer staging. Using the laparoscopic US probe on the surface of the kidney, small cauterization marks should be made on the surface of the kidney about 5 mm away from the tumor to provide safety margins. The depth of the tumor and its proximity to the renal collecting system should be also noted on the US images.

24.4.2.3.1
Clamping the Vessels and Excising the Tumor

Although small exophytic tumors may be enucleated without arterial clamping, most partial nephrectomies require clamping of the renal artery before excising the tumor. The kidney can sustain 30–40 min of warm time ischemia without permanent damage. Before clamping the vessels, the surgeon should prepare and check all necessary tools that are needed for excising the tumor, check the collecting system for leaks, repair the collecting system when necessary, and provide hemostasis to the renal surface. We usually prepare laparoscopic bulldog clamps, Surgicel, 5° and 0 Vicryl sutures, diluted methylene blue, and SurgiFoam (Johnson & Johnson) loaded in a 10-ml syringe, and a laparoscopic applicator for the SurgiFoam.

The patient is given 12.5 g of intravenous Mannitol a few minutes before clamping the vessels to improve the renal flow and reduce the effect of oxygen radicals after unclamping. The renal artery is temporarily occluded with a bulldog clamp. We prefer to occlude the vein with a separate clamp to reduce the back bleeding from the kidney surface (Fig. 24.5). The tumor with a rim of normal renal tissue is then excised under vision with laparoscopic scissors at the previously marked areas. The assistant should use suction to aspirate the blood leaking from the surface of the kidney to allow cutting under vision. This technique obviates cutting into the tumor and positive margins. The tumor is positioned behind the kidney in a visible area until it is extracted at the end of the procedure. Small biopsies are then excised from the kidney tissue at the tumor bed and are sent for frozen sections to rule out positive margins. The surgeon should continue to repair the kidney surface while waiting on the frozen sections.

The assistant injects 3–4 ml of the diluted methylene blue in the ureteric stent to check for leaks from the collecting system. If a leak exists, the collecting system should be repaired carefully with the 5° sutures until it is water tight (Fig. 24.6). The Flowcel is then applied to the tumor bed and covered with a Surgicel bolster (Ethicon). The edges of the tumor bed are then approximated tightly with the 0 Vicryl sutures (Fig. 24.7). We prefer to use Lapra-Ty clips (Ethicon) to secure the stitches and to apply tension to the kidney surface. They are quicker to use and less likely to cut through the kidney tissue than sur-

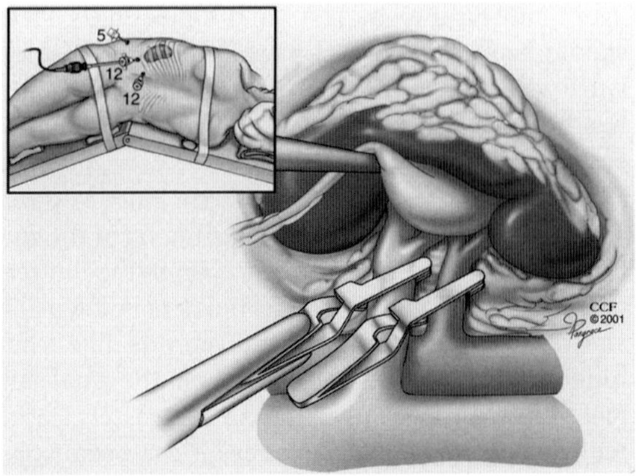

Fig. 24.5. Drawing showing clamping of the vessels during retroperitoneal laparoscopic partial nephrectomy. Because of limited operative space in the retroperitoneum, two laparoscopic bulldog clamps were used for individual control of the mobilized renal artery and vein instead of Satinsky clamps. *Inset* shows three-port retroperitoneal approach.

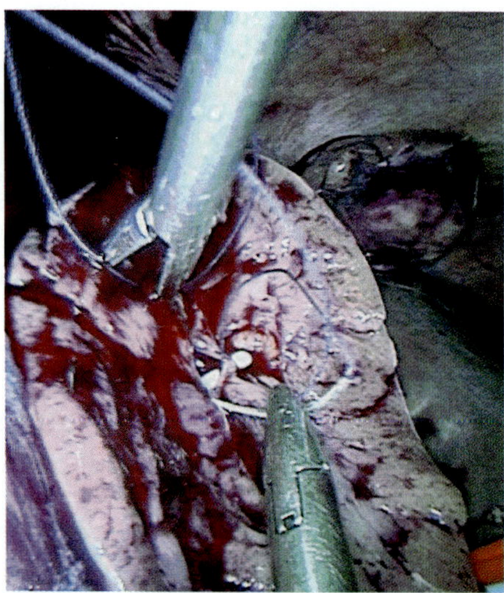

Fig. 24.6. Collecting system closure after tumor resection. Collecting system is identified by saline outflow and closed accurately with interrupted absorbable sutures.

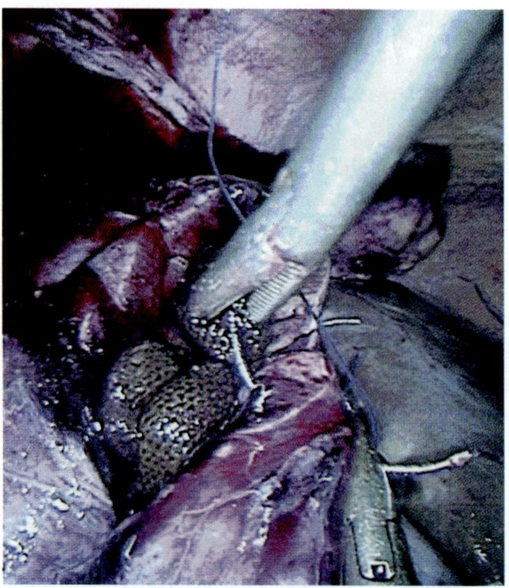

Fig. 24.7. Edges of renal parenchyma closure after tumor resection. Edges of renal parenchyma are approximated with absorbable sutures over hemostatic mesh.

gical knots. The vein is then unclamped followed by the artery. The kidney surface is observed carefully for bleeding. If bleeding occurs, extra sutures might be necessary.

24.4.2.3.2
Possible Surgical Complications

The surgeon should try to keep warm-time ischemia to the minimum in all cases. This is achieved by preparing the tools and materials in advance and by planning the excision before clamping. The excision of the tumor should be performed under vision to avoid cutting into it. The renal collecting system should be checked with a methylene blue injection since visual inspection is not reliable and could result in neglecting a perforation in the collecting system and a urine leak.

Some surgeons report using fibrin glues or other similar substances to control bleeding from the collecting system. In our experience, applying Flowcel to the tumor bed with Surgicel bolsters and tension sutures is the most reliable and reproducible technique for hemostasis. If bleeding from the renal surface continues after unclamping the vessels, more tension sutures should be taken in the tumor bed edges until hemostasis is secured.

Manipulation of the renal artery with the bulldog clamp should be gentle to avoid damage to the arterial wall. If the artery goes into spasm, applying a papaverine solution to the arterial wall using the cleaned SurgiFoam injector is usually helpful.

If the frozen sections are positive for tumor, a decision should be made to re-clamp the vessels and excise more of the kidney tissue, versus performing radical nephrectomy. Re-clamping the vessels carries more risk for permanent renal damage, however, in patients with impaired total renal function, partial nephrectomy is preferred.

24.4.3
Retroperitoneal Approach

For the retroperitoneal approach, the patient is usually positioned in a 90° flank position. An incision is made in the mid-axillary line under the costal margin long enough to admit the surgeon's index finger. The fat is separated and the abdominal wall fascia and muscles are perforated with the tip of a hemostat. The surgeon's finger is then admitted into the wound to palpate the retroperitoneal fat under the muscles. The insufflating trocar with an oval balloon at its tip is introduced with the laparoscope inserted in the port to allow insufflation of the retroperitoneum under vision. The retroperitoneal space is developed with the balloon and the balloon is kept inflated for 3 min to improve hemostasis. The port is then removed and a working port with a retention balloon is introduced (Hasson port). The retroperitoneum is then insufflated directly with CO_2 to a pressure of 15 mm Hg. A second 5-mm trocar is inserted under vision in the posterior axillary line. The fat and bowels are dissected with blunt dissection from the back of the abdominal muscles. A Kittner dissector is usually good for that purpose; if one is not available, the tip of the suction tube could be used. A third, 12-mm trocar is inserted medially in the anterior axillary line. The dissection should continue behind the kidney in front of the psoas muscle. The ureter is usually identified easily. The dissection continues cephalad looking for the artery. In most patients the pulsations of the renal artery are visible and the artery is dissected free. The renal vein is then displayed in front of the artery. The rest of the procedure is continued as in transperitoneal laparoscopy.

The patient selection for this approach is important. Patients with a significant amount of retroperitoneal fat and those with a short stature or back problems present difficulties for this procedure. The surgeon should be sure that the initial incision is through the abdominal fascia and his finger can feel the retroperitoneal fat before developing the space; otherwise, the developed space will be in the wrong level and the operation will become more complicated.

After insufflation, the iliopsoas muscle is an excellent landmark for the ureter and the renal hilum. Before inserting the medial port in the anterior axillary line, the surgeon should be sure to mobilize the fat completely to see the muscle fibers of the transversus abdominis muscle. Failure to do so risks transfixing the colon with the trocar, an injury that, if unnoticed, could result in serious consequences.

24.5
Hand-Assisted Laparoscopic Partial Nephrectomy

With a hand in the abdomen, it is easier to make the transition from traditional open surgery to laparoscopy. Hand-assisted laparoscopy provides more safety and security to the surgeon and patient. There are many commercially available hand ports. We prefer using the Gellport (Applied Medical) over other products because of its ease of use and lack of air leaks. The ideal hand port does not yet exist and we hope that better products become available.

This procedure is performed through a 6- to 8-cm incision in the midline where the surgeon's non-dominant hand is inserted in the abdomen to assist in the dissection. The position of the incision should be centered around the umbilicus in most patients; however, in large patients a paramedian incision

and laterally placed port incisions are more suitable. Some surgeons prefer to insert the hand port incision in the ipsilateral iliac region. It is important when fitting the hand port to make sure that none of the abdominal contents are trapped under the port collar. The abdomen should be insufflated with CO_2 and the camera should be introduced into the hand port to inspect the abdomen before placing the instrument ports. Three laparoscopic ports are inserted: 10 mm for the camera; 12 mm for large instruments; and 5 mm for assistance. On the right side, another 5-mm port under the xiphisternum is useful for liver retraction as mentioned above. The dissection should be continued as in full laparoscopy; however, having a hand in the abdomen allows for palpation and more flexibility in handling the tissues.

Hand-assisted laparoscopy has the advantages of a short learning curve and shorter operative time; however, most LPN can be performed with full laparoscopy where the tumor is extracted through a 2- to 3-cm incision, thus avoiding the 8-cm incision for hand-assisted surgery.

24.6
Challenges in Laparoscopic Partial Nephrectomy

Laparoscopic partial nephrectomy has proved to be a challenging technique for most urologists. Urinary leaks from the injured collecting system and difficulty achieving hemostasis from the renal surface are the two most common challenges. Water-tight sutures of the renal collecting system have proved to be the most reliable way of avoiding a urinary leak. The insertion of a ureteric catheter and injection of indigo carmine in the kidney identifies any urinary leak from the collecting system that needs to be sutured until completely sealed off.

Reliable hemostasis of the cut renal surface presents a challenge to the surgeon. The kidney is a highly vascular organ that receives half a liter of blood per minute. Several hemostatic techniques have been tried in LPN; these include the use of monopolar and bipolar electric coagulation, radiofrequency energy, laparoscopic harmonic scissors, fibrin glue, gelatin resorcinol formaldehyde glue, microwave coagulation, and laparoscopic sutures. The effectiveness of these techniques is not universally agreed upon. In our experience inserting compressing sutures that approximate the cut edges of the kidney on a Surgicel bolster is the most reproducible hemostatic technique. Table 24.1 summarizes some of the published results for LPN.

24.7
Results

The initial 50 patients undergoing laparoscopic partial nephrectomy at the Cleveland Clinic had a mean tumor size of 3 cm (1.7–7 cm), mean warm-ischemic time of 23 min, mean estimated blood loss of 270 ml, mean operative time of 3 h, and a median length of hospital stay of 2.2 days (GILL et al. 2002). Recently, the initial 200 patients undergoing laparoscopic partial nephrectomy were compared with a contemporary cohort of patients undergoing open NSS (GILL et al. 2003). The median tumor size was 2.8 cm in the laparoscopic group compared with 3.3 cm in the open group ($p=0.005$). When comparing the laparoscopic to open groups, the median surgical time was 3 vs 3.9 h ($p<0.001$), the estimated blood loss was 125 vs 250 ml ($p=0.001$), and the mean warm-ischemic time was 28 vs 18 min ($p=0.001$). The laparoscopic group required less postoperative analgesia and experienced a shorter hospital stay and a shorter period of convalescence ($p<0.001$ for all three comparisons). Although there were more intraoperative complications in the laparoscopic group (5% vs 0), the frequency of postoperative complications was similar (9 vs 14%; $p=0.27$). The specific complications occurring in the laparoscopic group are detailed in Table 24.2. There were three positive surgical margins in the laparoscopic group and none in the open group. One of these patients had an oncocytoma and the other two had renal cell carcinoma. At 2- and 3-year follow-up, both patients remained free of disease.

KIM et al. (2003) recently compared complications related to LPN and laparoscopic radical nephrectomy for tumors <4.5 cm at Johns Hopkins medical institution. Laparoscopic partial nephrectomy is associated with specific complications such as urine leak, pseudoaneurysm formation, and delayed hemorrhage. In the group of patients undergoing laparoscopic partial nephrectomy ($n=79$), mean surgical time was 181.9 min, mean warm-ischemic time 26.4 min (range 13–37 min), and the mean estimated blood loss was 391.2 ml with 4 patients (5.1%) requiring transfusion and one conversion to open surgery for bleeding problems. Specific complications included one ureteral injury managed laparoscopically, and persistent urine leak in 2 patients that resolved with conservative measures. Surgical margins were reported to be positive in 2 patients postoperatively, of whom 1 underwent laparoscopic radical nephrectomy while the other has remained free of disease after 26 months of follow-up. Table 24.3 summarizes some of the published results of LPN.

Table 24.1. Clinical laparoscopic partial nephrectomy series. *US* ultrasound, *RF* radiofrequency, *NR* not reported

Reference	Technique	Hemostasis	No. of patients	Mean tumor size (cm)	Positive margin	Tumor recurrence	Mean follow-up (months)
GILL et al. (2002)	Full laparoscopy		50	3.0	0	0	7.2
STIFELMAN et al. (2001)	Hand-assisted		11	1.9	0	0	8.0
HARMON et al. (2000)		US shears	15	2.3	0	0	8.0
GETTMAN et al. (2001)		RF coagulation	10	2.1	0	NR	NR
YOSHIMURA et al. (2001)		Microwave tissue coagulator	6	1.8	1	0	3.0

Table 24.2. Complications of laparoscopic partial nephrectomy ($n=100$)

Intraoperative complications ($n=5$)	Postoperative complications ($n=9$)	Late complications ($n=16$)
Bleeding (3)	Urine leak (3)	Delayed nephrectomy (1)
Bowel injury (1)	Pneumonia (1)	Wound infection (2)
Resected ureter (1)	Atelectasis (3)	Hematuria (1)
Convert to open surgery (0)	Arrhythmia (2)	Severe constipation (hospitalized) (1)
		Embolization (1)
		Chronic heart failure (hospitalized) (1)
		Wound dehiscence (1)
		Urine leak (1)
		Hematoma (1)
		Incisional hernia (1)
		Pneumonia after discharge (3)
		Pulmonary embolus/deep (1)
		Vein thrombosis (1)

Table 24.3. Published series of laparoscopic partial nephrectomy with at least ten patients treated

Reference	No. of patients	Mean tumor size (cm)	Hilar control	No. of pelvicalyceal repairs
JANETSCHEK et al. (2000)	25	1.9	No	0
HARMON et al. (2000)	15	2.3	No	3
RASSWEILER et al. (2000)	53	2.3	–	–
GILL et al. (2003)	100	2.8	Yes (91)	64
GUILLONNEAU et al. (2003)	28	1.9	No (12)	0
		2.5	Yes (16)	–
KIM et al. (2003)	79	2.5	Yes (52)	–
SIMON et al. (2003)	19	2.1	No	0

24.8
Conclusion

Laparoscopic partial nephrectomy is emerging as an attractive, minimally invasive nephron-sparing option for the management of select renal lesions. It is associated with less need for postoperative analgesia, earlier hospital discharge, and more rapid convalescence. Experience with LPN continues to grow. The technique is evolving and issues of hemostasis and renal ischemia are being further addressed in the laboratory. It should be performed by surgeons with considerable laparoscopic expertise at centers where there is frequent interaction between open and laparoscopic surgeons.

References

Assimos DG, Boyce H, Woodruff RD, Harrison LH, McCullough DL, Kroovand RL (1991) Intraoperative renal ultrasonography: a useful adjunct to partial nephrectomy. J Urol 146:1218–1220

Bosniak MA (1991) Difficulties in classifying cystic lesions of the kidney. Urol Radiol 13:91–93

Bosniak MA (1994) How does one deal with a renal cyst that appears to be Bosniak class II on a CT scan but that has sonographic features suggestive of malignancy (e.g., nodularity of wall or a nodular, irregular septum)? Am J Roentgenol 163:216

Bosniak MA (1986) The current radiological approach to renal cysts. Radiology 158:1–10

Bosniak MA (1997) The use of the Bosniak classification system for renal cysts and cystic tumors. J Urol 157:1852–1853

Coll DM, Uzzo RG, Herts BR, Davros WJ, Wirth SL, Novick AC (1999) Three-dimensional volume rendered computerized tomography for preoperative evaluation and intraoperative treatment of patients undergoing nephron sparing surgery. J Urol 161:1097–1102

Fergany AF, Hafez KS, Novick AC (2000) Long term results of nephron sparing surgery for localized renal cell carcinoma: 10-year followup. J Urol 163:442–445

Gettman MT, Bishoff JT, Su LM, Chan D, Kavoussi LR, Jarett TW, Cadeddu JA (2001) Hemostatic laparoscopic partial nephrectomy; initial experience with the radiofrequency coagulation-assisted technique. Urology 58:8–11

Gill IS, Desai MM, Kaouk JH, Meraney AM, Murphy DP, Sung GT, Novick AC (2002) Laparoscopic partial nephrectomy for renal tumor: duplicating open surgical techniques. J Urol 167:469–477

Gill IS, Matin SF, Desai MM, Kaouk JH, Steinberg A, Mascha E, Thornton J, Sherief MH, Strzempkowski B, Novick AC (2003) Comparative analysis of laparoscopic versus open partial nephrectomy for renal tumors in 200 patients. J Urol 170:64–68

Guillonneau B, Bermudez H, Gholami S, El Fettouh H, Gupta R, Adorno Rosa J, Baumert H, Cathelineau X, Fromont G, Vallancien G (2003) Laparoscopic partial nephrectomy for renal tumor: single center experience comparing clamping and no clamping techniques of the renal vasculature. J Urol 169:483–486

Harmon WJ, Kavoussi LR, Bishoff JT (2000) Laparoscopic nephron-sparing surgery for solid renal masses using the ultrasonic shears. Urology 56:754–759

Janetschek G, Jeschke K, Peschel R, Strohmeyer D, Henning K, Bartsch G (2000) Laparoscopic surgery for stage T1 renal cell carcinoma: radical nephrectomy and wedge resection. Eur Urol 38:131–138

Kim FJ, Rha KH, Hernandez F, Jarrett TW, Pinto PA, Kavoussi LR (2003) Laparoscopic radical versus partial nephrectomy: assessment of complications. J Urol 170:408–411

Koga S, Nishikido M, Inuzuka S, Sakamoto I, Hayashi T, Hayashi K, Saito Y, Kanetake H (2000) An evaluation of Bosniak's radiological classification of cystic renal masses. BJU Int 86:607–609

Mazer MJ, Quaife MA (1979) Hypertrophied column of Bertin pseudotumor: radionuclide investigation. Urology 14:210–211

McDougall EM, Elbahnasy AM, Clayman RV (1998) Laparoscopic wedge resection and partial nephrectomy: The Washington University experience and review of the literature. JSLS 2:15–23

Mevorach RA, Segal AJ, Tersegno ME, Frank IN (1992) Renal cell carcinoma: incidental diagnosis and natural history: review of 235 cases. Urology 39:519–522

Rassweiler JJ, Abbou C, Janetschek G, Jeschke K (2000) Laparoscopic partial nephrectomy. The European experience. Urol Clin North Am 27:721–736

Schatz SM, Lieber MM (2003) Update on oncocytoma. Curr Urol Rep 4:30–35

Shalhav Al, Leibovitch I, Lev R, Hoenig DM, Ramon J (1998) Is laparoscopic radical nephrectomy with specimen morcellation acceptable cancer surgery? J Endourol 12:255–257

Simon SD, Ferrigni RG, Novicki DE, Lamm DL, Swanson SS, Andrews PE (2003) Mayo Clinic Scottsdale experience with laparoscopic nephron sparing surgery for renal tumors. J Urol 169:2059–2062

Stifelman MD, Sosa RE, Nakada SY, Shichman SJ (2001) Hand-assisted laparoscopic partial nephrectomy. J Endoourol 15:161–164

Thornbury JR, McCormick TL, Silver TM (1980) Anatomic/radiologic classification of renal cortical nodules. Am J Roentgenol 134:1–7

Winfield HN, Donovan JF, Lund GO, Kreder KJ, Stanley KE, Brown BP, Loening SA, Clayman RV (1995) Laparoscopic partial nephrectomy: initial experience and comparison to the open surgical approach. J Urol 153:1409–1414

Yoshimura K, Okubo K, Ichioka K, Terada N, Matsua Y, Arai Y (2001) Laparoscopic partial nephrectomy with a microwave tissue coagulator for small renal tumor. J Urol 165:1893–1896

Subject Index

List of Contributors

RAID ABO-KAMIL, MD
Research fellow
Department of Surgery
Division of Urology
University of Alabama School of Medicine
at Birmingham
1530 3rd Avenue South, MEB 602
Birmingham, AL 35294-3296
USA

DAVID W. BARKER, MD
Senior Radiologist
Tennessee Cancer Specialists, PLLC
Medical Director
LifeCare Partners, LLC
1450 Dowell Springs Boulevard, Suite 230
Knoxville, TN 37909
USA

EMILY D. BILLINGSLEY, MD
Chief Resident
Department of Radiology
Louisiana State University Health Sciences Center
1542 Tulane Avenue
New Orleans, LA 70112
USA

JOCELYN A. S. BROOKES, MRCP, FRCR
Consultant Interventional Radiologist
Department of Radiology
The Middlesex Hospital, UCLH
Mortimer Street
London W1T 3AA, England
UK

RONAN F. J. BROWNE, MD
Fellow in Abdominal Imaging
Abdominal Division
Department of Radiology
Vancouver General Hospital
899 West 12th Avenue
Vancouver V5Z 1M9, British Columbia
Canada

JAE YOUNG BYUN, MD
Professor and Chairman
Department of Radiology
Kangnam St. Mary's Hospital
College of Medicine
The Catholic University of Korea
505 Banpo-Dong, Seocho-Ku
Seoul 137-040
South Korea

JUNG AH CHOI, MD, PhD
Instructor, Department of Radiology
Seoul National University
Bundang Hospital
College of Medicine
300 Gumi-dong
Bundang-gu, Seong Nam
Gyeonggi-Do 463-707
South Korea

JEAN-MICHEL CORREAS, MD, PhD
Associate Professor and Vice-Chairman
Department of Radiology
Necker University Hospital
149 rue de Sèvres
75743 Paris Cedex 15
France

NANCY S. CURRY, MD
Professor of Radiology and Urology
Department of Radiology
Medical University of South Carolina
169 Ashley Avenue
Charleston, SC 29425
USA

RIZK EL-GALLEY, MB BCH, FRCS
Associate Professor
Department of Surgery, Division of Urology
University of Alabama School of Medicine
at Birmingham
1530 3rd Avenue South
Birmingham, AL 35294-3296
USA

Iman El-Hariry, MD, PhD
Senior Director
Oncology Clinical Development
& Medical Affairs
Glaxo Smith Kline R&D
Greenford Road
Greenford
Middlesex UB6 0HE, England
UK

Elliot K. Fishman, MD, FACR
Professor of Radiology and Oncology
Johns Hopkins University School of Medicine
Director, Diagnostic Radiology and Body CT
Department of Radiology
Johns Hopkins Outpatient Center
601 North Caroline Street, Room 3254
Baltimore, MD 21287
USA

Takahiro Fujimori, MD, PhD
Professor and Chairman
Department of Surgical and Molecular Pathology
DOKKYO University School of Medicine
Director, Department of Surgical Pathology
DOKKYO University Hospital
880 Kitakobayashi
Mibu, Shimo-tsuga
Tochigi 321-0293
Japan

Debra A. Gervais, MD
Assistant Professor of Radiology
Harvard Medical School
Department of Radiology
Director of Interventional Radiology
Division of Abdominal Imaging
and Interventional Radiology
Massachusetts General Hospital
55 Fruit Street
Boston, MA 02114
USA

Ali Guermazi, MD
Senior Radiologist
Scientific Director, Oncology Services
Department of Radiology Services
Synarc Inc.
575 Market Street, 17th Floor
San Francisco, CA 94105
USA

Peter F. Hahn, MD, PhD
Associate Professor of Radiology
Harvard Medical School
Department of Radiology
Division of Abdominal Imaging
and Interventional Radiology
Massachusetts General Hospital
55 Fruit Street
Boston, MA 02114
USA

Olivier Hélénon, MD
Professor and Chairman
Department of Radiology
Necker University Hospital
149 rue de Sèvres
75743 Paris Cedex 15
France

Gary M. Israel, MD
Associate Professor
Department of Diagnostic Radiology
Yale University School of Medicine
PO Box 208042
333 Cedar Street
New Haven, CT 06520-8042
USA

Hisao Ito, MD
Professor and Chairman
Department of Radiology
Graduate School of Medicine
Chiba University
1-8-1 Inohana, Chuoh-ku
Chiba-city, Chiba 260-8670
Japan

Heung Sik Kang, MD, PhD
Professor
Department of Radiology
President, Seoul National University
Bundang Hospital
Seoul National University
College of Medicine
300 Gumi-dong
Bundang-gu, Seong Nam
Gyeonggi-Do 463-707
South Korea

Kyeong Ah Kim, MD
Assistant Professor
Department of Radiology
Korea University Guro Hospital
97 Gurodong-Gil, Guro-Ku
Seoul 152-703
South Korea

Lisa H. Lowe, MD, FAAP
Associate Professor of Pediatric Radiology
Children's Mercy Hospital and Clinics
University of Missouri-Kansas City
2401 Gillham Road
Kansas City, MO 64108
USA

Yves Miaux, MD, MSc
Senior Vice President, Radiology Services
Synarc Inc.
575 Market Street, 17th Floor
San Francisco, CA 94105
USA

Toshiyuki Miyazaki, MD
Chairman
Department of Radiology
Arao City Hospital
2600 Arao
Arao city 864-0041
Japan

Peter R. Mueller, MD
Professor of Radiology
Harvard Medical School
Department of Radiology
Division Head
Division of Abdominal Imaging
and Interventional Radiology
Massachusetts General Hospital
55 Fruit Street
Boston, MA 02114
USA

Clara G.C. Ooi, MD
Associate Professor and Honorary Consultant
Department of Diagnostic Radiology
Queen Mary Hospital
University of Hong Kong
Pokfulam Road, Room 405, Block K
Hong Kong SAR
China

Cheol Min Park, MD
Professor
Department of Radiology
Korea University Guro Hospital
97 Gurodong-Gil, Guro-Ku
Seoul 152-703
South Korea

Uday Patel, MRCP, FRCR
Consultant Interventional Radiologist
Department of Radiology
St George's Hospital and Medical School
Blackshaw Road
London SW17 0QT, England
UK

Jean-Pierre Pelage, MD, PhD
Associate Professor
Department of Radiology
Ambroise Paré University Hospital
9 avenue Charles de Gaulle
92104 Boulogne Billancourt
France

E. Scott Pretorius, MD
Wallace T. Miller Sr. Chair of Radiologic Education
Residency Program Training Director
MRI Section, Department of Radiology
University of Pennsylvania Medical Center
1 Silverstein, 3400 Spruce Street
Philadelphia, PA 19104
USA

Salah Dine Qanadli, MD, PhD
Associate Professor
Department of Radiology and Interventional
Radiology
Centre Hospitalier Universitaire Vaudois (CHUV)
46 rue du Bugnon
1011 Lausanne
Switzerland

Santiago Restrepo, MD
Associate Professor of Radiology
Vice Chairman of Research
Department of Radiology
Louisiana State University Health Sciences Center
1542 Tulane Avenue
New Orleans, LA 70112
USA

Seo Hee Rha, MD, PhD
Associate Professor
Department of Pathology
Dong-A University College of Medicine
1, 3-Ga, Dongdaesin-Dong, Seo-Gu
Busan 602-715
South Korea

Sung Eun Rha, MD
Assistant Professor
Department of Radiology
Kangnam St. Mary's Hospital College of Medicine
The Catholic University of Korea
505 Banpo-Dong, Seocho-Ku
Seoul 137-040
South Korea

Christiaan Schiepers, MD, PhD
Professor
Department of Molecular and Medical
Pharmacology
Professor
Department of Radiological Sciences
David Geffen School of Medicine at UCLA
10833 Le Conte Avenue
AR-144 CHS
Los Angeles, CA 90095-6942
USA

Sheila Sheth, MD
Associate Professor of Radiology and Pathology
Johns Hopkins University School of Medicine
Director, Biopsy Service
Department of Radiology
Johns Hopkins Hospital
600 North Wolfe Street
HAL B176D
Baltimore, MD 21287
USA

Ajay K. Singh, MD
Clinical Instructor of Radiology
Harvard Medical School
Department of Radiology
Division of Emergency Radiology
Massachusetts General Hospital
55 Fruit Street
Boston, MA 02114
USA

Eugenio M. Taboada, MD, FACP
Assistant Professor of Pathology
Director of Surgical Pathology
Children's Mercy Hospital and Clinics
University of Missouri-Kansas City
2401 Gillham Road
Kansas City, MO 64108
USA

Mutsumasa Takahashi, MD
Emeritus Professor
Department of Radiology
Kumamoto University
International Imaging Center
1-2-23 Kuhonji
Kumamoto city 862-0976
Japan

Shigeki Tomita, MD, PhD
Assistant Professor of Pathology
Department of Surgical and Molecular Pathology
DOKKYO University School of Medicine
Department of Surgical Pathology
DOKKYO University Hospital
880 Kitakobayashi, Mibu, Shimo-tsuga
Tochigi 321-0293
Japan

William C. Torreggiani, MD
Consultant Radiologist
Department of Radiology
Adelaide and Meath Hospital
Tallaght
Dublin 24
Ireland

Takuya Ueda, MD
Faculty Radiologist, Teaching Stuff
Department of Radiology
Graduate School of Medicine Chiba University
1-8-1 Inohana, Chuoh-ku
Chiba-city, Chiba 260-8670
Japan

Yoshihiko Ueda, MD, PhD
Professor and Chairman
Department of Pathology
Koshigaya Hospital
DOKKYO University School of Medicine
2-1-50 Minami-Koshigaya, Koshigaya
Saitama 343-8555
Japan

Seong Kuk Yoon, MD, PhD
Assistant Professor
Department of Diagnostic Radiology
Dong-A
University College of Medicine
1, 3-Ga, Dongdaesin-Dong
Seo-Gu
Busan 602-715
South Korea

Ronald J. Zagoria, MD, FACR
Professor of Radiology
Section Head of Abdominal Imaging
Vice Chairman for Clinical Affairs
Department of Radiology
Wake Forest University School of Medicine
Medical Center Boulevard
Winston-Salem, NC 27157
USA

MEDICAL RADIOLOGY Diagnostic Imaging and Radiation Oncology

Titles in the series already published

DIAGNOSTIC IMAGING

Innovations in Diagnostic Imaging
Edited by J. H. Anderson

Radiology of the Upper Urinary Tract
Edited by E. K. Lang

**The Thymus - Diagnostic Imaging,
Functions, and Pathologic Anatomy**
Edited by E. Walter, E. Willich,
and W. R. Webb

Interventional Neuroradiology
Edited by A. Valavanis

Radiology of the Pancreas
Edited by A. L. Baert,
co-edited by G. Delorme

Radiology of the Lower Urinary Tract
Edited by E. K. Lang

Magnetic Resonance Angiography
Edited by I. P. Arlart, G. M. Bongartz,
and G. Marchal

Contrast-Enhanced MRI of the Breast
S. Heywang-Köbrunner and R. Beck

Spiral CT of the Chest
Edited by M. Rémy-Jardin and J. Rémy

Radiological Diagnosis of Breast Diseases
Edited by M. Friedrich
and E.A. Sickles

Radiology of the Trauma
Edited by M. Heller and A. Fink

Biliary Tract Radiology
Edited by P. Rossi,
co-edited by M. Brezi

Radiological Imaging of Sports Injuries
Edited by C. Masciocchi

Modern Imaging of the Alimentary Tube
Edited by A. R. Margulis

Diagnosis and Therapy of Spinal Tumors
Edited by P. R. Algra, J. Valk,
and J. J. Heimans

**Interventional Magnetic
Resonance Imaging**
Edited by J.F. Debatin and G. Adam

Abdominal and Pelvic MRI
Edited by A. Heuck and M. Reiser

**Orthopedic Imaging
Techniques and Applications**
Edited by A. M. Davies
and H. Pettersson

**Radiology of the
Female Pelvic Organs**
Edited by E. K.Lang

**Magnetic Resonance of the Heart
and Great Vessels**
Clinical Applications
Edited by J. Bogaert, A.J. Duerinckx,
and F. E. Rademakers

Modern Head and Neck Imaging
Edited by S. K. Mukherji
and J. A. Castelijns

**Radiological Imaging
of Endocrine Diseases**
Edited by J. N. Bruneton
in collaboration with B. Padovani
and M.-Y. Mourou

Trends in Contrast Media
Edited by H. S. Thomsen,
R. N. Muller, and R. F. Mattrey

Functional MRI
Edited by C. T. W. Moonen
and P. A. Bandettini

Radiology of the Pancreas
2nd Revised Edition
Edited by A. L. Baert
Co-edited by G. Delorme
and L. Van Hoe

Emergency Pediatric Radiology
Edited by H. Carty

Spiral CT of the Abdomen
Edited by F. Terrier, M. Grossholz,
and C. D. Becker

**Liver Malignancies
Diagnostic and
Interventional Radiology**
Edited by C. Bartolozzi
and R. Lencioni

Medical Imaging of the Spleen
Edited by A. M. De Schepper
and F. Vanhoenacker

Radiology of Peripheral Vascular Diseases
Edited by E. Zeitler

Diagnostic Nuclear Medicine
Edited by C. Schiepers

Radiology of Blunt Trauma of the Chest
P. Schnyder and M. Wintermark

Portal Hypertension
Diagnostic Imaging-Guided Therapy
Edited by P. Rossi
Co-edited by P. Ricci and L. Broglia

**Recent Advances in
Diagnostic Neuroradiology**
Edited by Ph. Demaerel

**Virtual Endoscopy
and Related 3D Techniques**
Edited by P. Rogalla, J. Terwisscha
Van Scheltinga, and B. Hamm

Multislice CT
Edited by M. F. Reiser, M. Takahashi,
M. Modic, and R. Bruening

Pediatric Uroradiology
Edited by R. Fotter

**Transfontanellar Doppler Imaging
in Neonates**
A. Couture and C. Veyrac

**Radiology of AIDS
A Practical Approach**
Edited by J.W.A.J. Reeders
and P.C. Goodman

CT of the Peritoneum
Armando Rossi and Giorgio Rossi

Magnetic Resonance Angiography
2nd Revised Edition
Edited by I. P. Arlart,
G. M. Bongratz, and G. Marchal

Pediatric Chest Imaging
Edited by Javier Lucaya
and Janet L. Strife

**Applications of Sonography
in Head and Neck Pathology**
Edited by J. N. Bruneton
in collaboration with C. Raffaelli
and O. Dassonville

Imaging of the Larynx
Edited by R. Hermans

3D Image Processing
Techniques and Clinical Applications
Edited by D. Caramella
and C. Bartolozzi

**Imaging of Orbital and
Visual Pathway Pathology**
Edited by W. S. Müller-Forell

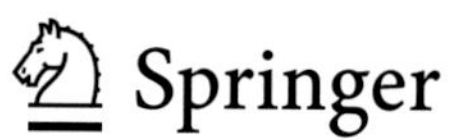

Springer

RADIATION ONCOLOGY

Lung Cancer
Edited by C.W. Scarantino

Innovations in Radiation Oncology
Edited by H. R. Withers
and L. J. Peters

**Radiation Therapy
of Head and Neck Cancer**
Edited by G. E. Laramore

**Gastrointestinal Cancer –
Radiation Therapy**
Edited by R.R. Dobelbower, Jr.

**Radiation Exposure
and Occupational Risks**
Edited by E. Scherer, C. Streffer,
and K.-R. Trott

Radiation Therapy of Benign Diseases
A Clinical Guide
S. E. Order and S. S. Donaldson

**Interventional Radiation
Therapy Techniques – Brachytherapy**
Edited by R. Sauer

Radiopathology of Organs and Tissues
Edited by E. Scherer, C. Streffer,
and K.-R. Trott

**Concomitant Continuous Infusion
Chemotherapy and Radiation**
Edited by M. Rotman
and C. J. Rosenthal

**Intraoperative Radiotherapy –
Clinical Experiences and Results**
Edited by F. A. Calvo, M. Santos,
and L.W. Brady

**Radiotherapy of Intraocular
and Orbital Tumors**
Edited by W. E. Alberti and
R. H. Sagerman

**Interstitial and Intracavitary
Thermoradiotherapy**
Edited by M. H. Seegenschmiedt
and R. Sauer

Non-Disseminated Breast Cancer
Controversial Issues in Management
Edited by G. H. Fletcher and
S.H. Levitt

**Current Topics in
Clinical Radiobiology of Tumors**
Edited by H.-P. Beck-Bornholdt

**Practical Approaches to
Cancer Invasion and Metastases**
A Compendium of Radiation
Oncologists' Responses to 40 Histories
Edited by A. R. Kagan with the
Assistance of R. J. Steckel

Radiation Therapy in Pediatric Oncology
Edited by J. R. Cassady

Radiation Therapy Physics
Edited by A. R. Smith

Late Sequelae in Oncology
Edited by J. Dunst and R. Sauer

Mediastinal Tumors. Update 1995
Edited by D. E. Wood
and C. R. Thomas, Jr.

**Thermoradiotherapy
and Thermochemotherapy**
Volume 1:
Biology, Physiology, and Physics
Volume 2:
Clinical Applications
Edited by M.H. Seegenschmiedt,
P. Fessenden, and C.C. Vernon

Carcinoma of the Prostate
Innovations in Management
Edited by Z. Petrovich, L. Baert,
and L.W. Brady

**Radiation Oncology
of Gynecological Cancers**
Edited by H.W. Vahrson

Carcinoma of the Bladder
Innovations in Management
Edited by Z. Petrovich, L. Baert,
and L.W. Brady

**Blood Perfusion and
Microenvironment of Human Tumors**
Implications for
Clinical Radiooncology
Edited by M. Molls and P. Vaupel

Radiation Therapy of Benign Diseases
A Clinical Guide
2nd Revised Edition
S. E. Order and S. S. Donaldson

**Carcinoma of the Kidney and Testis,
and Rare Urologic Malignancies**
Innovations in Management
Edited by Z. Petrovich, L. Baert,
and L.W. Brady

**Progress and Perspectives in the
Treatment of Lung Cancer**
Edited by P. Van Houtte,
J. Klastersky, and P. Rocmans

**Combined Modality Therapy of
Central Nervous System Tumors**
Edited by Z. Petrovich, L. W. Brady,
M. L. Apuzzo, and M. Bamberg

Age-Related Macular Degeneration
Current Treatment Concepts
Edited by W. A. Alberti, G. Richard,
and R. H. Sagerman

**Radiotherapy of Intraocular
and Orbital Tumors**
2nd Revised Edition
Edited by R. H. Sagerman,
and W. E. Alberti

Modification of Radiation Response
Cytokines, Growth Factors,
and Other Biolgical Targets
Edited by C. Nieder, L. Milas,
and K. K. Ang

Radiation Oncology for Cure and Palliation
R. G. Parker, N. A. Janjan,
and M. T. Selch

**Clinical Target Volumes in Conformal and
Intensity Modulated Radiation Therapy**
A Clinical Guide to Cancer Treatment
Edited by V. Grégoire, P. Scalliet,
and K. K. Ang

**Advances in Radiation Oncology
in Lung Cancer**
Edited by Branislav Jeremić

New Technologies in Radiation Oncology
Edited by W. Schlegel, T. Bortfeld,
and A.-L. Grosu

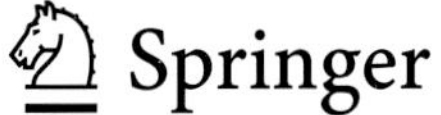

Printing and Binding: Stürtz GmbH, Würzburg